Glycobiology and Human Diseases

Glycobiology and Human Diseases

Editor

Gherman Wiederschain

Department of Biology
Boston College
Boston, MA
USA

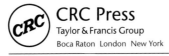

CRC Press

Taylor & Francis Group

Boca Raton London New York

CRC Press is an imprint of the
Taylor & Francis Group, an **informa** business

A SCIENCE PUBLISHERS BOOK

Cover Acknowledgement

· Upper left panel figure: reproduced by permission of Drs. Yi-Pin Lin, Marcia S. Osburne, Michael Pereira, Jenifer Coburn and John M. Leong (authors of Chapter 4)
· Upper right panel figure: reproduced by permission of Dr. Joseph Alroy (author of Chapter 6)
· Bottom left & right figures: reproduced by permission of Drs. Ida Annunziata and Alessandra d'Azzo (authors of Chapter 8)

CRC Press
Taylor & Francis Group
6000 Broken Sound Parkway NW, Suite 300
Boca Raton, FL 33487-2742

First issued in paperback 2021

© 2016 by Taylor & Francis Group, LLC
CRC Press is an imprint of Taylor & Francis Group, an Informa business

No claim to original U.S. Government works

Version Date: 20151209

ISBN 13: 978-0-367-78317-4 (pbk)
ISBN 13: 978-1-4987-0918-7 (hbk)

Library of Congress Cataloging-in-Publication Data

Names: Wiederschain, Gherman.
Title: Glycobiology and human diseases / [edited by] Gherman Wiederschain.
Description: Boca Raton : Taylor & Francis, 2016. | Includes bibliographical references and index.
Identifiers: LCCN 2015043262 | ISBN 9781498709187 (hardcover : alk. paper)
Subjects: LCSH: Glycoconjugates. | Epidemiology. | Inflammation--Mediators. | Glycosylation.
Classification: LCC QP702.G577 G5913 2016 | DDC 572/.567--dc23
LC record available at http://lccn.loc.gov/2015043262

Visit the Taylor & Francis Web site at
http://www.taylorandfrancis.com

and the CRC Press Web site at
http://www.crcpress.com

Preface

This book presents two important, closely connected and fundamental areas of research: glycobiology and human diseases. The field of glycobiology is focused upon understanding the chemical structure, metabolism and biological function of simple and complex carbohydrates (glycans) and their glycoconjugates: glycoproteins, glycosaminoproteoglycans and glycolipids. The last three groups of biopolymers are final products of post-translational modification of proteins and lipids and play a pivotal role in cellular homeostasis. Protein folding, intercellular communication, development, the immune system, various types of cell and molecular recognition and many others processes are characterized by close involvement of glycoconjugates. Major achievements in glycobiology have been obtained by the combined efforts of multiple investigators with a variety of backgrounds and expertise in carbohydrate chemistry, cell and molecular biology, enzymology and life sciences. Glycomics, younger than genomics and proteomics, deals with the analysis of glycan moieties of glycoconjugates and elucidation of their functional roles. Comprehensive glycomics methods has led to an understanding of not only many unknown earlier glycobiology processes in the normal state, but has also significantly expanded our knowledge of processes related to glycobiology in various human diseases. The contents of this book illustrate the research productivity of these two directions in glycobiology.

Chapter 1 (Wiederschain) presents an introduction to basic data about the peculiarity of simple and complex carbohydrates and glycoconjugates. Consideration of the unique structure, biosynthesis, degradation and function of glycans forms a basis for consideration of critical changes in many of these processes in disease, and lays the ground work for the chapters that follow. The reference list of this chapter includes many recently published reviews, monographs and collective comprehensive editions, and summarizes basic directions in glycobiology that may help readers expand their knowledge and skills in both theoretical and experimental areas of this science.

Methods of structural analysis of glycosaminoglycans (GAG), applications of these methods for identification of lysosomal storage diseases (LSD) and GAG participation in the development of Lyme disease are reviewed in Chapters 2 (Azadi and Heiss), 3 (Bruggink et al.) and 4 (Lin et al.), respectively. Various methodical approaches for GAG analysis are described as well as changes of these biopolymers in different types of LSD, and the role of GAG in tissue tropism for the Lyme disease spirochete.

Chapter 5 (Hartshorn) highlights the role of viral envelope protein glycosylation in pathogenesis of influenza A virus. In collaboration with experts in crystallography, molecular modeling, and molecular dynamics, the author and his colleagues have determined the molecular mechanism of binding of surfactant protein D (SP-D) to the influenza A virus hemagglutinin, and established the basis for increased inhibitory activity of mutant versions of SP-D. These studies provide the first detailed molecular mechanism for viral inhibition by an innate lectin inhibitor based on shared expertise in virology, structural biology, protein chemistry, and glycomics.

Chapter 6 (Alroy et al.) describes the application of lectin histochemistry for the diagnosis of LSD and Chapter 7 (Dingjan et al.) discusses computational approaches for studying carbohydrate-lectin interactions in infection. These two contributions illustrate the significance of lectinology in glycoscience pathology. Chapters 8 (Annunziata and d'Azzo) and 9 (Amith et al.), respectively, review pathogenic effects of altered sialylation (biosynthesis and degradation) of specific glycoconjugates in genetic diseases, as well as the role of Neu1 sialidase in the activation of toll-like receptors, their downstream signaling events, and effector functions. In both of these reviews various types of mammalian sialidases (neuraminidases) are discussed in the context of specificity and function.

Chapter 10 (Dimitroff) focuses on novel insights on sialyltransferase regulation of cancer-associated O-glycans. The importance and more recognizable roles of Galectin-binding cancer cell O-glycans continue to provide new paradigms for cancer research and development of novel cancer therapies. The future model of glycobiological development for the treatment of cancer is scientific partnership between industrial and academic scientists. Each entity can effectively leverage their scientific expertise, research tools and laboratory infrastructure to develop potent and specific glyco-therapeutics in a cost-efficient manner. This type of collaborative relationship provides an opportune circumstance to rapidly test lead candidates in biologically-relevant screening assays and translate their use *in vivo*—namely to humans.

Chapter 11 (Popov) summarizes the history of pectin study, chemistry and medicinal uses of pectin, including physiological effects of individual pectins in human studies, processes that underlay the action of pectins, and the beneficial effects of pectin consumption on human health.

Chapter 12 (He and Newburg) discuss the glycobiology of human milk in health and disease. New data presented in this review strongly support the unique properties of human milk glycans and glycoconjugates in various infant defense mechanisms against bacterial and virus infections, including interaction with gut microbiota and effects on human intestinal cells.

Chapter 13 (Maor and Horowitz) considers molecular mechanisms underlying the association between Gaucher's disease (GD) and Parkinson's disease (PD). Since carriers of GD mutations develop PD, a dominant effect of the GBA mutation should be considered to be mediated by either gain of function or haploinsufficiency. The data show that expression of a mutant GBA allele is enough to cause ER stress and ER stress response, which leads to degeneration of dopaminergic cells.

Chapter 14 (Schwarting) highlights expression and function of poly-N-acetyllactosamine (PLNs) glycans in the nervous system. PLNs interact with a large family of endogenous lectins, the galectins. A great deal of what we know about lactosamine function comes from studies of galectin-1, which preferentially binds to lactosamine on N- and O-glycans; PLNs can affect biological systems in two ways: by directly modulating properties of the proteins to which they are attached, and by interacting with galectins and other glycan binding proteins.

Chapter 15 (Conroy and Anthony) reviews the role of glycosylation in various types of immunoglobulins in health and disease. The authors analyze 5 major subtypes of immunoglobulins in mammals, namely IgG, IgA, IgM, IgD, and IgE, all of which are glycoproteins produced by B cells and responsible for protection against a wide spectrum of threats. There is evidence that the peculiarity of glycosylation, the number of glycosylation sites and the types of glycans attached play an important role in antibody function. Many autoimmune diseases, including rheumatoid arthritis, systemic lupus erythematosus, diabetes mellitus, thyroid disease and others, are triggered by antibodies erroneously targeted against host proteins. The intrinsic variable nature of antibodies, including their glycan parts, allow for specificity that can be engineered to meet a clinical need. The therapeutic role of antibodies through engineering modification methods is discussed. Antibody mediated immunotherapy is very promising for a wide range of diseases including cancer.

Chapter 16 (Sparks) highlights basic biochemical, genetic and clinical features of congenital disorders of glycosylation (CDG). Knowledge of glycosylation defects has been rapidly expanding due to improved clinical awareness and biochemical diagnostic techniques. This chapter deals with classification and modern nomenclature of known types of CDG, mechanisms of development of these diseases as a result of direct or indirect deficiency of enzymes involved in glycosylation processes, characterization of analytical techniques for CDG diagnosis, and possible approaches for treatment of these diseases. The clinical spectrum for defects in both N- and O-linked glycosylation is extremely broad, creating a challenge for clinicians to screen for these defects in a variety of settings and disciplines. Since there are some 500 genes involved in the synthesis and function of glycoproteins, it is likely that many more CDG defects will be identified in the future.

Chapter 17 (Ziganshina et al.) focuses on the immune response by human antibodies to hyaluronic acid in preeclampsia, one of the main causes of maternal and perinatal morbidity and mortality worldwide. The authors hypothesize a role for the glycocalyx in the pathogenesis of the disease and discuss the significance of autoantibodies directed against hyaluronic acid as a marker for diagnostics and clinical disease prognosis.

I wish to thank all the authors for their contributions, which made this book possible. I also express my gratitude to the Editorial staff of CRC/Taylor&Francis Group for their helpful support in book preparation and publication. We anticipate that a variety of readers, including glycobiologists, carbohydrate chemists, immunologists, cell- and molecular biologists as well as clinical physicians, will find this book as a useful source of information, ideas and productive speculation to take further steps forward in understanding the impact of glycobiology in human health and disease.

The book is dedicated to my wife Lyudmila (Mila) in appreciation of her loyal support, understanding, patience and generous love during all my years working in science.

Boston, Massachusetts, USA   **Gherman Wiederschain**
August, 2015

Contents

CHAPTER 1

Introduction to Glycobiology and Human Diseases

Gherman Wiederschain

Introduction

The recent several decades have provided outstanding information about glycoconjugates–biopolymers consisting of a carbohydrate (glycan) part covalently linked to protein or lipid. The major types of glycoconjugates are glycoproteins, glycolipids and proteoglycans. These biopolymers have an incredible structural complexity and diversity of the glycan moieties, huge heterogeneity and wide biological roles in living organisms. The addition of mono- or oligosaccharides to proteins and glycolipids is a significant posttranslational modification that modulates the structure and localization of biopolymers (Kannicht 2002).

Glycans present a difficult challenge in the analytical field because of the intricate dynamics of their synthesis as well as the complexity of the structures themselves. In addition to the role of glycans in development and disease, they are of great interest in the biotherapeutic industry where modification of glycosylation can alter efficacy and biological activity in a range of glycoconjugate products. Functional glycomics is emerging as a central field in systems biology and will continue to be a key focus in discerning health and disease (Lennarz and Hart 1994, Kamerling et al. 2007, Fraser-Reid et al. 2008, Varki et al. 2009a,b,c, Struwe et al. 2011, Taylor and Drickamer 2011, Narin and Moremen 2015, Taniguchi et al. 2015).

Glycans are vital for development in all eukaryotes and are centrally involved in a large number of human diseases, ranging from glycan genetic diseases to autoimmune disorders and cancer (Ohtsubo and Marth 2006, Taniguchi et al. 2015, Terao et al. 2015). Several recent reviews that appeared in a special issue of "Glycobiology" (vol. 24, no. 12, 2014) provide direct evidence that glycans and glycan-binding proteins play central roles in vascular biology, including endothelial cell signaling, angiogenesis, hemostasis, leukocyte trafficking and inflammation (Thijssen and Rabinovich 2014).

Data about structure and biological roles of glycoconjugates have led to the investigation and characterization of metabolic errors in the biosynthesis, degradation and functionality of these molecules in various pathological conditions of animals and humans and the development of approaches to corrections of some of these diseases.

Program in Glycobiology, Department of Biology, Boston College, 140 Commonwealth Ave, Chestnut Hill, MA, USA-02467.
  E-mail: Gherman.Wiederschain@bc.edu

This book highlights some of these diseases with presentations by leading experts in the field, who discuss the most recent scientific data, models, and hypotheses, as well as outlining future directions. It is obviously impossible in one monograph to cover the entire field of glycobiology and human disease that is currently available in scientific publications. However, it is hoped that this book will serve as a useful review of the presented topics, and that the provided reference lists will be a useful guide for additional information. This opening chapter discusses the structure, biosynthesis, degradation, and biological roles of glycoconjugates and describes mechanisms of certain pathological conditions that are related to glycobiology so as to lay the groundwork for the chapters that follow.

Unique Informational Structural Features of Simple and Complex Carbohydrates

Studies on the structures of simple carbohydrates, monosaccharides, started with E. H. Fischer near the end of the 19th century. All simple monosaccharides have the general empirical formula $C_x(H_2O)$ n, where n is an integer ranging from 3 to 9. As distinct from nucleic acids and proteins, which are linear polymers with the same type of bonds between monomers (phosphodiester bonds for nucleic acids and peptide bonds for proteins) in their structures, monosaccharides as a unit of carbohydrate chains can be D or L-sugars and with varieties of glycosidic linkage between carbohydrate monomers. Each individual carbohydrate moiety can be in a furanoside or pyranoside form bound to each other by α or β-glycosidic linkage between the most reactive hemiacetal hydroxyl group at the C1 of one monosaccharide and one of the hydroxyl groups at C2, C3, C4, or C6 of another monosaccharide, or also with the C1 atom of other monosaccharide in some cases (e.g., trehalose). Just as polypeptides have amino and carboxyl termini and polynucleotides have 5' and 3' termini, oligosaccharides, have a polarity that is defined by their *reducing* and *nonreducing termini*.

When a glycosidic bond is formed, its configuration is maintained indefinitely. The glycosidic linkage is the most flexible part of a disaccharide structure. Whereas the chair conformation of the constituent monosaccharides is relatively rigid, the torsion angles around the glycosidic bond can vary greatly (Bochkov and Zaikov 1979). Thus a disaccharide of well-defined primary structure can adopt multiple conformations in solution that differ in the relative orientation of the two monosaccharides. The combination of structural rigidity and flexibility is typical of complex carbohydrates, and, more than likely, essential to their biological functions. For example, two glucose residues can be joined together in numerous ways, as illustrated by two disaccharides: maltose (Glcα1-4Glc) and gentibiose (Glcβ1-6Glc).

These isomers have very different three-dimensional structures and biological activities. Also, a monosaccharide can be involved in more than two glycosidic linkages, thus serving as a branch point. The common occurrence of branched sequences (as opposed to the linear sequences that are found in almost all peptides) is unique to glycans and contributes to their structural diversity.

With the exception of hyaluronic acid, glycans are linked to other biomolecules, such as lipids or amino acids within polypeptides, through glycosidic linkages to form glycoconjugates. Glycans are often referred to as the *glycone* of a glycoconjugate and the noncarbohydrate component is called the *aglycone*.

The hydroxyl groups of both monosaccharides and oligosaccharides can be biochemically (by enzymes) or chemically modified without affecting the glycosidic linkages. Various chemical modifications of hydroxyl groups can take place: phosphorylation, methylation, esterification, and deoxygenation, when hydroxyl groups can be replaced with hydrogen atoms to form deoxysugars (e.g., L-fucose, L-rhamnose). Due to the nature of multi-functionality within a single carbohydrate moiety, all these possible connections between monosaccharides lead to the formation of complex carbohydrate structures.

For example, three identical monosaccharides of hexoses (e.g., D-glucopyranoside) can be theoretically jointed to produce 176 different linear trisaccharides, and three different monosaccharides (XYZ) can be connected to produce 1056 possible linear trisaccharides. These many possible trisaccharides include not only those arising from different glycosidic linkages between monosaccharides (i.e., 1–2, 1–3, 1–4, and 1–6), but also the carbohydrates containing different type of glycoside bonds at the anomeric positions (i.e., α, β, αα, αβ, or ββ). In contrast, three identical amino acid units can only be linked together to form one tripeptide, whereas three different amino acids can form only six different tripeptides (i.e., 3! = 6,

ABC, ACB, BCA, BAC, CAB, and CBA). The longer carbohydrate chains, including those of simple glycans, polysaccharides, and glycoconjugates, can also be branched. Such combinations significantly increase the number of possible carbohydrate structures having the same monosaccharide sequence. Thus, a pentasaccharide consisting of five different hexose units has 2,144,640 possible structural isomers, and a hexasaccharide consisting of six different hexoses has more than a trillion possible structural combinations (Sharon 1975, Varki and Sharon 2009). It seems that the spectrum of carbohydrate structures are expanding and yielding new combinations under the influence of various factors, including disease associated changes in the body. The tremendous diversity of glycoconjugates structures derives from many elements. The multiple monosaccharide building blocks can be linked to various regiochemistries and stereochemistries, and the resulting oligosaccharides can be assembled on protein or lipid scaffolds. Glycoconjugates therefore comprise an "information-rich" system capable of participating in a wide range of biological functions. Fortunately, the structures of natural glycans are not so enormously diversified due to limitations in the donor and acceptor specificity of glycosyl transferases.

One of these sugars, N-acetylneuraminate (N-acetylneuraminic acid, Neu5Ac, NANA, Sia, also called sialic acid) is unique and often found as a terminal residue of oligosaccharide chains of glycoproteins and glycolipids. Sialic acid imparts hydrophilicity and negative charge to glycoproteins and glycolipids, because its carboxyl group tends to dissociate a proton at physiological pH. Sialic acid is a generic term for the *N*- or *O*-substituted derivatives of neuraminic acid, a monosaccharide with a nine-carbon backbone. It is also the name for the most common member of this group, N-acetylneuraminic acid. In the human body, the highest concentration of sialic acid (as Neu5Ac) occurs in the brain where it participates as an integral part of glycolipids. Generally sialic acids comprise a family of more than 50 naturally occurring derivatives of the nine-carbon sugar neuraminic acid (5-amino-3,5-dideoxy-d-glycero-d-galacto-nonulsonic acid). *N*-acetylneuraminic acids, which are the most widespread form of sialic acid and almost the only form found in humans. The other form of sialic acid is based on *N*-glycolylneuraminic acids (Neu5Gc) which are common in many animal species, but not found in normal human tissues. Sialic acid molecules can be substituted in more than one position. *O*-substitution at C4, -7, -8 and -9 (O-acetyl, O-methyl, O-sulphate, and phosphate groups) or the introduction of a double bond between C-2 and C-3 can give rise to a wide variety of possible isomers. An unusual modification is an additional hydroxyl group present instead of the amino function at position 5 of the sugar, leading to 2-keto-3-deoxy-nonulosonic acid (Ketodeoxynonulosonic acid, Kdn). This component has been found in fish eggs (Caviar). Sialic acid in the form of polysialic acid is an unusual posttranslational modification that occurs on the neural cell adhesion molecules (NCAMs). In the synapse, the strong negative charge of the polysialic acid prevents NCAM cross-linking of cells. Due to their unique chemical and physical properties, diversity of structure and exposed position, sialic acids have been implicated in numerous essential biological processes, such as neural cell growth and embryogenesis, stem cell biology, immune system regulation, human evolution, cancer progression, and microbial pathogenesis (Varki 1992, Varki and Schauer 2009, Tiralongo and Martínez-Duncker 2013).

Another unusual monosaccharide is L-fucose (Fuc, 6-deoxy-L-galactose), that is a common component of many N- and O-linked glycans and glycolipids produced by mammalian cells. Two structural features distinguish fucose from other six-carbon sugars present in mammals. These include the lack of a hydroxyl group on the carbon at the C-6 position by replacement with a more hydrophobic CH_3–group, and this monosaccharide is also unusual in having an L-configuration. The location of fucose in carbohydrate chains of glycoconjugates is similar to that of Neu5Ac and both of these sugars very often exist as a terminal component of glycan structures. Moreover, there is some reciprocal relationship in glycoconjugate chains between these two terminal sugars, particularly in glycoproteins: more Fuc-residues leads to less Neu5Ac-residues, and vice versa (Dische 1963). Perhaps, this competition is the result of specific action of numerous types of sialyl- and fucosyltransferases during complex glycosylation processes. In mammals, fucose-containing glycans have important roles in blood transfusion reactions, selectin mediated leukocyte-endothelial adhesion, hostmicrobe interactions, and numerous ontogenic events, including signaling events by the Notch receptor family. Alterations in the expression of fucosylated oligosaccharides have also been observed in several pathological processes, including cancer and atherosclerosis. Fucose deficiency is accompanied by a complex set of phenotypes both in humans with leukocyte adhesion deficiency type II (LAD II; also known as congenital disorder of glycosylation type IIc) and in a recently generated strain of mice with a conditional defect in fucosylated glycan expression. Fucose is a fundamental sub-unit of the bioactive sulfated polysaccharide found mainly in various species of brown algae and brown seaweed (Becker and Lowe 2003, Cumashi et al. 2007, Ustyuzhanina et al. 2014, Anisimova et al. 2015).

The other naturally occurring deoxysugar is L-rhamnose (6-deoxy-L-mannose). Rhamnose is commonly bound to other sugars in nature. It is a usually a glycone component of plant glycosides (Larskaya and Gorshkova 2015). Rhamnose is also a component of the outer cell membrane of acid-fast bacteria in the Mycobacterium genus, which includes the organism that causes tuberculosis.

A limited number of other monosaccharide (all in D-configuration): glucose (Glc), galactose (Gal), galactosamine (GalN), galacturonic acid (GalA), glucosamine (GlcN), glucuronic acid (GlcA), mannose (Man), mannuronic acid (ManA), mannosamine (ManN), xylose (Xyl), N-acetylglucosamine (GlcNAc), N-acetylgalactosamine (GalNAc), potentially can provide a very large number of structures of carbohydrate chains in all types of glycoconjugates. Theoretically, the number of possible structural isomers both branched and linear based only on reducing hexasaccharides might be greater than 1.05×10^{12} (Laine 1994). The analysis of various types of protein glycosylation indicates that 13 different monosaccharides and 8 amino acids are involved in glycoprotein linkages leading to a total of at least 41 bonds, if the anomeric configurations, the phosphoglycosyl linkages, as well as the GPI (glycophosphatidylinositol) phosphoethanolamine bridge are also considered (Spiro 2002).

The conclusions to be drawn from this are obvious: carbohydrates are ideal for generating units with explicit informational properties, since the permutations of linkages are much larger than can be achieved with amino acids on proteins. Moreover, the oligosaccharide units are not flexible but exhibit highly specific structures with only limited degrees of freedom. Thus the different building blocks of glycans (the alphabet of the sugar code) and the way they can be linked to form oligo- and polysaccharides (words, messages) provide additional sequence and conformational information that transforms the two-dimensional biological code to three-dimensional structures and significantly increases the spectrum of biological specificity of glycoconjugates. Carbohydrates form the third alphabet of life. Compared to amino acids in proteins and nucleotides in nucleic acids, carbohydrate versatility for isomer formation is unsurpassed. The resulting high-density coding capacity of carbohydrate chains is established by variability in (i) anomeric status, (ii) linkage positions, (iii) ring size, (iv) by branching and (v) introduction of site-specific substitutions (Gabius 2009).

Cellular and Subcellular Localization of Glycoconjugates

We are still very far from a complete understanding of the construction of glycoconjugate molecules during their progress along the "assembly lines" within cells. Unique biosynthesis occurs on the way from the rough endoplasmic reticulum (RER), where glycosylation of proteins and lipids begins, and continue through the assembly line of smooth endoplasmic reticulum (SER) and different cisternae of the Golgi complex (GC) (Warren and Rothman 2011). The GC is the place of final construction of carbohydrate chains that modifies carbohydrates via sulfation, phosphorylation, acetylation, and many other changes under the influence of highly specific glycosyltransferases, processing glycosidases, sulfotransferases, and other modifying enzymes.

It should be reemphasized that various cells, tissues, and organs are characterized by specific sets of glycoconjugates. In turn, these glycoconjugates determine the specialized functions of cells, tissues, and organs, and the highly efficient function and cooperation of metabolic processes of the whole organism. The diversity and heterogeneity of glycoconjugates structures, as well as existence of their so-called "glycoforms", show that these molecules have virtually unlimited structural-functional abilities that are not inherent in any other class of compounds in living organisms (Rademacher et al. 1988, Bertozzi and Rabuka 2009).

The question arises of whether these unique varieties of structure of glycoconjugates are actually used in living organisms. The answer is affirmative, because nature has taken advantage of the offered possibilities during the long period of evolution. Glycosylation of different molecules of living systems is generally accepted to be the most frequent molecular modification. To some degree, this modification is found in various molecules of plant and bacterial cells, viruses, and fungi, and is most fully documented in molecules of eukaryote cells. Polysaccharides of plant cells form their envelopes and comprise their major nutritional stores. In bacteria and fungi, glycans are the most important structural elements of the cell walls responsible for intracellular homeostasis and protection against bacteriophages and antibiotics generated by other microorganisms (Dumitriu 2005, Hattrup and Gendler 2008).

Due to the combined features of their complex molecules–amphipathic (glycoproteins, glycolipids), conformational, neutral or negatively charged (sialobiopolymers and proteoglycans)–glycoconjugates can be located in membranes of all cells and subcellular organelles, including the nuclear membrane. Carbohydrate chains can be oriented both outside the membranes and inside the organelles and perform specific functions that include signal transduction and triggering of different processes under the influence of events on the cell surface or on the outer surface of organelles. Proteoglycans, some glycoproteins, and glycolipids occupy intercellular spaces in animals and plants and form a layer covering the plasma membrane known as the glycocalyx. The glycocalyx influences cell adhesion and protects cells against deleterious chemical influences and is involved in mineral and water metabolism of cells. The glycocalyx also mediates the immune response to a large spectrum of microorganisms, recognizes tumor cells, protects leukocyte movement in normal endothelium of blood vessels, and participates in fertilization and embryogenesis (Reitsma et al. 2007).

Thus, glycoconjugates occupy "strategic posts" in cellular communication, performing the important functions of intercellular interaction, signaling, stabilization, and protection of biologically active compounds against untimely proteolysis, as well as binding and neutralizing viruses and bacteria. Moreover, glycan-containing molecules of biological fluids, e.g., many glycoproteins of the bloodstream, various secreted molecules, and mobile cells in blood vessels can be recognized through their carbohydrate determinants by many animal lectins. High affinity binding with lectins often determines the lifetime and further fate of molecules and cells. It is relevant to the discussion to consider some functional features of glycoconjugates—their biosynthesis, degradation, and mechanisms of delivery to particular places in cells and tissues where these molecules "are in service" (Sansom and Markman 2007, Wiederschain 2013).

Biosynthesis and Degradation of Glycans and Glycoconjugates

Biosynthesis. Glycosylation in animal cells is initiated in the RER through the interaction of three main components: acceptors and donors of carbohydrate residues, and the highly specific glycosyltransferases located on the inner surface of the RER membranes and in different compartments of the Golgi complex.

Acceptors of carbohydrate residues can be proteins, lipids, or other simple or complex carbohydrates. Two classes of compounds can act as the donors of carbohydrate residues. The first class includes nucleoside diphosphate sugars (NDPS), which are α- or β-glycosyl esters of nucleotides (nucleotide sugars). These nucleoside diphosphate sugars contain adenine, guanine, cytosine, thymine, or uracil as nitrogenous bases. There are more than 50 different NDPSs, which are mainly produced during the interaction of nucleoside triphosphate and a phosphate sugar in the cell cytoplasm. In animal tissues, every monosaccharide is linked to a single, specific nucleoside diphosphate, more strictly to its heterocyclic base. For example, L-fucose is linked only to GDP-fucose, TDP-rhamnose is the donor of L-rhamnose, and UDP-glucose is the donor of D-glucose. Likewise, the activated form of sialic acids is CMP-sialic acid, which is the only nucleoside monophosphate sugar acting as a donor of sialic acids in animal cells.

By contrast, plants and bacteria contain multiple nucleoside diphosphates that can be the donors of the same sugar. For example, glucose binding with UDP, GDP, ADP or CDP can be the donor of glucose in plants. This is because plant cells contain a set of enzymes responsible for the production of different glucose-bound nucleotides that can serve as the donors of glucose residues during biosynthesis of more complex carbohydrates.

NDPSs function well as the donors of carbohydrate residues because they all contain a phosphoanhydride moiety with very high free energy that can be released during the glycosylation and used to lower the activation energy of the glycosylation. Also, each NDPS can be recognized by specific transferases during glycosylation (Wiederschain 1976).

The second class of carbohydrate donors includes lipid carriers, often polyprenol phosphate sugars, which are much more hydrophobic than NDPSs. The lipophilic moiety of these compounds is a polyunsaturated alcohol consisting of isoprene residues binding to carbohydrate residues through one or two phosphoric acid units.

In mammals, the most widely distributed polyprenol is dolichol. The term dolichol (from δολιχος– long, in Greek) has been proposed for all prenols having a saturated α-isoprene residue with a hydroxyl group to discriminate them from the bacterial polyprenols (i.e., undecaprenol) having an unsaturated α-terminal unit. The hydrophobic chain of dolichol consists of 80 to 125 carbon atoms and is one of the longest aliphatic molecules known. By contrast, the undecaprenol chain consists of 50 to 60 carbon atoms.

Dolichol can be converted into the ester of phosphoric acid by means of esterification at the terminal hydroxyl group, to form dolicholmonophosphate or dolicholpyrophosphate, respectively, to which sugar residues are bound via the phosphate or pyrophosphate bridge. The resulting dolicholmono- and dolicholdiphosphate sugars are known to be the main lipid carriers during the biosynthesis of carbohydrate chains of N-linked glycoproteins (Shibaev 1976, Snider 1984). The functional difference between these two types of activated donors of carbohydrate residues is that NDPSs donate only one monosaccharide residue to peptides, proteins, lipids, and carbohydrates. Dolicholmonophosphate sugars also donate their carbohydrate residues (monosaccharides) either directly to the peptide core of the synthesized glycoprotein molecule, the nonreducing end of the constructed oligosaccharide chain, or the dolicholpyrophosphate sugar (DPPS). In this case, the dolicholpyrophosphate sugar acts as an acceptor of carbohydrate residues so that its oligosaccharide chain can grow to contain up to 14 monosaccharide units in eukaryotes and more in prokaryotes. Upon completion, the entire oligosaccharide can be transferred to a protein or another acceptor of the carbohydrate component by the corresponding oligosaccharyltransferase. Thus, DPPSs act as the acceptors of carbohydrate residues at the first stage of glycosylation and as the donors at the second stage.

While some disaccharides and nucleotide trisaccharides have been detected in animals, their biological role is unclear as no enzyme systems capable of transferring oligosaccharide blocks from such donors to the corresponding acceptors are known. In addition, a potential role of some lipid soluble vitamins, such as vitamin A (i.e., retinol) and vitamin K, should be mentioned. From animal cells, retinylphosphate, retinylpyrophosphate galactose, and retinylphosphate mannose, as well as some sugars bound through phosphate or pyrophosphate with vitamin K have been isolated (Wolf 1984). It is still unclear whether sugars as components of phosphorylated lipid soluble vitamins act as the donors of carbohydrate residues during the biosynthesis of glycans, or if they play other roles in carbohydrate metabolism. Monosaccharides and their activated NDPSs can penetrate across the plasma and intracellular membranes through a series of specific transport proteins (Caffaro and Hirschberg 2006, Liu and Hirschberg 2010a,b, Xu et al. 2010).

Glycosyltransferases and specific glycosidases modify the structure of carbohydrate chains during their biosynthesis and maturation in the endoplasmic reticulum and the Golgi complex. Maturation is a very important step for determining the final structure of glycans. Glycosyltransferases are highly specific for nontemplate biosynthesis of glycan chains. These enzymes are specific for the nature of transported sugars and for the donor and acceptor structures, which join together to form a unique glycosidic linkage (via α or β glycosidic bond) at the anomeric positions (Sajdel-Sulkowska et al. 1997, Taniguchi et al. 2002, Wiederschain and Newburg 2002a,b, Cummings and Piers 2009). The known glycosyltransferases are classified into different families (EC 2.4.1 and EC 2.4.2) and subfamilies according to their specificities during glycan biosynthesis (at least 381 glycosyltransferases have been described). Most of these glycosyltransferases support the nontemplate biosynthesis postulate: "one enzyme–one type of glycosidic linkage", originally proposed by Hagopian and Eylar. However, an increasing number of glycosyltransferases have been discovered that fail to obey this hypothesis, using either the same glycosyl donor to make more than one type of glycosidic linkage or different glycosyl donors to make each distinct glycosidic linkage (Stick and Williams 2010).

Although many of these enzymes are membrane bound and are difficult to separate, modern methods of isolation and purification have allowed researchers to isolate these enzymes in homogenous states, and to crystallize them and study their structural features. Studies of the glycosyltransferases at the gene level have revealed that comparatively elongated regions (motifs) similar in structure and sequence in genes encode the same family of enzymes, e.g., galactosyl-, fucosyl-, or sialyltransferases, and also the short regions that constitute a common feature of the enzymes, e.g., glycosyltransferases of eukaryotes (Kapitonov and Yu 1999, Hu and Walker 2002, Qasba and Ramakrishnan 2007, Qasba 2012).

However, many factors related to the biosynthesis of carbohydrate chains need further clarification. These undetermined factors include time and space correlated interactions of glycosyltransferases with donors and acceptors, regulation of the growth and termination of the carbohydrate chain, the influence of metal ions, optimum pH, effective multi-enzyme complexes, energy and mechanics of mutual movements, and interactions of the complex biosynthetic assembly with carbohydrate chains (Lairson et al. 2008, Stanley et al. 2009, Wagner and Pesnot 2010).

This type of biosynthesis is rather accurate as shown by the structure of the resulting molecules, but synthesized molecules of the same type are often not identical even if their biosynthesis occurs in the same cell. Such microheterogeneity is inevitable in molecules produced by nontemplate biosynthesis. Minute changes in positions of one or two monosaccharide residues increase the heterogeneity of carbohydrate structures. Although the function of such structural diversity is still unknown, it may become apparent under certain conditions, including pathology.

The macro and microheterogeneity of glycoconjugate molecules make it difficult to establish the structure–function relationship. During their biosynthesis, these glycoconjugates molecules undergo multiple modifications due to many enzymatic systems operating at all stages of the intracellular assembly. For example, the activity of some glycosidases involved in creation of N-linked carbohydrate chains is to cleave the terminal glucose residues initially bound on the N-glycans with a branched chain of mannose on a dolicholphosphate acceptor: "cutting" or "trimming" by glucosidase 1 in the endoplasmic reticulum starts detachment of the initial glucose residue from the carbohydrate structure of $Glc_3Man_9GlcNAc_2$ that has already been transferred onto proteins and the remaining two glucose residues are subsequently removed by α-glucosidase 2.

Modification of the remaining part of the carbohydrate chain may continue upon its movement into the cisternae of the GC by a series of α-mannosidase, depending on glycan accessibility after protein folding. This processing specificity is influenced by a new GlcNAc-residue added during the penultimate stage of trimming.

The biological reason for the cooperation of glycosyltransferases and glycosidases during the biosynthesis of glycan chains is still unclear. Regulatory mechanisms responsible for the movement of glycoconjugates as they are constructed along the RER–ER–GC pathway are also unknown. Possibly, modification of molecules as they are constructed serves for their recognition by transport receptors responsible for their movement along the biological conveyer, including the delivery of glycoconjugates into the GC, from its *cis* to *trans* compartments, and further into other cellular organelles or for export.

The GC is a highly organized and multifunctional biological fabric producing various molecules when they move along a set of conveyer–cistern–domains during their structural completion, resulting in the ultimate subcellular orientation and localization. Glycosylation is a very common modification of proteins and lipids, and most glycosylation processes occur in the GC. Although the transfer of initial sugar(s) to glycoproteins or glycolipids occurs in the endoplasmic reticulum, subsequent addition of the many different sugars that make up a mature glycan is accomplished in the GC. Golgi membranes are studded with glycosyltransferases, glycosidases, and nucleotide sugar transporters arrayed in an ordered manner from the *cis*-Golgi to the *trans*-Golgi network (TGN), such that each activity is able to act on specific substrates generated earlier in the pathway. The spectrum of glycosyltransferases and other enzymes and cofactors that effect glycosylation may vary with cell type, and thus the final complement of glycans on glycoconjugates is variable. In addition, glycan synthesis is affected by Golgi membrane dynamics, and cellular stress. Knowledge of Golgi glycosylation has fostered the development of assays to identify mechanisms of intracellular vesicular trafficking with the goal of facilitating glycosylation engineering of recombinant glycoproteins. Further studies of this extremely complex cellular compartment seem hold promise for advances in our understanding of vital cellular activities. At present, some experimental and theoretical work analyzing the GC organization deserves the greatest attention (Pfeffer 2010, 2011a, Stanley 2011, Kamiya et al. 2012, Pasek et al. 2012).

In the past two decades, glycosylation of proteins has been detected in the cellular nucleus and cytoplasm of various living systems including fungi, protozoa, worms, insects, and humans. Yeast seems to be a rare exception from this list (Pfeffer 2011b). This type of glycosylation involves the transfer of only one N-acetylglucosamine residue (GlcNAc) from its activated form, UDP-GlcNAc, to the hydroxyl group of serine/threonine within fully folded proteins, resulting in a β-glycosidic bond. This type of glycosylation is distinct from all other common forms of protein glycosylation in several major respects. First, it occurs exclusively within the nuclear and cytoplasmic compartment of the cell. Second, the GlcNAc-residue is not elongated or modified to form more complex carbohydrate structures. Third, it is attached and removed multiple times in the life of polypeptide, often cycling rapidly and at different rates at different sites on a polypeptide. Researchers consider this feature of glycosylation involving UDP-GlcNAc to resemble protein phosphorylation and it is very different from the classic glycosylation within the endoplasmic reticulum and GC cisternae.

This dynamic modification of carbohydrates occurs by the action of just two enzymes: O-GlcNAc-transferase and O-GlcNAc-glycosidase (β-N-acetylglucosaminidase). These two enzymes with opposite activities coexist in the same complex and seem to be controlled by an as yet unknown regulatory system responsible for overseeing O-GlcNAc-glycosylation and deglycosylation.

O-GlcNAc-glycosylation occurs in many compartments of eukaryotic cells and has been found to glycosylate proteins including chromatin, cytoskeleton proteins, and other relevant proteins in this structure. This type of glycosylation has been shown in membrane proteins, proteins of nuclear pores, RNA-processing proteins, and protein regulatory factors involved in protein translation. During the past two decades, it has become clear that O-GlcNAc-glycosylation is one of the most abundant posttranslational modifications within nucleocytoplasmic compartments of all metazoans including plants, animals, and the viruses that infect them.

The number of known proteins that can be the targets for O-GlcNAc-glycosylation continues to increase, and this type of glycosylation/deglycosylation seems to compete with phosphorylation/dephosphorylation of proteins by a plethora of specific kinases/phosphatases. All of these enzymes seem to be part of multi-enzyme complexes. It has been suggested that altered O-GlcNAc-glycosylation takes place in some neurodegenerative diseases such as Alzheimer's disease, diabetes, and various stresses, but details of these changes are still unclear (Zachara and Hart 2004).

Glycoconjugates with a more complex structure than that of the above described O-GlcNAc-glycoproteins are found in the plasma membrane and in most cellular organelles, including the nucleus, mitochondria, and lysosomes (Rondanino et al. 2003, Hart and Akimoto 2009). These molecules may originate from the biosynthesis in the RER and GC and are subsequently transferred into other compartments. Glycosylation can also occur in places that glycoconjugates localize, including the outer surface of plasma membrane. This glycosylation process is now intensively studied (Burnham-Marusich and Berninson 2012).

The detection of glycosyltransferases in many biological fluids and secretions, and in the cytoplasm and on the cell membrane surface suggests that glycosylation of molecules and their partial deglycosylation are dynamic processes that can only be better understood after further study. Modern mass spectrometric approaches for screening potential carbohydrate acceptors and analyzing the glycosylation products may lead to the discovery of novel glycosyltransferases with unique specificities (Lairson et al. 2008, Varki et al. 2009a,b,c). New effective approaches for measurement of the activity of glycosyltransferase based on the highly sensitive fluorometry, mass spectrometry (Ban et al. 2012) and electrochemical detection should increase the numbers of enzymes of this type (Luzhetskyy et al. 2005, Kohler and Patrie 2013). Special synthetic glycoconjugates allow researchers to obtain data on the activity and substrate specificity of previously unknown glycosyltransferases, in particular, of xylosyltransferases involved in biosynthesis of carbohydrate chains of O-glycoproteins (Wongkongkatep et al. 2006, Krylov et al. 2007, Gerardy-Schahn and Bakker 2010, Sethi et al. 2010, 2012).

Degradation of glycan chains. Enzymatic degradation of the carbohydrate moiety of glycoconjugate molecules in living organisms is catalyzed by a large group of hydrolytic enzymes—the glycosidases. Glycosidases catalyze the degradation of O-, N-, or S-glycosidic bonds in different glycosides, oligosaccharides, polysaccharides and glycoconjugates. It should be pointed out that the N- and S-glycosidases are represented by only a few enzymes, whereas O-glycosidases (carbohydrases) are much more common and degrade the O-glycosidic bonds, the major glycosidic linkages in most common glycans. For convenience, we shall use the term "glycosidases" instead of "O-glycosidases".

In addition to hydrolytic activity, many glycosidases can catalyze transglycosylation as well, i.e., the transfer of a glycosyl residue onto another acceptor to produce a new glycoside or oligosaccharide. It has been proposed that all reactions catalyzed by glycosylhydrolases and glycosyltransferases involve the same mechanism of glycosyl proton exchange and both types of enzymes should be categorized under the general name "glycosylases" (Henrissat et al. 2008, Vocadlo and Davies 2008). The enzymatic activity of glycosidases on natural substrates has been characterized by the identification and quantitative determination of a carbohydrate residue or an oligosaccharide fragment of a carbohydrate chain removed as a result of the enzymatic hydrolysis, using various physicochemical methods. The use of synthetic substrates significantly simplifies the determination of glycosidase activities and makes the determination very much more sensitive because in this case not only the carbohydrate moiety of the substrates but also its detached aglycone part can be identified. The aglycone moiety is a free chromogenic or fluorogenic product, such as phenol, 2- or 4-nitrophenol, 4-methylumbellipherone, α or β-naphthol, and derivatives of these molecules (Tsvetkova et al. 1991, Voznyi et al. 1993, Tsvetkova et al. 1996, Wiederschain and Newburg 2002a,b, Bojarova and Kren 2009). For example, the rate of hydrolysis of some synthetic substrates by certain glycosidases, e.g., hexosaminidase, is 10^3–10^5 times higher than the rate of hydrolysis of natural substrates. As of today, the number of synthetic substrates of glycosidases is still growing, and many of these synthetic substrates are readily available from various sources.

Notwithstanding the abovementioned advantages, the structure of synthetic substrates does not always satisfy the specificity requirements of a particular glycosidase (Bakh et al. 1980, 1981, Shapiro et al. 1991). There are glycosidases with tenfold lower affinity for synthetic substrates than for natural ones. In such cases, further efforts need to be made to synthesize substrates with an aglycone moiety that more closely mimics the structure of natural substrates. Fluorogenic glycolipids have been successfully used as the substrates of glycolipidhydrolases for determining the activities of such enzymes in the normal state and in some glycolipidoses (Wiederschain et al. 1992a,b). The structure of so-called semisynthetic substrates is closer to that of natural substrates for some glycosidases. For example, in a special case of glycolipids initially isolated from particular sources, the fatty acid is detached from ceramide by alkaline hydrolysis and substituted with a fluorophore labeled fatty acid. The resulting glycolipid is very similar to the original glycolipid substrate. One such compound (Gal-A-sphinganine) is an effective substrate for galactocerebrosidase (Semenyuk and Wiederschain 1984). The use of a wide spectrum of synthetically modified analogs of different sugars, in particular, of iminosugars, as inhibitors of glycosidases has enabled researchers to obtain new data on the specificity and catalytic mechanisms of these enzymes (Stütz 1999, Rye and Withers 2000).

Since the discovery of lysosomes by De Duve in 1955, many studies have shown that glycosidases are mainly located in such cellular organelles, which together with other hydrolytic enzymes—proteases, nucleases, lipases, and some other enzymes—degrade virtually all components of living cells (De Duve 2005). Many of the lysosomal glycosidases, both soluble and bound within the lysosomal membrane, are specific to the structure of monosaccharide residues and to the linkage and anomericity of glycosidic bonds.

In addition to their function as an "intracellular stomach", lysosomes are now considered as organelles involved in various processes in living organisms: processing of proteins, degradation of extra and intracellular waste structures (autophagy), initiation of apoptosis, import of cytoplasmic proteins, and export of products degraded in the lysosomes (Saftig and Klumperman 2009, Luzio et al. 2014).

Glycosidases are N-glycoproteins synthesized on ribosomes as precursors whose molecular weights are higher than that of the mature enzymes in the lysosomes. The enzyme precursors contain a signaling peptide responsible for penetration of the enzyme across the RER membrane that is detached from the enzyme by a corresponding protease after entering the RER. Subsequent glycosylation and maturation occur in the SER and GC cisternae. Then, a unique phosphorylation process comes into play. Hydroxyl groups of certain mannose residues are phosphorylated by an N-acetylglucosaminyltransferase as follows: the enzyme transfers a GlcNAcP from UDP-GlcNAc to the hydroxyl group at C6 of specific mannoses in the oligosaccharide chain of lysosomal enzyme. The Man6P-determinant is then exposed upon release of GlcNAc by another enzyme, i.e., GlcNAc-1-phosphodiester-α-N-acetylglucosaminidase, which is different from lysosomal α-N-acetylglucosaminidase in specificity and immunological and catalytic properties (Figura and Hasilik 1986, Kornfeld and Mellman 1989).

It should be noted that the phosphorylation enzymes are highly specific for the carbohydrate and the protein moieties of lysosomal hydrolases. Other glycoproteins processed in the SER and GC cisternae are not phosphorylated under the influence of phosphotransferase. Lysosomal hydrolases, including glycosidases, have certain carbohydrate and peptide sequences that determine enzymatic phosphorylation. The uniqueness of phosphorylation of each hydrolase is determined by the high order conformation of the enzyme.

Phosphorylation of carbohydrate chains of lysosomal hydrolases seems to prevent their further processing but is a prerequisite for binding of these molecules with the two mannose-6-phosphate receptors (Man-6-P-R) recognizing the Man-6-P-groups of the enzymes. Upon binding with the receptor in the *cis* compartments of the GC where the hydrolase concentration is highest, the hydrolases are packed into vesicles and delivered into lysosomes. The acidic medium in the lysosomes, provided by an ATP-driven proton pump, promotes dissociation of the Man-6-P-R—hydrolase complex, whereupon the receptor returns to the GC and onto surface of plasma membranes for recycling. A Man-6-P-R with molecular weight of about 300 kDa has been isolated in a homogenous state, and is known to be an integral glycoprotein as a component of intracellular vesicles, with its C-terminal of polypeptide inserted into the membrane and into the cytoplasm. Such Man-6-P-R organization seems to promote receptor recycling and prevents its movement into the interior of the lysosome. The receptor is a protein kinase with the ability to phosphorylate its own serine and tyrosine residues, which reduces its ability to bind lysosomal enzymes. This modification probably promotes the dissociation of receptor–ligand complex and receptor recycling.

On binding with lysosomal hydrolases, the 300 kDa Man-6-P-R does not need Mn^{2+} like cations, and thus it is designated as a cation-independent Man-6-P-R (CIM6PR). Some data indicate that CIM6PR is involved in regulation of cellular growth and mobility (Ghosh et al. 2003). Cells also have another M6PR with a molecular weight of 46 kDa that does require cations for the binding of lysosomal hydrolases. This cation-dependent Man6PR (CDM6PR) also participates in intracellular transfer of lysosomal hydrolases into particular lysosomes, but is inactive on the plasma membrane. Regulatory systems that determine the specialization of both cation-dependent and cation-independent receptors have not been characterized yet despite very intensive studies (Braulke and Bonifacino 2009, Fontes and Gilbert 2010, McMahon and Boucrot 2011).

The system of intracellular transport of hydrolases described above is not universal for all enzymes of this type. Some of these hydrolases, e.g., acidic phosphatase and β-glucocerebrosidase of fibroblasts and also lysosomal enzymes in other type of cells and tissues, are delivered to lysosomes by transport systems independent of Man-6-P-receptors that involve Man rather than Man-6 receptors. One such receptor for membrane bound β-glucocerebrosidase is more likely the lysosomal integral membrane protein 2 (LIMP2). Further studies will help us understand the delivery of glycosidases into various lysosomes and should significantly expand our ideas about this complicated system of enzyme delivery between cellular compartments and its targeting into different organelles.

Glycoconjugates, as natural substrates of glycosidases, enter lysosomes by receptor mediated endocytosis, which accomplishes the delivery of many biopolymers into cells (Schmid et al. 2014). In the first stage of this process, the terminal carbohydrate residues of glycoconjugates are bound to plasma membrane receptors, which recognize individual sialic acid, galactose, fucose, and mannose residues, with rather high specificity. Then, the receptor–ligand complex is packed into a vesicle produced by the plasma membrane intrusion, and the vesicle is separated from the plasma membrane by covering with the fibrillar protein clathrin. After that, the clathrin cover is discarded, the separated vesicle is acidified by a proton pump, and is converted into an endosome. In the next segregation stage, the receptor–ligand complex dissociates, and the receptor returns to the plasma membrane (recycling). The ligand containing vesicle fuses with the primary lysosomes and produces secondary lysosomes, which contain the previously delivered enzymes and the corresponding substrates. Only in the secondary lysosomes are glycoconjugates degraded by glycosidases, proteases, sulfatases, phosphatases, and lipases (McMahon and Boucrot 2011). The carbohydrate chains are degraded by both exoglycosidases and endoglycosidases. Exoglycosidases successively detach monosaccharide units from the non-reducing end of the carbohydrate chain and are specific for the monosaccharide residue, the anomeric configuration of the glycoside bond, and the distinct features of the structure and conformation of the aglycone moiety of the substrate. By contrast, endoglycosidases catalyze the detachment of an oligosaccharide block that is further degraded to monosaccharides by the successive action of exoglycosidases. The glycosidases have another specific feature of heterocatalytic enzymes that are capable of cleaving the same carbohydrate residues from different classes of carbohydrate containing compounds. Thus, some β-D-galactosidases cleave galactose from glycoproteins, glycolipids, and proteoglycans but the enzyme affinity for various substrates and the rate of their degradation can differ tenfold.

Whereas the chemistry of catalytic processes that determine the activity and specificity of many isolated glycosidases is well studied, their intralysosomal organization still remains poorly understood. Glycosidases, similarly to glycosyltransferases, can exist as multi-enzyme complexes as exemplified by the giant cellulosomal multi-enzyme complex of many bacteria that hydrolyzes plant polysaccharides of high molecular weight (Fontes and Gilbert 2010) or by the galactosialidase complex of animals (Hiraiwa et al. 1997). However, these enzymes need stabilizing proteins, or activator proteins to act as the biological detergents that help the glycolipid hydrolases catalyze the degradation of the carbohydrate moiety of glycolipids (Kolter and Sandhoff 2005).

An important and still unsolved problem is the interaction of glycosidases with the lysosomal membrane and other components of the intralysosomal matrix that seems to inhibit the action of glycosidases against each other and with proteases. Certainly, this does not mean an absolute stability of glycosidases within the lysosomes. Every glycosidase is characterized by its half-life, many glycosidases undergo partial proteolysis and deglycosylation within the lysosomes, although the degree of proteolysis and deglycosylation varies from enzyme to enzyme. It is noteworthy that some glycosidases, e.g., β-glucuronidase, are actually located on the outer surface of the lysosomal membrane, and these contribute to the modification of the surface of different subcellular organelles and pinocytotic vesicles as they translocate within the cell. These glycosidases also trigger certain signaling mechanisms. Glycosidases and glycosyltransferases located on the outer surface of the plasma membrane play an important role in intercellular interactions and in cell defense against bacteria and viruses (Aureli et al. 2012). Glycosidases are also found in the soluble cytoplasmic and microsomal fractions, in GC membranes, and in fractions of cellular nuclei. Some of these enzymes are different from the similarly named lysosomal enzymes in properties and substrate specificity for the glycan chains of different molecules, whereas other glycosidases have similar features but are different in composition of carbohydrates and amino acids as shown in β-glucuronidase of lysosomes and microsomes from rat liver.

In most cases, the nature of factors that determine the localization of glycosidases in a particular subcellular compartment is still not known. However, in the case of β-glucuronidase, certain anchoring egasin-like proteins determine the localization of the enzyme (Brown et al. 1987). It is reasonable to suggest that glycosidases of non-lysosomal origin, together with glycosyltransferases, contribute to the modifications of glycan chains of glycoconjugates in virtually all cellular compartments and membrane formations. Such modifications seem to "switch on", "turn off", or "redirect" certain metabolic pathways and be an integral system of an organism's general homeostasis. This standpoint is consistent with the existence of multiple forms of glycosidases that detach the same glycan moiety of the substrate, but with different physicochemical features, dependence on activators and inhibitors, subcellular localization, and substrate specificity (Wiederschain and Rosenfeld 1971, Wiederschain and Prokopenkov 1973, Wiederschain et al. 1973). Molecular forms of glycosidases have intraspecies, interspecies, and organ dependent differences. Studies on molecular forms of α-L-fucosidase in human kidney, placenta, liver, and blood serum revealed a polymorphic isoenzyme spectrum (Wiederschain et al. 1981, Wiederschain 1982, Beyer and Wiederschain 1982a,b).

In addition to the intracellular degradation of glycans, glycosidases are involved in numerous other biological processes. Firstly, they are essential for autolysis and autophagy, the processes of cellular elimination of "garbage" and preventing irreversible changes during starvation and under other unfavorable conditions. Secondly, glycosidases contribute to cell division, cell transformation during malignant growth, fertilization through acrosomal enzymes of spermatozoa, and the subsequent division of the fertilized oocyte under the influence of cortical granules located on the oocyte surface. Thirdly, glycosidases, in particular β-glucuronidase and hyaluronidase, are involved in embryogenesis, growth and differentiation of organs of insects and birds, and in wound epitheliation in mammals. Fourthly, exo and endo glycosidases of phages and also viral neuraminidase play an important role during infection of cells, from the interaction of influenza viruses with the cell surface to leaving the host cells and entering the bloodstream. Lastly, some glycosidases, in particular a highly specific N-glycosidase, are involved in the repair of DNA molecules damaged by mutagenic factors (Pearl 2000, Zharkov et al. 2010).

In summary, it is necessary to accentuate the importance of combined synthetic and enzymological approaches for the biosynthesis and degradation of glycans, which allow researchers to purposefully create substrates with desired structures. Studies on enzymatic modifications of such substrates containing carbohydrate chains and noncarbohydrate groups (sulfates, phosphates, acyl groups) that often influence the biological activity of the whole molecule are continuously expanding. This is exemplified in the studies of fucosidases and fucosyltransferases using synthetic substrates and acceptors and also in the study of the sulfotransferase that terminates biosynthesis of the glycan chain of the HNK1 antigen (Wiederschain 1979, Bakker et al. 1997, Wiederschain et al. 1998, 2000, Jungalvala 2005).

Biological Role of Glycoconjugates

Four decades ago, information about the biological role of carbohydrates was quite limited, and most research groups devoted their energies to studying problems associated with nucleic acids and proteins. Great advances were made in these fields, and it seemed that nucleic acids and proteins were responsible for all vital cellular processes. However, notwithstanding the great significance of molecular biology and proteomics, it has now been shown that the control of processes in living organisms is also dependent on an extremely diverse arsenal of simple and complex carbohydrates and glycoconjugates.

Examples of the biological significance of carbohydrates have already been presented in the introduction to this chapter. The biological importance of glycosylation is not only relevant to glycobiology, but also directly impacts the fields of molecular and cellular biology, proteomics and medicine, because disorders in these processes lead to severe diseases.

Glycan labeling in determination of the fate of molecules. Although the glycan content in glycoconjugates is relatively low, it frequently endows unique properties to these molecules that elucidate the biological functions of glycoconjugates.

In 1965, Eylar proposed a most interesting hypothesis concerning the role of the carbohydrate component in proteins. He suggested that the carbohydrate component is a special "passport" that determines the movement of glycosylated molecules from cells to various biological fluids: saliva, blood and others. Eylar analyzed data on the distribution of glycoproteins, and found that at least 100 glycoproteins were located outside cells and were components of different biological fluids including blood, saliva, milk, and other secretions. According to Eylar's hypothesis, the carbohydrate component was a kind of "chemical passport", which provided a signal for the protein molecule to leave the cell (Eylar 1965). Later, many intracellular glycoproteins were found and, on the contrary, many nonglycosylated proteins, including albumin, α-lactalbumin, and chymotrypsinogen were found in blood and various secretions. Thus, the hypothesis about the role of carbohydrate components failed to be universally applicable, but it did contain a farsighted idea about particular carbohydrate labeling determining the fate of the whole molecule.

Experimental data indicating the key role of the carbohydrate component in determining the half-life of serum glycoproteins were obtained nearly 10 years later from the group of Ashwell and Morell and their coworkers during their study of the mechanisms responsible for the development of Wilson–Konovalov disease (Ashwell and Harford 1982). This hereditary disease is associated with disorders in copper metabolism due to a decreased level of ceruloplasmin and asialoglycoproteins in blood that are the main carriers of copper in the human body.

In order to label the carbohydrate moiety of ceruloplasmin with radioactive tritium, it was necessary to cleave the terminal residues of neuraminic acid so that the penultimate galactose residues of the remaining glycans became accessible for labeling with tritium. Upon finishing this modification, the fate of the tritium labeled asialoceruloplasmin in rabbit blood was monitored. Surprisingly, human asialoceruloplasmin disappeared from the blood in a few minutes, whereas the half-life of native ceruloplasmin under the same conditions was about 56 hours. The same effect on removal of the neuraminic acid exposing galactose as the terminal residues in the glycan chains was also observed with other serum glycoproteins, such as haptoglobin, fetuin, and orosomucoid. All these glycoproteins left the bloodstream within a few minutes after the injection, and their half-life became normal upon the further removal of galactose residues or after modification with galactose oxidase (Ashwell and Harford 1982). Subsequent studies by many groups have demonstrated that the surface of the parenchymal cells in mammalian liver contains receptors capable of binding asialoglycoproteins with high affinity. This receptor protein was termed Hepatic Binding Protein (HBP). HBP is the first mammalian lectin that has been characterized in detail, with known amino acid and carbohydrate sequences in its protein and glycan moieties, subunit and domain structure, features of biosynthesis as a phosphorylated glycoprotein, and its subcellular localization in the GC and on the surface of plasma membrane of liver parenchymal cells. The orientation of this protein on the surface of liver parenchymal cells is different from other human receptors. In addition to its recognition of terminal galactose residues in the glycan chains of glycoproteins, HBP is also specific for terminal N-acetylgalactosamine residues in asialoglycoproteins, as exemplified by asialomucin from bovine submandibular glands.

After the discovery of HBP, a lectin with different specificity was found in chicken liver that binds glycoproteins with a terminal N-acetylglucosamine residue, but does not bind to galactose like HBP (Stockert 1995).

For some time it was believed that the main role of HBP, now known as the Ashwell-Morell Receptor (AMR) or Mammalian Asialoglycoprotein Receptor (ASGPR) in the literature, was to bind desialylated glycoproteins resulting from the action of blood sialidases, and also some cells, including desialylated erythrocytes, thus determining the lifetimes of these cells under physiological conditions. But there is no direct proof to support this viewpoint. Recently, the AMR was shown to be involved in the binding of some glycoproteins and regulatory participants of blood coagulation and thrombogenesis, including von Willebrand factor and platelets. Infection with *Streptococcus pneumoniae* is associated with accumulation of a great number of desialylated platelets in blood under the influence of bacterial neuraminidase. Such platelets are dangerous because they promote thrombosis in blood vessels. These desialylated platelets are removed by AMR into lysosomes of the liver parenchymal cells where they are destroyed, resulting in the prevention of general sepsis and increasing the survival of infected animals (Crewal et al. 2008, Veer and van der Poll 2008).

HBP/AMR is a member of the C-family of lectins capable of binding asialoglycoproteins. This ability is used for the development of effective approaches for creating new pharmaceuticals by directing some drugs with terminal galactose into the liver from the blood. The discovery of HBP/AMR triggered many studies that lead to the discovery of new mammalian lectins specific for terminal residues of galactose, fucose, mannose, and N-acetylglucosamine in glycan chains of different glycoproteins. In some cases, different lectins are specific for different organs and cell types. For example, a lectin specific for mannose/N-acetylglucosamine residue was isolated from the plasma membrane of Kupffer cells of rabbit liver. The same receptor was found on the surface of alveolar macrophages but had an additional specificity to terminal fucose. Receptor-lectin systems with different specificities determine important but yet undefined functions that may be present in the majority of, if not all, organs of mammals. Overall, liver parenchymal cells carry HBR/AMR on their membrane as an integral component, whereas the reticulo-endothelial cells of this organ (macrophages, endothelial, and Kupffer cells) contains receptors recognizing mannose/N-acetylglucosamine/fucose.

The number of human and animal lectins with different cellular and organ specificities has significantly increased, and the functions of many of these lectins are well understood (Vasta and Ahmed 2009). The mannose binding lectin (MBL) of blood serum specifically binds glycan chains on the surface of some microorganisms and thus prevents infection by helping macrophages attack pathogens. Various selectins participate in the regulation of protective reactions of mobile blood cells, lymphocytes and neutrophils, on their movement towards inflammation foci. C-Type lectins are involved in presentation of antigens that will be neutralized. Lectins of the Siglec family are signal receptors on immune system cells that recognize sialic acid residues on target cells. Extracellular galectins recognizing β-galactose residues are involved in cell adhesion and cell signaling (Rapoport and Bovin 2015). Moreover, lectins of this class modulate T-cell activation and controls cell survival by inhibiting apoptosis. Galectin1 and Galectin3 are found in the cell nucleus. Galectin3 is distributed between the cytoplasm and the nucleus depending on the stage of cell proliferation. The concentration of nuclear lectins is increased in the nuclei of virus transformed fibroblasts, suggesting a possible contribution of these proteins to cell proliferation and transformation. Although some lectins, e.g., calnexin and calreticulin, are not integral components of plasma or intracellular membranes, they are present as soluble proteins in the endoplasmic reticulum cisternae and are involved in the control of normal folding of mature glycoprotein molecules during their biosynthesis. Under disturbances of normal folding, other types of lectins are involved in degradation of such "improper" molecules (Haltiwanger et al. 1986, Varki 1993, Issitt and Anstee 1998, Cummings and Piers 2009, Moran et al. 2009, Fukuda 2010).

Glycoconjugates as biological antifreezes. Many plants, insects, animals and other organisms have evolved with unique adaptive mechanisms that allow them to survive in harsh environments at the extremes of temperature. Nearly two-thirds of the surface of earth is comprised of water, with the average surface temperature of seas and oceans varying from 2°C to 30°C depending on latitude. Within the Polar Regions, seawater temperatures are consistently below the freezing point of physiological solutions, which themselves have freezing points below the freezing point of pure water, i.e., 0°C at 1 atmosphere, due to the dissolved sugars and salts. The effect of these subzero temperatures on the cells of plants, animals, bacteria and fungi can be extremely harmful, if not deadly. Analysis of the blood plasma of fish showed that while the concentrations of salts and small ions in body fluids of polar fish are somewhat higher than that of fish in temperate water, these salts are only responsible for 40–50% of the observed freezing point depression. The remainder of the protective effect is attributed to the presence of a series of glycoproteins and proteins with relatively high molecular mass. 'Antifreeze' proteins (AFPs) and 'antifreeze' glycoproteins (AFGPs) have since been identified in the body fluids of many species of polar fish. Four classes of structurally diverse AFPs, classified as type I, type II, type III and type IV have now been identified along with a single class of glycosylated protein denoted as AFGP. Antifreeze glycoproteins (AFGPs) constitute the major fraction of proteins in the blood serum of Antarctic notothenioids and Arctic cod. Each AFGP consists of a varying number of repeating units of $(Ala-Ala-Thr)_n$, with minor sequence variations, and the disaccharide β-D-galactosyl-(1-3)-α-N-acetyl-D-galactosamine joined as a glycoside to the hydroxyl group of Thr residues. These compounds allow the fish to survive in subzero ice-laden polar oceans by kinetically depressing the temperature at which ice grows in a noncolligative manner. In contrast to the more widely studied antifreeze proteins, little is known about the mechanism for the inhibition of ice growth by AFGPs. So far, there is no definitive model that explains these properties (Harding et al. 2003).

Role of glycoconjugates in the immune system and cell malignancy. Studies in this field started with Landsteiner in 1900, who considered the carbohydrates as specific markers of antigenic molecules. At the beginning, blood group substances (BGS)—carbohydrate-containing biopolymers of glycoprotein or glycolipid from blood or different secretions of humans and other animals were thought to determine the blood group (Derevitskaya 1988, Hakomori 2008). The antigenic specificity of BGS is determined by a sequence of only a few terminal monosaccharides of these glyco-polymers. In the ABO(H) system of human blood classification, the specificity of type A blood antigen depends on a determinant oligosaccharide GalNAcα1,3(Fucα1,2)Galβ1,4GlcNAc with the key GalNAc residue; the B-antigen specificity is established by Galα1,3(Fucα1,2)Galβ1,4GlcNAc with the key Gal-residue; the H-antigen specificity is determined by Fucα1,2Galβ1,4GlcNAc with the key Fuc-residue. By contrast, in the MNSs system of blood groups, the specificity of N- and M-antigens are determined by one or two residues of N-acetylneuraminic acid, respectively. For each determinant oligosaccharide, only one rather rigid conformation created by noncovalent interactions of carbohydrate residues is preeminent. This results in the maximum accessibility of the determinant residues (Fuc, Gal, and GalNAc) for intermolecular interactions with corresponding antibodies (Issitt and Anstee 1998).

Carbohydrate determinants of various BGSs have been characterized in detail. These carbohydrate determinants can also be detached or added using specific glycosidases and glycosyltransferases to change the antigenic specificity of erythrocytes or soluble BGSs of biological fluids. For example, the carbohydrate determinants can be specifically cleaved with bacterial preparations of glycosidases that allow researchers to transform the A or B-type antigen containing erythrocytes into H (O) type cells of the universal blood group (Henrissat and Clausen 2007). This is especially important for blood transfusion (Issitt and Anstee 1998). Glycosidases of animal origin are inefficient for the BGS transformation. α-L-Fucosidase of animal origin could not cleave the L-fucose from native molecules of BGSs, but this monosaccharide is released from low-molecular weight glycopeptides fragments of these molecules (Wiederschain and Rosenfeld 1969).

In most cases, histocompatibility antigens responsible for the immune response upon transplantation of organs or tissues are glycoproteins, of which many of the carbohydrate antigenic determinants have been identified, such as the mouse H2 complex. T-lymphocyte receptors in charge of immunological control and recognition of foreign antigens are also often glycoproteins (Brondz 1987).

Major cell surface antigens are glycoconjugates, whose composition changes during the growth and tissue differentiation of cells and during tumor transformation. In distinction to normal cells, membrane glycosphingolipids are accumulated in tumor cells. Excretion of these tumor glycolipids, in particular gangliosides, into the extracellular medium changes the composition of glycolipid in the serum of cancer patients compared to normal serum. Gangliosides are suggested to suppress immune competent cells by decreasing antitumor immunity (Dyatlovitskaya and Bergelson 1987, Feizi and Childs 1987).

Glycolipids of tumor cell membranes are associated with the production of new fucolipids and simplification of corresponding structures. Fucolipids are synthesized due to activation of fucosyltransferases in the transformed cells. Fucolipids are rarely found in normal cells and seem to be important during the invasion and metastasis of tumors due to the presence of a fucose binding protein in some tissues. The composition of glycolipids in tumor cell membranes is simplified as a result of the production of shorter oligosaccharide chains. Among these abnormal oligosaccharides, the simplest gangliosides (GM3, GD3) and lactosylceramide become prevalent (Daniels and Withers 2007, Liu et al. 2010). Gangliosides are essential compounds of the plasma membrane involved in cell adhesion, proliferation, and recognition processes, as well as in the modulation of signal transduction pathways. These functions are mainly supported by the glycan moiety, and changes in the structure of gangliosides occur under pathological conditions including cancers. With progress in mass spectrometric analysis of gangliosides, the role of gangliosides in breast cancer progression and new perspectives in breast cancer therapy targeting gangliosides were also reviewed recently (Groux-Degroote et al. 2015).

There is no questions that a large number of glycoconjugates, particularly glycoproteins and glycolipids, are altered in primary cancerous and metastatic tissues. These changes have found differences in cell surface glycoconjugates accompanying malignant transformation in animals and humans both in cell culture (*in vitro*) and in solid tissues (*in vivo*). As was noted in the excellent review by Jack Alhadeff 25 years ago (Alhadeff 1989), these findings are significant since the cell surface is concerned with many normal physiological properties related to neoplastic transformation and the metastatic spread of malignancy: cell shape, growth, division, and differentiation; cellular recognition, communication, adhesiveness, and migration; contact inhibition of growth and immunological competence. Although current methodical level is much higher, there are still many unsolved old and new questions related to specificity of these changes in cancer cells, and it is still unclear whether these changes are epiphenomena or an integral part of the process of malignancy. New data reveal a close connection between tumor metabolism and Golgi function (Karsten and Goletz 2015).

A similar situation exists for sialomucins of tumor cells. Sialomucins are O-glycoproteins with sialic acid as terminal residue in glycan chains. These biopolymers are present in both mucous secretions and on the surface of many cells. For example, glycophorin is a sialomucin on the surface of erythrocytes. It has been suggested that sialomucins are antirecognition factors favorable for the protection of the tumor cells against the host. Sialomucins exfoliated from the surface of tumor cell bind with antisialomucins and produce a complex named blocking factor. It has also been proposed that sialomucins on the cell surface mask the cell antigens against the immune system of the body (Caraway and Spielman 1986).

Genetic alteration allow malignant cells to over-express growth signals and become indifferent to the inhibitory effects of tumor suppressor gene products such as Rb and p53. Certain genetic changes further allow the reactivation of telomerase activity creating an extensive replication potential. In addition to genetic alterations, phenotypic alterations also provide malignant cells the ability to escape tissue boundaries through engulfment, invasion and angiogenesis. Other phenotypic changes provide malignant cells with mechanisms to escape immunosurveillance (Couldrey and Green 2000, Schwartz-Albiez et al. 2008, Ghazarian et al. 2011, Stowell et al. 2015).

Some pathogenic microbes and viruses have specific proteins on their surface that are capable of recognizing accessible host sialoglycan chains and binding to them. These pathogens include human influenza viruses A and B, A-type virus of avian influenza, Vibrio cholera, Plasmodium falciparum, Clostridium botulinum, and Helicobacter pylori. Binding to such sialylated glycans is the first and very important step for the subsequent invasion of a pathogen into the body. Many vaccines developed against pathogenic bacteria and viruses have been strategically designed to contain the active moiety of a sialo-containing determinant that is capable of binding the pathogen and preventing its "landing" on the surface of host target cells (Varki and Gagneux 2012).

Also, it has been found that carbohydrates play an important role in the transport and secretion of glycosylated immunoglobulins by maintaining the conformation of the domains necessary for proper function of immunoglobulins, and protecting the sensitive regions of these molecules from proteolysis (Benjamini et al. 2000). The involvement of two typical terminal sugars in glycans, i.e., neuraminic acid and fucose, during the interaction between antigen sensitized T-lymphocytes and macrophages is exemplified by the function of a lymphocyte mediator that is a glycoprotein. It loses its ability to inhibit the migration of macrophages upon the removal of its neuraminic acid component by treatment with neuraminidase. The receptor of this mediator on the macrophage surface is a glycolipid with a terminal fucose. Cleavage of this fucose by α-L-fucosidase completely abolishes the effect of the mediator (macrophage inhibition factor, MIF) because of its inability to bind with the membrane of macrophages (Liu et al. 1982).

Another important role of glycoconjugates in immune system is demonstrated by activation of an alternative pathway of complement activation and establishment of glycoprotein moiety of many surface antigens of T- and B-lymphocytes, soluble immune mediators, lymphokines, monokines, suppressors, and other immune factors. During the recirculation of lymphocytes, carbohydrate specific receptor systems play an important role that determine the binding of lymphocytes to the surface of venules and peripheral lymphatic nodes (Stolman 1989).

The role, specificity and application of broad range of natural antibodies to glycans are discussed in several recent reviews (Bovin 2013, Bello-Gil and Manez 2015, Khasbiullina and Bovin 2015).

Glycoconjugates as Components of Receptor Systems

Most known receptors are glycoconjugates that selectively recognize the corresponding ligands. Some of these receptors have already been characterized. Examples of glycoconjugates as receptors that bind toxins, viruses, hormones, and other biologically active compounds, will be briefly discussed below.

Carbohydrate receptor systems that recognize toxins are exemplified, in particular, by the well-studied multistage binding of cholera toxin with GM1 ganglioside on the target cell plasma membranes. The same glycolipid attracts the toxin of *E. coli* but with lower specificity. Other gangliosides with additional residues of neuraminic acid in the structure, such as GD1b, GT1, and GT1b, are receptors of tetanus and botulism toxins. The ricin toxin penetrates into macrophages only upon binding with a mannose specific receptor on the cell surface. The binding of some pathogenic bacteria with terminal mannose in glycan chains of glycoproteins of target cell plasma membranes has already been mentioned. Specific receptor interactions can be realized by the glycoproteins on the oral cavity and Streptococcus sanguinis bacteria that bind to salivary glycoproteins via their terminal residue of N-acetylneuraminic acid and cause dental caries. The same residue, as a part of the carbohydrate chains of glycophorin on erythrocyte membrane, is involved in the binding of influenza myxoviruses and paramyxoviruses, e.g., Sendai virus to the surface of erythrocyte (Morris and McBride 1984, Haywood 1994, Plummer et al. 2006, Nobbs et al. 2007).

The hormonal system for regulating metabolism uses glycoconjugates of intercellular space (glycocalyx) of plasma membranes of target cells for recognition and signal transduction. There is a specific glycoprotein receptor capable of binding insulin on the surface of liver cells, adipocytes and lymphocytes. Treatment of this receptor with neuraminidase and galactosidase abolishes its binding ability. The transduction of the receptor signal is a very complex multistage process.

Hereditary Disorders in Degradation and Biosynthesis of Glycans

The famous British physician William Harvey (1 April, 1578–3 June, 1657) discovered the blood circulation. More than three centuries ago Harvey pointed out the importance of studying rare forms of diseases for a better understanding of many medical problems. He wrote: "Nature is nowhere accustomed more openly to display her secret mysteries than in cases where she shows traces of her workings apart from the beaten path; nor is there any better way to advance the proper practice of medicine than to give our minds to the discovery of the usual law of nature by careful investigation of cases of rarer forms of disease". The perfect examples of such types of diseases are lysosomal storage diseases and diseases developing as a result of hereditary errors of glycosylation.

Glycosidoses are the main group of lysosomal storage diseases. The term "glycosidoses" refers to those diseases caused by the storage of complex carbohydrates and carbohydrate-containing compounds. The glycosidoses as the main group of lysosomal storage diseases (LSD), develop as a result of the hereditary deficiency of any glycosidases/hydrolases that are associated with the catabolism of carbohydrate-containing products in lysosomes. Some types of mucopolysaccharidoses are associated with an insufficiency of sulfatases that are not formally glycosidases, leading to the defective detachment of sulfate residues on the ends of carbohydrate chains of glycoconjugates. As a result, glycosaminoglycans are accumulated due to the blocked action of other enzymes responsible for sequential detachments of monosaccharide units from the nonreducing end of the glycan chains. Thus, the term "glycosidoses" is sufficiently broad and convenient to classify a large group of diseases based on two parameters: the enzyme insufficiency (most frequently of a glycosidase) and the nature of the primary storage product—glycan/glycoconjugate (Wiederschain 1980, 1986).

Glycosidoses were initially observed by clinicians before the molecular mechanisms of their development had been elucidated. Therefore, many of these diseases are named after the clinicians who were the first to report the severe clinical symptoms of these human pathologies. Examples are Tay–Sachs, Gaucher, Fabry, and Hurler diseases, Hunter and Sanfilippo syndromes, and others. These diseases are accompanied by disorders in the nervous, muscular, and bone systems, by mental retardation, and other disturbances that finally lead to the death of patients at an early age (Hers and van Hoof 1973, Callachan and Lowden 1981, Durand and O'Brien 1982, Barranger and Brady 1984, Scriver et al. 2001, Futerman and van Meer 2004). A few LSDs are now treatable by enzyme replacement therapy.

Interpretation of the molecular bases of glycosidoses started a half century ago when Hers found in 1963 that in the second type of glycogenosis (Pompe's disease), lysosomes of various cells did not contain acidic α-glucosidase resulting in glycogen accumulation in these cells (Rosenfeld and Popova 1989). Pompe's disease was the first glycosidosis that was shown to develop owing to the insufficiency of a glycosidase. Later Hers formulated a concept of hereditary LSDs characterized by four main features: (1) the pathology is a storage disease; (2) the storage products are always located in lysosomes; (3) the accumulated compounds can be homogenous or heterogeneous depending on the specificity of the deficient enzyme; and (4) LSDs are a monogenic group of diseases characterized by deficiency of a single enzyme.

Since the formulation of hereditary LSDs by Hers, the types and subtypes of these molecular disorders have approached 50 in number. Their inheritance is mainly autosomal recessive and less frequently the recessive X-chromosome linked type. Although each of these diseases is relatively rare, in total LSDs contribute significantly to human pathology and attract the attention of clinicians and researchers as unique models for studying the aberrant metabolism induced by deficiency of a single enzyme from a multi enzyme group. The cellular responses to events resulting in the storage of uncleavable products in lysosomes are also nontrivial and help to understand previously unknown processes in the body.

Glycosidoses are divided into four major types: mucopolysaccharidoses, glycolipidoses, mucolipidoses, and glycoproteinoses.

In the past several decades, these human diseases have attracted the attention of many research groups. The accumulated experimental data have been summarized in hundreds of papers and tens of monographs (Kleta et al. 2004, Platt and Walkley 2004, Futerman and Zimran 2007, Freeze 2009, Mehta and Winchester 2012, Sandhoff and Harzer 2013) and certainly cannot be fully covered in this chapter.

However, it is reasonable to emphasize some recent scientific data and ideas obtained as a result of studies on glycosidoses and the approaches for their treatments using enzyme replacement therapy to remedy the metabolic problems of pathological cells.

Receptors responsible for enzyme uptake and delivery into lysosomes have been identified. In galactosialidosis, a glycosidase complex is found in the lysosomes. In some other diseases (Sanfilippo C, mucolipidoses), the successive degradation of glycan chains is inefficient if the biogenesis of an enzyme involved in this degradation is disturbed because of an insufficiency of certain transferases normally responsible for processing of glycoconjugates. Alternatively, these diseases can also be caused by disorders in the biogenesis of lysosomal enzymes. Lysosomal membranes contain some transporters of free sugars that are cleaved during degradation, especially the transporter of sialic acids. The insufficiency of such transporters on the lysosomal membranes is also associated with an LSD, e.g., Salla disease (Wiederschain 1977, Aula and Aula 2006).

Metabolic rearrangements in glycosidoses lead to an appearance of glycans with unusual structure and unusual location in tissues. "Chemical dedifferentiation" of tissues and organs can occur and be followed by secondary negative influences on biochemical processes (Beyer et al. 1993).

Products stored in lysosomes change the spectrum of secreted enzymes and their molecular forms, the value of the intralysosomal pH, and organization of components of the cytoskeleton system (Ivleva and Wiederschain 1994, Beyer et al. 1995). Attempts to correct glycosidoses by substitutive enzymatic and gene therapy gave important information about the organism's immune response, the efficiency of enzyme delivery in different formulations including liposomes (Pabst et al. 2014), and the function of genes incorporated into regions of the genome controlling biosynthesis of glycosidases. During the treatment of glycosidoses, a new strategy was developed for decreasing the accumulation of glycoconjugates by suppressing their biosynthesis. This strategy has been tested on animal models in a few cases.

It seems that in the very near future further studies of glycosidoses will result in elucidation of mechanisms for triggering a cellular response to the overload of accumulated compounds. There is a pronounced activation of some lysosomal enzymes that are unrelated to the primary genetic deficiency related to biosynthesis of lysosomal enzymes and factors responsible for their activity in the cells. As an example, in fucosidosis there is more than a 7-fold increase of α-galactosidase activity, a 6-fold increase of β-xylosidase activity, and a 5-fold increase of α-glucosidase activity. Such hyperactivations are observed in LSDs not only relating to glycosidases, but also other lysosomal hydrolytic enzymes, such as cathepsin D, acidic phosphatase, and others. Besides the increase in the total activity of some lysosomal enzymes, in glycosidoses the concentration of protein activators/chaperones that are components of the intralysosomal matrix is also significantly increased. Based on these data, we propose that the hyperactivation of the lysosomal hydrolytic system could be a protective reaction of the cell with respect to product accumulation. The elucidation of systems that regulate these processes possibly through certain signaling messengers of lysosomes–cytoplasm–nucleus–cell membranes may lead to the discovery of other important pathways of intracellular communication.

These abnormal changes due to an LSD lead to numerous metabolic and morphological changes such as the storage of non-degradable metabolic products, impaired uptake, sorting, digesting of cellular and extracellular substances and defective release of the digestion products. Interruption of biomolecule recycling results in a variety of pathogenic cascades including alteration of calcium homeostasis, oxidative stress, inflammation, altered lipid trafficking, autophagy, endoplasmic reticulum stress and autoimmune responses. The progressive lysosomal accumulation of non-degradable metabolites results in generalized dysfunction of cell and tissue and multi-systemic pathology (Alroy et al. 2014). LSDs are now in the focus of a few biotech companies specialized in creating preparations for correcting glycosidoses (Hopwood et al. 2006).

Genetic Diseases Developing from Disorders in Glycosylation

Although the genes encoding the enzymes involved in biosynthesis of glycans comprise about 1–2% of the human genome, knowledge of hereditary disorders in this area was obtained relatively recently, beginning in the 1980s. Such knowledge concerns virtually all stages and forms of glycosylation. Some studies have been mentioned already as shown in the previous case of glycosidoses with deficient glycosylation of glycosidases during their maturation and processing. Initially, these pathologies only included the biosynthesis of N-glycoproteins, but the number of such known diseases significantly increased after extensive patient studies. Now, they form a large group of hereditary disorders in virtually all aspects of the biosynthesis of glycoproteins, glycolipids and proteoglycans. As in the case of glycosidoses, a disturbance in only one link of glycosylation may lead to severe manifestations in various diseases (Sandhoff and Harzer 2013).

Classification and biochemical characterization of genetic diseases associated with the disorders in glycosylation were recently reviewed by Freeze (Freeze 2013) and are discussed by Susan Sparks in a special chapter of this book. Data on relationships of glycans with more general human diseases, such as cancer and infectious and viral diseases have been summarized (Litwack 2008, Nizet and Esko 2009, Varki and Freeze 2009, Varki et al. 2009a,b,c).

To study and treat the whole spectrum of hereditary and nonhereditary diseases related to disorders in the metabolism of glycans and glycoconjugates, a huge arsenal of highly efficient approaches and medications produced by many pharmacological and biotechnological companies is available (Townsend and Hotchkiss 1997, Hounsell 1998, McGrath and Walsh 2006, Brockhausen 2006, Packer and Karlsson 2009, Struwe et al. 2011, Han and Costello 2013, Yuriev and Ramsland 2013). These trends have provided a powerful stimulus to the development of analytical and synthetic chemistry of carbohydrates. Clearly, the number of patients with any single condition will be a key determinant in whether a company will be willing to make the necessary investment in pursuing an appropriate treatment.

Glycobiology is now a mature field for chemical synthesis and structural analysis now capable of producing glycans with complicated structures, different degrees of polymerization, and modified with other biologically important groups (Shibaev 1985, Hanessian 1997, Large and Warren 1997, Withczak and Nieforth 1997, Iozzo 2001, Wang and Bertozzi 2001, Thibault and Honda 2002, Volpe 2002, Garg et al. 2005, Yarema 2005, Plou et al. 2007, Taniguchi et al. 2008, Liu et al. 2009, Li 2010, Musto and Suslick 2010, Redini 2012, Rohrer et al. 2013, Severov et al. 2015). Chemical glycobiology brings a huge impact to the understanding of the role of simple and complex sugars and glycoconjugates in an additional "language of life" in various biological process. The isolation of biologically active glycans of plant and animal origin from the World's Oceans create huge stores of novel glycans from natural algal and animal sources (Cumashi et al. 2007, Kiessling and Splain 2010, Croci et al. 2011, Usov 2011, Kiessling and Splain 2013, Dwek 2014, Wang and Amin 2014). A new line of science that can be termed "glycopharmacology" and "glycobiopharmaceutical engineering" has already appeared and is developing successfully (Pomin and Mourao 2008, Ghosh et al. 2009, Sola and Griebenow 2010, Beck 2013, Hudak and Bertozzi 2014).

Conclusions

In human health, glycans are involved in myriad processes that are part of normal physiology, development, and cell signaling, along with the development of hereditary, chronic and infectious diseases. Much of the information content in cells is encompassed in the glycome. Glycans contain key biological information that complements the information stored in DNA to help complete the link between genotype and phenotype or between the genome and expressed traits. Many advances in understanding human health and diseases are the result of current knowledge about nucleic acids, proteins, and glycans and how these vary in different circumstances and in different people. However, much is still unknown. Continued advances in understanding the biological roles played by glycans, along with the factors that influence or alter their functions, will have consequences for the fundamental understanding of biology and will contribute to the development of new therapeutic medicines (See in Reference List: Transforming Glycoscience: A Roadmap for the Future 2012). Publication of new results of intensive studies in glycobiology is burgeoning. The interest in better comprehension of molecular processes underlying human diseases is obviously displayed in many of these theoretical and experimental studies. Naturally, this interest is not casual. Detection of any deviation from normal cells leads to an understanding of many underlying processes in normally functioning living organisms. In turn, this helps to elaborate efficient approaches to correct metabolic disorders at every level. These two trends are inseparable and mutually enriched with new ideas and methods. Glycobiology is becoming a science of the structure, function, and metabolism of carbohydrate-containing compounds in humans under normal and pathological conditions. Possibly, the term "glycobiomedicine" will better reflect advances in this field in the near future.

Periodic scientific journals and virtually all major publishers are increasing the publications of new results of intensive studies in glycobiology and glycoscience. The great success in this field is based on the most effective analytical approaches for studies of the structures of simple and complex glycans and glycoconjugates, the discovery of new sources for isolation of unique bioactive carbohydrates from marine hydrobionts and plants, and a deep understanding of cell and subcellular events with carbohydrate involvement. Many of these discoveries were reviewed recently (Beck 2013, Wiederschain 2013, Newburg and Grave 2014, Wang and Amin 2014, Knirel et al. 2015, Larskaya and Gorshkova 2015, Tang et al. 2015).

Acknowledgement

I kindly thank Dr. Peter Daniel for his critical reading manuscript and excellent editorial help.

Keywords: glycobiology, glycoscience, glycomics, Golgi complex, lysosomes, glycoconjugates, glycosyltransferases, glycosidases, glycosidoses, lysosomal storage diseases (LSD), glycans and cancer

References

Alhadeff, J. A. 1989. Malignant cell glycoproteins and glycolipids. CRC Critical Reviews in Oncology/Hematology 9: 37–107.

Alroy, J., C. Garganta and G. Wiederschain. 2014. Secondary biochemical and morphological consequences in lysosomal storage diseases. Biochemistry (Moscow) 79: 619–636.

Anisimova, N. Yu., N. E. Ustyuzhanina, F. V. Donenko, M. I. Bilan, N. A. Ushakova, A. I. Usov et al. 2015. Influence of fucoidans and their derivatives on antitumor and phagocytic activity of human blood leucocytes. Biochemistry (Moscow) 80: 925–933.

Ashwell, G. and J. Harford. 1982. Carbohydrate-specific receptors of the liver. Annual Review of Biochemistry 51: 531–554.

Aula, N. and P. Aula. 2006. Prenatal diagnosis of free sialic acid storage disorders (SASD). Prenatal Diagnosis 26: 655–658.

Aureli, M., R. Bassi, N. Loberto, S. Regis, A. Prinetti, V. Chigorno et al. 2012. Cell surface associated glycohydrolases in normal and Gaucher disease fibroblasts. J Inherit Metab Dis 35: 1081–1091.

Bakh, N. L., E. M. Beyer, N. V. Bovin, S. E. Zurabyan and G. Ya. Wiederschain. 1980. Specificity and properties of multiple forms of human α-L-fucosidase. Doklady Academy of Sciences USSR (Russ) 255: 996–999.

Bakh, N. L., E. M. Beyer, G. Ya. Wiederschain, N. V. Bovin and S. E. Zurabyan. 1981. A study of properties and substrate specificity of human α-L-fucosidase multiple forms using natural and synthetic fucose-containing oligosaccharides. Bioorganic Chemistry (Russ) 7: 1024–1033.

Bakker, H., I. Friedmann, S. Oka, T. Kawasaki, N. Nifant'ev, M. Schachner et al. 1997. Expression Cloning of a cDNA encoding a sulfotransferase involved in the biosynthesis of the HNK-1 carbohydrate epitope. J Biol Chem 272: 29942–29946.

Ban, L., N. Pettit, L. Li, A. D. Stuparu, L. Cai, W. Chen et al. 2012. Discovery of glycosyltransferases using carbohydrate arrays and mass spectrometry. Nat Chem Biol 8: 769–773.

Barranger, J. A. and R. O. Brady (eds.). 1984. Molecular Basis of Lysosomal Storage Disorders, Academic Press, Orlando-San Diego-New York-London.

Beck, A. (ed.). 2013. Glycosylation Engineering of Biopharmaceuticals. Methods and Protocols. Humana Press, Springer, New York, pp. 355.

Becker, D. J. and J. B. Lowe. 2003. Fucose: biosynthesis and biological function in mammals. Daniel Glycobiology 13(7): 41R–53R.

Bello-Gil, D. and R. Manez. 2015. Exploiting natural anti-carbohydrate antibodies for therapeutic purposes. Biochemistry (Moscow) 80: 836–845.

Benjamini, E., R. Coico and G. Sunshine. 2000. Immunology. A Short Course, 4th ed., Wiley-Liss, New York-Toronto.

Bertozzi, C. R. and D. Rabuka. 2009. Structural basis of glycan diversity. pp. 23–36. In: Varki, A., R. D. Cummings, J. D. Ensco, H. Freeze, P. Stanley, C. R. Bertozzi et al. (eds.). Essentials of Glycobiology 2nd ed. Cold Spring Harbor Laboratory Press, New York.

Beyer, E. M. and G. Ya. Wiederschain. 1982a. Human and animal fucosidases (Review). Uspechi Biological Khimii (Russ) 23: 103–122.

Beyer, E. M. and G. Ya. Wiederschain. 1982b. Further evidence of human α-L-fucosidase polymorphism. Clin Chim Acta 123: 251–259.

Beyer, E. M., T. S. Ivleva, G. T. Artykova and G. Ya. Wiederschain. 1993. Comparative studies of intracellular activity, secretion and multiple forms spectra of human skin fibroblast α-L-fucosidase in the normal and after sucrose load. Biochem Molec Biol Intrnational 30: 367–375.

Beyer, E. M., T. S. Ivleva, G. T. Artykova and G. Ya. Wiederschain. 1995. Change of isoforms' spectra of α-L-fucosidase from human skin fibroblasts in intracellular storage of nonhydrolyzable substances. Biochem Molec Biol Intrnational 1270: 7–11.

Bochkov, A. F. and G. E. Zaikov. 1979. Chemistry of the O-Glycosidic Bond: Formation and Cleavage. Pergamon Press, New York.

Bojarova, P. and V. Kren. 2009. Glycosidases: a key to tailored carbohydrates. Trends in Biotechnology 27: 199–209.

Bovin, N. V. 2013. Natural antibodies to glycans. Biochemistry (Moscow) 78: 786–797.

Braulke, T. and J. S. Bonifacino. 2009. Sorting of lysosomal proteins. Biochimica Biophysica Acta 1793: 605–614.

Brockhausen, I. (ed.). 2006. Glycobiology Protocols. Humana Press, Totowa, NJ, USA.

Brondz, B. D. 1987. T-Lymphocytes and Their Receptors in Immunological Recognition [in Russian], Nauka, Moscow.

Brown, J., E. K. Novak, K. Takeuchi, K. Moore, S. Medda and R. Swank. 1987. Lumenal location of the microsomal β-glucuronidase-egasyn complex. J Cell Biol 105: 1571–1578.

Burnham-Marusich, A. R. and P. M. Berninson. 2012. Multiple proteins with essential mitochondrial functions have glycosylated isoforms. Mitochondrion 12: 423–427.

Caffaro, C. E. and C. B. Hirschberg. 2006. Nucleotide sugar transporters of the Golgi apparatus: from basic science to diseases. Accounts of Chemical Research 39: 805–812.

Callachan, J. W. and J. A. Lowden (eds.). 1981. Lysosomes and Lysosomal Storage Disease. Raven Press, New York.

Caraway, K. L. and J. Spielman. 1986. Structural and functional aspects of tumor cell surface sialomucins. Mol Cell Biochem 72: 108–120.

Couldrey, C. and J. E. Green 2000. Metastases: the glycan connection. Breast Cancer Res 2: 321–323.

Crewal, P. K., S. Uchiyama, D. Ditto, N. Varki, D. T. Le, V. Nizet et al. 2008. The Ashwell receptor mitigates the lethal coagulopathy of sepsis. Nat Medicine 14: 648–655.

Croci, D. O., A. Cumashi, N. A. Ushakova, M. E. Preobrazhenskaya, A. Piccoli, L. Totani et al. 2011. Fucans, but not fucomannoglucuronans, determine the biological activities of sulfated polysaccharides from Laminaria saccharina brown Seaweed. PLoS ONE 6(2): e17283.

Cumashi, A., N. A. Ushakova, M. E. Preobrazhenskaya, A. D'Incecco, A. Piccoli, L. Totani et al. 2007. A comparative study of the anti-inflammatory, anticoagulant, antiangiogenic, and antiadhesive activities of nine different fucoidans from brown seaweeds. Glycobiology 17: 541–552.

Cummings, R. D. and J. M. Piers (eds.). 2009. Handbook of Glycomics. Elsevier, Academic Press, Amsterdam-Boston-Heidelberg-London-New York-Oxford-Tokyo.

Daniels, G. and S. G. Withers. 2007. Towards universal red blood cells. Nature Biotechnology 25: 427–428.

De Duve, C. 2005. The lysosome turns fifty. Nat Cell Biol 7: 847–849.

Derevitskaya, V. A. 1988. Biosynthesis of carbohydrate chains of glycoproteins and their heterogeneity. Bioorganic Chemistry (Russian) 14: 1605–1625.

Dische, Z. 1963. Reciprocal relation between fucose and sialic acid in mammalian glycoproteins. Ann NY Acad Sci 106: 259–270.

Dumitriu, N. (ed.). 2005. Polysaccharides. Structural Diversity and Functional Versatility, 2nd ed. Marcel Dekker, New York.

Durand, P. and J. S. O'Brien (eds.). 1982. Genetic Errors of Glycoprotein Metabolism, Edi-Ermes, Milano, Springer-Verlag, Berlin, Heidelberg, New York.

Dwek, R. A. 2014. Journeys in Science: Glycobiology and other paths. Annual Review of Biochemistry 83: 1–44.

Dyatlovitskaya, E. V. and L. D. Bergelson. 1987. Glycosphingolipids and antitumor immunity. Biochim Biophys Acta 907: 125–143.

Eylar, E. 1965. On the biological role of glycoproteins. J Theoretical Biol 10: 89–113.

Feizi, T. and R. A. Childs. 1987. Carbohydrates as antigenic determinants of glycoproteins. Biochemistry Journal 245: 1–11.

Figura, K. V. and A. Hasilik. 1986. Lysosomal enzymes and their receptors. Ann Rev Biochem 55: 167–193.

Fontes, C. M. G. A. and H. J. Gilbert. 2010. Cellulosomes: highly efficient nanomachines designed to deconstruct plant cell wall complex carbohydrates. Annual Review of Biochemistry 79: 655–681.

Fraser-Reid, B. O., K. Tatsuta and J. Thiem (eds.). 2008. Glycoscience. Chem and Chem Biol, 2nd ed. Springer-Verlag, Tokyo-Berlin-Heidelberg-New York.

Freeze, H. 2009. Genetic disorders of glycan degradation. pp. 567–583. *In*: Varki, A., R. D. Cummings, J. D. Esko, H. Freeze, P. Stanley, C. R. Bertozzi et al. (eds.). Essentials of Glycobiology 2nd ed. Cold Spring Harbor Laboratory Press, Cold Spring Harbor, New York.

Freeze, H. 2013. Understanding human glycosylation disorders: Biochemistry leads the charge. J Biol Chem 288: 6936–6945.

Fukuda, M. (ed.). 2010. Methods in Enzymology, v. 478 (Glycomics); v. 479 (Functional Glycomics); v. 480 (Glycobiology). Elsevier Inc., Academic Press.

Futerman, A. H. and G. van Meer. 2004. The cell biology of lysosomal storage disorders. Nat Rev Mol Cell Biol 5: 554–565.

Futerman, A. H. and A. Zimran (eds.). 2007. Gaucher Disease, CRC, Taylor and Francis Group, Boca Raton, FL, USA.

Gabius, H. -J. (ed.). 2009. The Sugar Code. Fundamentals of Glycoscience. Wiley-VCH Verlag, GmbH and Co, KGaA, Weinheim.

Garg, H., R. Linchardt and C. A. Hales (eds.). 2005. Chemistry and Biology of Heparin and Heparan Sulfate. Elsevier, Amsterdam-Boston-New York-London.

Gerardy-Schahn, R. and H. Bakker. 2010. Identification of glycosyltransferase 8 family members as xylosyltransferases acting on O-glucosylated notch epidermal growth factor repeats. J Biol Chem 285: 1582–1586.

Ghazarian, H., B. Idoni and S. B. Oppenheimer. 2011. A glycobiology review: carbohydrates, lectins, and implications in cancer therapeutics. Acta Histochem 113: 236–247.

Ghosh, P., N. M. Dahms and S. Kornfeld. 2003. Mannose 6-phosphate receptors: new twists in the tale. Nature Reviews Molecular and Cell Biology 4: 202–212.

Ghosh, T., K. Chattopadhyay, M. Marshall, P. Karmakar, P. Mandal and B. Ray. 2009. Focus on antivirally active sulfated polysaccharides: From structure-activity analysis to clinical evaluation. Glycobiology 19: 2–15.

Groux-Degroote, S., Y. Guérardel, S. Julien and P. Delannoy. 2015. Gangliosides in breast cancer: New perspectives. Biochemistry (Moscow) 80: 808–819.

Hakomori, S. -I. 2008. Structure and function of glycosphingolipids and sphingolipids: Recollections and future trends. Biochim Biophys Acta 1780: 325–346.

Haltiwanger, R. S., M. A. Lehrman, A. E. Eckhardt and R. L. Hill. 1986. The distribution and localization of the fucose-binding lectin in rat tissues and the identification of a high affinity form of the mannose/N-acetylglucosamine-binding lectin in rat liver. J Biol Chem 261: 7433–7439.

Han, L. and C. Costello. 2013. Mass spectrometry of glycans. Biochemistry (Moscow) 78: 710–720.

Hanessian, S. (ed.). 1997. Preparative Carbohydrate Chemistry. Marcel Dekker, New York.

Harding, M. M., P. I. Anderberg and A. D. J. Haymet. 2003. "Antifreeze" glycoproteins from polar fish. European Journal of Biochemistry 270: 1381–1392.

Hart, G. W. and Y. Akimoto. 2009. The O-GlcNAc modification. pp. 263–279. In: Varki, A., R. D. Cummings, J. D. Esko, H. Freeze, P. Stanley, C. R. Bertozzi et al. (eds.). Essentials of Glycobiology, 2nd ed. Cold Spring Harbor Laboratory Press, Cold Spring Harbor, New York.

Hattrup, C. L. and S. J. Gendler. 2008. Structure and function of the cell surface (Tethered) mucins. Annu Rev Physiol 70: 431–457.

Haywood, A. M. 1994. Virus receptors: Binding, adhesion strengthening, and changes in viral structure. Journal of virology 68(1): 1–5.

Henrissat, B. and H. Clausen. 2007. Bacterial glycosidases for the production of universal red blood cells. Nature Biotechnology 25: 454–464.

Henrissat, B., G. Sulzenbacher and Y. Bourne. 2008. Glycosyltransferases, glycoside hydrolases: Surprise, surprise! Cur Opin Struct Biol 18: 527–533.

Hers, H. G. and F. van Hoof (eds.). 1973. Lysosomes and Storage Diseases. Academic Press, New York-London.

Hiraiwa, M., M. Saitoh, N. Arai, T. Shiraishi, S. Odani, Y. Uda et al. 1997. Protective protein in the bovine lysosomal β-galactosidase complex. Biochimica Biophysica Acta 1341: 189–199.

Hopwood, J., G. Bate and P. Kirkpatrick. 2006. Galsulfase. Nature Reviews Drug Discovery 5: 101–102.

Hounsell, E. (ed.). 1998. Glycoanalysis Protocols, 2nd ed. Humana Press, Totowa, NJ, USA.

Hu, Y. and S. Walker. 2002. Remarkable structural similarities between diverse glycosyltransferases. Chem and Biol 9: 1287–1296.

Hudak, J. E. and C. R. Bertozzi. 2014. Glycotherapy: New advances inspire a reemergence of glycans in medicine. Chem and Biol 21: 16–37.

Iozzo, R. (ed.). 2001. Proteoglycan Protocols. Humana Press, Totowa, NJ, USA.

Issitt, P. D. and D. J. Anstee. 1998. Applied Blood Group Serology, 4th ed. Montgomery Scientific Publications, Durham, North Carolina, USA.

Ivleva, T. S. and G. Ya. Wiederschain. 1994. Reversible rearrangement of vimentin-type intermediate filaments in cultured human skin fibroblasts from patients with lysosomal storage diseases. Cell Biol Int 18: 647–653.

Jungalvala, F. B. 2005. Biosynthesis and function of HNK-1 glycans. pp. 59–94. In: Fukuda, M., U. Rutishauser and R. Schnaar (eds.). Neuroglycobiology (Molecular and Cellular Neurobiology). Oxford University Press, Oxford, United Kingdom.

Kamerling, J. P., G. -J. Boons, Y. C. Lee, A. Suzuki, N. Taniguchi and A. G. J. Voragen (eds.). 2007. Comprehensive Glycoscience. From Chemistry to System Biology, Vol. 14. Elsevier, Amsterdam-Boston-New York-London.

Kamiya, Y., T. Satoh and K. Kato. 2012. Molecular and structural basis for N-glycan-dependent determination of glycoprotein fates in cells. Biochim Biophys Acta 1820: 1327–1337.

Kannicht, C. (ed.). 2002. Posttranslational Modifications of Proteins: Tools for Functional Proteomics. Humana Press, Totowa, NJ, USA.

Kapitonov, D. and R. K. Yu. 1999. Conserved domains of glycosyltransferases. Glycobiology 9: 961–978.

Karsten, U. and S. Goletz. 2015. What controls the expression of the core_1 (Thomsen–Friedenreich) glycotope on Tumor Cells? Biochemistry (Moscow) 80: 801–807.

Khasbiullina, N. R. and N. V. Bovin. 2015. Hypotheses of the origin of natural antibodies: A Glycobiologist's opinion. Biochemistry (Moscow) 80: 820–835.

Kiessling, L. L. and R. A. Splain. 2010. Chemical approaches to glycobiology. Annu Rev Biochem 79: 619–653.

Kiessling, L. L. and B. G. Splain. 2013. Realizing the promise of chemical glycobiology. Chem Sci 4: 3381–3394.

Kleta, R., R. P. Morse, E. Orvisky, D. Krasnewich, J. Alroy, A. A. Ucci et al. 2004. Clinical, biochemical, and molecular diagnosis of a free sialic acid storage disease patient of moderate severity. Mol Genet Metabolism 82: 137–143.

Knirel, Y. A., Q. Sun, S. N. Senchenkova, A. V. Perepelov, A. S. Shashkov and J. Xu. 2015. O-Antigen modifications providing antigenic diversity of *Shigella flexneri* and underlying genetic mechanisms. Biochemistry (Moscow) 80: 901–914.

Kohler, J. J. and S. M. Patrie (eds.). 2013. Mass Spectrometry of Glycoproteins: Methods and Protocols. Humana Press, Springer Science, New York-Heidelberg-Dordrecht-London.

Kolter, T. and K. Sandhoff. 2005. Lysosomal glycosphingolipid storage diseases. pp. 199–223. *In*: Fukuda, M., U. Rutishauser and R. L. Schnaar (eds.). Neuroglycobiology (Molecular and Cellular Neurobiology). Oxford University Press, Oxford, United Kingdom.

Kornfeld, S. and I. Mellman. 1989. The biogenesis of lysosomes. Annu Rev Cell Biol 5: 483–526.

Krylov, V., N. Ustyuzhanina, H. Bakker and N. Nifantiev. 2007. Stereoselective synthesis of the 3-aminopropyl glycosides of α-D-Xyl-(1→3)β-D-Glc and α-D-Xyl-(1→3)-α-D-Xyl-(1→3)-β-D-Glc and of their corresponding *N*-octanoyl derivatives. Synthesis 3147–3154.

Laine, R. A. 1994. A calculation of all possible oligosaccharide isomers both branched and linear yields 1.05 x 10^{12} structures for reducing hexasaccharide: The Isomer Barrier to development of single-method saccharide sequence or synthetic system. Glycobiology 4: 759–767.

Lairson, L. L., B. Henrissat, G. J. Davies and S. G. Withers. 2008. Glycosyltransferases: Structures, functions, and mechanisms. Annu Rev Biochem 77: 521–555.

Large, D. G. and C. D. Warren (eds.). 1997. Glycopeptides and Related Compounds. Synthesis, Analysis, and Applications, Marcel Dekker, New York.

Larskaya, I. A. and T. A. Gorshkova. 2015. Plant oligosaccharides—outsiders among elicitors? Biochemistry (Moscow) 80: 881–900.

Lennarz, W. and G. Hart (eds.). 1994. Methods in Enzymology, Guide to Techniques in Glycobiology. Academic Press, San Diego-New York-Boston-London, Vol. 230.

Li, J. (ed.). 2010. Functional Glycomics. Methods and Protocols. Humana Press, Springer Science, New York.

Litwack, G. 2008. Human Biochemistry and Disease. Elsevier, Amsterdam-Boston-New York-London.

Liu, D. Y., K. D. Petschek, H. G. Remold and J. R. David. 1982. Isolation of guinea pig macrophage glycolipid with the properties of the putative migration inhibitory factor receptor. J Biol Chem 257: 159–162.

Liu, L. and C. B. Hirschberg. 2010a. The role of nucleotide sugar transporters in development of eukaryotes. Seminars in Cell Develop Biol 21: 600–608.

Liu, L. and C. B. Hirschberg. 2010b. Developmental diseases caused by impaired nucleotide sugar transporters. Glycoconjugate Journal 30: 5–10.

Liu, Y., A. S. Palma and T. Feizi. 2009. Carbohydrate microarrays: Key developments in glycobiology. Biological Chemistry 390: 647–656.

Liu, Y., S. Yan, A. Wondimu, D. Bob, M. Weiss, K. Sliwinski, J. Villar, V. Notario, M. Sutherland, A. M. Colberg-Poley and S. Ladisch. 2010. Oncogene 29: 3297–3306.

Luzhetskyy, A., A. Vente and A. Bechtold. 2005. Glycosyltransferases involved in the biosynthesis of biologically active natural products that contain oligosaccharides. Mol Biol System 1: 117–126.

Luzio, J. P., Y. Hackmann, N. M. G. Dieckmann and G. M. Griffiths. 2014. The Biogenesis of lysosomes and lysosome-related organelles. pp. 227–243. *In*: Schmid, S., A. Sorkin and M. Zerial (eds.). Endocytosis. Cold Spring Harbor Laboratory Press, Cold Spring Harbor, NY.

McGrath, B. M. and G. Walsh (eds.). 2006. Directory of Therapeutic Enzymes. CRC Press, Taylor and Francis Group, Boca Raton-London-New York-Washington.

McMahon, H. T. and E. Boucrot. 2011. Molecular mechanism and physiological functions of clathrin-mediated endocytosis. Nat Rev Mol Cell Biol 12: 517–533.

Mehta, A. and B. Winchester (eds.). 2012. Lysosomal Storage Disorders: a Practical Guide. Wiley Blackwell.

Moran, A. P., O. Holst, P. J. Brennan and von M. Itzstein (eds.). 2009. Microbial Glycobiology. Structures, Relevance and Applications. Elsevier, Academic Press, Amsterdam-Boston-Heidelberg-London-New York-Oxford-Tokyo.

Morris, E. J. and B. C. McBride. 1984. Adherence of Streptococcus sanguis to saliva-coated hydroxyapatite: Evidence for two binding sites. Infection and Immunity 43: 656–663.

Musto, C. J. and K. Suslick. 2010. Differential sensing of sugars by colorimetric arrays. Curr Opin Chem Biol 14: 758–766.

Narin, A. and K. Moremen. 2015. Glycotranscriptomics. pp. 1475–1482. *In*: Taniguchi, N., T. Endo, G. W. Hart, P. H. Seeberger and C. -H. Wong (eds.). Glycoscience: Biology and Medicine. Springer, Tokyo-Berlin-Heidelberg-New York.

Newburg, D. and G. Grave. 2014. Recent advance in human milk glycobiology. Pediatric Res 75: 675–679.

Nizet, V. and J. D. Esko. 2009. Bacterial and viral infection. pp. 537–551. *In*: Varki, A., R. D. Cummings, J. D. Esko, H. Freeze, P. Stanley, C. R. Bertozzi et al. (eds.). Essentials of Glycobiology, 2nd ed. Cold Spring Harbor Laboratory Press, Cold Spring Harbor, New York.

Nobbs, A. H., Y. Zhang, A. Khammanivong and M. C. Herzberg. 2007. Streptococcus gordonii has environmentally constrains competitive binding by Streptococcus sanguinis to saliva-coated hydroxyapatite. J Bacteriol 189: 3106–3114.

Ohtsubo, K. and J. D. Marth. 2006. Glycosylation in cellular mechanisms of health and disease. Cell 126: 855–867.

Pabst, G., N. Kucerka, M. -P. Nieh and J. Katsaras (eds.). 2014. Liposomes, Lipid Bilayers and Model Membranes: From Basic Research to Application. CRC Press, Taylor & Francis Group, Boca Raton-London-New York.

Packer, N. H. and N. G. Karlsson (eds.). 2009. Glycomics. Methods and Protocols. Humana Press, Springer Science, New York.

Pasek, M., B. Ramakrishnan, E. Boeggeman, N. Mercer, A. E. Dulcey, G. L. Griffiths and P. K. Qasba. 2012. The N-Acetyl-binding pocket of N-acetylglucosaminyl-transferases also accommodates a sugar analog with a chemical handle at C2. Glycobiology 22: 379–388.

Pearl, L. H. 2000. Structure and function in the uracil-DNA glycosylase superfamily. Mutation Research/DNA Repair 460: 165–181.

Pfeffer, S. 2010. How the Golgi works: A cisternal progenitor model. Proceedings of National Academy of Science USA 107: 19614–19618.

Pfeffer, S. 2011a. Cold Spring Harbor Perspective in Biology, 3, a005272, 1–11.

Pfeffer, S. 2011b. Entry at the trans-face of the Golgi. pp. 183–193. *In*: Warren, G. and J. Rothman (eds.). The Golgi. Cold Spring harbor Lab Press, Cold Spring Harbor, New York.

Platt, F. M. and S. U. Walkley (eds.). 2004. Lysosomal Disorders of the Brain. Recent Advances in Molecular and Cellular Treatment, Oxford University Press, Oxford.

Plou, F. J., A. G. de Segura and A. Ballesteros. 2007. Application of glycosidases and transglycosidases in the synthesis of oligosaccharides. pp. 141–160. *In*: Polaina, J. and A. P. MacCabe (eds.). Industrial Enzymes Structure, Function and Applications. Springer, Dordrecht, The Netherlands.

Plummer, C., C. William and I. Douglas. 2006. Relationship between the ability of oral streptococci to interact with platelet glycoprotein Ibα and with the salivary low-molecular-weight mucin, MG2. FEMS Immunology and Medical Microbiology 48: 390–399.

Pomin, V. H. and P. A. S. Mourao. 2008. Structure, biology, evolution, and medical importance of sulfated fucans and galactans. Glycobiology 18: 1016–1027.

Qasba, P. K. and B. Ramakrishnan. 2007. X-ray crystal structures of glycosyltransferases. pp. 251–281. *In*: Kamerling, J. P., G. J. Boons, Y. C. Lee, A. Suzuki, N. Taniguchi and A. G. J. Voragen (eds.). Comprehensive Glycoscience. From Chemistry to System Biology, Vols. 1–4. Elsevier Ltd., Amsterdam-Boston-New York-London.

Qasba, P. K. 2012. The N-acetyl-binding pocket of N-acetylglucosaminyltransferases also accommodates a sugar analog with a chemical handle at C2. Glycobiology 22: 379–388.

Rademacher, T. W., R. B. Parekh and R. A. Dwek. 1988. Glycobiology. Annu Rev Biochem 57: 785–838.

Rapoport, E. M. and N. V. Bovin. 2015. Specificity of human galectins on cell surfaces. Biochemistry (Moscow) 80: 846–856.

Redini, F. (ed.). 2012. Proteoglycans. Methods and Protocols. Humana Press, Springer Science, New York.

Reitsma, S., D. W. Slaaf, H. Vink, M. A. M. J. van Zandvoort and Mirjam G. A. oude Egbrink. 2007. The endothelial glycocalyx: Composition, functions, and visualization. Pflugers Arch - Eur J Physiol 454: 345–359.

Rohrer, J. S., L. Basumallick and D. Hurum. 2013. High-performance anion-exchange chromatography with pulsed amperometric detection for carbohydrate analysis of glycoproteins. Biochemistry (Moscow) 78: 697–709.

Rondanino, C., M. T. Bousser, M. Monsigni and A. C. Roche. 2003. Sugar dependent nuclear import of glycosylated proteins in living cells. Glycobiology 13: 509–519.

Rosenfeld, E. L. and I. A. Popova. 1989. Inborn Disorders in Glycogen Metabolism [in Russian]. Meditsina, Moscow.

Rye, C. S. and S. G. Withers. 2000. Glycosidase mechanisms. Current Opinion in Chemical Biology 4: 573–580.

Saftig, P. and J. Klumperman. 2009. Lysosome biogenesis and lysosomal membrane proteins: Trafficking meets function. Nat Rev Mol Cell Biol 10: 623–635.

Sajdel-Sulkowska, E. M., F. I. Smith, G. Y. Wiederschain and R. H. McCluer. 1997. Cloning of a rat α1,3-fucosyltransferase gene: A member of the fucosyltransferase IV family. Glycocon J 14: 249–258.

Sandhoff, K. and K. Harzer. 2013. Gangliosides and gangliosidoses: Principles of molecular and metabolic pathogenesis. The Journal of Neuroscience 33: 10195–10208.

Sansom, S. and O. Markman (eds.). 2007. Glycobiology. Scion Publishing Ltd. Bloxham , Oxfordshire, United Kingdom.

Schmid, S., A. Sorkin and M. Zerial (eds.). 2014. Endocytosis. Cold Spring Harbor Laboratory Press, Cold Spring Harbor, NY.

Schwartz-Albies, R., A. Eichmuller and M. Kirschfink. 2008. Cytotoxic natural antibodies against human tumours: an option for anti-cancer immunotherapy? Autoimmun Rev 7: 491–495.

Scriver, C. R., A. L. Beaudet, W. S. Sly and D. Valle (eds.). 2001. Lysosomal disorders. pp. 3371–3894. *In*: The Metabolic and Molecular Bases of Inherited Disease, 8th ed., McGrawHill, Vol. III, Part 16, Chapters 134–154.

Semenyuk, E. P. and G. Ya. Wiederschain. 1984. The use of the fluorescently labelled cerebroside as a substrate for galactosylceramidase from human skin fibroblasts. Biokhimiya 49: 1556–1560.

Sethi, M. K., F. F. R. Buettner, V. B. Krylov, H. Takeuchi, N. E. Nifantiev, R. S. Haltiwanger et al. 2010. Molecular cloning of a xylosyltransferase that transfers the second xylose to O-glucosylated epidermal growth factor repeats of Notch. J Biol Chem 285: 1582–1586.

Sethi, M. K., F. F. R. Buettner, A. Ashikov, V. B. Krylov, H. Takeuchi, N. E. Nifantiev et al. 2012. Molecular cloning of a xylosyltransferase that transfers the second xylose to O-glucosylated epidermal growth factor repeats of Notch. Journal of Biological Chemistry 287: 2739–2748.

Severov, V. V., G. V. Pazynina, T. V. Ovchinnikova and N. V. Bovin. 2015. The synthesis of oligosaccharides containing internal and terminal Galβ1-3GlcNAcβ fragments. Russian Journal of Bioorganic Chemistry 41: 147–160.

Shapiro, E., L. Lockman, W. Kennedy, D. Zimmerman, E. Kolodny, S. Raghavan et al. 1991. Bone marrow transplantation as treatment for globoid cell leukodystrophy. pp. 223–238. *In*: Desnick, R. J. (ed.). Treatment of Genetic Diseases. Churchill Livingstone, New York.

Sharon, N. 1975. Complex Carbohydrates. Their Chemistry, Biosynthesis, and Functions. Addison-Wesley Publishing, Company, London.

Shibaev, V. N. 1976. Uspechi Biologicheskoy Khimii (Russ) 17: 187–216.

Shibaev, V. N. 1985. *In*: Progress in Chemistry of Carbohydrates [in Russian], Nauka, Moscow 149–173.

Snider, M. D. 1984. Biosynthesis of glycoproteins: formation of N-linked oligosaccharides. pp. 163–198. *In*: Ginsburg, V. and P. W. Robbins (eds.). Biology of Carbohydrates, Vol. 2. Wiley, New York.

Sola, R. J. and K. Griebenow. 2010. Glycosylation of therapeutic proteins: an effective strategy to optimize efficacy. BioDrugs 24: 9–20.

Spiro, R. G. 2002. Protein glycosylation: Nature, distribution, enzymatic formation, and disease implications of glycopeptide bonds. Glycobiology 12: 43R–56R.

Stanley, P., H. Schachter and N. Taniguchi. 2009. N-Glycans. pp. 101–114. *In*: Varki, A., R. D. Cummings, J. D. Esko, H. Freeze, P. Stanley, C. R. Bertozzi et al. (eds.). Essentials of Glycobiology, 2nd ed. Cold Spring Harbor Laboratory Press, Cold Spring Harbor, New York.

Stanley, P. 2011. Golgi glycosylation. pp. 21–33. *In*: Warren, G. and J. Rothman (eds.). The Golgi. Cold Spring Harbor Laboratory Press. Cold Spring Harbor, New York.

Stick, R. V. and S. Williams. 2010. Carbohydrates: The Essential Molecules of Life, 2nd edition. Elsevier, Amsterdam, The Netherlands.

Stockert, R. J. 1995. The Asialoglycoprotein receptor: relationships between structure, function, and expression. Physiol Rev 75: 591–609.

Stolman, L. M. 1989. Adhesion molecules controlling lymphocyte migration. Cell 56: 907–910.

Stowell, S. R., T. Ju and R. D. Cummings. 2015. Protein glycosylation in cancer. Annu Rev Pathol 10: 473–510.

Struwe, W. B., J. C. Byrne, R. Saldova and P. M. Rudd. 2011. Therapeutic proteins: facing the challenges of glycobiology pp. 1–38. *In*: Owens, R. J. and J. E. Nettleship (eds.). Glycoproteomics in Health and Disease. In Functional and Structural Proteomics of Glycoproteins, Springer Netherlands.

Stütz, A. E. (ed.). 1999. Iminosugars as Glycosidase Inhibitors. Nojirimycin and Beyond. Wiley-VCH, Weinheim-New York-Toronto.

Tang, H., P. Hsue, D. Kletter, M. Bern and B. Haab. 2015. The detection and discovery of glycan motifs in biological samples using lectins and antibodies: new methods and opportunities. Adv Cancer Res 126: 167–202.

Taniguchi, N., K. Honke and M. Fukuda (eds.). 2002. Handbook of Glycosyltransferases and Related Genes. Springer-Verlag, Tokyo.

Taniguchi, N., A. Suzuki, Y. Ito, H. Narimatsu, T. Kawasaki and S. Hase (eds.). 2008. Experimental Glycoscience. Glycochemistry. Springer, Tokyo-Berlin-Heidelberg-New York.

Taniguchi, N., T. Endo, G. W. Hart, P. H. Seeberger and C. -H. Wong (eds.). 2015. Glycoscience: Biology and Medicine. Springer, Tokyo-Berlin-Heidelberg-New York.

Taylor, M. E. and K. Drickamer. 2011. Introduction to Glycobiology, 3rd ed. Oxford University Press, Oxford, New York.

Terao, N., S. Takamatsu, T. Minehira, T. Sobajima, K. Nakayama, Y. Kamada et al. 2015. Fucosylation is a common glycosylation type in pancreatic cancer stem cell-like phenotypes. World J Gastroenterol 21: 3876–3887.

Thibault, P. and S. Honda (eds.). 2002. Capillary Electrophoresis of Carbohydrates. Humana Press, Totowa, NJ, USA.

Thijssen, V. L. and G. A. Rabinovich. 2014. Glycans in vascular biology. Glycobiology 24: 1235–1236.

Tiralongo, J. and I. Martínez-Duncker (eds.). 2013. Sialobiology: Structure, Biosynthesis and Function. Sialic Acid Glycoconjugates in Health and Disease. Bentham Science Publishers, Sharjah, United Arab Emirates.

Townsend, R. R. and A. T. Hotchkiss, Jr. (eds.). 1997. Techniques in Glycobiology. Marcel Dekker, New York.

Transforming Glycoscience: A Roadmap for the Future. 2012. Committee on Assessing the Importance and Impact of Glycomics and Glycosciences; Board on Chemical Sciences and Technology; Board on Life Sciences; Division on Earth and Life Studies; National Research Council, National Academies Press online, National Academies Press, Washington, DC, USA.

Tsvetkova, I. V., E. A. Karpova, Y. V. Voznyi, T. V. Zolotukhina, V. V. Biryukov and A. N. Semyachkina. 1991. Use of 4-trifluoromethylumbelliferyl-α-L-iduronide as a new substrate for detection of α-L-iduronidase deficiency in human tissues and for rapid prenatal diagnosis of Hurler disease. J Inher Metab Diseases 14: 134–139.

Tsvetkova, I. V., E. A. Karpova, T. V. Dudukina and Y. V. Voznyi. 1996. 4-Penta-fluoroethylumbelliferyl-β-D-glucoside as a new fluorogenic substrate for acid β-D-glucosidase. Clin Chim Acta 248: 125–133.

Usov, A. 2011. Polysaccharides of the red algae. Advances in Carbohydrate Chemistry and Biochemistry 65: 115–217.

Ustyuzhanina, N. E., M. I. Bilan, N. A. Ushakova, A. I. Usov, M. V. Kiselevskiy and N. E. Nifantiev. 2014. Fucoidans: Pro- or antiangiogenic agents? Glycobiology 24: 1265–1274.

Varki, A. 1992. Diversity in the sialic acids. Glycobiology 2: 25–40.

Varki, A. 1993. Biological roles of oligosaccharides: all of the theories are correct. Glycobiology 3: 97–130.

Varki, A. and R. Schauer. 2009. Sialic acids. pp. 199–217. *In*: Varki, A., R. D. Cummings, J. D. Esko, H. Freeze, P. Stanley, C. R. Bertozzi et al. (eds.). Essentials of Glycobiology, 2nd ed. Cold Spring Harbor Laboratory Press, Cold Spring Harbor, New York.

Varki, A. and N. Sharon. 2009. Historical background and overview. pp. 1–22. *In*: Varki, A., R. D. Cummings, J. D. Esko, H. Freeze, P. Stanley, C. R. Bertozzi et al. (eds.). Essentials of Glycobiology, 2nd ed. Cold Spring Harbor Laboratory Press, Cold Spring Harbor, New York.

Varki, A. and H. Freeze. 2009. Glycans in acquired human diseases. pp. 601–615. *In*: Varki, A., R. D. Cummings, J. D. Esko, H. Freeze, P. Stanley, C. R. Bertozzi et al. (eds.). Essentials of Glycobiology, 2nd ed. Cold Spring Harbor Laboratory Press, Cold Spring Harbor, New York.

Varki, A., R. Kangxi and B. Toole. 2009a. Glycosylation changes in cancer. pp. 617–632. *In*: Varki, A., R. D. Cummings, J. D. Esko, H. Freeze, P. Stanley, C. R. Bertozzi et al. (eds.). Essentials of Glycobiology, 2nd ed. Cold Spring Harbor Laboratory Press, Cold Spring Harbor, New York.

Varki, A., J. D. Esko and K. Colley. 2009b. Cellular organization of glycosylation. pp. 37–46. *In*: Varki, A., R. D. Cummings, J. D. Esko, H. Freeze, P. Stanley, C. R. Bertozzi et al. (eds.). Essentials of Glycobiology, 2nd ed., Cold Spring Harbor Laboratory Press, Cold Spring Harbor, New York.

Varki, A., R. D. Cummings, J. D. Ensco, H. Freeze, P. Stanley, C. R. Bertozzi et al. (eds.). 2009c. Essentials of Glycobiology, 2nd ed. Cold Spring Harbor Laboratory Press, Cold Spring Harbor, New York.

Varki, A. and P. Gagneux. 2012. Multifarious roles of sialic acids in immunity. Annals of the New York Academy of Sciences 1253: 16–36.

Vasta, G. R. and H. Ahmed (eds.). 2009. Animal Lectins. A Functional View, CRC Press, Taylor and Frances Group, Boca Raton, FL, USA.

Veer, C. and T. van der Poll. 2008. Keeping blood clots at bay in sepsis. Nat Med 14: 606–608.

Vocadlo, D. J. and G. Davies. 2008. Mechanistic insights into glycosidase chemistry. Current Opinion in Chemical Biology 12: 539–555.

Volpe, N. (ed.). 2002. Capillary Electrophoresis of Carbohydrates. From Monosaccharides to Complex Carbohydrates, Humana Press, Springer Science, New York.

Voznyi, Y. V., E. A. Karpova, T. V. Dudukina, I. V. Tsvetkova, A. M. Boer, H. C. Janse et al. 1993. A fluorimetric enzyme assay for the diagnosis of Sanfilippo disease C (MPS III C). J Inherit Metab Disease 16: 465–472.

Wagner, G. K. and T. Pesnot. 2010. Glycosyltransferases and their assays. ChemBioChem 11: 1939–1949.

Wang, L. -X. and M. N. Amin. 2014. Chemical and chemoenzymatic synthesis of glycoproteins for deciphering functions. Chem and Biol 21: 51–66.

Wang, P. G. and C. R. Bertozzi (eds.). 2001. Glycochemistry, Principles, Synthesis, and Applications. Marcel Dekker, New York.

Warren, G. and J. Rothman (eds.). 2011. The Golgi. Cold Spring Harbor Laboratory Press, Cold Spring Harbor, New York.

Wiederschain, G. Ya. and E. L. Rosenfeld. 1969. Specificity of pig kidney fucosidase and its action on different fragments of blood group (A+H) substance. Bull Soc Chim Biol, Paris 51: 1075–1084.

Wiederschain, G. Ya. and E. L. Rosenfeld. 1971. Two forms of α-L-fucosidase from pig kidney and their action on natural oligosaccharides. Biochemistry and Biophysics Research Communications 44: 1008–1014.

Wiederschain, G. Ya. and A. S. Prokopenkov. 1973. β-D-Galactosidase and β-D-fucosidase of pig kidney. Arch Biochem Biophys 158: 539–543.

Wiederschain, G. Ya., E. L. Rosenfeld and L. G. Kolibaba. 1973. Human α-L-fucosidases. Clinic Chim Acta 46: 305–310.

Wiederschain, G. Ya. 1976. Molecular Biology (Moscow) 10: 957–980.

Wiederschain, G. Ya. 1977. Glycosidases in normal cell and in hereditary disorders in degradation of carbohydrate-containing compounds. Adv Biol Chem (Russ) 18: 185–210.

Wiederschain, G. Ya. 1979. Carbohydrate-containing biopolymers in the recognition processes of molecules and cells (Review). Advances of Biological Chemistry (Russ) 20: 46–70.

Wiederschain, G. Ya. 1980. Biochemical Basis of Glycosidoses [in Russian], Meditsina, Moscow, pp. 286.

Wiederschain, G. Ya., E. M. Beyer, B. A. Klyashchitsky and A. S. Shashkov. 1981. Specificity patterns of different types of human fucosidase. Recognition by enzymes of a certain region of the pyranose ring in sugars. Bioch Biophys Acta 659: 434–444.

Wiederschain, G. Ya. 1982. Multiple forms of human glycosidases and their role in glycoconjugates degradation. Adv Clin Enzymol 2: 150–157.

Wiederschain, G. Ya. 1986. Aspects of glycolipid metabolism in normal state and glycolipidoses (Review). Adv Biol Chem (Russ) 27: 117–135.

Wiederschain, G. Ya., S. Raghavan and E. Kolodny. 1992a. Characterization of 6-hexadecanoylamino-4-methylumbelliferyl-ß-D-galactopyranoside as fluorogenic substrate of galactocerebrosidase for the diagnosis of Krabbe disease. Clin Chim Acta 205: 87–96.

Wiederschain, G. Ya., I. K. Kozlova, G. S. Ilyina, M. A. Mikhaylova and E. M. Beyer. 1992b. The use of glycosides of 6- and 8-acylamino-4 methylumbelliferone in studies of the specificity and properties of human lysosomal glycolipid hydrolases. Carbohydrate Res 224: 255–272.

Wiederschain, G. Ya., O. Koul, J. Aucoin, F. I. Smith and R. H. McCluer. 1998. α1,3 Fucosyltransferase, α-L-fucosidase, α-D-galactosidase, β-D-galactosidase, and Le^x glycoconjugates in developing rat brain. Glycoconj J 15: 379–388.

Wiederschain, G. Ya., O. Koul, N. V. Bovin, N. E. Nifantiev and R. H. McCluer. 2000. The study of the substrate specificity of rat-brain fucosyltransferase using synthetic acceptors. Russian Journal of Bioorganic Chemistry 26: 403–406.

Wiederschain, G. Ya. and D. S. Newburg. 2002a. Fucosyltransferases. pp. 1335–1338. *In*: Creighton, T. E. (ed.). Wiley Encyclopedia of Molecular Medicine. J Wiley & Sons Press, New York.

Wiederschain, G. Ya. and D. S. Newburg. 2002b. α-Fucosidases. pp. 133–136. *In*: Creighton, T. E. (ed.). Wiley Encyclopedia of Molecular Medicine. J Wiley & Sons Press, New York.

Wiederschain, G. 2013. Glycobiology: Progress, problems, and perspectives. Biochemistry (Moscow) 78: 679–696.

Withczak, Z. and K. A. Nieforth (eds.). 1997. Carbohydrates in Drug Design. Marcel Dekker, New York.

Wolf, G. 1984. Multiple functions of vitamin A. Physiology Review 64: 873–931.

Wongkongkatep, J., Y. Miyahara, A. Ojida and I. Hamachi. 2006. Label-free, real-time glycosyltransferases assay based on fluorescent artificial chemosensor. Angw Chemie 45: 665–668.

Xu, Y. X., L. Liu, C. E. Caffaro and C. B. Hirschberg. 2010. J Biol Chem 285: 24600–24608.

Yarema, K. (ed.). 2005. Handbook of Carbohydrate Engineering. CRC Press, Taylor and Francis Group, Boca Raton, FL, USA.

Yuriev, E. and P. A. Ramsland (eds.). 2013. Structural Glycobiology. CRC Press, Taylor and Francis Group, Boca Raton, FL, USA.

Zachara, N. E. and G. W. Hart. 2004. O-GlcNAc a sensor of cellular state: The role of nucleocytoplasmic glycosylation in modulating cellular function in response to nutrition and stress. Biocim Biophys Acta 1673: 12–28.

Zharkov, D. O., G. V. Mechetin and G. A. Nevinsky. 2010. Uracil-DNA glycosylase: Structural, thermodynamic and kinetic aspects of lesion search and recognition. Mutation Research/Fundamental and Molecular Mechanisms of Mutagenesis 685: 11–20.

CHAPTER 2

Structural Analysis of Glycosaminoglycans—An Indispensable Tool for the Diagnosis, Treatment and Prevention of Human Disease

Christian Heiss and *Parastoo Azadi**

Introduction

Virtually all cells produce proteoglycans, which are macromolecules consisting of a protein core and one or more polysaccharide side chains. The polysaccharides are made up of unbranched chains of disaccharide repeats termed "glycosaminoglycans" (GAGs). Proteoglycans are either excreted into the extracellular matrix, installed into the cell membrane facing outward, or stored in vesicles inside the cell. The GAG portions of proteoglycans are able to interact with a myriad of proteins and thus are involved in a great number of physiological processes, including cell/matrix interactions (Monslow et al. 2015), angiogenesis (van Wijk and van Kuppevelt 2014), axon guidance (Rowlands et al. 2015), embryogenesis (Xiong et al. 2014), bone formation (Jochmann et al. 2014), coagulation, and many more. GAGs have been implicated in a number of pathologies, including cancer (Basappa et al. 2014), inflammation (Pomin 2015), rheumatoid arthritis (Zhou et al. 2010), Alzheimer's disease (Ariga et al. 2010), Parkinson's disease (Lehri-Boufala et al. 2015), and infection (Kamhi et al. 2013). There are also several hereditary illnesses that are caused by defects in GAG degradation. These are collectively called mucopolysaccharidoses (MPS) (Cimaz and La Torre 2014), and it is estimated that one out of every 25,000 children born in the U.S. have an MPS.

The GAG-protein interactions that are the basis for GAG function are determined by the three-dimensional structure of GAGs, which in turn is a consequence of their primary monosaccharide sequence. Although only five different monosaccharide types make up the disaccharide repeats of GAGs, variations in their connectivities and especially in their sulfation pattern impart to them an immense variability in primary structure. This structural abundance allows the manifold interactions of GAGs with protein ligands but also makes their molecular characterization extremely challenging.

Analytical Services & Training Laboratory, Complex Carbohydrate Research Center, The University of Georgia, 315 Riverbend Road, Athens, GA 30602, USA.
  E-mail: cheiss@uga.edu
* Corresponding author: azadi@uga.edu

The GAG polysaccharides consist of a disaccharide repeating unit comprising a 2-aminohexose and a uronic acid. The 2-aminohexose is galactosamine (GalN) inchondroitin (CN), chondroitin sulfate (CS), dermatan sulfate (DS), and keratan sulfate (KS) and glucosamine (GlcN) in hyaluronic acid (HA), heparin (Hp), and heparan sulfate (HS). The GlcN residues in Hp and HS can be N-acetylated or N-sulfated, whereas GlcN in HA and GalN in CN, CS, DS, and KS are always N-acetylated. The uronic acid can either be glucuronic acid (GlcA) or iduronic acid (IdoA). The proportions of these two uronic acids vary according to GAG type. HA has only GlcA, CN, CS and HS have mostly GlcA, while DS and Hp have mostly IdoA. In KS theuronic acid is replaced by galactose (Gal). All GAGs with the exception of HA and CN are O-sulfated to varying degrees. The structures of the different GAG types are pictured in Fig. 1.

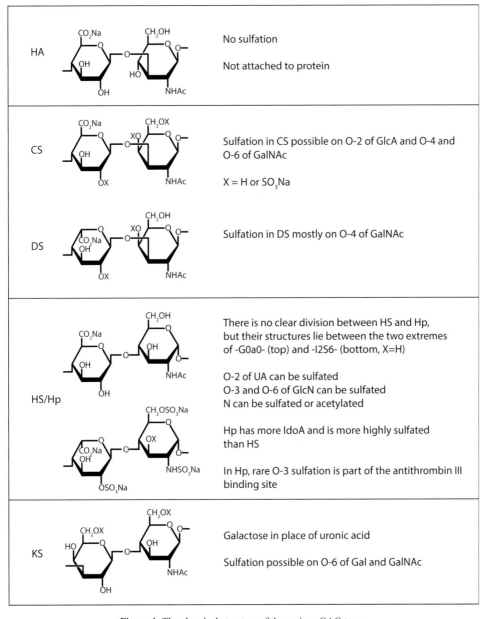

Figure 1. The chemical structure of the various GAG types.

Many of the analytical methods routinely used for the structural elucidation of neutral polysaccharides are not easily applicable to GAGs. Monosaccharide analysis, for instance, relies on acid catalyzed cleavage of all of the glycosidic bonds present in the polymer. While neutral polysaccharides are readily depolymerized with this method, GAGs show considerable recalcitrance toward acid catalyzed depolymerization. Linkage analysis of GAGs is complicated by the presence of sulfated positions, which cannot readily be distinguished from linkage positions. Mass spectrometry of GAGs is hampered by their high charge density and their propensity to lose sulfate groups, which are structure-defining. NMR spectroscopy is limited by its low sensitivity, requiring large amounts of material, and these are usually not available for GAGs. For these reasons, GAG analysis has necessitated significant modification of the existing methods and development of new methods unique to GAGs.

This chapter is meant as a "handbook" for those who encounter GAGs in their research and are not experts in structural analysis of carbohydrates. It is not an exhaustive list of every advance that has been made recently in GAG analysis, but summarizes the most commonly used and most reliable methods to elucidate GAG structure. We have endeavored to include selected references that provide the researcher with clearly written and reproducible protocols. Only methods for the determination of primary structure ("sequence") are included, whereas conformation of GAG molecules (Rudd et al. 2010, Pomin 2014) and binding to protein ligands (Silva et al. 2011, Tocchi and Parks 2013, Wang et al. 2013, Xu and Esko 2014) are not covered.

Isolation of GAGs

Generally, the isolation of GAGs consists of the sequential removal of contaminating substances (lipids, protein, nucleic acids, salt) from the biological material. Although there are numerous different protocols described in the literature for the isolation of GAGs from biological samples, all these procedures are variations of a general scheme. Figure 2 shows the most general isolation scheme for GAGs. The tissue is first homogenized, then dried by acetone extraction or lyophilization and delipidated by extraction with chloroform-methanol (Ledin et al. 2004). Protein digestion can be accomplished with actinase E (Warda et al. 2006), pronase (Anno et al. 1964, Ledin et al. 2004), papain (Volpi 1994), papain followed by pronase (Kanwar and Farquhar 1979), or proteinase K (Huynh et al. 2012). If needed, nucleic acids can be degraded with benzonase (Sakai et al. 2003) or DNAse I (Huynh et al. 2012). Separation of the GAG, which at this point still is attached to a small peptide fragment, from the mixture of free peptides, nucleic acid oligomers, and other low-molecular weight contaminants is accomplished in one of three ways, namely precipitation with a cationic detergent, such as cetylpyridinium chloride (CPC) (Anno et al. 1964), precipitation with an organic solvent, such as acetone (Camara et al. 2011), or anion exchange chromatography (Ledin et al. 2004), which can also be considered a type of precipitation. Each of these can be carried out in ways that not only remove contaminants, but also separate different GAGs from each other (Schiller et al. 1961, Blumenkrantz and Asboe-Hansen 1976, Volpi 1994, Ramachandra et al. 2014). The GAG-peptide bond can be cleaved by alkaline β-elimination in the presence of sodium borohydride, which prevents degradation of the GAG by the peeling reaction due to high pH (Sakai et al. 2003). The β-elimination step may be carried out before or after the precipitation, depending on what precipitation method is used. In the case of anion exchange chromatography, β-elimination can be done afterwards to avoid wasting reducing agent on reducible contaminants. Elution from the anion exchange column requires high concentrations of salt, which can be removed together with the reducing agent in a subsequent desalting step. When CPC or acetone are used for precipitation, β-elimination is usually done first. The final desalting is accomplished by gel filtration (Deakin and Lyon 2008) or acetone precipitation (Osborne et al. 2008). The concentration of purified GAG can at this point be determined using a colorimetric assay specific for uronic acid (Taylor and Buchanan-Smith 1992), hexosamine (Reissig et al. 1955), or hexose (KS only) (Wessler 1971).

Not all types of samples require every step in this general scheme. Nuclease digestion is often omitted from the isolation (Takegawa et al. 2011). Some samples, such as cultured cells, may have low levels of lipid, so that the drying and lipid extraction steps may be omitted (Deakin and Lyon 2008, Murali et al. 2009). Additionally, liquid samples, such as some biological fluids, may not even require protein digestion (Buzzega et al. 2010).

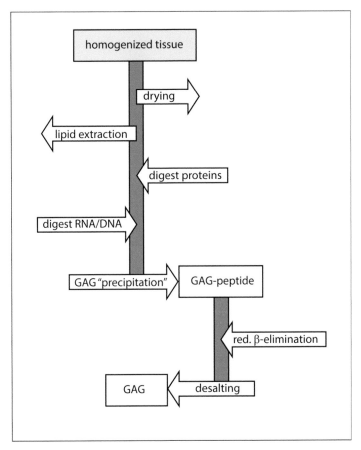

Figure 2. General flow diagram outlining the sequence of steps in GAG isolation.

Depolymerization of GAGs

The great complexity of GAGs has historically necessitated breaking up the polysaccharide into its constituent pieces for the purpose of structural characterization. Although recent developments in methodology and instrumentation have allowed great progress in the structural analysis of native GAG samples, complete or partial depolymerization are still the mainstay of GAG analysis.

Acid-Catalyzed Glycosidic Bond Cleavage

Acid-catalyzed depolymerization is of limited value for GAG structural characterization because it also cleaves off all sulfate groups, which are a critical factor in the biological activity of GAGs. Nevertheless, there is useful information that can be obtained by acidic depolymerization of GAGs. One of these is the monosaccharide composition of the polymer or the mixture of polymers. Accurate knowledge of the quantities of constituent monosaccharides present in GAG samples can be beneficial for several reasons. It serves to quantify the total amount of GAG and provides an estimation of the different types of GAGs. For example, Gal is diagnostic for KS, IdoA occurs only in DS, HS, and Hp, and GalN only in CN, CS, and DS. An important application of these differences is the detection of oversulfated CS in Hp, a contaminant that has been responsible for over 100 deaths (Pan et al. 2010). Most of the enzymes capable of depolymerizing GAGs effect a loss of the distinction between iduronic and glucuronic acid, necessitating an independent method to assess the ratios between these monosaccharides. Furthermore, the production processes of some low-molecular weight heparins entail formation of unnatural monosaccharides. Thus, enoxaparin contains mannosamine, galacturonic acid, and $\Delta^{4,5}$-unsaturated uronic acid ($\Delta^{4,5}$-UA), while dalteparin contains 2,5-anhydromannitol (Linhardt and Gunay 1999). Reliable monosaccharide analysis is thus profitable for the structural characterization and quality control of important drug products.

The acid-catalyzed depolymerization of GAGs is challenging because the glycosidic bonds of uronic acids and hexosamines are resistant to acid, both in water (Zhang et al. 2012) and in methanol (Dierckxsens et al. 1983). The glycosidic linkages of most hexuronic acids are stable to acid due to the inductive effect of the carboxyl group on C-5. Only IdoA presents an exception, its rate of glycosidic bond hydrolysis being roughly equivalent to that of neutral sugars (Conrad 1980). Unfortunately, the released IdoA monosaccharide is readily degraded by the acid, leading to recoveries of less than 75% (Zanetta et al. 1999).

The glycosidic bonds of N-acetylglucosamine (GlcNAc) and N-acetylgalactosamine (GalNAc) are easily hydrolyzed, but the N-acetyl group is also removed under acidic conditions, resulting in an ammonium substituent at C-2, and if this happens before glycosyl hydrolysis, the adjacent glycosidic bond becomes almost completely inert to cleavage by mild to moderately strong acid (Shively and Conrad 1970), so that hydrolysis of the aminosugar glycosidic linkage remains incomplete. Very strong acid leads to further complications, including sugar degradation and epimerization (Whitfield et al. 1991). The problem is still more pronounced in the case of N-sulfoglucosamine (GlcNS) because the N-sulfate is even more labile to acid than the N-acetyl group.

The resistance of aminosugars to acid has been addressed by Dierckxens et al. who followed up a first methanolysis step by re-N-acetylation and a second methanolysis (Dierckxsens et al. 1983). This procedure increased the yield of monosaccharides to a useful level. Toida et al. (Toida et al. 1992), following work by Shively and Conrad (Shively and Conrad 1976) further improved GC-MS quantification of GAGs by dealing with the recalcitrance of the uronic acids through reducing their carboxyls to hydroxymethyl groups, resulting in the conversion of the uronic acids to the corresponding neutral sugars, which were much more easily deglycosylated. The IdoA to GlcA acid ratios of DS, HS, and Hp measured with this method were in excellent agreement with NMR values. Zanetta et al. (Zanetta et al. 1999) have shown that the presence of barium acetate reduces monosaccharide degradation under acidic conditions by removing sulfuric acid, which is formed from sulfate groups that are liberated from the GAGs.

Although both uronic acids and aminosugars tend to resist glycosidic bond cleavage under acidic conditions, one of the residues in any given disaccharide subunit is usually more easily cleaved than the other. This leads to the release of disaccharides as major product under certain conditions. Which of the glycosidic bonds is broken preferentially depends on the type of GAG that is analyzed. For example, CS consists only of GlcA, which is inherently hard to cleave, and GalNAc, which is susceptible to cleavage, as long as the N-acetyl group remains. Thus, acidic methanolysis of CS releases a significant amount of GlcA-GalNAc disaccharide. On the other hand, Hp is made up largely of the acid labile IdoA and GlcNS, which immediately loses the N-sulfate group and thereby becomes highly resistant to acid. Accordingly, the main disaccharide product is GlcN-IdoA. DS and KS, consisting of IdoA and GalNAc, respectively, give very little disaccharide product (Zanetta et al. 1999). The disaccharides produced from the different GAGs can be separated, identified, and quantified by ESI-LC-MS. Although the mechanistic details of this method are not entirely clear, it can be used diagnostically to detect the presence of excessive levels of GAGs in the urine (Auray-Blais et al. 2011, 2012, Zhang et al. 2013, 2015) and cerebrospinal fluid (Zhang et al. 2011) of patients suffering from various mucopolysaccharidoses (MPS).

Enzymatic Depolymerization

Multiple specific enzymes exist that are able to digest GAGs into oligosaccharides. The individual enzymes are specific for the different classes of GAGs and more or less specific for certain sulfation, acetylation, or epimerization patterns and thus can be used to great advantage in the identification and quantification of different GAG types. The GAG degrading enzymes are divided into two major classes, GAG lyases and GAG hydrolases (Fig. 3). GAG lyases cleave GAG chains at C-4 of the uronic acid residue via β-elimination and produce oligosaccharides with a double bond between C-4 and C-5 of the

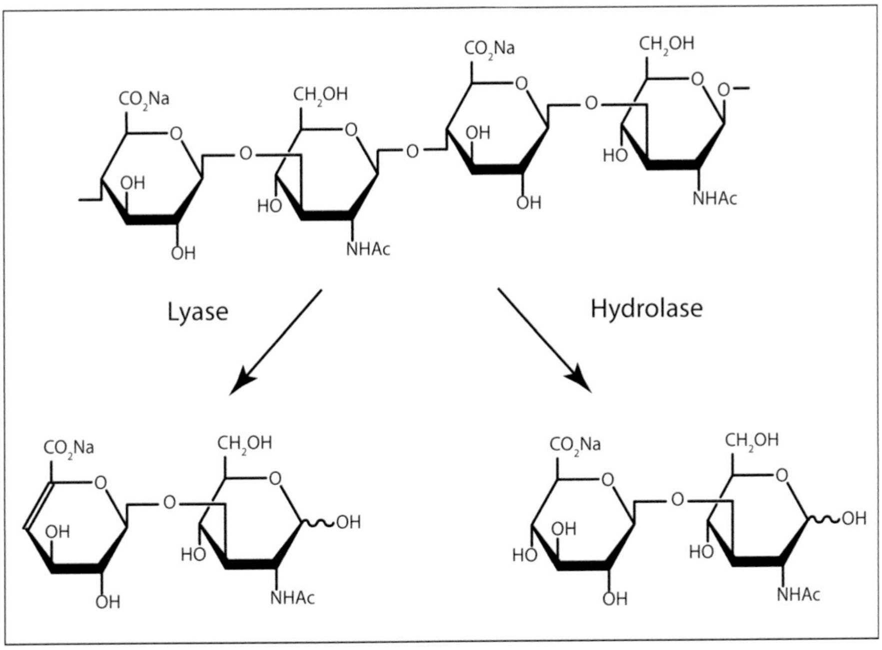

Figure 3. Reactions catalyzed by GAG lyases and GAG hydrolases.

uronic acid ($\Delta^{4,5}$-unsaturated oligosaccharides). The main drawback of lyase digestion is the destruction of the stereochemistry of the uronic acid, so that the GlcA and IdoA content and ratio cannot, at least not directly, be determined with this method.

The properties relevant to GAG analysis of common, commercially available GAG-degrading enzymes are summarized in Table 1. The main concern for the enzymes with respect to GAG analysis is the type of product that they make. The products are characterized by their degree of polymerization (dp), referring to the number of monosaccharides comprising the chain. A disaccharide has dp2, a tetrasaccharide dp4, etc. The enzyme specificity is also reflected in the sulfation pattern of the reducing-end (RE) and non-reducing-end (NRE) residues of the product oligosaccharide. Substrate identity further characterizes enzyme specificity. Thus, for example, chondroitinase AC-I can only cleave CS and HA, indicating that it is able to cleave next to GlcA, but not next to IdoA.

The enzyme characteristics tend not to be absolute, but describe their most prevalent behavior. For instance, chondroitinases AC, ABC, and B produce 80–85 wt.% dp2 (Pomin et al. 2012a), but leave behind a significant amount of larger oligosaccharides. This should always be taken into consideration when reporting the results of a disaccharide analysis.

Three heparin lyase enzymes exist, heparinase I, heparinase II, and heparinase III. Each of these have slightly different specificities. Although results from different groups are partially contradicting (Desai et al. 1993, Nader et al. 1999), a rule of thumb is that heparinase I digests Hp, heparinase III digests HS, and heparinase II digests both Hp and HS (Bohlmann et al. 2015). Individually, these enzymes produce mixtures of di-, tetra- and larger oligosaccharides, but they can be used together to maximize the depolymerization. However, even a "complete" digestion using all three enzymes results in mixtures containing only ~70 mol% (~50 wt.%) disaccharides (Ziegler and Zaia 2006).

There exists no GAG lyase for KS, as it does not contain a uronic acid residue. However, keratan sulfate can be cleaved by keratanase II from *bacillus* sp. and partially cleaved by β-galactosidase, which is unable to cleave galactose residues bearing a sulfate group in the 6-position. Unlike the GAG lyases, β-galactosidase produces oligosaccharides with the aminosugar at the non-reducing end. Both keratanase and β-galactosidase, as well as testicular hyaluronidase, which cleaves hyaluronic acid and chondroitin

Table 1. Overview of commonly available GAG-degrading enzymes and their most abundant products.

Enzyme	Source	Type	Substrate	Product dp	NRE residue	RE residue	Ref.	Action pattern
Hyaluronidase	*bovine testes*	hydrolase	HA, CS	4^a	GlcA(2S)^b	3-GlcNAc, 3-GalNAc(4S,6S)	(1)	*exo* (2)
Hyaluronidase	*Streptomyces hyalurolyticus*	lyase	HA	4, 6	$\Delta^{4,5}$-UA	3-GlcNAc	(3)	*endo* (4)
Hyaluronidase	*Streptococcus dysgalactiae*	lyase	HA, CN	2	$\Delta^{4,5}$-UA	3-GlcNAc, 3-GalNAc	(5)	*endo-exo*^{c} (6)
Chondroitinase AC-I	*Flavobacterium heparinum*	lyase	CS, HA	2	$\Delta^{4,5}$-UA	3-GalNAc(4S,6S)	(7)	*endo* (8)
Chondroitinase AC-II	*Arthrobacter aurescens*	lyase	CS, HA	2	$\Delta^{4,5}$-UA	3-GalNAc(4S,6S)	(9)	*exo* (8)
Chondroitinase ABC	*Proteus vulgaris*	lyase	CS, DS, HA	2	$\Delta^{4,5}$-UA(2S)	3-GalNAc(4S,6S)	(9)	*endo*^{d} (10)
Chondroitinase C	*Flavobacterium heparinum*	lyase	CS, HA	2	$\Delta^{4,5}$-UA(2S)	3-GalNAc(6S)	(11)	
Chondroitinase B	*Flavobacterium heparinum*	lyase	DS	2	$\Delta^{4,5}$-UA(2S)	3-GalNAc4S	(12)	*endo* (7)
Heparinase I	*Flavobacterium heparinum*	lyase	Hp	2, 4	$\Delta^{4,5}$-UA2S	4-GlcNS(3S,6S)	(7)	*endo* (7)
Heparinase II	*Flavobacterium heparinum*	lyase	Hp, HS	2, 4	$\Delta^{4,5}$-UA(2S)	4-GlcN(Ac,S,6S)	(7)	*endo* (7)
Heparinase III	*Flavobacterium heparinum*	lyase	HS	2	$\Delta^{4,5}$-UA	4-GlcN(Ac,S,6S)	(7)	*endo* (7)
Keratanase	*Pseudomonas* sp.	hydrolase	KS	2, 4	GlcNAc6S	Gal	(13)	*endo* (14)
Keratanase II	*Bacillus* sp.	hydrolase	KS	2, 4	Gal(6S)	GlcNAc6S	(15)	*endo*^{e} (16)
β-Galactosidase	*Escherichia freundii*	hydrolase	KS	2	GlcNAc(6S)	Gal	(13, 16)	*endo* (17)

^{a} Although *bovine testes* hyaluronidase processively cleaves disaccharides from the non-reducing end of hyaluronan, it also acts as glycosyltransferase, adding a disaccharide unit to this product, resulting in the tetrasaccharide final product.

^{b} The number(s) with the letter S indicates the O-sulfate position(s). If they are in parentheses, sulfate presence is optional, otherwise it is required.

^{c} Hyaluronidase from *Streptococcus dysgalactiae* cleaves first in an *endo*-pattern, followed by processive *exo*-cleavage from the NRE.

^{d} The commercial preparation of *Proteus vulgaris* chondroitinase ABC contains about 10% of an *exo*-lyase with similar substrate specificity.

^{e} *exo*-galactosidase activity was also detected in the same preparation, but it was not clear whether or not it originated from the keratanase II protein.

(1) (Knudson et al. 1984); (2) (Takagaki et al. 1994); (3) (Payan et al. 1993); (4) (Park et al. 1997); (5) (Saad et al. 2005b); (6) (Baker and Pritchard 2000); (7) (Jandik et al. 1994); (8) (Zhang et al. 2009); (9) (Toyoda et al. 1991); (10) (Hamai et al. 1997); (11) (Michelacci and Dietrich 1976); (12) (Oguma et al. 2007); (13) (Ito et al. 1986); (14) (Nakazawa and Suzuki 1975); (15) (Yamagishi et al. 2003); (16) (Plaas et al. 2001); (17) (Fukuda and Matsumura 1976).

sulfate into tetrasaccharides, work by a hydrolytic mechanism that yields saturated products in contrast to the GAG lyases, which use a β-eliminative mechanism that produces $\Delta^{4,5}$-unsaturated disaccharides.

GAG-degrading enzymes can also be distinguished by their action pattern, i.e., whether they cleave off individual monosaccharides processively from the NRE (*exo*) or cut the GAG somewhere along the chain between two internal residues (*endo*). If enzymes are to be used to produce GAG-OS of intermediate size, by lowering the enzyme concentration or shortening the reaction time, then it is important to choose from those that have an *endo*-action pattern.

Nitrous Acid Deamination

Nitrous acid is unstable at low pH and forms the nitrosyl cation, which in turn reacts with any free amino groups present, but not with amino groups that are acetylated or sulfated. However, at low pH, sulfated amino groups are readily desulfated, and become susceptible to nitrous acid deamination. N-acetylated sugar residues can only be deaminated by nitrous acid after a separate preparative step of de-N-acetylation with anhydrous hydrazine (Shaklee and Conrad 1984, Guo and Conrad 1989). Optimal conditions for the de-N-acetylation reaction have been worked out for various GAGs (Edge and Spiro 1985, Zhao et al. 2013). If N-sulfates are present in the de-N-acetylated GAG, they can either be deaminated by performing the nitrous acid reaction at pH 1.5 or be protected from the deamination by keeping the solution at pH 4, under which conditions the N-sulfates are stable (Conrad 2001).

The mechanism of the deamination reaction is outlined in Fig. 4. The free amino group reacts with the nitrosyl ion and is converted into a diazonium ion, which quickly releases molecular nitrogen, leaving behind a carbocation. The sugar residue then rearranges to form a 5-membered ring, and in the process the glycosidic bond is broken. The newly created reducing end residue is either 2,5-anhydromannose (from GlcN) or 2,5-anhydrotalose (from GalN).

Since free amino sugars do not naturally occur in GAGs, nitrous acid degradation at pH 1.5 can be used to distinguish between heparin/heparan sulfate, which are degraded under these conditions, and the other GAGs, which are not.

One of the main advantages of this method is that the uronic acid epimerization is preserved in the depolymerization, permitting the determination of IdoA to GlcA ratios (Gill et al. 2012). Careful control of reaction time in the nitrous acid deamination allows the partial depolymerization of GAGs to produce oligomers of intermediate size (Zhao et al. 2013). Another application of this method is the estimation of the degree of sulfation in heparin or heparin sulfate. This is accomplished by nitrous acid digestion at pH 1.5 and subsequent sizing of the resulting fragments by gel filtration (Hiscock et al. 1995). Similarly, nitrous acid deamination can also be used to determine the position of N-acetyl groups in HS oligosaccharides (Mason et al. 2006).

Nitrous acid degradation is also part of a sequencing strategy (see below) relying on glycosidase digests and analysis by PAGE (Turnbull et al. 1999) or SAX-HPLC (Stringer et al. 2003).

Oxidative Cleavage

GAGs can also be depolymerized by an oxidative free radical process (Uchiyama et al. 1990, Vismara et al. 2007, Beccati et al. 2012), but the reaction is not structurally specific and therefore introduces additional heterogeneity into the structures. Although this chemistry is useful for the synthesis of low-molecular weight heparins, it has not been used for structural analysis. Oxidative cleavage can also be accomplished with periodic acid, which has been used to make "glycol-split" heparin (Casu et al. 2004), but in spite of the fact that some structural characterization of this product has been achieved (Alekseeva et al. 2013, 2014), this method has not been used for GAG analysis.

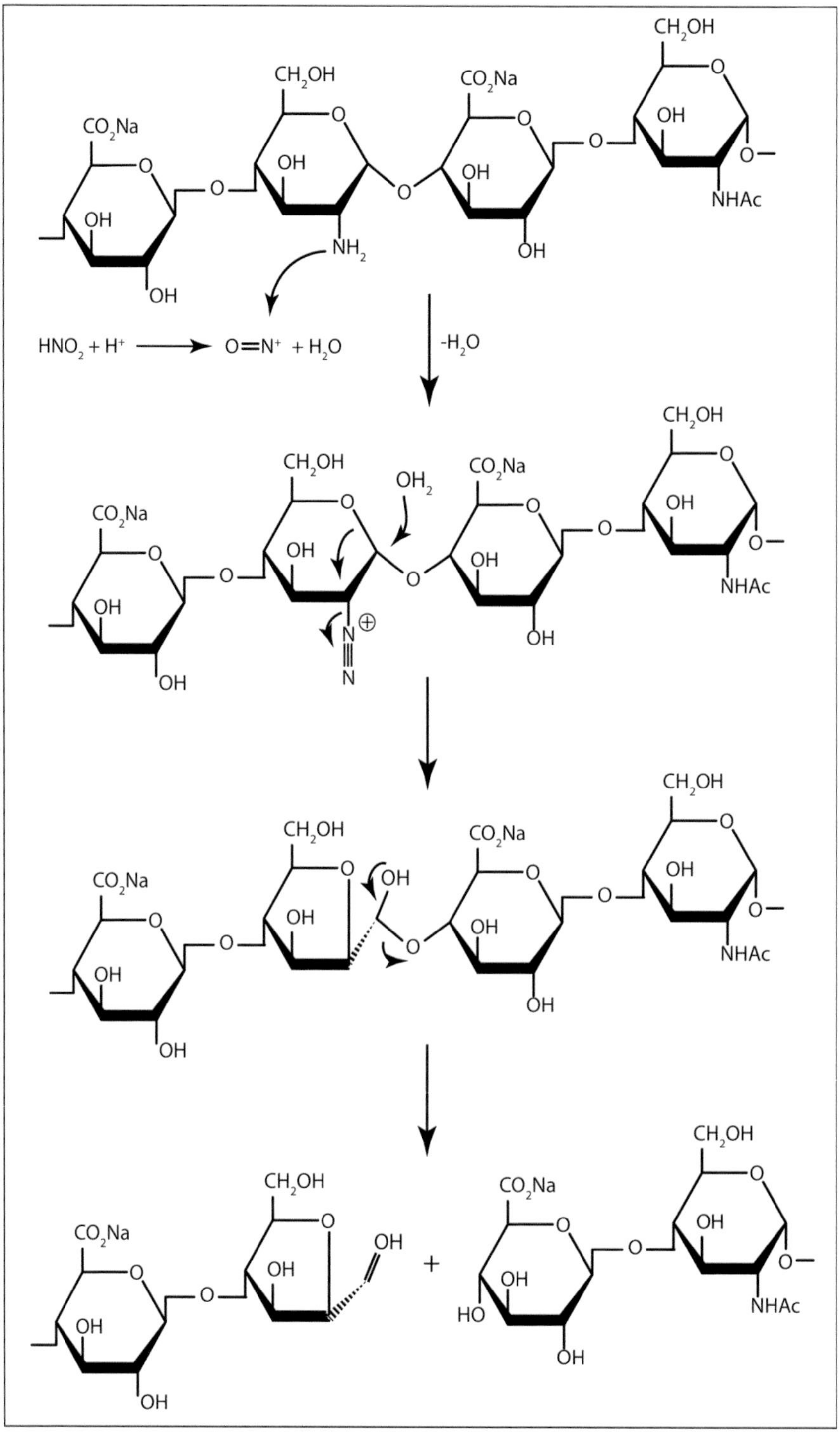

Figure 4. Mechanism of nitrous acid deamination.

Analytical Methods for Depolymerized GAGs

Monosaccharides

Gas Chromatography-Mass Spectrometry (GC-MS)

Gas chromatography is the classical method to quantify monosaccharides after suitable chemical derivatization of all the hydroxyls, most commonly by acetyl or a combination of methyl and trimethylsilyl (TMS) groups, the latter being the more generally applicable derivatization method, allowing simultaneous quantification of neutral sugars, aminosugars, and uronic acids. For this purpose, the products of hydrolysis or, more commonly, methanolysis are re-N-acetylated and derivatized with TMS (Dierckxsens et al. 1983, Toida et al. 1992) or heptafluorobutyryl (Zanetta et al. 1999) groups. Non-polar columns with dimethylpolysiloxane stationary phases are used for separation. MS ionization is either by electron impact (EI) or chemical ionization (CI). Carbohydrate peaks in GC-MS are recognized by characteristic peaks. For example, TMS-derivatized monosaccharides have peaks at 204 and 217 u. Ions at 230 and 234 u are diagnostic for uronic acid derivatives, and ions at 173 and 186 u indicate aminosugar derivatives. Quantification by mass spectrometric detection (MSD) is not as accurate as by flame ionization detection (FID), but because of its power in monosaccharide identification, MSD is the most widely used method for monosaccharide analysis. If very accurate quantification is needed, FID gas chromatograms can be acquired also, but they should not be solely relied upon for peak identification.

High pH Anion Exchange Chromatography with Pulsed Amperometric Detection (HPAEC-PAD)

An alternative analytical method for monosaccharide quantification is HPAEC-PAD (Zhang et al. 2012), which has the advantage that it does not require derivatization of monosaccharides and allows more accurate quantification than GC-MS. However, it is somewhat difficult to obtain consistent data with this method as retention times tend to change. Since retention time is the only identifying quantity in HPAEC, this can sometimes lead to wrong peak assignments. This is in contrast to GC-MS, where compounds are identified by mass spectral data and retention times.

Disaccharides

Nomenclature

Until 2008, when a unified nomenclature for all GAG di- and oligosaccharides was proposed (Lawrence et al. 2008), the naming of GAG oligomers was inconsistent between GAG types, unwieldy for oligosaccharides with dp > 2, and not or not entirely related to the structure. The new "disaccharide structure code" (DSC) by Lawrence et al. describes each monosaccharide by a letter, representing the monosaccharide identity, and a number, representing the sulfation positions. If a monosaccharide is substituted by more than one sulfate, the numbers of the positions are added together to form a single number. For example, disulfation on O-4 and O-6 is indicated by the number 10. Figure 5 shows how the code works. Table 2 lists the structure, previous name(s), and new nomenclature of several disaccharides.

High-Performance Liquid Chromatography (HPLC)

HPLC is the most widely used analytical method to identify and quantify GAG fragments from both chemical and enzymatic depolymerization. The hydrophilic character of GAG oligosaccharides (GAG-OS), which is a result of the abundance of hydroxyl, carboxylate and sulfate groups, leads to special challenges in the HPLC separation of these molecules. Nevertheless, a number of separation modes have been developed for GAG-OS, so that it is now possible to separate, identify, and quantify GAG-OS efficiently and with high sensitivity.

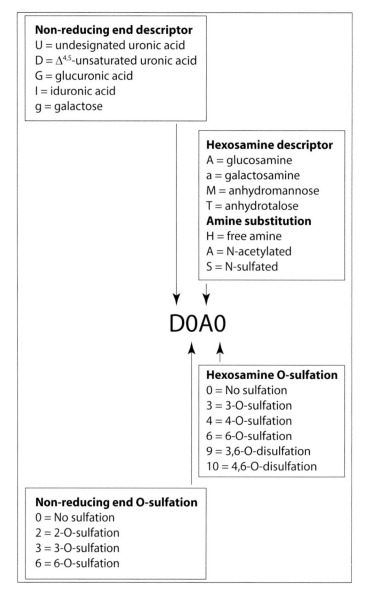

Figure 5. Structural code for the naming of GAG-OS, adapted from Lawrence et al. (2008).

Strong Anion Exchange HPLC (SAX-HPLC). Due to the abundance of charged sulfates and carboxylates in GAGs, the SAX-HPLC technique is well suited for the separation of GAG-OS. The column stationary phases include tertiary alkyl ammonium-functionalized silica gel or latex. The silica-based columns require that the pH remain below 7, while the latex-based columns tolerate any pH. Elution of oligosaccharides is accomplished by an increasing salt gradient, so that the retention time of disaccharides correlates with the number of sulfates they carry.

SAX-HPLC is routinely used for quantitative disaccharide analysis after exhaustive GAG lyase digestion (Linhardt et al. 1988, Lee et al. 1998). Disaccharide analysis by SAX-HPLC is not only able to quantify the disaccharide components of native GAGs, but also the unusual disaccharides of chemically modified GAGs such as low molecular weight heparins and is thus very important in the pharmaceutical

Table 2. Old and new nomenclature of HS and CS disaccharides and tetrasaccharides.

Structure	Old	New (DSC)
ΔUA2S-GlcNS6S	Is	D2S6
ΔUA-GlcNS6S	IIs	D0S6
ΔUA2S-GlcNS	IIIs	D2S0
ΔUA-GlcNS	IVs	D0S0
ΔUA2S-GlcNAc6S	Ia	D2A6
ΔUA-GlcNAc6S	IIa	D0A6
ΔUA2S-GlcNAc	IIIa	D2A0
ΔUA-GlcNAc	IVa	D0A0
ΔUA2S-GlcN6S	Ih	D2H6
ΔUA-GlcN6S	IIh	D0H6
ΔUA2S-GlcN	IIIh	D2H0
ΔUA-GlcN	IVh	D0H0
ΔUA-GalNAc	ΔDi-0S	D0a0
ΔUA-GalNAc4S	ΔDi-4S	D0a4
ΔUA-GalNAc6S	ΔDi-6S	D0a6
ΔUA2S-GalNAc	ΔDi-UA2S	D2a0
ΔUA2S-GalNAc4	ΔDi-S$_B$	D2a4
ΔUA2S-GalNAc6	ΔDi-S$_D$	D2a6
ΔUA-GalNAc4S,6S	ΔDi-S$_E$	D0a10
ΔUA2S-GalNAc4S,6S	ΔDiTriS	D2a10
ΔUA-GlcNAc6S-GlcA-GlcNS3S6S	ΔIIa-IIs$_{glu}$	D0A6G0S9
ΔUA-GlcNAc6S-GlcA-GlcNS3S	ΔIIa-IVs$_{glu}$	D0A6G0S3

industry. It may be advantageous to reduce the disaccharides to the corresponding alditols in order to eliminate the presence of anomeric mixtures and to achieve separation of all components (Mourier and Viskov 2005).

Detection is most commonly carried out by UV absorbance, taking advantage of the presence of the $\Delta^{4,5}$-UA chromophore produced by the action of the GAG lyases. Use of a diode array detector enables the distinction between N-acetylated and N-sulfated disaccharides (Mourier and Viskov 2005). Fluorescence detection can achieve much greater sensitivity but requires either pre- (Skidmore et al. 2010) or post-column derivatization (Fig. 6).

Reverse-Phase Ion-Pairing HPLC (RPIP-HPLC). Because of the highly charged nature of GAGs, their underivatized oligosaccharide fragments do not bind to reverse phase HPLC columns. However, if the mobile phase contains a sufficient concentration of an appropriate alkylamine and an acid, ion pairs can form between the negatively charged sulfate groups of the GAG-OS and the positively charged alkylammonium ions, dramatically increasing lipophilicity and binding to a reverse phase stationary phase. Common ion-pairing reagents include dibutylamine (Kuberan et al. 2002), tributylamine (Jones et al. 2010), hexylamine (Solakyildirim et al. 2010), and tetrabutylammonium bisulfate (Galeotti and Volpi 2013). Jones et al. found that a combination of tributylamine and ammonium acetate resulted in optimal peak resolution (Jones et al. 2010). As long as the ion pairing reagent is volatile, coupling to MS for detection is straightforward, and this combination of the high resolution of RPIP separation with the high information content of modern MS instruments offers the greatest promise for the detailed analysis of complex GAG oligosaccharide mixtures. For applications that require extreme sensitivity or greater quantitative accuracy (Toyoda et al. 1997, 1999) fluorescence detection can also be coupled to RPIP, with derivatization either before or after separation (Toyoda et al. 1999).

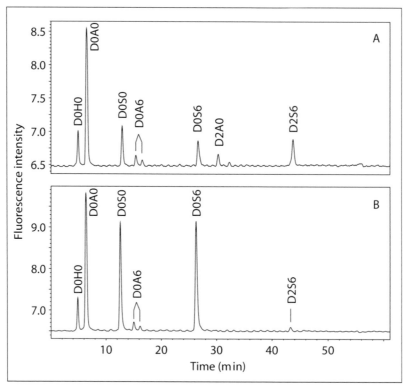

Figure 6. SAX-HPLC separation with post-column derivatization and fluorescence detection of HS from control mice (A) and mice deficient in heparan sulfate 2-O-sulfotransferase enzyme (B).

The RPIP method offers very good resolution and does not require any derivatization of the sample. Although coupling to MS is possible and frequently done, the high concentration of ion-pairing reagents reduces overall sensitivity and contaminates the MS instrument.

Reverse Phase HPLC (RP-HPLC). Reverse-phase columns, although not retentive of underivatized GAG-OS, are nevertheless effective in the separation of derivatized or reducing-end labeled GAG-OS (Deakin and Lyon 2008). For example, AMAC-labeled di- and oligosaccharides generated from low-molecular weight heparins by GAG lyase digestion are baseline separated on a C18 column (Wang et al. 2014) and detected by MS. The advantage of this method is the universal detection of reducing-end labeled oligosaccharides together with those that have a non-reactive reducing end, such as 1,6- or 2,5-anhydro structures and therefore do not carry the label. Yang et al. were able to separate the disaccharides generated from HS, CS, and HA simultaneously using this method (Yang et al. 2012).

Size-Exclusion Chromatography (SEC). Although SEC of GAGs is primarily used for the size determination of polysaccharides and the isolation of oligosaccharides, it is also suitable for disaccharide analysis (Shao et al. 2013). However, due to the inherently inferior resolving power of SEC, this method has not been widely used for disaccharide analysis.

Hydrophilic Interaction Chromatography (HILIC). Hydrophilic interaction chromatography is a separation mode that was originally developed by running normal phase columns (i.e., underivatized silica gel) with acetonitrile-water or methanol-water mixtures. When the silica gel is exposed to the water-organic mixture, a thin water layer binds tightly to the very polar solid surface, and this water layer then becomes the stationary phase. The sample is loaded onto the column in a solvent high in organic solvent content so that polar analytes, such as carbohydrates, partition into the water layer. Over time, the water content of the eluent is increased, shifting the partitioning into the mobile phase and eluting the carbohydrates in order of increasing polarity. Since the time that HILIC was first introduced, a great number of modified silica gel and other supports have been developed (Buszewski and Noga 2012). The amide functionality (e.g., TSK Amide-80 and Waters BEH HILIC) has been the most widely used chemistry for HILIC of carbohydrates in general (Zauner et al. 2011) and GAGs in particular (Zaia 2009). Some less common stationary phases used for GAGs include cross-linked diols (Phenomenex Luna HILIC) (Li et al. 2014b) and zwitterionic surfaces (ZIC-HILIC) (Takegawa et al. 2011). Cationic solid supports, including amine-bound silica gel, are not recommended for highly anionic analytes, such as GAGs, as these tend to be irreversibly bound to such columns. HILIC has been used for disaccharide analysis with online MS detection of CS and HS disaccharides from lyase digestion and nitrous acid degradation (Gill et al. 2013). ZIC-HILIC (Fig. 7) has been used with pre-column fluorescent labeling for the simultaneous quantification of CS, HS, and HA disaccharides (Takegawa et al. 2011).

HILIC is compatible with most detection methods, including post-column (Toyoda et al. 1997) and pre-column fluorescence labeling (Kitagawa et al. 1995). However, in the latter case, the label may reduce the retention of analytes, especially if it is large and hydrophobic. Coupling with MS is straightforward since no salt or other additives are required for elution or retention, as is the case with SAX-HPLC and RPIP-HPLC.

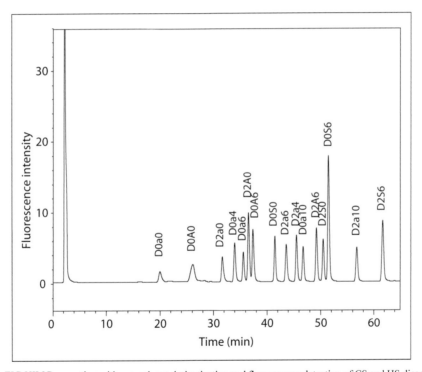

Figure 7. ZIC-HILIC separation with pre-column derivatization and fluorescence detection of CS and HS disaccharides.

Fluorescent Labeling

Pre-column. Most fluorescent labeling prior to HPLC separation ("pre-column labeling") is done by reductive amination (Anumula 2006). In this reaction, a fluorescent primary amine initially makes a Schiff base with the aldehyde form of the glycan reducing end. In aqueous conditions, Schiff bases are usually not stable, but revert back to the unlabeled sugar. However, if sodium cyanoborohydride is added to the reaction mixture, the Schiff base is reduced to a stable secondary amine incorporating the fluorescent tag. Sodium cyanoborohydride is not able to reduce the unlabeled reducing end, and therefore the tagging reaction can be very efficient. Unfortunately, in the normal equilibrium only a very small proportion of the reducing end is in the open-chain, aldehydic form, and the acid required to activate the sugar tends to deactivate the amine by turning it into an ammonium salt. As a result, reductive amination is a slow reaction, potentially giving rise to side reactions and low yield. For this reason, reductive aminations are often carried out in DMSO-acetic acid mixtures. An exception is anthranilic acid, whose adjacent carboxyl group participates as intramolecular acid catalyst and vastly accelerates the reaction, so that it can be carried out in water-methanol solution at slightly acidic pH (Anumula 2014). Reductive amination can also be done with fluorescent hydrazides, which form more stable Schiff bases with carbohydrates (Skidmore et al. 2006).

Advantages of pre-column labeling include that one can choose from a wide variety of available fluorescent tags, according to one's specific needs (high sensitivity, introduction of charges for MS or CE, optimization of HPLC separation). Fluorescent hydrazides especially are offered commercially with fluorophores for many wavelengths and extreme fluorescence emission intensities. Pre-column labeling is can often be achieved with near quantitative yield, further enhancing sensitivity. Drawbacks include the need to remove all other amine containing contaminations (proteins, peptides, buffers). Pre-column labeling requires at least one additional derivatization step, and sometimes it is necessary to further clean the sample from the derivatizing agent, reducing analysis speed.

Post-column. Reducing carbohydrates can also be labeled after HPLC separation ("post-column labeling"). Although several reagents have been proposed for post-column derivatization of carbohydrates (Honda 1996), one compound that has found major acceptance as post-column labeling reagent for GAGs is 2-cyanoacetamide. In the optimized instrumental setup (Schlabach and Robinson 1983), a 1% solution of 2-cyanoacetamide, which itself is not fluorescent, is mixed by a reagent pump with 0.5 M NaOH, and introduced into the eluent of the HPLC column via a tee. From there, the eluent is passed through a long (~10 m) coil of tubing, and placed inside an oven set at 110–130°C (Toyoda et al. 1997). During the time that the mixture spends in the oven, a complex reaction (Honda et al. 1988) takes place between the 2-cyanoacetamide and the reducing end of the carbohydrate, forming a fluorescent derivative, which is subsequently detected.

An obvious advantage of the post-column labeling method is its ease and speed, allowing high-throughput analysis. There is no need for sample preparation or cleanup, as the method is very specific for reducing sugars and other aldehydes, and because the reagent is non-fluorescent, so that it does not interfere with the detection of analytes.

Disadvantages include the need for specialized equipment, loss of resolution, which is a result of band broadening due to the long reaction coil, and lower sensitivity than pre-column labeling caused by low efficiency of the 2-cyanoacetamide labeling reaction (Honda et al. 1988).

Both labeling approaches are compatible with most HPLC separation modes.

Direct Infusion Electrospray Ionization Mass Spectrometry (ESI-MS). GAG disaccharide mixtures do not necessarily have to be separated to be quantitatively analyzed. Electrospray ionization mass spectrometry, together with application of an internal standard, allow the quantification of heparin disaccharides, whereby isobaric species are teased apart by two- and three-stage MS (MS2 and MS3) (Saad and Leary 2003, Saad et al. 2005a). Figure 8 shows the MS2 spectra that are used for the quantification of the isobaric pair D0A6 and D2A0. The individual quantification of D0S6 and D2S0 requires MS3 spectra, but is done analogously (not shown). CS disaccharides have been quantified without an internal standard by direct infusion MS and MS2 (Desaire and Leary 2000).

CE. As a result of their highly charged nature, GAGs are excellent candidates for capillary electrophoresis, and this method has been used successfully for GAG disaccharide analysis. There are two principles that determine the overall movement of analytes in CE, electrophoretic mobility (EM) and electroosmotic flow (EOF). The EM determines how fast an ion will migrate under the influence of a given electric field, and the EOF is the flow of the bulk solution toward the cathode. The net velocity of any particle inside the capillary is the vector sum of EM and EOF. Accordingly, positively charged ions move faster and negatively charged ions more slowly than the EOF. The efficiency of CE separations can be manipulated either by changing the magnitude of the EOF, usually via buffer pH, additives, or capillary coating, or by changing

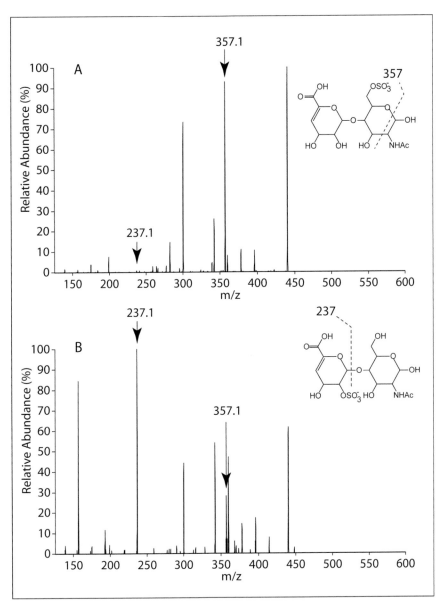

Figure 8. Relative quantification of a pair of isobaric HS disaccharides by ESI-ion trap tandem MS. CID of the molecular ion of D0A6 (A) and D2A0 (B) at m/z 458 yields fragments of identical mass (labeled peaks), but different intensity. These intensities can be used to quantify each disaccharide in a mixture (Saad and Leary 2003).

the EM by derivatization with charged covalent labels or by adding complexing agents, such as borate, to the solution. In the separation of negatively charged analytes the EOF can be reduced to be lower in absolute value than the EM, and then the net migration of analyte ions goes toward the anode. In that case, the polarity of the setup must be reversed for detection at the capillary outlet. The unique mechanism of CE is contrasted to HPLC, in that the EOF generates a much flatter flow profile, which results in greater resolution. Additionally, the small diameter of the capillaries used leads to minute injection volumes and greatly reduced solvent consumption.

CE of GAG disaccharides can be accomplished without labeling using reverse polarity and UV detection at 200 nm (Bendazzoli et al. 2010). Separations can be optimized by experimenting with borate complexation and addition of surfactants (Yang et al. 2005). Most CE disaccharide analyses are performed with pre-column fluorescent labeling and laser-induced fluorescence (LIF) detection. Using this technique, CE was able to separate and quantify all the disaccharides released by exhaustive enzymatic digestion of CS, DS, HS, Hp, KS, and HA from bovine cornea after labeling with 2-aminoacridone (AMAC) (Chang et al. 2012, Ucakturk et al. 2014).

Fluorophore-Assisted Carbohydrate Electrophoresis (FACE). Polyacrylamide gel electrophoresis of fluorescently labeled carbohydrates is known by its commercial name of "fluorophore-assisted carbohydrate electrophoresis" and has been used for GAG disaccharide analysis. It was found to provide quantitative results that agreed well with CE data of the same samples (Karousou et al. 2014). FACE has the decided advantage that up to 20 samples can be analyzed simultaneously, depending on the number of lanes present in the gel. Quantification is performed by measuring the pixel intensity of the bands photographed under UV light.

Oligosaccharides

While the disaccharide composition is a critical piece of information in the structural analysis of GAGs, it is not sufficient to fully characterize a GAG molecule or to understand its interaction with proteins. For this purpose, it is further necessary to know the sequence of more extended GAG structures, i.e., GAG-OS. The classic example is the heparin pentasaccharide motif that binds to antithrombin III. There are numerous GAG-protein interactions, but for most of them, the sequence specifications for binding are not known (Hileman et al. 1998, Hamel et al. 2009, Gesslbauer et al. 2013). To better understand the interactions between GAGs and proteins, it is essential to be able to completely characterize individual active oligosaccharide species out of a complex mixture of inactive structures or, if active fractions have been enriched by affinity chromatography, out of a number of other active structures. This bottom-up approach could be called "needle in a haystack" (NH). On the other hand, one may want to characterize a complex mixture of oligosaccharides and obtain a fingerprint for comparative purposes, e.g., to compare different lots of a low-molecular weight heparin. This top-down approach could be called "bird's-eye" (BE). The reason we use the terms NH and BE instead of bottom-up and top-down is that we want to emphasize the scope rather than the direction of the approach. Considering the fact that analytical and instrumental capabilities are constantly increasing, the NH and BE approaches may eventually move closer to each other, eventually coinciding in a comprehensive characterization of a GAG mixture.

Needle-in-a-Haystack Approach (NH)

The NH approach usually begins with separation of the partially depolymerized GAG mixture into dp-homogeneous fractions by semi-preparative SEC. The fractions of interest are then further divided into their individual components by one of the HPLC methods discussed above. Due to the rich diversity of structures, especially in the larger sized fractions, one may be limited to obtain pure samples only of the major oligosaccharides, while many of the minor ones can only be partially purified. At the end of the purification, and before they can be structurally characterized, the fractions may have to be freed of salt and other contaminations.

Size-Exclusion Chromatography. SEC is used advantageously to isolate oligosaccharide products obtained by partial depolymerization using enzymes or nitrous acid. SEC of highly charged analytes such as GAGs is commonly done at high ionic strengths of the buffer, which weaken the repulsive electrostatic interactions between negatively charged groups on the stationary phase and the sulfates and carboxylates present in GAGs (Ziegler and Zaia 2006). SEC is most typically used for the isolation of pools of dp-homogeneous fractions, i.e., for the separation of di-, tetra-, hexasaccharides, etc. (Pomin et al. 2012a).

Depending on the chemistry of the depolymerization process, detection of eluates can be accomplished by UV absorption (Fig. 9), fluorescence, refractive index, light scattering, and MS. For preparative purposes, non-destructive detection methods are preferred. If such a detection method is not available, it is necessary to install a split that diverts a small percentage of the eluent into the detector and directs the bulk of it into a fraction collector.

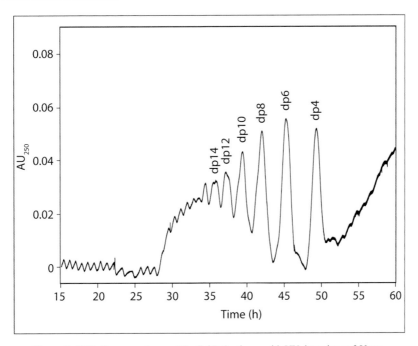

Figure 9. SEC of enoxaparin on a Bio-Gel P-6 column with UV detection at 250 nm.

Strong Anion Exchange HPLC. Like disaccharides, larger oligosaccharides, obtained by partial GAG lyase digestion can also be separated (Cesaretti et al. 2004) or isolated (Ozug et al. 2012, Pomin et al. 2012a, Shastri et al. 2013) with SAX-HPLC. The main advantages of SAX-HPLC for the purpose of purifying individual oligosaccharides are its great resolving power and large capacity, which allows isolation of quantities sufficient for NMR analysis. The main drawback is that the eluent contains a lot of salt, so that detection by MS is difficult, and isolation of oligosaccharides requires an additional desalting step. Lower salt concentrations in the fractions may be obtained by using weak-anion exchange resins (e.g., amine-bound silica gel), at the expense of somewhat lower resolution. However, desalting is still necessary before further analysis (Mizumoto et al. 2013). Desalting is usually achieved by gel permeation chromatography (Larnkjaer et al. 1995, Sugahara et al. 1995, Mourier and Viskov 2004) or ethanol precipitation (Larnkjaer et al. 1995).

Molecular Weight Determination of Purified GAG-OS. The molecular weight of a GAG oligosaccharide can be estimated by SEC or FACE, but accurate masses require the use of mass spectrometry. In order to avoid premature fragmentation, ionization methods have to be soft. Today, only two types of ionization are in use for GAG-OS, matrix-assisted laser desorption ionization (MALDI) and electrospray ionization (ESI). Due to the anionic character of GAGs, negative ion mode is used most of the time, unless the GAG oligosaccharide is first derivatized.

Matrix-Assisted Laser Desorption Ionization-Time-of-Flight MS (MALDI-TOF-MS). In MALDI-TOF MS, the sample is mixed with a solution of an organic acid ("matrix"), co-crystallized by drying on a stainless steel plate, and, after introduction into the mass spectrometer, irradiated with short, high-energy laser pulses. The matrix absorbs the laser energy and transfers it to the sample, which is thus vaporized and ionized.

The resulting ions of both matrix and sample are introduced into a flight tube by an electric field, and the time it takes them to reach the detector is recorded and converted into mass by the instrument software. Although MALDI-TOF-MS is very straightforward, highly sensitive, reasonably accurate (0.1–1 u), and reliable for N- and O-glycans and glycolipids, it is problematic for the use with GAGs. The large number of negative charges make GAGs rather hard to vaporize, and the sulfates are so labile that they are easily lost during ionization. Juhasz and Biemann found that the use of short basic peptides can overcome both of these problems by complexing with the sulfate groups, making the GAG-OS more volatile and more stable (Juhasz and Biemann 1995). The resulting mass spectrum records the masses of the adducts, so that the mass of the peptide has to subtracted to obtain the mass of the oligosaccharide. Unfortunately, the basic peptides are not readily commercially available, so that their use has been rather limited. More recently, liquid ionic matrices have been found to allow effective and mild ionization of GAG-OS (Laremore and Linhardt 2007, Laremore et al. 2007, Przybylski et al. 2010). Application of this type of matrix allows detection of intact molecular ions, but is still associated with significant loss of sulfates (Tissot et al. 2007). Infrared-MALDI in combination with frozen ice as matrix has been shown to almost completely suppress sulfate loss (Witt et al. 2014).

Electrospray Ionization Mass Spectrometry. ESI is able to ionize GAG oligosaccharides from aqueous-organic (acetonitrile or methanol) solutions without the need for additives, although ammonium (Saad et al. 2005b) or alkali metal hydroxides can be added to provide counter ions for sulfates and carboxylates (Kailemia et al. 2013). By choosing appropriate conditions, it is usually possible to obtain molecular ions with minimal loss of sulfates (McClellan et al. 2002). An example is shown in Fig. 10.

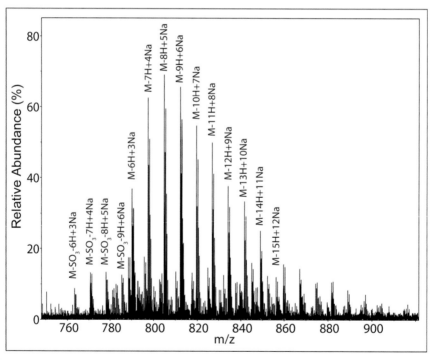

Figure 10. ESI-Fourier-transform ion cyclotron resonance MS (see below) of a heparin octasaccharide, showing the various sodiation states and minor loss of sulfate.

Sequencing of Isolated Oligosaccharides. Sequencing can be done by one of two approaches. The first of these works by dissecting the oligosaccharide with an assortment of specific methods that require certain structural elements for cleavage and observing their effect on the sample. The second leaves the oligosaccharide intact and uses sophisticated instrumentation to elucidate the structure, which includes the sequence.

Dissecting Approach for GAG Oligosaccharide Sequencing. As described in detail above in the section entitled "Depolymerization of GAGs", several methods exist for the cleavage of GAGs in well-defined positions. Each of these have specific structural requirements for the vicinity of the cleavage site. Knowledge of these requirements can be used to deduct the presence or absence of certain structural elements, based on how each site responds to the treatment. The methods include chemical and enzymatic degradations. In addition to the depolymerizing enzymes, there are exo-glycosidases that remove single residues from the NRE and sulfatases that remove sulfate from specific positions. Chemical means include nitrous acid degradation, treatment with mercuric acetate, which reacts with the double bond of $\Delta^{4,5}$-UA at the NRE and leads to loss of that whole residue, and RE mass tags, which add a specified mass rather than cleaving off a group or residue. A list of available treatments is given in Table 3. The choice of treatments and their order best suited for the sequencing of a specific oligosaccharide have to be tailored for the particular structure at hand, and no universal protocol is available. After each step, the sample is analyzed to observe the effect that the treatment had on the individual fragments. Every time, those GAG-OS structures that are inconsistent with the results are eliminated from the set of theoretically possible structures for a particular dp. The dp is determined prior to digestion by MS or FACE. In order to simplify the comparison of theoretical structures with the data, a system of "Property-Encoded Nomenclature" (PEN) (Shriver et al. 2000) has been developed. The products obtained from each treatment are analyzed by MALDI-MS (Shriver et al. 2000), FACE (Turnbull et al. 1999), SAX-HPLC (Vives et al. 1999, Kreuger et al. 2001), weak anion exchange HPLC (Liu et al. 2002), or CE (Guerrini et al. 2002).

Table 3. Available treatments for the selective degradation of GAG-OS and the structural elements they require for cleavage.

Degradant	Structural requirement
Nitrous acid pH 1.5	GlcNS
Heparinase I	*endo*-IdoA(2S)
Heparinase III	*endo*-GlcA
Iduronidase	*exo*-IdoA
Iduronate 2-O-sulfatase + iduronidase	*exo*-IdoA(2S)
Glucosamine 6-O-sulfatase	6-O-Sulfate
Glucuronidase	*exo*-GlcA
N-Acetylglucosaminidase	*exo*-GlcNAc
Sulfamidase	N-Sulfate
Δ-Glycuronidase	*exo*-$\Delta^{4,5}$-UA
Mercuric acetate	*exo*-$\Delta^{4,5}$-UA
Mass tag	RE

Intact Approach for GAG Oligosaccharide Sequencing. Recent advances in analytical instrumentation, especially in mass spectrometry and NMR, have brought about great progress in the sequencing of intact oligosaccharides, without the need for laborious and non-standard degradation schemes.

GAG Oligosaccharide Sequencing by Tandem-MS. The mass of a molecular ion found in a mass spectrum may be used to obtain a composition comprising the number of uronic acids, hexosamines, sulfates and acetates, but to determine the sulfate positions and the sequence of monosaccharides requires that the oligosaccharide ion is fragmented in tandem-MS. If the sulfation pattern is not uniform, it is also necessary that the resulting fragments do not arise solely from glycosidic bond cleavages, but that there is a sufficient number of cross-ring scissions. Furthermore, it is important that the sulfates are stable under the fragmentation conditions. Although recently there have been some advances in MALDI-MS/ MS in obtaining cross-ring cleavages, these have been accompanied by sulfate loss (Tissot et al. 2007) or have only been achieved in disaccharides (Witt et al. 2014). On the other hand, electrospray ionization has enjoyed greater success in breaking molecular ions with abundant cross-ring cleavages and minimal loss of sulfate. This is due to ESI's softness as an ion source, its capability of producing multiply charged ions, and its flexibility in allowing combination with various fragmentation methods and mass analyzers.

Fourier-Transform Ion Cyclotron Resonance Mass Spectrometry (FT-ICR). A lot of work has been done with ESI in combination with FT-ICR instruments. The most successful fragmentation method for GAG-OS using this type of instrument has turned out to be electron detachment dissociation (EDD). In this technique, the negatively charged GAG ion is bombarded with moderately energetic electrons (16–20 eV) (Leach et al. 2008), detaching an electron from the ion, and converting it into an unstable radical that then breaks at a bond that is near to the radical, and not necessarily the weakest bond. This is called a "non-ergodic" process and stands in contrast to ergodic processes where the energy supplied by a collision is randomly distributed within the ion and causes breakage of the weakest bond. The result of the non-ergodic nature of EDD fragmentation is that sulfate loss and glycosidic bond cleavage are minimized, and cross-ring scissions are maximized. The greatest such effect was observed when the number of sodium atoms plus the charge state was one greater than the number of sulfate groups (Wolff et al. 2008). However, this is hard to achieve for highly sulfated oligosaccharides where complete deprotonation leads to increased charge repulsion. Addition of sodium can reduce this repulsion, but has its own problems as it increases the heterogeneity of ions due to Na/H exchange and causes buildup of salts in the MS instrument. Nevertheless, Huang et al. were able to elucidate all the sulfate positions on a highly sulfated pentasaccharide and two hexasaccharides using EDD (Huang et al. 2013b). Furthermore, EDD can be used to distinguish GlcA from IdoA residues (Wolff et al. 2007, Leach et al. 2012).

Ion Trap Mass Spectrometry. The most common and accessible mass spectrometers today are ion-trap instruments, where ions are stored in a quadrupole ion trap and fragmented by collision-induced dissociation (CID), higher-energy collisional dissociation (HCD), or electron-transfer dissociation (ETD). In the negative ion mode, the latter is called negative ETD (nETD). Being an ergodic process, CID fragmentation always breaks the weakest bonds first, and accordingly is always associated with sulfate loss and predominant glycosidic bond cleavage (Zaia and Costello 2003). However, some sequencing of underivatized CS and DS has been achieved with this method (Zamfir et al. 2011), although sulfate positions were not determined. Amster and Linhardt were able to sequence several whole GAG chains with dp between 27 and 43 from the simple proteoglycan bikunin and found that they all had the same sequence pattern (Ly et al. 2011). What made this remarkable achievement possible was the fact that the bikunin GAG is sparsely sulfated and only on O-4 of GalNAc, and all the uronic acids are in the gluco-configuration. Therefore, cross-ring cleavages were not necessary to obtain the sequence.

The abundance of fragment ions resulting from glycosidic bond cleavage is related to the sulfate positions and C-5 epimerization state of the involved residues, so long as the charge state is greater than the number of sulfates present (Zaia et al. 2003). Sulfate migration has been shown to be common in CID of sulfated oligosaccharides and should be taken into consideration when interpreting spectra (Kenny et al. 2011).

Ion-trap CID has also been proposed for sequencing of GAG-OS after extensive derivatization (Huang et al. 2013a), consisting of a sequence of permethylation (Heiss et al. 2011), desulfation (Nagasawa et al. 1979), and O-acetylation (Bendiak et al. 2002). In that report, sulfate loss was dealt with by replacing all the sulfates with acetates in the derivatization scheme.

Although HCD has not yet been applied to the fragmentation of GAG-OS, it is expected to show similar behavior as CID, both being ergodic processes. ETD, on the other hand, is a non-ergodic process that leads to fragmentations that are complimentary to CID or HCD. In ETD, an electron is transferred from a radical anion or cation (for nETD), produced in an ETD source by electron irradiation of an ETD reagent, such as anthracene, fluoranthene, or xenon. Fragmentation does not involve the weakest bond, but occurs near the site of electron capture. nETD has been demonstrated to give rich fragmentation of GAG-OS, and many cross ring cleavages were observed (Wolff et al. 2010). nETD is roughly equivalent to EDD in the fragmentation pattern it causes in GAG ions. The main advantage of nETD over EDD is that it is a more efficient process because the reagent ion is positively charged and therefore is attracted to the negatively charged analyte ions. In EDD, on the other hand, the electrons are repelled by the ions they are supposed to activate, and most of them fail to interact, leading to the need for large amounts of sample. Conversely, nETD is more sensitive and gives less sulfate loss, and can be implemented on the more common ion trap instruments, while EDD requires an FT-ICR. These factors make nETD better suited for GAG oligosaccharide sequencing, and this has been demonstrated in the structural characterization of heparin oligosaccharides with the help a computer program designed for this purpose (Huang et al. 2013b). Unfortunately, nETD is not yet implemented as part of the standard functionality of most commercial ion trap instruments, but requires customization by the manufacturer.

GAG Oligosaccharide Sequencing by Nuclear Magnetic Resonance Spectroscopy (NMR). NMR is an enormously powerful technique for the structural characterization of purified GAG-OS, as long as sufficient material is available. A one-dimensional (1D) proton spectrum can provide the number of anomeric protons and with that the number of residues in the oligosaccharide. It can also determine how many of the glucosamine residues in Hp or HS are N-acetylated. Furthermore, it can differentiate between IdoA and GlcA residues, based on the chemical shift of the anomeric protons. However, two-dimensional (2D) methods are necessary for determination of sulfate positions and connectivities between residues. Two different 2D experiments, total correlation spectroscopy (TOCSY) and nuclear Overhauser effect spectroscopy (NOESY), are the minimum needed to sequence a small oligosaccharide, but additional experiments, such as correlation spectroscopy (COSY), heteronuclear single-quantum coherence (HSQC), and heteronuclear multiple-bond correlation (HMBC) may be required for a complete structure elucidation. A special version of NOESY, known as rotating frame NOESY (ROESY) is better suited for compounds of about 1,000 Da, and many GAG-OS fall in this range, for which NOESY gives weak or no signals. Even with all these experiments, it may not be possible to completely define the structure, especially for larger oligosaccharides. Currently, the limit in size of oligosaccharides to be sequenced by NMR alone is dp8–dp10.

The TOCSY experiment visualizes all or most of the chemical shifts of protons belonging to the same monosaccharide residue (Fig. 11A). Because the anomeric protons are attached to carbons bonded to two oxygen atoms, they are chemically and magnetically unique among all the protons in sugars and therefore resonate in a region of the spectrum separated from the rest of the protons. Consequently, the anomeric protons experience much less signal overlap in the spectra, and the different monosaccharides can often be observed separately in a TOCSY spectrum. Peaks that correlate two different nuclei in a 2D spectrum a called cross peaks, and each anomeric proton usually has a number of cross peaks, all of which belong to protons within the same residue. Therefore, the chemical shifts of the TOCSY signals can frequently identify the individual monosaccharide residues, especially in GAGs, where there is a limited number of possible constituent sugars. Such an identification may in certain cases still be difficult, but COSY can be used to show which protons are on neighboring carbons, and HSQC provides the chemical shifts of the carbons to which the protons are attached (Fig. 11B), further defining each monosaccharide. Once each residue is identified, NOESY or ROESY can be used to determine the sequence of monosaccharides. These experiments visualize through-space interactions between protons and usually give a cross peak whenever the distance between two protons is less than about 5 Å. The distance between an anomeric proton and the proton of the linking position in the next residue is usually around 2.5 Å and therefore gives rise to a NOESY cross peak, which reveals the connection between two sugar residues (Fig. 11A). If NOESY cross peaks can be found for each glycosidic bond, then the sequence is completely defined. Frequently, the unambiguous sequence assignment is hindered by overlapping signals, and sometimes unusual conformations (often seen with IdoA) may give rise to NOESY correlations between anomeric protons and protons in other positions of the adjacent residue, which further hampers definitive sequencing. The connectivities between monosaccharide residues can also be determined by an HMBC spectrum. HMBC is similar to HSQC in that it shows correlations between protons and nearby carbons, but in HMBC, conditions are optimized to show correlations to carbons that are two or three bonds removed, while those to the directly bonded carbon are filtered out. Since anomeric protons are three bonds removed from the linking carbon of the next sugar, interglycosidic connections can be visualized by HMBC. However, HMBC and HSQC experiments require much more material than TOCSY, COSY, and NOESY, and are often not feasible on biological samples because of the small amounts of carbohydrates available.

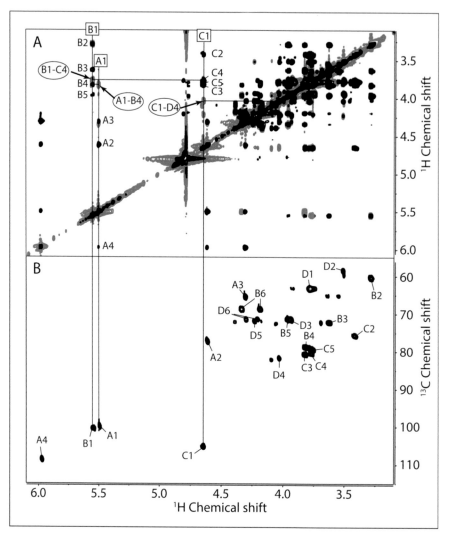

Figure 11. Two-dimensional NMR spectroscopy of the reduced heparin tetrasaccharide D2A6G0A6-ol. The monosaccharide residues are re-labeled for the sake of clarity as A (=D2), B (=A6), C (=G0), and D (=A6-ol). The numbers in the figure refer to the atom positions in each monosaccharide, with 1 being the anomeric position. Three anomeric signals are observed, for residues A, B, and C. Residue D is reduced and has no anomeric carbon. Panel A show an overlay of a 2D-TOCSY spectrum (black) and a 2D-ROESY spectrum (gray). The circled labels indicate ROESY cross peaks that reveal the connections between residues therefore monosaccharide sequence. Panel B shows the 2D-^{1}H-^{13}C HSQC spectrum.

Structural analysis and sequencing of GAG oligosaccharide requires high resolution in the spectra, because the presence of several similar residues can lead to significant overlap even of the anomeric signals. If slight differences in chemical shift cannot be distinguished, sequence information becomes inaccessible. Resolution can be improved by factors involving the instrument, the sample, and data processing. Instrument factors include the strength of the magnetic field strength, where stronger fields lead to higher dispersion of signals, the acquisition time, which is directly related to digital resolution, and the homogeneity of the magnetic field, which is achieved by careful shimming. Samples should be free of particulates and paramagnetic substances, which can be removed by addition of EDTA. It is also important that samples have a length that is substantially greater than the sensitive area of the probe, and sufficient time is allowed for temperature equilibration before collecting data. Resolution can also be enhanced by data processing (e.g., by zero filling, linear prediction, or Lorentz-to Gauss resolution enhancement). Rabenstein and colleagues (Chuang et al. 2001, Nguyen and Rabenstein 2011) proposed the use of band-selective homonuclear decoupling (BASHD) to significantly increase the resolution of 2-dimensional spectra of heparin oligosaccharides and demonstrated its use for the unambiguous sequencing of an octasaccharide. The method works by eliminating the splitting of peaks caused by homonuclear spin coupling in a narrow area of the spectra, namely the anomeric region and is able to allow distinction of spin systems with anomeric protons that are only 0.002 ppm apart.

The difference in energy between different nuclear spin states is very small, and therefore the higher energy state is only slightly less occupied than the lower state. Consequently, it takes a large number of nuclei to produce a measurable signal, which explains why NMR is an inherently insensitive technique. For elements where only rare isotopes have a magnetic moment (e.g., carbon or nitrogen), sensitivity is even lower. These nuclei also have lower gyromagnetic ratios than protons, and this further reduces sensitivity. The energy difference between spin states increases with the strength of the applied magnetic field (by a factor of 2.8 when doubling the field), which makes the use of high-field instruments desirable. However, other factors have an even greater impact on the signal-to-noise ratio (S/N) in NMR experiments. These include the use of narrow-bore tubes (~50% improvement when using 3-mm instead of 5-mm tube), special NMR tubes with solvent-matched magnetic susceptibility plugs (~3-fold improvement), and cryogenically cooled probes (~2–4-fold improvement) (Styles et al. 1984). A significant gain in sensitivity was achieved with the use of a capillary flow probe with which it was possible to sequence as little as 20 μg of tetrasaccharides in a volume of 3 μL (Limtiaco et al. 2011).

Bird's Eye Approach (BE)

In the BE approach, emphasis is laid on the mixture of GAG-OS as a whole, instead of on precise structure elucidation of single oligosaccharide species. Although this approach cannot provide the level of detail in structural information, it is nevertheless a valid and necessary concept because of the complexity and diversity encountered in real life, whether in biology or pharmacy. Practically, the comprehensive approach is most applicable in the realm of GAG-based drug products, and most of the work done in this area has been in the context of low-molecular weight heparins (LMWH), and specifically for the purpose of demonstrating the overall structural equivalence of generic versions and innovator drugs. The idea is that if one can show that a generic drug is chemically equivalent it follows that it is also functionally equivalent and equally safe (Lee et al. 2013). A central part of this proof of "sameness" is "chain mapping", i.e., the chromatographic separation and detection of all the oligosaccharide chains present in the LMWH and comparison of the chromatogram with that of the innovator drug. Chain mapping of the LMWH enoxaparin was first achieved by cetyltrimethylammonium dynamically coated stationary phases (CTA-SAX) (Mourier and Viskov 2004). This method is reminiscent of RPIP-HPLC in that it uses a cationic surfactant to establish retention of GAG-OS on a reverse-phase column. However, instead of simply adding the surfactant to the eluent, in CTA-SAX the reverse-phase column is first coated with surfactant in a preparatory step, effectively turning it into a SAX-column with immobilized quaternary ammonium groups. Elution of GAG-OS is accomplished by an increasing salt gradient. The advantage of CTA-SAX over regular SAX-HPLC is the fact that retention properties of the column are readily tunable by varying the composition of the coating solution. It was found that the higher the concentration of methanol in the coating solution, the higher the loading with quaternary ammonium groups. This is essential for the analysis of highly charged molecules like enoxaparin, which would be difficult to elute completely from a regular SAX-HPLC column. Limitations of CTA-SAX include the low resolution (only about 20 peaks are resolved in CTA-SAX of enoxaparin) and the need for optical detection, which does not provide detailed structural information. Due to the high salt concentration in the eluate, CTA-SAX cannot easily be combined with MS detection. Therefore, other chromatographic methods are needed in order to take advantage of the additional dimension of mass spectrometry in the profiling of GAG oligosaccharide mixtures. These include HILIC and RPIP, whose combinations with MS are described below.

HILIC-LC-MS. The principle of HILIC, including the ease with which it can be coupled to MS, has been discussed under the heading of disaccharide analysis. Although resolution in HILIC-HPLC tends to be inferior to that of SAX-HPLC or RPIP-HPLC, much greater resolution can be achieved by coupling this separation technique to MS, because components that are not baseline-separated in the chromatogram can be deconvoluted based on their mass spectra (Li et al. 2012). Mass spectral identification of peaks also delivers greater reliability in equivalency tests. However, the demands on the spectral interpretation and deconvolution become very high, especially for larger oligosaccharides, making the analysis quite time-consuming.

RPIP-LC-MS. RPIP is superior to HILIC in resolution, not least because the choice of ion-pairing reagent provides flexibility in the optimization of the method for specific applications. Using n-pentylamine as ion-pairing reagent and negative ion mode MS, separation of enoxaparin oligosaccharides up to dp14 was achieved (Langeslay et al. 2013). Another group, using the same ion-pairing reagent, achieved mass spectrometric compositional identification of 143 individual enoxaparin oligosaccharides up to dp22 (Li et al. 2014a). An example with dibutylamine as ion-pairing reagent is shown in Fig. 12.

It is very difficult to efficiently ionize and detect large oligosaccharides in MS, and therefore one has to be aware of the bias in MS for smaller ions. The adverse effect of sulfation on the detection of large oligosaccharides in illustrated by the fact that hyaluronan oligosaccharides up to dp40 could be detected with RPIP-LC-MS (Volpi and Linhardt 2010) under similar conditions. As a result of its high resolution, which is enhanced by the second dimension of MS, RPIP-LC-MS is a valuable tool for the fingerprinting of complex GAG oligosaccharide mixtures for comparison purposes. The interpretation of the complex mass spectra observed in LC-MS of GAGs requires the development of data analysis software, and some approaches have been published (Saad and Leary 2005, Tissot et al. 2008, Maxwell et al. 2012, Chiu et al. 2015), but these are not yet at a stage to allow full automation. Work in this area is currently underway in the Zaia, Amster, and Linhardt labs. Due to the analytical power of modern MS instruments, including advanced fragmentation modes, RPIP-LC-MS promises to bring us closer to the ideal of comprehensively characterizing complex GAG-OS mixtures. One can envision LC-MS runs where each fraction is not only compositionally defined by its mass, but also sequenced by appropriate, consecutive MSn fragmentations using advanced MS interpretation software.

NMR. One-dimensional proton and carbon NMR can be used as a fingerprinting method for GAG-OS mixtures in a straightforward manner by visual inspection. More quantitative comparisons can be achieved by statistical analysis (Guerrini et al. 2015). Knowledge of typical chemical shifts may also help gain insights into the potential origin of any differences encountered between samples. The increasing body of literature values for the chemical shifts of the various monosaccharide residues found in GAGs is very helpful in this regard for HS (Yamada et al. 1995, Limtiaco et al. 2011, Xiao et al. 2011) CN and HA (Sattelle et al. 2010), CS (Kinoshita-Toyoda et al. 2004, Huckerby et al. 2005, Blanchard et al. 2007), DS (Yamada et al. 1998, Ueoka et al. 1999), and KS (Brown et al. 1994, Huckerby et al. 1995). Simple 1-D NMR suffers from limited resolution and extensive signal overlap. This problem is partially overcome by 2-D NMR methods, where different 2-D experiments provide additional separation of signals (Oliveira et al. 2015). The general algorithm by which structural characterization is accomplished is similar to the one described under the heading of specific oligosaccharide characterization. However, in general, only monosaccharide assignment and sometimes the identity of the nearest neighboring residue can be achieved on mixtures, whereas complete sequencing is precluded by spectral complexity in most cases. Nearest neighbor identification is performed by chemical shift analysis through comparison with the chemical shifts of isolated oligosaccharides or chemically modified polysaccharides. The success of this method is based on the fact that chemical changes in the neighboring residue affect chemical shifts of the observed residue in rather consistent manner (Yates et al. 2000, Alekseeva et al. 2014).

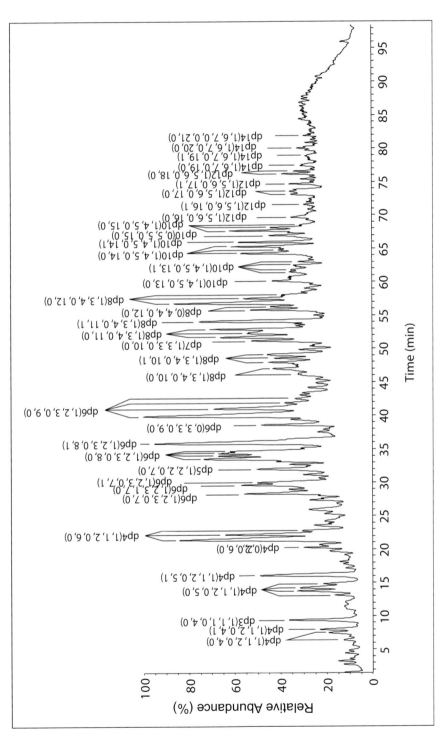

Figure 12. ESI-Ion trap RPIP-LC-MS chromatogram of enoxaparin with dibutylamine as ion-pairing reagent. The peak labels indicate dp, followed (in parentheses) by the number of ΔUA, UA, hexosamine, acetate, sulfate, and 1,6-anhydrohexosamine, in that order.

Polysaccharides

Analysis of unfractionated GAG polysaccharides is mostly limited to GAG type identification and the determination of bulk properties, such as concentration, average molecular weight, and degree of sulfation. NMR analysis of polysaccharides can give some structural information, in that it can be used to estimate sulfation levels, the ratio of GlcA and IdoA, and the percentage of N-acetylation.

SEC

The number- and weight average molecular weights of GAGs can be determined by SEC with commonly available detectors as long as calibration standards of known and narrow molecular weight distribution are available (Ahsan et al. 1995, Guo et al. 2003). Static light scattering detectors can obviate the need for calibration standards (Bertini et al. 2005, Beirne et al. 2011). When performing SEC on highly anionic polymers, one must take into consideration their electrostatic interactions with the resin (Wang et al. 2012). These interactions can be minimized by the addition of salt to the elution buffer.

Electrophoresis

Gel electrophoresis can be used to identify the types of GAGs present in a proteoglycan sample (Schmidtchen et al. 1990). This is accomplished by subjecting the sample to the different GAG degrading enzymes and running the reaction mixtures together with undigested proteoglycan on the same gel. Because the enzymes are specific, the identity of GAGs present can be determined by which enzyme treatments resulted in reduction of molecular weight and polydispersity. Released GAGs can also be distinguished and their molecular weights estimated by gel electrophoresis with agarose (Wang et al. 1997, Pomin et al. 2012b) or polyacrylamide (Edens et al. 1992). Intact GAGs can also be separated and identified with capillary electrophoresis and UV detection at low wavelength (200 nm) (Malavaki et al. 2008, Volpi et al. 2012).

NMR

The NMR spectra of whole glycosaminoglycan polymers usually show broader signals and diminished resolution when compared to the spectra of oligosaccharides and their mixtures. Nevertheless, NMR can still be used as a rich source of GAG polysaccharide structural information. For example, one can compare GAGs from different species based on their 1D proton spectra and identify structural differences on the monosaccharide level (Aquino et al. 2010). Although 1D spectra of unfractionated GAGs are characterized by extensive signal overlap, some signals are well enough separated to allow integration and quantification of residues of a certain substitution pattern. Accordingly, the degree of sulfation of heparin can be estimated by measuring the intensity of anomeric signals in the 1D proton spectra and of C6 signals in the 1D carbon spectra (Casu et al. 1996). The relative proportion of IdoA and GlcA can be determined by 1D proton NMR after first removing all the sulfate groups and re-N-acetylating the glucosamine residues (Sudo et al. 2001). Detection and quantification of impurities in GAG-based drugs has seen dramatically increased activity after the heparin contamination crisis of 2008 (Alban et al. 2011, Rudd et al. 2011, Zang et al. 2011). The approximate proportions of different GAGs and their monosaccharide constituents can also be estimated by 1D proton and carbon NMR, although some 2D spectra may be needed for identification of some of the signals (Volpi and Maccari 2009, Parra et al. 2012, Tovar et al. 2012). Detailed quantification of variously substituted monosaccharides in heparin has been accomplished by volume integration of 2D ^{1}H-^{13}C-HSQC NMR spectra (Guerrini et al. 2005). Since the protons in each position have varying one-bond coupling constants with the carbons to which they are attached, accurate quantification may require recording the spectra with a few different input values for this parameter. The ^{1}H-^{13}C HSQC spectra provide a lot of structural information, but because of the multitude of signals present, interpretation of the spectra can be a difficult task. The spectra produced with ^{1}H-^{15}N-HSQC are much simpler than ^{1}H-^{13}C HSQC spectra, and this has resulted in a number of useful applications for GAG analysis, including rapid identification of GAG types and the estimation of GlcNAc residues in Hp and HS. The reader is referred to Pomin's recent review for details (Pomin 2013).

Degree of Sulfation

Several methods are available to determine the degree of sulfation of GAG polysaccharides. Besides the two methods already described in previous sections (nitrous acid degradation, followed by SEC and 1-D NMR), the number of sulfates per disaccharide can also be measured by elemental analysis (Morimoto et al. 2014), ion chromatography (Bürgermeister et al. 2002), conductimetric titration (Casu and Gennaro 1975), or by precipitation of sulfate with barium chloride in gelatin solution and measuring the optical density of the resulting suspension (Saito et al. 1968). Saito et al. measured the sulfate released by sulfatases, but the method works equally well if the sulfates are released by acid hydrolysis (1.5 M HCl at 80ºC overnight, unpublished data).

GAG Assays

Sulfated GAGs can be quantified with a colorimetric dye-binding assay, taking advantage of the hypsochromic shift of 1,9-dimethylmethylene blue (DMB) upon binding to a sulfated GAG. Other polyanions, such as DNA, as well as proteins interfere with the assay and should be removed prior to analysis (Farndale et al. 1986). Alcian blue has been used as alternative to DMB in the assay, and it was found that the response was equal for all GAG types with Alcian blue, but differed significantly with DMB (Bjornsson 1998). Equal response is a decided advantage when dealing with GAG mixtures. Both assays have been performed in microplate format (Bjornsson 1998, Luhn et al. 2010), and sensitivity was greatly improved by measuring reflectance rather than absorbance (Bjornsson 1998).

Conclusions

Although heparin, which has been widely used as anti-coagulant for the past 80 years, is the most well-known GAG, it is by far not the only GAG with a role in human disease. The treatment of diseases related to GAGs has experienced tremendous progress in recent years. Enzyme replacement therapies (Sands 2014, Coutinho et al. 2015) now are used successfully to make up for the lack of GAG-degrading enzymes for the management of mucopolysaccharidoses. Administration of GAG preparations are used to treat various disorders, including bladder diseases (Bassi et al. 2011, Cicione et al. 2014), arthritis (Bannuru et al. 2015), and renal disease (Gambaro and Van der Woude 2000, Masola et al. 2014), and to prevent pregnancy loss (de Jong et al. 2013) and metastasis (Basappa et al. 2014). These, and the new treatments and preventions that are emerging for cancer (Afratis et al. 2012, Jordan et al. 2015), malaria (Gamain et al. 2007), and neurological disorders, including brain and spinal cord injury, stroke, epilepsy, and Alzheimer's disease (Soleman et al. 2013), are all a result of our increased understanding of GAG structure. It is all but certain that continued work in GAG structural analysis will further accelerate our knowledge of many disease processes and lead to new diagnostic tests and treatments for human disease. It is the purpose of this chapter to make the best currently available GAG analysis methods easily accessible to the medical community, in the hope to make a connection to the biochemical knowledge needed to unlock GAG structure.

Acknowledgements

The GAG research in the Analytical Service & Training Laboratory is supported by funding from the National Institutes of Health directly and by the U.S. Department of Energy through support of the scientific infrastructure. The authors wish to express their gratitude to Prof. Vitor H. Pomin for carefully reviewing the manuscript.

Keywords: Glycosaminoglycans (GAGs), Depolymerization, GAG Nomenclature, Heparinase, Enoxaparin, SAX-HPLC, RPIP-LC-MS, HSQC NMR, Sequencing

References

Afratis, N., C. Gialeli, D. Nikitovic, T. Tsegenidis, E. Karousou, A. D. Theocharis et al. 2012. Glycosaminoglycans: key players in cancer cell biology and treatment. FEBS J 279: 1177–1197.

Ahsan, A., W. Jeske, D. Hoppensteadt, J. C. Lormeau, H. Wolf and J. Fareed. 1995. Molecular profiling and weight determination of heparins and depolymerized heparins. J Pharm Sci 84: 724–727.

Alban, S., S. Luhn, S. Schiemann, T. Beyer, J. Norwig, C. Schilling et al. 2011. Comparison of established and novel purity tests for the quality control of heparin by means of a set of 177 heparin samples. Anal Bioanal Chem 399: 605–620.

Alekseeva, A., B. Casu, G. Torri, S. Pierro and A. Naggi. 2013. Profiling glycol-split heparins by high-performance liquid chromatography/mass spectrometry analysis of their heparinase-generated oligosaccharides. Anal Biochem 434: 112–122.

Alekseeva, A., B. Casu, G. Cassinelli, M. Guerrini, G. Torri and A. Naggi. 2014. Structural features of glycol-split low-molecular-weight heparins and their heparin lyase generated fragments. Anal Bioanal Chem 406: 249–265.

Anno, K., Y. Kawai and N. Seno. 1964. Isolation of chondroitin from squid skin. Biochim Biophys Acta 83: 348–349.

Anumula, K. R. 2006. Advances in fluorescence derivatization methods for high-performance liquid chromatographic analysis of glycoprotein carbohydrates. Anal Biochem 350: 1–23.

Anumula, K. R. 2014. Single tag for total carbohydrate analysis. Anal Biochem 457: 31–37.

Aquino, R. S., M. S. Pereira, B. C. Vairo, L. P. Cinelli, G. R. Santos, R. J. Fonseca et al. 2010. Heparins from porcine and bovine intestinal mucosa: Are they similar drugs? Thromb Haemost 103: 1005–1015.

Ariga, T., T. Miyatake and R. K. Yu. 2010. Role of proteoglycans and glycosaminoglycans in the pathogenesis of Alzheimer's disease and related disorders: amyloidogenesis and therapeutic strategies—a review. J Neurosci Res 88: 2303–2315.

Auray-Blais, C., P. Bherer, R. Gagnon, S. P. Young, H. H. Zhang, Y. An et al. 2011. Efficient analysis of urinary glycosaminoglycans by LC-MS/MS in mucopolysaccharidoses type I, II and VI. Mol Genet Metab 102: 49–56.

Auray-Blais, C., P. Lavoie, H. Zhang, R. Gagnon, J. T. Clarke, B. Maranda et al. 2012. An improved method for glycosaminoglycan analysis by LC-MS/MS of urine samples collected on filter paper. Clin Chim Acta 413: 771–778.

Baker, J. R. and D. G. Pritchard. 2000. Action pattern and substrate specificity of the hyaluronan lyase from group B streptococci. Biochem J 348 Pt 2: 465–471.

Bannuru, R. R., C. H. Schmid, D. M. Kent, E. E. Vaysbrot, J. B. Wong and T. E. McAlindon. 2015. Comparative effectiveness of pharmacologic interventions for knee Osteoarthritis a systematic review and network meta-analysis pharmacologic interventions for knee OA. Ann Int Med 162: 46–54.

Basappa, K., S. Rangappa and K. Sugahara. 2014. Roles of glycosaminoglycans and glycanmimetics in tumor progression and metastasis. Glycoconj J 31: 461–467.

Bassi, P. F., E. Costantini, S. Foley and S. Palea. 2011. Glycosaminoglycan therapy for bladder diseases: Emerging new treatments. Eur Urol Suppl 10: 451–459.

Beccati, D., S. Roy, M. Lech, J. Ozug, J. Schaeck, N. S. Gunay et al. 2012. Identification of a novel structure in heparin generated by sequential oxidative-reductive treatment. Anal Chem 84: 5091–5096.

Beirne, J., H. Truchan and L. Rao. 2011. Development and qualification of a size exclusion chromatography coupled with multiangle light scattering method for molecular weight determination of unfractionated heparin. Anal Bioanal Chem 399: 717–725.

Bendazzoli, C., L. Liverani, F. Spelta, M. Prandi, J. Fiori and R. Gotti. 2010. Determination of dermatan sulfate and chondroitin sulfate as related substances in heparin by capillary electrophoresis. J Pharm Biomed Anal 53: 1193–1200.

Bendiak, B., T. T. Fang and D. N. M. Jones. 2002. An effective strategy for structural elucidation of oligosaccharides through NMR spectroscopy combined with peracetylation using doubly 13C-labeled acetyl groups. Can J Chem 80: 1032–1050.

Bertini, S., A. Bisio, G. Torri, D. Bensi and M. Terbojevich. 2005. Molecular weight determination of heparin and dermatan sulfate by size exclusion chromatography with a triple detector array. Biomacromolecules 6: 168–173.

Bjornsson, S. 1998. Quantitation of proteoglycans as glycosaminoglycans in biological fluids using an alcian blue dot blot analysis. Anal Biochem 256: 229–237.

Blanchard, V., F. Chevalier, A. Imberty, B. R. Leeflang, Basappa, K. Sugahara et al. 2007. Conformational studies on five octasaccharides isolated from chondroitin sulfate using NMR spectroscopy and molecular modeling. Biochemistry 46: 1167–1175.

Blumenkrantz, N. and G. Asboe-Hansen. 1976. Micromethod for fractionation of acid mucopolysaccharides. Clin Biochem 9: 9–15.

Bohlmann, L., C. W. Chang, I. Beacham and M. von Itzstein. 2015. Exploring bacterial heparinase II activities with defined substrates. ChemBioChem 16: 1205–1211.

Brown, G. M., T. N. Huckerby, H. G. Morris, B. L. Abram and I. A. Nieduszynski. 1994. Oligosaccharides derived from bovine articular cartilage keratan sulfates after keratanase II digestion: Implications for keratan sulfate structural fingerprinting. Biochemistry 33: 4836–4846.

Bürgermeister, J., D. H. Paper, H. Vogl, R. J. Linhardt and G. Franz. 2002. LaPSvS1, a (1→3)-β-galactan sulfate and its effect on angiogenesis *in vivo* and *in vitro*. Carbohydr Res 337: 1459–1466.

Buszewski, B. and S. Noga. 2012. Hydrophilic interaction liquid chromatography (HILIC)—a powerful separation technique. Anal Bioanal Chem 402: 231–247.

Buzzega, D., F. Pederzoli, F. Maccari, D. Aslan, M. Turk and N. Volpi. 2010. Comparison of cetylpyridinium chloride and cetyltrimethylammonium bromide extractive procedures for quantification and characterization of human urinary glycosaminoglycans. Clin Chem Lab Med 48: 1133–1139.

Camara, R. B., L. S. Costa, G. P. Fidelis, L. T. Nobre, N. Dantas-Santos, S. L. Cordeiro et al. 2011. Heterofucans from the brown seaweed Canistrocarpus cervicornis with anticoagulant and antioxidant activities. Mar Drugs 9: 124–138.

Casu, B. and U. Gennaro. 1975. A conductimetric method for the determination of sulphate and carboxyl groups in heparin and other mucopolysaccharides. Carbohydr Res 39: 168–176.

Casu, B., M. Guerrini, A. Naggi, G. Torri, L. De-Ambrosi, G. Boveri et al. 1996. Characterization of sulfation patterns of beef and pig mucosal heparins by nuclear magnetic resonance spectroscopy. Arzneim Forsch 46: 472–477.

Casu, B., M. Guerrini, S. Guglieri, A. Naggi, M. Perez, G. Torri et al. 2004. Undersulfated and glycol-split heparins endowed with antiangiogenic activity. J Med Chem 47: 838–848.

Cesaretti, M., E. Luppi, F. Maccari and N. Volpi. 2004. Isolation and characterization of a heparin with high anticoagulant activity from the clam Tapes phylippinarum: Evidence for the presence of a high content of antithrombin III binding site. Glycobiology 14: 1275–1284.

Chang, Y., B. Yang, X. Zhao and R. J. Linhardt. 2012. Analysis of glycosaminoglycan-derived disaccharides by capillary electrophoresis using laser-induced fluorescence detection. Anal Biochem 427: 91–98.

Chiu, Y., R. Huang, R. Orlando and J. S. Sharp. 2015. GAG-ID: Heparan Sulfate (HS) and Heparin Glycosaminoglycan high-throughput identification software. Mol Cell Proteomics 14: 1720–1730.

Chuang, W. -L., M. D. Christ and D. L. Rabenstein. 2001. Determination of the primary structures of heparin- and heparan sulfate-derived oligosaccharides using band-selective homonuclear-decoupled two-dimensional 1H NMR Experiments. Anal Chem 73: 2310–2316.

Cicione, A., F. Cantiello, G. Ucciero, A. Salonia, I. Madeo, I. Bava et al. 2014. Restoring the glycosaminoglycans layer in recurrent cystitis: experimental and clinical foundations. Int J Urol 21: 763–768.

Cimaz, R. and F. La Torre. 2014. Mucopolysaccharidoses. Curr Rheumatol Rep 16: 389.

Conrad, H. E. 1980. The acid lability of the glycosidic bonds of L-iduronic acid residues in glycosaminoglycans. Biochem J 191: 355–363.

Conrad, H. E. 2001. Nitrous acid degradation of glycosaminoglycans. Curr Prot Mol Biol Unit 17.22A.

Coutinho, M. F., L. Matos and S. Alves. 2015. From bedside to cell biology: A century of history on lysosomal dysfunction. Gene 555: 50–58.

de Jong, P. G., M. Goddijn and S. Middeldorp. 2013. Antithrombotic therapy for pregnancy loss. Hum Reprod Update 19: 656–673.

Deakin, J. A. and M. Lyon. 2008. A simplified and sensitive fluorescent method for disaccharide analysis of both heparan sulfate and chondroitin/dermatan sulfates from biological samples. Glycobiology 18: 483–491.

Desai, U. R., H. M. Wang and R. J. Linhardt. 1993. Specificity studies on the heparin lyases from Flavobacterium heparinum. Biochemistry 32: 8140–8145.

Desaire, H. and J. A. Leary. 2000. Detection and quantification of the sulfated disaccharides in chondroitin sulfate by electrospray tandem mass spectrometry. J Am Soc Mass Spectrom 11: 916–920.

Dierckxsens, G. C., L. de Meyer and G. J. Tonino. 1983. Simultaneous determination of uronic acids, hexosamines, and galactose of glycosaminoglycans by gas-liquid chromatography. Anal Biochem 130: 120–127.

Edens, R. E., A. al-Hakim, J. M. Weiler, D. G. Rethwisch, J. Fareed and R. J. Linhardt. 1992. Gradient polyacrylamide gel electrophoresis for determination of molecular weights of heparin preparations and low-molecular-weight heparin derivatives. J Pharm Sci 81: 823–827.

Edge, A. S. B. and R. G. Spiro. 1985. Structural elucidation of glycosaminoglycans through characterization of disaccharides obtained after fragmentation by hydrazine-nitrous acid treatment. Arch Biochem Biophys 240: 560–572.

Farndale, R. W., D. J. Buttle and A. J. Barrett. 1986. Improved quantitation and discrimination of sulphated glycosaminoglycans by use of dimethylmethylene blue. Biochim Biophys Acta 883: 173–177.

Fukuda, M. N. and G. Matsumura. 1976. Endo-beta-galactosidase of Escherichia freundii. Purification and endoglycosidic action on keratan sulfates, oligosaccharides, and blood group active glycoprotein. J Biol Chem 251: 6218–6225.

Galeotti, F. and N. Volpi. 2013. Novel reverse-phase ion pair-high performance liquid chromatography separation of heparin, heparan sulfate and low molecular weight-heparins disaccharides and oligosaccharides. J Chromatogr A 1284: 141–147.

Gamain, B., J. D. Smith, N. K. Viebig, J. Gysin and A. Scherf. 2007. Pregnancy-associated malaria: parasite binding, natural immunity and vaccine development. Int J Parasitol 37: 273–283.

Gambaro, G. and F. J. Van der Woude. 2000. Glycosaminoglycans: Use in treatment of diabetic nephropathy. J Am Soc Nephrol 11: 359–368.

Gesslbauer, B., M. Theuer, D. Schweiger, T. Adage and A. J. Kungl. 2013. New targets for glycosaminoglycans and glycosaminoglycans as novel targets. Expert Rev Proteomics 10: 77–95.

Gill, V. L., Q. Wang, X. Shi and J. Zaia. 2012. Mass spectrometric method for determining the uronic acid epimerization in heparan sulfate disaccharides generated using nitrous acid. Anal Chem 84: 7539–7546.

Gill, V. L., U. Aich, S. Rao, C. Pohl and J. Zaia. 2013. Disaccharide analysis of glycosaminoglycans using hydrophilic interaction chromatography and mass spectrometry. Anal Chem 85: 1138–1145.

Guerrini, M., R. Raman, G. Venkataraman, G. Torri, R. Sasisekharan and B. Casu. 2002. A novel computational approach to integrate NMR spectroscopy and capillary electrophoresis for structure assignment of heparin and heparan sulfate oligosaccharides. Glycobiology 12: 713–719.

Guerrini, M., A. Naggi, S. Guglieri, R. Santarsiero and G. Torri. 2005. Complex glycosaminoglycans: profiling substitution patterns by two-dimensional nuclear magnetic resonance spectroscopy. Anal Biochem 337: 35–47.

Guerrini, M., T. R. Rudd, L. Mauri, E. Macchi, J. Fareed, E. A. Yates et al. 2015. Differentiation of generic enoxaparins marketed in the United States by employing NMR and multivariate analysis. Anal Chem Jul 19 [Epub ahead of print].

Guo, X., M. Condra, K. Kimura, G. Berth, H. Dautzenberg and P. L. Dubin. 2003. Determination of molecular weight of heparin by size exclusion chromatography with universal calibration. Anal Biochem 312: 33–39.

Guo, Y. and H. E. Conrad. 1989. The disaccharide composition of heparins and heparan sulfates. Anal Biochem 176: 96–104.

Hamai, A., N. Hashimoto, H. Mochizuki, F. Kato, Y. Makiguchi, K. Horie et al. 1997. Two distinct chondroitin sulfate ABC lyases: an endoeliminase yielding tetrasaccharides and an exoeliminase preferentially acting on oligosaccharides. J Biol Chem 272: 9123–9130.

Hamel, D. J., I. Sielaff, A. E. I. Proudfoot and T. M. Handel. 2009. Interactions of chemokines with glycosaminoglycans. Methods Enzymol 461: 71–102.

Heiss, C., Z. Wang and P. Azadi. 2011. Sodium hydroxide permethylation of heparin disaccharides. Rapid Commun Mass Spectrom 25: 774–778.

Hileman, R. E., J. R. Fromm, J. M. Weiler and R. J. Linhardt. 1998. Glycosaminoglycan-protein interactions: definition of consensus sites in glycosaminoglycan binding proteins. Bioessays 20: 156–167.

Hiscock, D. R., A. Canfield and J. T. Gallagher. 1995. Molecular structure of heparan sulphate synthesised by bovine aortic endothelial cells. Biochim Biophys Acta 1244: 104–112.

Honda, S., K. Kakehi, K. Fujikawa, Y. Oka and M. Takahashi. 1988. Mechanism of the reaction of reducing carbohydrates with 2-cyanoacetamide, used for postcolumn labeling in high performance liquid chromatography for photometric, fluorimetric and electrochemical detection. Carbohydrate Research 183: 59–69.

Honda, S. 1996. Postcolumn derivatization for chromatographic analysis of carbohydrates. J Chromatogr 720: 183–199.

Huang, R., J. Liu and J. S. Sharp. 2013a. An approach for separation and complete structural sequencing of heparin/heparan sulfate-like oligosaccharides. Anal Chem 85: 5787–5795.

Huang, Y., X. Yu, Y. Mao, C. E. Costello, J. Zaia and C. Lin. 2013b. *De novo* sequencing of heparan sulfate oligosaccharides by electron-activated dissociation. Anal Chem 85: 11979–11986.

Huckerby, T. N., G. M. Brown, J. M. Dickenson and I. A. Nieduszynski. 1995. Spectroscopic characterisation of disaccharides derived from keratan sulfates. Eur J Biochem 229: 119–131.

Huckerby, T. N., I. A. Nieduszynski, M. Giannopoulos, S. D. Weeks, I. H. Sadler and R. M. Lauder. 2005. Characterization of oligosaccharides from the chondroitin/dermatan sulfates. 1H-NMR and 13C-NMR studies of reduced trisaccharides and hexasaccharides. FEBS J 272: 6276–6286.

Huynh, M. B., C. Morin, G. Carpentier, S. Garcia-Filipe, S. Talhas-Perret, V. Barbier-Chassefiere et al. 2012. Age-related changes in rat myocardium involve altered capacities of glycosaminoglycans to potentiate growth factor functions and heparan sulfate-altered sulfation. J Biol Chem 287: 11363–11373.

Ito, M., Y. Hirabayashi and T. Yamagata. 1986. Substrate specificity of endo-beta-galactosidases from Flavobacterium keratolyticus and Escherichia freundii is different from that of Pseudomonas sp. J Biochem 100: 773–780.

Jandik, K. A., K. Gu and R. J. Linhardt. 1994. Action pattern of polysaccharide lyases on glycosaminoglycans. Glycobiology 4: 289–296.

Jochmann, K., V. Bachvarova and A. Vortkamp. 2014. Heparan sulfate as a regulator of endochondral ossification and osteochondroma development. Matrix Biol 34: 55–63.

Jones, C. J., N. Membreno and C. K. Larive. 2010. Insights into the mechanism of separation of heparin and heparan sulfate disaccharides by reverse-phase ion-pair chromatography. J Chromatogr A 1217: 479–488.

Jordan, A. R., R. R. Racine, M. J. Hennig and V. B. Lokeshwar. 2015. The role of CD44 in disease pathophysiology and targeted treatment. Front Immunol 6: 182.

Juhasz, P. and K. Biemann. 1995. Utility of non-covalent complexes in the matrix-assisted laser desorption ionization mass spectrometry of heparin-derived oligosaccharides. Carbohydr Res 270: 131–147.

Kailemia, M. J., L. Li, Y. Xu, J. Liu, R. J. Linhardt and I. J. Amster. 2013. Structurally informative tandem mass spectrometry of highly sulfated natural and chemoenzymatically synthesized heparin and heparan sulfate glycosaminoglycans. Mol Cell Proteomics 12: 979–990.

Kamhi, E., E. J. Joo, J. S. Dordick and R. J. Linhardt. 2013. Glycosaminoglycans in infectious disease. Biol Rev Camb Philos Soc 88: 928–943.

Kanwar, Y. S. and M. G. Farquhar. 1979. Isolation of glycosaminoglycans (heparan sulfate) from glomerular basement membranes. Proc Natl Acad Sci USA 76: 4493–4497.

Karousou, E., A. Asimakopoulou, L. Monti, V. Zafeiropoulou, N. Afratis, P. Gartaganis et al. 2014. FACE analysis as a fast and reliable methodology to monitor the sulfation and total amount of chondroitin sulfate in biological samples of clinical importance. Molecules 19: 7959–7980.

Kenny, D. T., S. M. Issa and N. G. Karlsson. 2011. Sulfate migration in oligosaccharides induced by negative ion mode ion trap collision-induced dissociation. Rapid Commun Mass Spectrom 25: 2611–2618.

Kinoshita-Toyoda, A., S. Yamada, S. M. Haslam, K. -H. Khoo, M. Sugiura, H. R. Morris et al. 2004. Structural determination of five novel tetrasaccharides containing 3-O-sulfated d-glucuronic acid and two rare oligosaccharides containing a β-d-glucose branch isolated from squid cartilage chondroitin sulfate E†. Biochemistry 43: 11063–11074.

Kitagawa, H., A. Kinoshita and K. Sugahara. 1995. Microanalysis of glycosaminoglycan-derived disaccharides labeled with the fluorophore 2-aminoacridone by capillary electrophoresis and high-performance liquid chromatography. Anal Biochem 232: 114–121.

Knudson, W., M. W. Gundlach, T. M. Schmid and H. E. Conrad. 1984. Selective hydrolysis of chondroitin sulfates by hyaluronidase. Biochemistry 23: 368–375.

Kreuger, J., M. Salmivirta, L. Sturiale, G. Giménez-Gallego and U. Lindahl. 2001. Sequence analysis of heparan sulfate epitopes with graded affinities for fibroblast growth factors 1 and 2. J Biol Chem 276: 30744–30752.

Kuberan, B., M. Lech, L. Zhang, Z. L. Wu, D. L. Beeler and R. D. Rosenberg. 2002. Analysis of heparan sulfate oligosaccharides with ion pair-reverse phase capillary high performance liquid chromatography-microelectrospray ionization time-of-flight mass spectrometry. J Am Chem Soc 124: 8707–8718.

Langeslay, D. J., E. Urso, C. Gardini, A. Naggi, G. Torri and C. K. Larive. 2013. Reversed-phase ion-pair ultra-high-performance-liquid chromatography-mass spectrometry for fingerprinting low-molecular-weight heparins. J Chromatogr A 1292: 201–210.

Laremore, T. N. and R. J. Linhardt. 2007. Improved matrix-assisted laser desorption/ionization mass spectrometric detection of glycosaminoglycan disaccharides as cesium salts. Rapid Commun Mass Spectrom 21: 1315–1320.

Laremore, T. N., F. Zhang and R. J. Linhardt. 2007. Ionic liquid matrix for direct UV-MALDI-TOF-MS analysis of dermatan sulfate and chondroitin sulfate oligosaccharides. Anal Chem 79: 1604–1610.

Larnkjaer, A., S. H. Hansen and P. B. Ostergaard. 1995. Isolation and characterization of hexasaccharides derived from heparin. Analysis by HPLC and elucidation of structure by 1H NMR. Carbohydr Res 266: 37–52.

Lawrence, R., H. Lu, R. D. Rosenberg, J. D. Esko and L. Zhang. 2008. Disaccharide structure code for the easy representation of constituent oligosaccharides from glycosaminoglycans. Nat Methods 5: 291–292.

Leach, F. E., 3rd, J. J. Wolff, T. N. Laremore, R. J. Linhardt and I. J. Amster. 2008. Evaluation of the experimental parameters which control electron detachment dissociation, and their effect on the fragmentation efficiency of glycosaminoglycan carbohydrates. Int J Mass Spectrom 276: 110–115.

Leach, F. E., 3rd, M. Ly, T. N. Laremore, J. J. Wolff, J. Perlow, R. J. Linhardt et al. 2012. Hexuronic acid stereochemistry determination in chondroitin sulfate glycosaminoglycan oligosaccharides by electron detachment dissociation. J Am Soc Mass Spectrom 23: 1488–1497.

Ledin, J., W. Staatz, J. -P. Li, M. Götte, S. Selleck, L. Kjellén et al. 2004. Heparan sulfate structure in mice with genetically modified heparan sulfate production. J Biol Chem 279: 42732–42741.

Lee, K., J. Kim, S. Kwak, W. Sim, J. Kwak and Y. Kim. 1998. Isolation and identification of chondroitin sulfates from the mud snail. Arch Pharm Res 21: 555–558.

Lee, S., A. Raw, L. Yu, R. Lionberger, N. Ya, D. Verthelyi et al. 2013. Scientific considerations in the review and approval of generic enoxaparin in the United States. Nat Biotechnol 31: 220–226.

Lehri-Boufala, S., M. O. Ouidja, V. Barbier-Chassefiere, E. Henault, R. Raisman-Vozari, L. Garrigue-Antar et al. 2015. New roles of glycosaminoglycans in alpha-synuclein aggregation in a cellular model of Parkinson disease. PLoS One 10: e0116641.

Li, D., L. Chi, L. Jin, X. Xu, X. Du, S. Ji et al. 2014a. Mapping of low molecular weight heparins using reversed phase ion pair liquid chromatography-mass spectrometry. Carbohydr Polym 99: 339–344.

Li, G., J. Steppich, Z. Wang, Y. Sun, C. Xue, R. J. Linhardt et al. 2014b. Bottom-up low molecular weight heparin analysis using liquid chromatography-Fourier transform mass spectrometry for extensive characterization. Anal Chem 86: 6626–6632.

Li, L., F. Zhang, J. Zaia and R. J. Linhardt. 2012. Top-down approach for the direct characterization of low molecular weight heparins using LC-FT-MS. Anal Chem 84: 8822–8829.

Limtiaco, J. F., S. Beni, C. J. Jones, D. J. Langeslay and C. K. Larive. 2011. The efficient structure elucidation of minor components in heparin digests using microcoil NMR. Carbohydr Res 346: 2244–2254.

Linhardt, R. J., K. G. Rice, Y. S. Kim, D. L. Lohse, H. M. Wang and D. Loganathan. 1988. Mapping and quantification of the major oligosaccharide components of heparin. Biochem J 254: 781–787.

Linhardt, R. J. and N. S. Gunay. 1999. Production and chemical processing of low molecular weight heparins. Semin Thromb Hemost 25 Suppl 3: 5–16.

Liu, J., Z. Shriver, R. M. Pope, S. C. Thorp, M. B. Duncan, R. J. Copeland et al. 2002. Characterization of a heparan sulfate octasaccharide that binds to herpes simplex virus type 1 glycoprotein D. J Biol Chem 277: 33456–33467.

Luhn, S., T. Schrader, W. Sun and S. Alban. 2010. Development and evaluation of a fluorescence microplate assay for quantification of heparins and other sulfated carbohydrates. J Pharm Biomed Anal 52: 1–8.

Ly, M., F. E. Leach, T. N. Laremore, T. Toida, I. J. Amster and R. J. Linhardt. 2011. The proteoglycan bikunin has a defined sequence. Nat Chem Biol 7: 827–833.

Malavaki, C. J., A. P. Asimakopoulou, F. N. Lamari, A. D. Theocharis, G. N. Tzanakakis and N. K. Karamanos. 2008. Capillary electrophoresis for the quality control of chondroitin sulfates in raw materials and formulations. Anal Biochem 374: 213–220.

Masola, V., G. Zaza and G. Gambaro. 2014. Sulodexide and glycosaminoglycans in the progression of renal disease. Nephrol Dial Transplant 29: i74–i79.

Mason, K. E., P. J. Meikle, J. J. Hopwood and M. Fuller. 2006. Characterization of sulfated oligosaccharides in mucopolysaccharidosis type IIIA by electrospray ionization mass spectrometry. Anal Chem 78: 4534–4542.

Maxwell, E., Y. Tan, Y. Tan, H. Hu, G. Benson, K. Aizikov et al. 2012. GlycReSoft: A software package for automated recognition of glycans from LC/MS data. PLoS One 7: e45474.

McClellan, J. E., C. E. Costello, P. B. O'Conno and J. Zaia. 2002. Influence of charge state on product ion mass spectra and the determination of 4S/6S sulfation sequence of chondroitin sulfate oligosaccharides. Anal Chem 74: 3760–3771.

Michelacci, Y. M. and C. P. Dietrich. 1976. Chondroitinase C from flavobacterium heparinum. J Biol Chem 251: 1154–1158.

Mizumoto, S., S. Murakoshi, K. Kalayanamitra, S. S. Deepa, S. Fukui, P. Kongtawelert et al. 2013. Highly sulfated hexasaccharide sequences isolated from chondroitin sulfate of shark fin cartilage: Insights into the sugar sequences with bioactivities. Glycobiology 23: 155–168.

Monslow, J., P. Govindaraju and E. Pure. 2015. Hyaluronan—a functional and structural sweet spot in the tissue microenvironment. Front Immunol 6: 231.

Morimoto, M., M. Takatori, T. Hayashi, D. Mori, O. Takashima, S. Yoshida et al. 2014. Depolymerization of sulfated polysaccharides under hydrothermal conditions. Carbohydr Res 384: 56–60.

Mourier, P. A. and C. Viskov. 2004. Chromatographic analysis and sequencing approach of heparin oligosaccharides using cetyltrimethylammonium dynamically coated stationary phases. Anal Biochem 332: 299–313.

Mourier, P. and C. Viskov. 2005. Method for determining specific groups constituting heparins or low molecular weight heparins, U.S. Patent Application 20050119477 A1.

Murali, S., K. J. Manton, V. Tjong, X. Su, L. M. Haupt, S. M. Cool et al. 2009. Purification and characterization of heparan sulfate from human primary osteoblasts. J Cell Biochem 108: 1132–1142.

Nader, H. B., E. Y. Kobayashi, S. F. Chavante, I. L. Tersariol, R. A. Castro, S. K. Shinjo et al. 1999. New insights on the specificity of heparin and heparan sulfate lyases from Flavobacterium heparinum revealed by the use of synthetic derivatives of K5 polysaccharide from *E. coli* and 2-O-desulfated heparin. Glycoconj J 16: 265–270.

Nagasawa, K., Y. Inoue and T. Tokuyasu. 1979. An improved method for the preparation of chondroitin by solvolytic desulfation of chondroitin sulfates. J Biochem 86: 1323–1329.

Nakazawa, K. and S. Suzuki. 1975. Purification of Keratan Sulfate-endogalactosidase and its action on keratan sulfates of different origin. J Biol Chem 250: 912–917.

Nguyen, K. and D. L. Rabenstein. 2011. Determination of the primary structure and carboxyl pK (A)s of heparin-derived oligosaccharides by band-selective homonuclear-decoupled two-dimensional (1)H NMR. Anal Bioanal Chem 399: 663–671.

Oguma, T., S. Tomatsu, A. M. Montano and O. Okazaki. 2007. Analytical method for the determination of disaccharides derived from keratan, heparan, and dermatan sulfates in human serum and plasma by high-performance liquid chromatography/turbo ionspray ionization tandem mass spectrometry. Anal Biochem 368: 79–86.

Oliveira, S. N., G. R. Santos, B. F. Glauser, N. V. Capillé, I. N. Queiroz, M. S. Pereira et al. 2015. Structural and functional analyses of biosimilar enoxaparins available in Brazil. Thromb Haemost 113: 53–65.

Osborne, S. A., R. A. Daniel, K. Desilva and R. B. Seymour. 2008. Antithrombin activity and disaccharide composition of dermatan sulfate from different bovine tissues. Glycobiology 18: 225–234.

Ozug, J., S. Wudyka, N. Gunay, D. Beccati, J. Lansing, J. Wang et al. 2012. Structural elucidation of the tetrasaccharide pool in enoxaparin sodium. Anal Bioanal Chem 403: 2733–2744.

Pan, J., Y. Qian, X. Zhou, A. Pazandak, S. B. Frazier, P. Weiser et al. 2010. Identification of chemically sulfated/desulfated glycosaminoglycans in contaminated heparins and development of a simple assay for the detection of most contaminants in heparin. Glycobiol Insights 2010: 1–12.

Park, Y., S. Cho and R. J. Linhardt. 1997. Exploration of the action pattern of streptomyces hyaluronate lyase using high-resolution capillary electrophoresis. Biochim Biophys Acta 1337: 217–226.

Parra, A., N. Veraldi, M. Locatelli, M. Fini, L. Martini, G. Torri et al. 2012. Heparin-like heparan sulfate from rabbit cartilage. Glycobiology 22: 248–257.

Payan, E., J. Y. Jouzeau, F. Lapicque, N. Muller and P. Netter. 1993. Hyaluronidase degradation of hyaluronic acid from different sources: influence of the hydrolysis conditions on the production and the relative proportions of tetra- and hexasaccharide produced. Int J Biochem 25: 325–329.

Plaas, A. H., L. A. West and R. J. Midura. 2001. Keratan sulfate disaccharide composition determined by FACE analysis of keratanase II and endo-beta-galactosidase digestion products. Glycobiology 11: 779–790.

Pomin, V. H., Y. Park, R. Huang, C. Heiss, J. S. Sharp, P. Azadi et al. 2012a. Exploiting enzyme specificities in digestions of chondroitin sulfates A and C: production of well-defined hexasaccharides. Glycobiology 22: 826–838.

Pomin, V. H., A. A. Piquet, M. S. Pereira and P. A. S. Mourão. 2012b. Residual keratan sulfate in chondroitin sulfate formulations for oral administration. Carbohydr Polym 90: 839–846.

Pomin, V. H. 2013. Advances in glycosaminoglycanomics by 15N-NMR spectroscopy. Anal Bioanal Chem 405: 3035–3048.

Pomin, V. H. 2014. Solution NMR conformation of glycosaminoglycans. Prog Biophys Mol Biol 114: 61–68.

Pomin, V. H. 2015. Sulfated glycans in inflammation. Eur J Med Chem 92: 353–369.

Przybylski, C., F. Gonnet, D. Bonnaffe, Y. Hersant, H. Lortat-Jacob and R. Daniel. 2010. HABA-based ionic liquid matrices for UV-MALDI-MS analysis of heparin and heparan sulfate oligosaccharides. Glycobiology 20: 224–234.

Ramachandra, R., R. B. Namburi, O. Ortega-Martinez, X. Shi, J. Zaia, S. T. Dupont et al. 2014. Brittlestars contain highly sulfated chondroitin sulfates/dermatan sulfates that promote fibroblast growth factor 2-induced cell signaling. Glycobiology 24: 195–207.

Reissig, J. L., J. L. Strominger and L. F. Leloir. 1955. A modified colorimetric method for the estimation of n-acetylamino sugars. J Biol Chem 217: 959–966.

Rowlands, D., K. Sugahara and J. C. Kwok. 2015. Glycosaminoglycans and glycomimetics in the central nervous system. Molecules 20: 3527–3548.

Rudd, T. R., M. A. Skidmore, M. Guerrini, M. Hricovini, A. K. Powell, G. Siligardi et al. 2010. The conformation and structure of GAGs: recent progress and perspectives. Curr Opin Struct Biol 20: 567–574.

Rudd, T. R., D. Gaudesi, M. A. Lima, M. A. Skidmore, B. Mulloy, G. Torri et al. 2011. High-sensitivity visualisation of contaminants in heparin samples by spectral filtering of 1H NMR spectra. Analyst 136: 1390–1398.

Saad, O. M. and J. A. Leary. 2003. Compositional analysis and quantification of heparin and heparan sulfate by electrospray ionization ion trap mass spectrometry. Anal Chem 75: 2985–2995.

Saad, O. M. and J. A. Leary. 2005. Heparin sequencing using enzymatic digestion and ESI-MSn with HOST: a heparin/HS oligosaccharide sequencing tool. Anal Chem 77: 5902–5911.

Saad, O. M., H. Ebel, K. Uchimura, S. D. Rosen, C. R. Bertozzi and J. A. Leary. 2005a. Compositional profiling of heparin/heparan sulfate using mass spectrometry: assay for specificity of a novel extracellular human endosulfatase. Glycobiology 15: 818–826.

Saad, O. M., R. A. Myers, D. L. Castleton and J. A. Leary. 2005b. Analysis of hyaluronan content in chondroitin sulfate preparations by using selective enzymatic digestion and electrospray ionization mass spectrometry. Anal Biochem 344: 232–239.

Saito, H., T. Yamagata and S. Suzuki. 1968. Enzymatic methods for the determination of small quantities of isomeric chondroitin sulfates. J Biol Chem 243: 1536–1542.

Sakai, S., W. S. Kim, I. S. Lee, Y. S. Kim, A. Nakamura, T. Toida et al. 2003. Purification and characterization of dermatan sulfate from the skin of the eel, Anguilla japonica. Carbohydr Res 338: 263–269.

Sands, M. S. 2014. Mucopolysaccharidosis type VII: A powerful experimental system and therapeutic challenge. Pediatr Endocrinol Rev 12 Suppl 1: 159–165.

Sattelle, B. M., J. Shakeri, I. S. Roberts and A. Almond. 2010. A 3D-structural model of unsulfated chondroitin from high-field NMR: 4-sulfation has little effect on backbone conformation. Carbohydr Res 345: 291–302.

Schiller, S., G. A. Slover and A. Dorfman. 1961. A method for the separation of acid mucopolysaccharides: Its application to the isolation of heparin from the skin of rats. J Biol Chem 236: 983–987.

Schlabach, T. D. and J. Robinson. 1983. Improvements in sensitivity and resolution with the cyanoacetamide reaction for the detection of chromatographically separated reducing sugars. J Chromatogr 282: 169–177.

Schmidtchen, A., I. Carlstedt, A. Malmstrom and L. A. Fransson. 1990. Inventory of human skin fibroblast proteoglycans. Identification of multiple heparan and chondroitin/dermatan sulphate proteoglycans. Biochem J 265: 289–300.

Shaklee, P. N. and H. E. Conrad. 1984. Hydrazinolysis of heparin and other glycosaminoglycans. Biochem J 217: 187–197.

Shao, C., X. Shi, M. White, Y. Huang, K. Hartshorn and J. Zaia. 2013. Comparative glycomics of leukocyte glycosaminoglycans. FEBS J 280: 2447–2461.

Shastri, M. D., C. Johns, J. P. Hutchinson, M. Khandagale and R. P. Patel. 2013. Ion exchange chromatographic separation and isolation of oligosaccharides of intact low-molecular-weight heparin for the determination of their anticoagulant and anti-inflammatory properties. Anal Bioanal Chem 405: 6043–6052.

Shively, J. E. and H. E. Conrad. 1970. Stoichiometry of the nitrous acid deaminative cleavage of model amino sugar glycosides and glycosaminoglycuronans. Biochemistry 9: 33–43.

Shively, J. E. and H. E. Conrad. 1976. Nearest neighbor analysis of heparin: identification and quantitation of the products formed by selective depolymerization procedures. Biochemistry 15: 3943–3950.

Shriver, Z., R. Raman, G. Venkataraman, K. Drummond, J. Turnbull, T. Toida et al. 2000. Sequencing of 3-O sulfate containing heparin decasaccharides with a partial antithrombin III binding site. Proc Natl Acad Sci USA 97: 10359–10364.

Silva, J. L., T. C. Vieira, M. P. Gomes, L. P. Rangel, S. M. Scapin and Y. Cordeiro. 2011. Experimental approaches to the interaction of the prion protein with nucleic acids and glycosaminoglycans: Modulators of the pathogenic conversion. Methods 53: 306–317.

Skidmore, M. A., S. E. Guimond, A. F. Dumax-Vorzet, A. Atrih, E. A. Yates and J. E. Turnbull. 2006. High sensitivity separation and detection of heparan sulfate disaccharides. J Chromatogr A 1135: 52–56.

Skidmore, M. A., S. E. Guimond, A. F. Dumax-Vorzet, E. A. Yates and J. E. Turnbull. 2010. Disaccharide compositional analysis of heparan sulfate and heparin polysaccharides using UV or high-sensitivity fluorescence (BODIPY) detection. Nat Protocols 5: 1983–1992.

Solakyildirim, K., Z. Zhang and R. J. Linhardt. 2010. Ultraperformance liquid chromatography with electrospray ionization ion trap mass spectrometry for chondroitin disaccharide analysis. Anal Biochem 397: 24–28.

Soleman, S., M. A. Filippov, A. Dityatev and J. W. Fawcett. 2013. Targeting the neural extracellular matrix in neurological disorders. Neuroscience 253: 194–213.

Stringer, S. E., B. S. Kandola, D. A. Pye and J. T. Gallagher. 2003. Heparin sequencing. Glycobiology 13: 97–107.

Styles, P., N. F. Soffe, C. A. Scott, D. A. Crag, F. Row, D. J. White et al. 1984. A high-resolution NMR probe in which the coil and preamplifier are cooled with liquid helium. J Magn Res (1969) 60: 397–404.

Sudo, M., K. Sato, A. Chaidedgumjorn, H. Toyoda, T. Toida and T. Imanari. 2001. 1H nuclear magnetic resonance spectroscopic analysis for determination of glucuronic and iduronic acids in dermatan sulfate, heparin, and heparan sulfate. Anal Biochem 297: 42–51.

Sugahara, K., H. Tsuda, K. Yoshida, S. Yamada, T. de Beer and J. F. Vliegenthart. 1995. Structure determination of the octa- and decasaccharide sequences isolated from the carbohydrate-protein linkage region of porcine intestinal heparin. J Biol Chem 270: 22914–22923.

Takagaki, K., T. Nakamura, J. Izumi, H. Saitoh, M. Endo, K. Kojima et al. 1994. Characterization of hydrolysis and transglycosylation by testicular hyaluronidase using ion-spray mass spectrometry. Biochemistry 33: 6503–6507.

Takegawa, Y., K. Araki, N. Fujitani, J. Furukawa, H. Sugiyama, H. Sakai et al. 2011. Simultaneous analysis of heparan sulfate, chondroitin/dermatan sulfates, and hyaluronan disaccharides by glycoblotting-assisted sample preparation followed by single-step zwitter-ionic-hydrophilic interaction chromatography. Anal Chem 83: 9443–9449.

Taylor, K. A. and J. G. Buchanan-Smith. 1992. A colorimetric method for the quantitation of uronic acids and a specific assay for galacturonic acid. Anal Biochem 201: 190–196.

Tissot, B., N. Gasiunas, A. K. Powell, Y. Ahmed, Z. L. Zhi, S. M. Haslam et al. 2007. Towards GAG glycomics: analysis of highly sulfated heparins by MALDI-TOF mass spectrometry. Glycobiology 17: 972–982.

Tissot, B., A. Ceroni, A. K. Powell, H. R. Morris, E. A. Yates, J. E. Turnbull et al. 2008. Software tool for the structural determination of glycosaminoglycans by mass spectrometry. Anal Chem 80: 9204–9212.

Tocchi, A. and W. C. Parks. 2013. Functional interactions between matrix metalloproteinases and glycosaminoglycans. FEBS J 280: 2332–2341.

Toida, T., G. Qiu, T. Matsunaga, Y. Sagehashi and T. Imanari. 1992. Gas chromatography-mass spectrometric determinations of iduronic and glucuronic acids in glycosaminoglycans after reduction of carboxylic group using sodium borodeuteride. Anal Sci 8: 799–804.

Tovar, A. M., N. V. Capille, G. R. Santos, B. C. Vairo, S. N. Oliveira, R. J. Fonseca et al. 2012. Heparin from bovine intestinal mucosa: glycans with multiple sulfation patterns and anticoagulant effects. Thromb Haemost 107: 903–915.

Toyoda, H., K. Motoki, M. Tanikawa, K. Shinomiya, H. Akiyama and T. Imanari. 1991. Determination of human urinary hyaluronic acid, chondroitin sulphate and dermatan sulphate as their unsaturated disaccharides by high-performance liquid chromatography. J Chromatogr 565: 141–148.

Toyoda, H., T. Nagashima, R. Hirata, T. Toida and T. Imanari. 1997. Sensitive high-performance liquid chromatographic method with fluorometric detection for the determination of heparin and heparan sulfate in biological samples: application to human urinary heparan sulfate. J Chromatogr B: Biomed Sci Appl 704: 19–24.

Toyoda, H., H. Yamamoto, N. Ogino, T. Toida and T. Imanari. 1999. Rapid and sensitive analysis of disaccharide composition in heparin and heparan sulfate by reversed-phase ion-pair chromatography on a 2 μm porous silica gel column. J Chromatogr 830: 197–201.

Turnbull, J. E., J. J. Hopwood and J. T. Gallagher. 1999. A strategy for rapid sequencing of heparan sulfate and heparin saccharides. Proc Nat Acad Sci USA 96: 2698–2703.

Ucakturk, E., C. Cai, L. Li, G. Li, F. Zhang and R. J. Linhardt. 2014. Capillary electrophoresis for total glycosaminoglycan analysis. Anal Bioanal Chem 406: 4617–4626.

Uchiyama, H., Y. Dobashi, K. Ohkouchi and K. Nagasawa. 1990. Chemical change involved in the oxidative reductive depolymerization of hyaluronic acid. J Biol Chem 265: 7753–7759.

Ueoka, C., S. Nadanaka, N. Seno, K. -H. Khoo and K. Sugahara. 1999. Structural determination of novel tetra- and hexasaccharide sequences isolated from chondroitin sulfate H (oversulfated dermatan sulfate) of hagfish notochord. Glycoconj J 16: 291–305.

van Wijk, X. M. and T. H. van Kuppevelt. 2014. Heparan sulfate in angiogenesis: A target for therapy. Angiogenesis 17: 443–462.

Vismara, E., M. Pierini, S. Guglieri, L. Liverani, G. Mascellani and G. Torri. 2007. Structural modification induced in heparin by a Fenton-type depolymerization process. Semin Thromb Hemost 33: 466–477.

Vives, R. R., D. A. Pye, M. Salmivirta, J. J. Hopwood, U. Lindahl and J. T. Gallagher. 1999. Sequence analysis of heparan sulphate and heparin oligosaccharides. Biochem J 339: 767–773.

Volpi, N. 1994. Fractionation of heparin, dermatan sulfate, and chondroitin sulfate by sequential precipitation: A method to purify a single glycosaminoglycan species from a mixture. Anal Biochem 218: 382–391.

Volpi, N. and F. Maccari. 2009. Structural characterization and antithrombin activity of dermatan sulfate purified from marine clam Scapharca inaequivalvis. Glycobiology 19: 356–367.

Volpi, N. and R. J. Linhardt. 2010. High-performance liquid chromatography-mass spectrometry for mapping and sequencing glycosaminoglycan-derived oligosaccharides. Nat Protocols 5: 993–1004.

Volpi, N., F. Maccari, J. Suwan and R. J. Linhardt. 2012. Electrophoresis for the analysis of heparin purity and quality. Electrophoresis 33: 1531–1537.

Wang, L., R. Malsch and J. Harenberg. 1997. Heparins, low-molecular-weight heparins, and other glycosaminoglycans analyzed by agarose gel electrophoresis and azure A-silver staining. Semin Thromb Hemost 23: 11–16.

Wang, X., J. S. Sharp, T. M. Handel and J. H. Prestegard. 2013. Chemokine oligomerization in cell signaling and migration. Prog Mol Biol Transl Sci 117: 531–578.

Wang, Z., F. Zhang, J. S. Dordick and R. J. Linhardt. 2012. Molecular mass characterization of glycosaminoglycans with different degrees of sulfation in bioengineered heparin process by size exclusion chromatography. Curr Anal Chem 8: 506–511.

Wang, Z., D. Li, X. Sun, X. Bai, L. Jin and L. Chi. 2014. Liquid chromatography–diode array detection–mass spectrometry for compositional analysis of low molecular weight heparins. Anal Biochem 451: 35–41.

Warda, M., T. Toida, F. Zhang, P. Sun, E. Munoz, J. Xie and R. J. Linhardt. 2006. Isolation and characterization of heparan sulfate from various murine tissues. Glycoconj J 23: 555–563.

Wessler, E. 1971. The nature of the non-ultrafilterable glycosaminoglycans of normal human urine. Biochem J 122: 373–384.

Whitfield, D. M., S. Stojkovski, H. Pang, J. Baptista and B. Sarkar. 1991. Diagnostic methods for the determination of iduronic acid in oligosaccharides. Anal Biochem 194: 259–267.

Witt, L., A. Pirkl, F. Draude, J. Peter-Katalinic, K. Dreisewerd and M. Mormann. 2014. Water ice is a soft matrix for the structural characterization of glycosaminoglycans by infrared matrix-assisted laser desorption/ionization. Anal Chem 86: 6439–6446.

Wolff, J. J., L. Chi, R. J. Linhardt and I. J. Amster. 2007. Distinguishing glucuronic from iduronic acid in glycosaminoglycan tetrasaccharides by using electron detachment dissociation. Anal Chem 79: 2015–2022.

Wolff, J. J., T. N. Laremore, A. M. Busch, R. J. Linhardt and I. J. Amster. 2008. Influence of charge state and sodium cationization on the electron detachment dissociation and infrared multiphoton dissociation of glycosaminoglycan oligosaccharides. J Am Soc Mass Spectrom 19: 790–798.

Wolff, J. J., F. E. Leach, T. N. Laremore, D. A. Kaplan, M. L. Easterling, R. J. Linhardt et al. 2010. Negative electron transfer dissociation of glycosaminoglycans. Anal Chem 82: 3460–3466.

Xiao, Z., W. Zhao, B. Yang, Z. Zhang, H. Guan and R. J. Linhardt. 2011. Heparinase 1 selectivity for the 3,6-di-O-sulfo-2-deoxy-2-sulfamido-α-D-glucopyranose (1,4) 2-O-sulfo-α-L-idopyranosyluronic acid (GlcNS3S6S-IdoA2S) linkages. Glycobiology 21: 13–22.

Xiong, A., S. Kundu and K. Forsberg-Nilsson. 2014. Heparan sulfate in the regulation of neural differentiation and glioma development. FEBS J 281: 4993–5008.

Xu, D. and J. D. Esko. 2014. Demystifying heparan sulfate-protein interactions. Annu Rev Biochem 83: 129–157.

Yamada, S., T. Murakami, H. Tsuda, K. Yoshida and K. Sugahara. 1995. Isolation of the porcine heparin tetrasaccharides with glucuronate 2-O-sulfate. Heparinase cleaves glucuronate 2-O-sulfate-containing disaccharides in highly sulfated blocks in heparin. J Biol Chem 270: 8696–8705.

Yamada, S., Y. Yamane, K. Sakamoto, H. Tsuda and K. Sugahara. 1998. Structural determination of sulfated tetrasaccharides and hexasaccharides containing a rare disaccharide sequence, -3GalNAc(4,6-disulfate)beta1-4IdoAalpha1-, isolated from porcine intestinal dermatan sulfate. Eur J Biochem 258: 775–783.

Yamagishi, K., K. Suzuki, K. Imai, H. Mochizuki, K. Morikawa, M. Kyogashima, K. Kimata and H. Watanabe. 2003. Purification, characterization, and molecular cloning of a novel keratan sulfate hydrolase, endo-beta-N-acetylglucosaminidase, from Bacillus circulans. J Biol Chem 278: 25766–25772.

Yang, B., Y. Chang, A. M. Weyers, E. Sterner and R. J. Linhardt. 2012. Disaccharide analysis of glycosaminoglycan mixtures by ultra-high-performance liquid chromatography–mass spectrometry. J Chromatogr 1225: 91–98.

Yang, Y., M. C. Breadmore and W. Thormann. 2005. Analysis of the disaccharides derived from hyaluronic acid and chondroitin sulfate by capillary electrophoresis with sample stacking. J Sep Sci 28: 2381–2389.

Yates, E. A., F. Santini, B. De Cristofano, N. Payre, C. Cosentino, M. Guerrini et al. 2000. Effect of substitution pattern on 1H, 13C NMR chemical shifts and 1JCH coupling constants in heparin derivatives. Carbohydr Res 329: 239–247.

Zaia, J. and C. E. Costello. 2003. Tandem mass spectrometry of sulfated heparin-like glycosaminoglycan oligosaccharides. Anal Chem 75: 2445–2455.

Zaia, J., X. -Q. Li, S. -Y. Chan and C. Costello. 2003. Tandem mass spectrometric strategies for determination of sulfation positions and uronic acid epimerization in chondroitin sulfate oligosaccharides. J Am Soc Mass Spectrom 14: 1270–1281.

Zaia, J. 2009. On-line separations combined with MS for analysis of glycosaminoglycans. Mass Spectrom Rev 28: 254–272.

Zamfir, A. D., C. Flangea, E. Sisu, D. G. Seidler and J. Peter-Katalinic. 2011. Combining size-exclusion chromatography and fully automated chip-based nanoelectrospray quadrupole time-of-flight tandem mass spectrometry for structural analysis of chondroitin/dermatan sulfate in human decorin. Electrophoresis 32: 1639–1646.

Zanetta, J. P., P. Timmerman and Y. Leroy. 1999. Determination of constituents of sulphated proteoglycans using a methanolysis procedure and gas chromatography/mass spectrometry of heptafluorobutyrate derivatives. Glycoconj J 16: 617–627.

Zang, Q., D. A. Keire, L. F. Buhse, R. D. Wood, D. P. Mital, S. Haque et al. 2011. Identification of heparin samples that contain impurities or contaminants by chemometric pattern recognition analysis of proton NMR spectral data. Anal Bioanal Chem 401: 939–955.

Zauner, G., A. M. Deelder and M. Wuhrer. 2011. Recent advances in hydrophilic interaction liquid chromatography (HILIC) for structural glycomics. Electrophoresis 32: 3456–3466.

Zhang, H., S. P. Young, C. Auray-Blais, P. J. Orchard, J. Tolar and D. S. Millington. 2011. Analysis of glycosaminoglycans in cerebrospinal fluid from patients with mucopolysaccharidoses by isotope-dilution ultra-performance liquid chromatography-tandem mass spectrometry. Clin Chem 57: 1005–1012.

Zhang, H., S. P. Young and D. S. Millington. 2013. Quantification of glycosaminoglycans in urine by isotope-dilution liquid chromatography-electrospray ionization tandem mass spectrometry. Curr Protoc Hum Genet Chapter 17: Unit 17 12.

Zhang, H., T. Wood, S. P. Young and D. S. Millington. 2015. A straightforward, quantitative ultra-performance liquid chromatography-tandem mass spectrometric method for heparan sulfate, dermatan sulfate and chondroitin sulfate in urine: an improved clinical screening test for the mucopolysaccharidoses. Mol Genet Metab 114: 123–128.

Zhang, Z., Y. Park, M. M. Kemp, W. Zhao, A. R. Im, D. Shaya et al. 2009. Liquid chromatography-mass spectrometry to study chondroitin lyase action pattern. Anal Biochem 385: 57–64.

Zhang, Z., N. M. Khan, K. M. Nunez, E. K. Chess and C. M. Szabo. 2012. Complete monosaccharide analysis by high-performance anion-exchange chromatography with pulsed amperometric detection. Anal Chem 84: 4104–4110.

Zhao, L., S. Lai, R. Huang, M. Wu, N. Gao, L. Xu et al. 2013. Structure and anticoagulant activity of fucosylated glycosaminoglycan degraded by deaminative cleavage. Carbohydr Polym 98: 1514–1523.

Zhou, X., P. Weiser, J. Pan, Y. Qian, H. Lu and L. Zhang. 2010. Chondroitin sulfate and abnormal contact system in rheumatoid arthritis. Prog Mol Biol Transl Sci 93: 423–442.

Ziegler, A. and J. Zaia. 2006. Size-exclusion chromatography of heparin oligosaccharides at high and low pressure. J Chromatogr B Analyt Technol Biomed Life Sci 837: 76–86.

CHAPTER 3

Identifying Urinary Glycans is a Suitable Approach for the Diagnosis of Lysosomal Storage Diseases

Cees Bruggink,[1,]* Jeffrey S. Rohrer[2] and Manfred Wuhrer[3]

Introduction

Many cell components are digested in the lysosome, a cell organelle. The mechanisms behind the lysosomal digestion of glycoconjugates and transport of the products are well understood. When the complete breakdown of glycoconjugates to monomers is not obtained in the lysosome, and fragments as small as dimers are left undigested, a lysosomal disorder may arise (Aronson and Kuranda 1989). If this degradation process to monosaccharides is disturbed, the oligosaccharides or glycoconjugates will be stored in the lysosome and will eventually be excreted into the extracellular space and appear in bodily fluids such as urine (Vellodi 2005, Winchester 2005). Many lysosomal storage diseases lead to increased level of glycoconjugates and oligosaccharides in different bodily fluids.

Fucosidosis, α-mannosidosis, G_{M1}-gangliosidosis, G_{M2}-gangliosidosis, and sialidosis are examples of autosomal recessive inherited lysosomal storage diseases (LSD). Defects in one or more enzymes or cofactors involved in the catabolism of glycoconjugates cause these LSDs.

A deficiency in lysosomal α-L-fucosidase (EC 3.2.1.51) causes fucosidosis and results in secretion of fucosyl-oligosaccharides (Lundblad et al. 1978, Cantz and Ulrich-Bott 1990, Michalski and Klein 1999). α-Mannosidosis is caused by a deficiency in lysosomal α-D-mannosidase (EC 3.2.1.24) and excessive urinary excretion of oligomannosidic glycans (Ockerman 1969, Ockerman et al. 1973, Michalski and Klein 1999, Winchester 2005). A deficiency in acid exo-α-sialidase (EC 3.2.1.18) (Cantz et al. 1977, Achyuthan and Achyuthan 2001) causes sialidosis. The excretion of urinary sialyloligosaccharides is the same as that found for galactosialidosis (Cantz and Ulrich-Bott 1990, van Pelt et al. 1991). G_{M1}-gangliosidosis is a neurosomatic disease due to deficient activity of β-galactosidase (EC 3.2.1.23)

[1] Thermo Fisher Scientific, Takkebijsters 1, 4817 BL Breda, The Netherlands.
[2] Thermo Fisher Scientific, 1214 Oakmead Parkway, B-10, Sunnyvale, CA 94085, USA.
   E-mail: jeff.rohrer@thermofisher.com
[3] Leiden University Medical Center, Center for Proteomics and Metabolomics, Albinusdreef 2, 2333 ZA Leiden, The Netherlands.
   E-mail: m.wuhrer@lumc.nl
* Corresponding author: cees.bruggink@thermofisher.com; Orc.bruggink@lumc.nl

(Landing et al. 1964, Takahashi and Orii 1989). In patients' urine, G_{M1}-gangliosides and glycoconjugates with β-galactose at the non-reducing end are increased. G_{M2}-gangliosidosis consist of a group of three disorders (1) Tay-Sachs disease, (2) Sandhoff disease, and (3) AB variant. The major neural storage compound is ganglioside G_{M2} for all variants of G_{M2}-gangliosidosis (Hoffman et al. 1977, Rubin et al. 1988, Mahuran 1999). Due to the deficiency of β-hexosaminidase A in addition to the (functional) deficiency of β-hexosaminidase B, only in Sandhoff disease do oligosaccharides from glycoproteins accumulate (Hou et al. 1996). In Sandhoff disease patients, oligosaccharides with a single *N*-acetylglucosamine residue at the non-reducing end accumulate in tissue and urine (Strecker et al. 1977, Warner et al. 1986, Kolter and Sandhoff 2006).

Urine is a non-invasive sample to obtain, relatively easy to collect from a new born, and is available at regular intervals. To identify free glycans in body fluids, such as urine, from lysosomal storage diseased patients, several analytical methods are available. A commonly used technique for screening is thin-layer chromatography (TLC) (Sewell 1979, Kin 1987, Schindler et al. 1990), as TLC is relatively easy to perform and does not require expensive equipment. However, interpretation and identifying excreted glycans from a TLC pattern requires significant experience. In modern times TLC is often successfully replaced by liquid chromatography (LC) combined with UV absorbance (An et al. 2000) or fluorescence (Neville et al. 2009) detection. LC-based methods are easier to reproduce, interpret, and are capable of (semi)quantitative measurements (Warner et al. 1986, Peelen et al. 1994). When LC is hyphenated with mass spectrometry (MS) detailed glycan characterization is possible and this combination enhances the selectivity compared to the previously discussed chromatography techniques (Wuhrer 2013).

In this chapter on-line hyphenation of MS to high performance anion-exchange (HPAE) chromatography with integrated pulsed amperometric detection (IPAD) has been used to identify and characterize urinary glycans in samples from lysosomal (LSD) storage diseased individuals. This combination of HPAE, IPAD, and MS detection allows detailed glycan analysis, when compared with TLC, HPLC, or HPAEC-IPAD without MS, and is an effective extra tool in diagnosing lysosomal storage disorders.

Mechanism of Separation

The dominant retention factor in ion-exchange chromatography is charge followed by analyte size and polarity (Weiss 2004). Neutral carbohydrates are very weak acids with a dissociation constants in the range of pKa 12–12.5 (Dean 1999) and therefore will dissociate at elevated pH in a sodium hydroxide mobile phase (Lee 1990). This dissociation is required for binding to the anion-exchange stationary phase. Carbohydrates possessing an anionic group, such as a carboxylate, phosphate, or sulfate, do not need high pH for ionization for binding to the stationary phase. These natively charged glycans have a high affinity for the stationary phase, and thus a stronger mobile phase is required for their elution. Typically a sodium acetate gradient in sodium hydroxide will be used for natively charged and large neutral glycans (Hardy and Townsend 1988). The feasibility of HPAE chromatography to separate isomeric glycans in their native state is very attractive (Hardy and Townsend 1988, Bruggink et al. 2005). The mechanism behind the separation of isomeric glycans with HPAE chromatography is not well understood.

Detection

Underivatized (native) carbohydrates are sensitively detected with integrated pulsed amperometric detection (IPAD) using a gold working electrode at high pH (Rocklin et al. 1998). IPAD under these conditions detects alcohol, aldehyde, and ketone groups and therefore IPAD does not depend on the presence of a reducing end, or whether a carbohydrate is a ketose or aldose. IPAD does not provide structural information of the eluting glycans and therefore tandem mass spectrometric detection is indispensable (Wuhrer 2013). To convert the eluent used for HPAE chromatography into a compatible composition for an electro-spray ionization (ESI) interface an online desalter is installed between the column and the ESI interface. The desalter, often named suppressor, is equipped with cation-exchange membranes kept continuously in the acidic form by electrolysis of water as regenerant (Rabin et al. 1993, Thayer et al. 1998). The desalter exchanges the sodium ions for hydronium ions and in this way sodium acetate is converted into volatile acetic acid and sodium hydroxide into water. To enhance spray formation and ionization efficiency, a makeup solution is added between the desalter and entrance of the ESI interface via a tee, see Fig. 1. The makeup solution contains acetonitrile and a very small amount of sodium ions. The sodium ions in the makeup solution serve to form a positively charged adduct with glycans to assist MS detection. Glycan-sodium adducts are stable enough to prevent in-source decay and do not need a high collision energy for collision induced dissociation (CID) for tandem MS to obtain structural information (Mohr et al. 1995, Penn et al. 1996). Moreover sodium adduct formation prevents glycan rearrangements in contrast to proton adducts (Wuhrer et al. 2011). This is especially important in case of structure elucidation of fucosyloligosaccharides in the disorder fucosidosis.

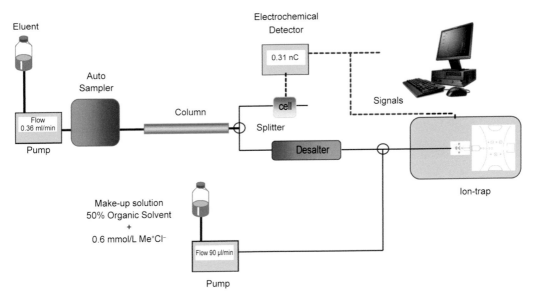

Figure 1. Instrumental setup for on-line HPAEC-PAD-MS. The figure is modified from (Bruggink 2012) and reprinted with permission.

Structural Information of Glycans by Tandem MS Detection

The first piece of information from the MS is the mass of the glycan from which the contribution of the monosaccharide constituents can be calculated (Table 1).

Table 1. Monoisotopic masses of some carbohydrates.

Water	18.0106
Sodium	22.9892
Fucose (deoxyhexose)	146.0579
Hexose	162.0528
Hexosamine	161.0688
Uronic acid	176.0321
N-acetylhexosamine	203.0794
N-acetylneuraminic acid	291.0954
N-glycolylneuraminic acid	307.0903

Prior knowledge of the monosaccharide composition, possible types of glycans in the sample, and retention time can help either identify the glycan from its mass or at minimum, reduce the number of possible structures. The second part of additional information is obtained with tandem MS detection where CID causes glycosidic cleavages and the presence or absence of ring-fragmentations. Glycosidic cleavages reveal the kind of monosaccharides that the glycan is comprised of, and in which order they are linked. Ring fragmentation uncovers the linkage positions between the different monosaccharides (Table 2). The broadly accepted nomenclature for fragmentation of carbohydrates was proposed by Domon and Costello 1988 and is depicted in Fig. 2.

Table 2. Mass loss values. Nomenclature belongs to cross-ring fragmentation of hexose (Hex) or *N*-acetylhexosamine (HexNAc) revealing their different linkage positions between carbohydrate units in the positive ion mode (Weiskopf et al. 1998, Harvey 2000, Mechref et al. 2003, Spina et al. 2004). Reprinted with permission (Bruggink et al. 2012).

Hex	HexNAc	1–6	1–4	1–3	1–2
−60	−101	$^{0,2}A$	$^{0,2}A$		
−90	−131	$^{0,3}A$			
−120	−161	$^{0,4}A$	$^{2,4}A$		$^{1,3}A$
−106	−147	$^{3,5}A$	$^{3,5}A$		
−78		$^{0,4}A$-H_2O			$^{0,4}A$-H_2O

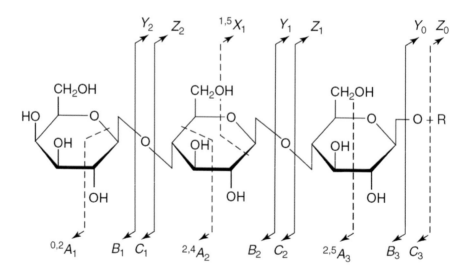

Figure 2. Glycan fragmentation types and their nomenclature as proposed by Domon and Costello (1988) reprinted with permission.

The non-reducing end of the glycan is at the left side of the figure, while the reducing end is at the right side. Glycosidic cleavages containing the non-reducing end are called B and C fragments while Y and Z fragments contain the reducing end. Cross-ring fragments containing the non reducing part of the oligosaccharide are A-ions, while X-ions are cross-ring fragments including the reducing part. These cross-ring fragment ions are accompanied by a subscript indicating the position of cleavage relative to the termini and a superscript in front indicating the cleavage position in the ring, starting with bond zero between the ring oxygen and the anomeric carbon with further counting in the clockwise direction (Fig. 2). Linkage position information between the different sugar constituents is derived from cross-ring fragments. Table 2 lists mass losses observed depending on cross-ring fragmentation when tandem MS is used in the positive mode.

Results and Discussion

Urine samples of patients suffering from fucosidosis, α-mannosidosis, G_{M1}-gangliosidosis, G_{M2}-gangliosidosis, and sialidosis were analyzed to study disease related free oligosaccharides by HPAEC-IPAD-MS. The obtained MS data were investigated for oligosaccharides targeting the aforementioned lysosomal storage disorders against a database (has also been referred to as unknown knowns analysis). Thus, the originally used extended mass list could be reduced to the lysosomal storage disease related masses listed in Table 3.

Table 3. Mass list of disease related glycans. H = hexose, N = *N*-acetylhexosamine, F = fucose, S = *N*-acetylneuraminic acid, SO3 = sulfate. Modified from Bruggink et al. 2012 and reprinted with permission.

m/z	Glycan	m/z	m/z	m/z	m/z	Disorder
390.2	NF					Fucosidosis
478.3	H_3N_2	933.5				G_{M1}-gangliosidosis
552.5	HNF					Fucosidosis
568.4	H_2N					α-Mannosidosis
580.0	H_3N_3	1136.5				G_{M2}-gangliosidosis
624.1	H_3N_2S	635.1	1224.5	1246.8		Sialidosis
635.1	H_3N_2S	624.1	1224.5	1246.8		Sialidosis
660.9	H_4N_3	1298.5				G_{M1}-gangliosidosis
664.0	$H_3SO_3N_2S$	674.5	685.8	1304.3	1348.2	Sialidosis
674.5	$H_3SO_3N_2S$	664.0	685.8	1304.3	1348.2	Sialidosis
681.2	H_3N_4	1339.4				G_{M2}-gangliosidosis
685.8	$H_3SO_3N_2S$	664.0	674.5	1304.3	1348.2	Sialidosis
697.6	HNS	719.5				Sialidosis
700.9	H_7N	1378.5				α-Mannosidosis
714.5	H_2NF					Fucosidosis
719.5	HNS	697.6				Sialidosis
730.4	H_3N					α-Mannosidosis
742.1	H_5N_3	1460.6				G_{M1}-gangliosidosis
771.5	H_2N_2					G_{M2}-gangliosidosis
782.0	H_8N	1540.4				α-Mannosidosis
863.0	H_9N	1702.8				α-Mannosidosis

Table 3. contd....

Table 3. contd.

m/z	Glycan	m/z	m/z	m/z	m/z	Disorder
865.4	HNSF					Fucosidosis
887.6	H_5N_3S	898.3				Sialidosis
892.4	H_4N					α-Mannosidosis
898.3	H_5N_3S	887.6				Sialidosis
924.5	H_6N_4					G_{M1}-gangliosidosis
927.2	$H_5SO_3N_3S$	938.3	949.4	1854.3	1876.3	Sialidosis
933.5	H_3N_2	478.3				G_{M1}-gangliosidosis
938.3	$H_5SO_3N_3S$	927.2	949.4	1854.3	1876.3	Sialidosis
949.4	$H_5SO_3N_3S$	927.2	938.3	1854.3	1876.3	Sialidosis
974.6	H_2N_3					G_{M2}-gangliosidosis
1033.1	$H_5N_3S_2$	1044.1	1055.1			Sialidosis
1044.1	$H_5N_3S_2$	1033.1	1055.1			Sialidosis
1054.5	H_5N					α-Mannosidosis
1055.1	$H_5N_3S_2$	1033.1	1044.1			Sialidosis
1079.4	H_3N_2F					Fucosidosis
1083.6	$H_5SO_3N_3S_2$	2166.6				Sialidosis
1095.5	H_4N_2					G_{M1}-gangliosidosis
1107.0	H_7N_5					G_{M1}-gangliosidosis
1136.5	H_3N_3	580.0				G_{M2}-gangliosidosis
1216.5	H_6N					α-Mannosidosis
1224.5	H_3N_2S	624.1	635.1	1246.8		Sialidosis
1237.4	$H_6N_4S_2$					Sialidosis
1246.8	H_3N_2S	624.1	635.1	1224.5		Sialidosis
1298.5	H_4N_3	660.9				G_{M1}-gangliosidosis
1304.3	$H_3SO_3N_2S$	664.0	674.5	685.8	1348.2	Sialidosis
1339.4	H_3N_4	681.2				G_{M2}-gangliosidosis
1348.2	$H_3SO_3N_2S$	664.0	674.5	685.8	1304.3	Sialidosis
1378.5	H_7N	700.9				α-Mannosidosis
1460.6	H_5N_3	742.1				G_{M1}-gangliosidosis
1540.4	H_8N	782.0				α-Mannosidosis
1702.8	H_9N	863.0				α-Mannosidosis
1854.3	$H_5SO_3N_3S$	927.2	938.3	949.4	1876.3	Sialidosis
1876.3	$H_5SO_3N_3S$	927.2	938.3	949.4	1854.3	Sialidosis
2166.6	$H_5SO_3N_3S_2$	1083.6				Sialidosis

Histogram A in Fig. 3 shows the found carbohydrates and their relative abundance for the disorder fucosidosis.

The disease related fucosyloligosaccharides are shown up with relative high abundance and are reported in Table 4.

In addition to disease related glycans, $Hex_1HexNAc_1Fuc_1$ is recorded in the table because this trisaccharide shows up significantly in the principal component analysis (PCA). A possible explanation for disease associated of this trisaccharide may be found in the fact that it is a blood group related saccharide (Ferreira et al. 2009). These fucosyloligosaccharides elute in the 8–10 min time window with the exception of the two isomers $Neu5Ac_1Hex_1HexNac_1Fuc_1$ eluting at 22.7 and 24 min, see Fig. 4.

This late elution is caused by the negative charge of sialic acid. The first eluting isomer is most likely the Neu5Ac(α2-6) version while the last eluting one is the most likely Neu5Ac(α2-3) version (Townsend et al. 1988, 1989).

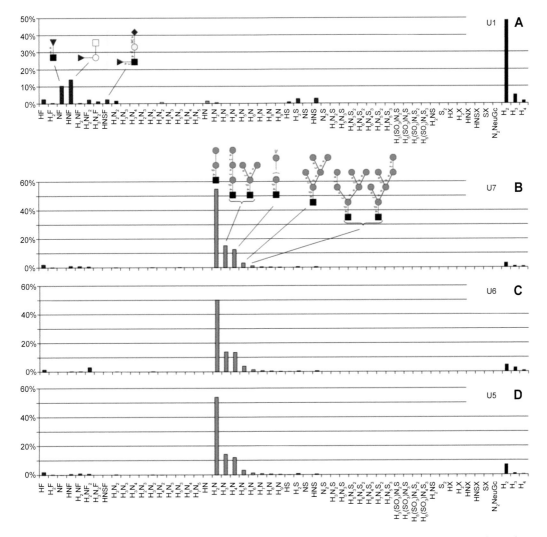

Figure 3. contd....

Figure 3. contd.

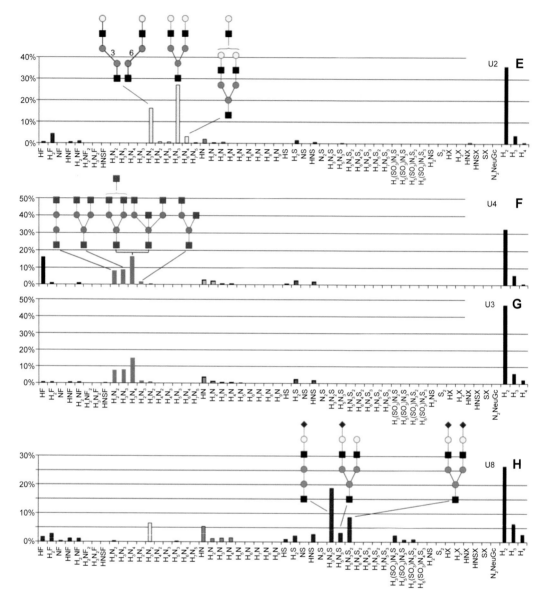

Figure 3. Histograms showing the relative abundance of the detected glycans in urine samples of lysosomal storage disorders fucosidosis (A), α-mannosidosis (B, C, and D), G_{M1}-gangliosidosis (E), G_{M2}-gangliosidosis (F and G), and sialidosis (H). H or white circle = hexose, N or white square = *N*-acetylhexosamine, F or triangle = fucose, S or diamond = *N*-acetylneuraminic acid, NeuGc = *N*-glycolylneuraminic acid, X = hexonic acid, SO3 = sulfate, white circle = galactose, grey circle = mannose, black square = *N*-acetylglucosamine. Reprinted with permission (Bruggink et al. 2012).

Table 4. Disease related glycans of fucosidosis. Modified from Bruggink et al. 2012 and reprinted with permission.

Composition	m/z	Charge	Ret. time (min)	Fragment ions
NF	390.2	[M+Na]$^+$	8.8	244.0 N; 226.0 N; 187.2 F; 169.1 F-18
H$_2$NF	714.5	[M+Na]$^+$	9.1	
H$_3$N$_2$F	1079.4	[M+Na]$^+$	9.2	
HNSF	865.4	[M-H+2Na]$^+$	22.7	719.5 HNS; 552.4 HNF; 534.3 HNF-18; 516.2 HS; 498.0 HS-18; 405.9 HN; 388.1 HN-18; 336.0 S-18; 318.1 S-2x18
			24.0	552.2 HNF; 534.1 HNF-18; 516.0 HS; 498.2 HS-18; 354.2 S; 336.0 S-18
HNF	552.5	[M+Na]$^+$	8.9	406.1 HN; 388.1 HN-18; 372.1 NF-18; 244.0 N; 226.0 N-18; 208.0 N-2x18; 203.0 H; 187.1 F; 185.0 H-18; 169.0 F-18

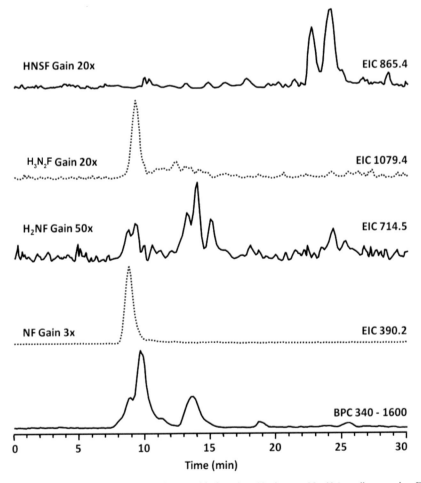

Figure 4. Separation of oligosaccharides in urine of a Fucosidosis patient. H = hexose, N = *N*-Acetylhexosamine, F = Fucose. Reprinted with permission (Bruggink et al. 2012).

For evaluation of α-mannosidosis there were three samples from three individuals from two different families. The histograms B, C, and D in Fig. 3 reveal the high abundance of the eight disease related glycans and are reported in Table 5.

Table 5. Disease related glycans of α-mannosidosis. Modified from Bruggink et al. 2012 and reprinted with permission.

Composition	m/z	Charge	Ret. time (min)	Fragment ions
H_2N	568.4	$[M+Na]^+$	5.8	406.2 HN; 388.1 HN-18; 365.2 H_2; 347.2 H_2-18; 244.1 N; 226.0 N-18; 203.1 H
H_3N	730.4	$[M+Na]^+$	8.1	568.3 H_2N; 550.3 H_2N-18; 527.3 H_3; 509.2 H_3-18; 388.2 HN-18; 365.1 H_2; 347.2 H_2-18; 329.0 H_2-2x18; 244.1 N; 226.0 N-18
		$[M+Na]^+$	8.9	527.2 H_3; 509.2 H_3-18; 406.2 HN; 388.1 HN-18; 365.3 H_2; 347.2 H_2-18; 329.2 H_2-2x18; 244.2 N; 226.2 N-18
H_4N	892.5	$[M+Na]^+$	10.6	730.2 H_3N; 712.3 H_3N-18; 689.4 H_4; 671.3 H_4-18; 527.1 H_3; 509.3 H_3-18; 406.3 HN; 347.1 H_2-18
			12.8	730.2 H_3N; 712.3 H_3-18; 689.3 H_4; 671.3 H_4-18; 568.4 H_2N; 550.3 H_2N-18; 527.2 H_3; 509.3 H_3-18; 491.3 H_3-2x18; 406.2 HN; 388.3 HN-18; 365.3 H_2; 347.2 H_2-18; 329.2 H_2-2x18; 244.2 N
			15.4	730.2 H_3N; 712.3 H_3N-18; 689.3 H_4; 671.3 H_4-18; 568.2 H_2N; 527.3 H_3; 509.2 H_3-18; 491.1 H_3N-2x18; 406.0 HN; 388.1 HN-18; 365.1 H_2; 347.2 H_2-18
H_5N	1054.5	$[M+Na]^+$	15.9	874.5 H_4N-18; 851.3 H_5; 833.4 H_5-18; 712.8 H_3N-18; 689.3 H_4; 671.3 H_4-18; 568.3 H_2N; 550.2 H_2N-18; 527.1 H_3; 509.3 H_3-18; 491.2 H_3-2x18
			16.7	851.4 H_5; 833.4 H_5-18; 712.3 H_3N-18; 689.4 H_4; 671.3 H_4-18; 653.4 H_4-2x18; 568.3 H_2N; 527.1 H_3; 509.3 H_3-18; 365.1 H_2; 347.1 H_2-18
			18.6	892.3 H_4N; 851.3 H_5; 833.1 H_5-18; 730.3 H_3N; 689.3 H_4; 671.4 H_4-18; 568.4 H_2N; 550.0 H_2N-18; 509.2 H_3-18; 491.1 H_3-2x18; 365.1 H_2; 346.9 H_2-18
H_6N	1216.5	$[M+Na]^+$	19.2	1054.3 H_5N; 1036.4 H_5N-18; 1013.4 H_6; 995.4 H_6-18; 892.4 H_4N; 874.4 H_4N-18; 851.3 H_5; 833.3 H_5-18; 730.3 H_3N; 671.4 H_4-18; 653.3 H_4-2x18; 568.3 H_2N; 527.3 H_3; 509.3 H_3-18; 491.2 H_3-2x18
			19.9	1054.5 H_5N; 1036.4 H_5N-18; 1013.3 H_6; 995.4 H_6-18; 892.3 H_4N; 851.3 H_5; 833.4 H_5-18; 730.2 H_3N; 689.3 H_4; 671.4 H_4-18; 527.5 H_3; 509.1 H_3-18; 347.1 H_2-18
			21.4	
H_7N	700.9/1378.5	$[M+2Na]^{2+}$	21.7	1198.3 H_6N-18; 1175.4 H_7; 1157.3 H_7-18; 1054.5 H_5N; 1036.4 H_5N-18; 1013.2 H_6; 995.4 H_6-18; 892.3 H_4N; 874.3 H_4N-18; 851.2 H_5; 833.1 H_5-18; 712.4 H_3N; 689.4 H_4; 671.4 H_4-18; 509.1 H_3-18; 491.3 H_3-2x18
H_8N	782.0/1540.4	$[M+2Na]^{2+}$	15.8	
			23.9	671.1 H_4-18; 346.9 H_2-18
			25.5	
H_9N	863.0/1702.8	$[M+2Na]^{2+}$	25.8	

The abundance decreases with increasing glycan size. From the oligosaccharides $Hex_{3-6\,and\,8}HexNAc_1$ two or more isotopes were separated. All the disease related glycans elute in the 5–30 min time window.

Table 6 lists G_{M1}-gangliosidosis disorder related glycans and those that have significant abundance in histogram E of Fig. 3.

Table 6. Disease related glycans of G_{M1}-gangliosidosis. Modified from Bruggink et al. 2012 and reprinted with permission.

Composition	m/z	Charge	Ret. time (min)	Fragment ions
H_3N_2	933.5/478.3	$[M+Na]^+/[M+2Na]^{2+}$	8.8	730.4 H_3N; 712.3 H_3N-18; 568.3 H_2N; 550.3 H_2N-18; 406.2 HN; 388.2 HN-18; 365.2 H_2; 347.2 H_2-18
	933.5/478.3	$[M+Na]^+/[M+2Na]^{2+}$	12.8	730.4 H_3N; 712.4 H_3N-18; 568.3 H_2N; 550.3 H_2N-18; 406.2 HN; 388.2 HN-18; 365.1 H_2; 347.2 H_2-18
H_4N_2	1095.5	$[M+Na]^+$	15.0	933.3 H_3N_2; 915.1 H_4N_2-18; 892.2 H_4N; 874.3 H_4N-18; 753.4 H_3N_2-18; 730.3 H_3N; 712.1 H_3N-18; 568.2 H_2N; 550.3 H_2N-18; 532.2 H_2N-2x18; 527.3 H_3; 509.0 H_3-18; 406.4 HN; 388.2 HN-18; 365.1 H_2
	1095.5	$[M+Na]^+$	16.1	933.3 H_3N_2; 892.2 H_4N; 874.4 H_4N-18; 730.3 H_3N; 568.2 H_2N; 550.3 H_2N-18; 509.2 H_3-18; 388.1 HN-18
	1095.5	$[M+Na]^+$	21.0	
H_4N_3	1298.5/660.9	$[M+Na]^+/[M+2Na]^{2+}$	15.8	
	1298.5/660.9	$[M+Na]^+/[M+2Na]^{2+}$	17.3	1077.7/550.3 H_4N_2-18; 933.3 H_3N_2; 550.3 H_2N-18 or H_4N_2-9; 388.1 HN-18 or H_2N_2-9
H_5N_3	1460.6/742.1	$[M+Na]^+/[M+2Na]^{2+}$	20.9	1298.6 H_4N_3; 1280.5 H_4N_3-18; 1257.6 H_5N_2; 1239.6 H_5N_2-18; 1095.6 H_4N_2; 1077.6 H_4N_2-18; 1059.6 H_4N_2-2x18; 933.5 H_3N_2; 915.4 H_3N_2-18; 892.5 H_4N; 874.6 H_4N-18; 771.4 H_3N_2; 730.5 H_3N; 712.4 H_3N-18; 694.3 H_3N-2x18; 568.4 H_2N; 550.3 H_2N-18; 532.4 H_2N-2x18; 527.3 H_3; 514.1 H_2N-3x18; 509.3 H_3-18; 405.9 HN; 388.2 HN-18; 370.2 HN-2x18; 365.3 H_2; 347.2 H_2-18; 329.2 H_2-2x18; 244.0 N; 226.0 N-18; 208.1 N-2x18
H_6N_4	924.5	$[M+2Na]^{2+}$	22.7	1442.7 H_5N_3-18; 1257.4 H_5N_2; 1239.5 H_5N_2-18; 892.3 H_4N; 651.7 H_4N_3-9; 570.8 H_3N_3-9; 388.2 HN-18
	924.5	$[M+2Na]^{2+}$	24.4	1622.4 H_6N_3; 1501.4 H_4N_4; 1460.5 H_5N_3; 1442.5 H_5N_3-18; 1424.4 H_5N_3-2x18; 1303.6 H_3N_4-2x18; 1298.6 H_4N_3; 1280.6 H_4N_3-18; 1257.6 H_5N_2; 1239.5 H_5N_2-18; 1118.5 H_3N_3-18; 1095.4 H_4N_2; 1077.6 H_4N_2-18; 1059.3 H_4N_2-2x18; 915.4 H_3N_2-18; 892.2 H_4N; 874.4 H_4N-18; 843.4 H_5N_4; 838.2 H_4N-3x18; 822.9 H_6N_3; 813.7 H_6N_3-9; 762.4 H_4N_4; 753.2 H_3N_2-18, H_4N_4-9; 741.9 H_5N_3; 735.2 H_3N_2-2x18; 732.9 H_5N_3-9; 730.2 H_3N; 712.3 H_3N-18; 660.8 H_4N_3; 640.3 H_5N_2; 570.3 H_3N_3; 568.3 H_2N; 559.3 H_4N_2; 552.6 H_3N_3-3x9; 550.2 H_2N-18; 406.2 HN; 388.2 HN-18; 347.2 H_2; 329.2 H_2-18
	924.5	$[M+2Na]^{2+}$	25.7	1604.5 H_6N_3-18; 1442.4 H_5N_3-18; 1257.4 H_5N_2; 1239.2 H_5N_2-18; 1095.4 H_4N_2; 1077.5 H_4N_2-18; 892.5 H_4N 874.4 H_4N-18; 822.8 H_6N_3; 753.3 H_3N_2-18; 730.3 H_3N; 550.2 H_4N_2; 388.2 HN-18
H_7N_5	1107.0	$[M+2Na]^{2+}$	25.9	1825.7 H_6N_3; 1807.6 H_6N_3-18; 1663.6/843.4 H_5N_4; 1627.5 H_6N_4-2x18; 1622.6/822.7 H_6N_3; 1501.9 H_4N_4; 1460.6/741.7 H_5N_3; 1442.5 H_5N_3-18; 1298.5 H_4N_3; 1257.7 H_5N_2; 1239.5/631.4 H_5N_2-18; 1095.5 H_4N_2; 1077.4 H_4N_2-18; 1059.3 H_4N_2-2x18; 1016.9 H_6N_5-9; 1005.3 H_7N_4; 933.4/478.1 H_3N_2; 924.3 H_6N_4; 915.4 H_6N_4-9; 813.8 H_6N_3-9; 804.8 H_6N_3-2x9; 771.1 H_3N_2; 753.3 H_2N_2-18; 550.4 H_2N-18; 388.2 HN-18

These G_{M1}-gangliosidosis related glycans elutes in the 8–28 min time window as shown in Fig. 5.

The extracted ion chromatogram (EIC) of m/z 933.5 shows a perfect separation of the two isomeric monoantennary glycans with the composition $Hex_3HexNAc_2$. The first eluting peak is the version Gal(β1-4)GlcNAc(β1-2)Man(α1-6)Man(β1-4)GlcNAc and the second eluting glycan is Gal(β1-4)GlcNAc(β1-2)Man(α1-3)Man(β1-4)GlcNAc (Bruggink et al. 2005).

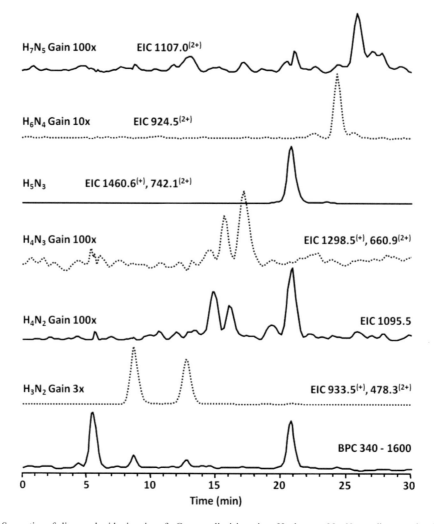

Figure 5. Separation of oligosaccharides in urine of a G_{M1}-gangliosisis patient. H = hexose, N = *N*-acetylhexosamine. Reprinted with permission (Bruggink et al. 2012).

Histograms F and G in Fig. 3 belong to the disorder G_{M2}-gangliosidosis. The reported disease related glycans $Hex_{2,3}HexNAc_{2-4}$ in Table 7 show a high abundance in the samples of diseased individuals.

These glycans elutes in the time window 10–20 min and EICs are shown in Fig. 6.

Another example of an isomer separation is shown in Fig. 6 EIC m/z 771.5 ($Hex_2HexNAc_2$) and EIC 1136.5 ($Hex_3HexNAc_3$). The interpretation of the first example is depicted in Fig. 7 (Bruggink et al. 2012).

In Table 8 the disease related glycans are reported for sialidosis.

The abundances of these eight disease related sialylglycans are shown in histogram H of Fig. 3. With this disease related glycans three sulfated sialyloligosaccharides are elevated which were earlier detected in urine samples of patients suffering from galactosialidosis (Bruggink et al. 2010). The sialyloligosaccharides

Table 7. Disease related glycans of G_{M2}-gangliosidosis. Modified from Bruggink et al. 2012 and reprinted with permission.

Composition	m/z	Charge	Ret. time (min)	Fragment ions
H_2N_2	771.5	$[M+Na]^+$	10.3	568.3 H_2N; 550.3 H_2N-18; 406.1 HN; 388.1 HN-18; 365.1 H_2; 347.1 H_2-18
	771.5	$[M+Na]^+$	11.9	568.3 H_2N; 550.3 H_2N-18; 406.1 HN; 388.1 HN-18; 365.1 H_2; 347.1 H_2N-18; 244.0 N; 226.0 N-18
H_3N_3	1136.5/580.0	$[M+Na]^+/[M+2Na]^{2+}$	15.1	933.4 H_3N_2; 915.3 H_3N_2-18; 771.5 H_3N_2; 730.4 H_3N; 712.3 H_3N-18; 568.2 H_2N; 550.2 H_2N-18
	1136.5/580.0	$[M+Na]^+/[M+2Na]^{2+}$	16.8	933.4 H_3N_2; 915.3 H_3N_2-18; 730.5 H_3N; 712.4 H_3N-18; 550.3 H_2N-18
	1136.5/580.0	$[M+Na]^+/[M+2Na]^{2+}$	18.1	933.5 H_3N_2; 915.3 H_3N_2-18; 730.5 H_3N; 712.3 H_3N-18; 568.3 H_2N; 550.2 H_2N-18; 347.1 H_2-18
H_3N_4	681.2	$[M+2Na]^{2+}$	10.0	
	1339.4/681.2	$[M+Na]^+/[M+2Na]^{2+}$	12.9	1136.4 H_3N_3; 1118.5 H_3N_3-18; 974.6 H_2N_3; 933.3 H_3N_2; 915.4 H_3N_2-18; 730.6 H_3N; 712.3 H_3N-18; 568.4 H_2N; 550.4 H_2N-18; 532.3 H_2N-2x18; 406.1 HN; 387.9 HN-18
	681.2	$[M+2Na]^{2+}$	14.0	1136.4/579.8 H_3N_3; 1118.5/570.9 H_3N_3-18; 974.3 H_2N_3; 933.4/478.2 H_3N_2; 915.3 H_3N_2-18; 897.4 H_3N_2-2x18; 771.3 H_2N_2; 753.4 H_2N_2-18; 712.2 H_3N-18; 591.4 HN_2-18; 568.4 H_2N; 388.2 HN-18; 244.0 N; 226.0 N-18
	681.2	$[M+2Na]^{2+}$	17.5	1136.4/579.8 H_3N_3; 1118.4/570.8 H_3N_3-18; 974.3 H_2N_3; 933.3/478.2 H_3N_2; 915.3/469.2 H_3N_2-18; 771.5 H_2N_2; 730.4 H_3N; 591.3 HN_2-18; 489.7 H_2N_3-9; 388.1 HN-18; 364.8 H_2; 347.1 H_2-18; 226.0 N-18
	1339.4/681.2	$[M+Na]^+/[M+2Na]^{2+}$	20.0	1136.4 H_3N_3; 1118.5 H_3N_3-18; 974.3 H_2N_3; 933.4 H_3N_2; 915.3 H_3N_2-18; 897.4 H_3N_2-2x18; 771.3 H_2N_2; 753.4 H_2N_2-18; 712.2 H_3N-18; 591.4 HN_2-18; 568.4 H_2N; 388.2 HN-18; 244.0 N; 226.0 N-18
H_2N_3	974.6	$[M+Na]^+$	11.1	771.4 H_2N_2; 753.4 H_2N_2-18; 609.4 HN_2; 568.3 H_2N; 550.3 H_2N-18; 365.0 H_2; 347.1 H_2-18

elutes in the time window 20–35 min. The urine of the sialidosis patient has been detected with the MS in the positive mode. As reported in Table 8, different proton and sodium adducts were observed from one component. This can complicate the interpretation of the MS spectra. Using the MS in the negative mode allows for easier interpretation of sialyloligosaccharides as previous shown for galactosialidosis (Bruggink et al. 2010).

The eight glycan fingerprints obtained for the five different LSDs were subjected to a hierarchical cluster analysis (Fig. 8).

The three α-mannosidosis samples were found to cluster together. Likewise, the two G_{M2}-gangliosidosis samples were grouped together. Moreover, G_{M1}- and G_{M2}-gangliosidosis samples were found in the same branch, whilst fucosidosis and sialidosis formed another group.

In addition, principal component analysis (PCA) was applied to the MS profiles of the different diseases in order to confirm the differences between the urinary oligosaccharides and to pinpoint the main structures responsible for those differences. Score plots using the first two PC's were used to present a 2D representation of variation among the spectra. Figure 9A shows a separation of the α-mannosidosis samples from the other four LSDs along PC1 (54 percentage of the variance is explained by the first PC).

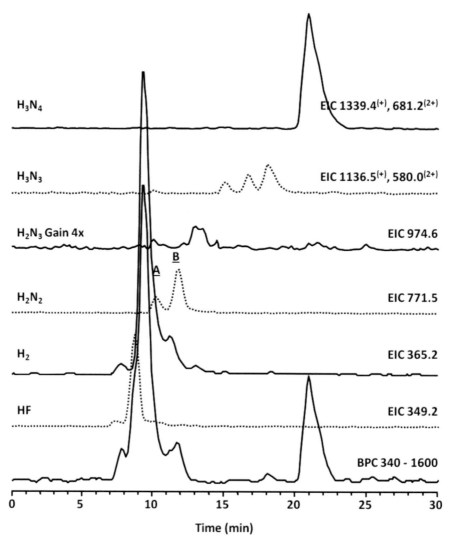

Figure 6. Separation of oligosaccharides in urine of a G_{M2}-gangliosisis patient. Fragment ion spectra of the species A and B is shown in Fig. 7. H = hexose, N = *N*-acetylhexosamine. Reprinted with permission (Bruggink et al. 2012).

The oligosaccharides contributing to the separation can be distinguished in the corresponding loadings plot, as the position of the samples in a given direction in the scores plot is determined by the structures lying in the same direction in the loadings plot. Accordingly, the loadings plot corresponding to PC1 *vs.* PC2 reveals an increase in H_2N, H_3N and H_4N (Fig. 9B) in the urine of patients suffering from α-mannosidosis.

While PC1 and PC2 showed little separation between fucosidosis, sialidosis, G_{M1}- and G_{M2}-gangliosidosis, such a separation was observed within the PCA analysis based on PC3 *vs.* PC4 (Fig. 9C). The corresponding loadings plot (Fig. 9D) shows high amounts of H_3N_2S and $H_5N_3S_2$ for sialidosis, for G_{M1}-gangliosidosis an increased amount of H_5N_3 and H_3N_2, an increased amount of H_3N_4, H_3N_3, and H_2N_2 for G_{M2}-gangliosidosis, and the amount of NF as well as HNF is increased in the case of fucosidosis. Although the number of samples used for the PCA analysis is limited, the results point to the major disease-related glycans described before (see, e.g., Fig. 3).

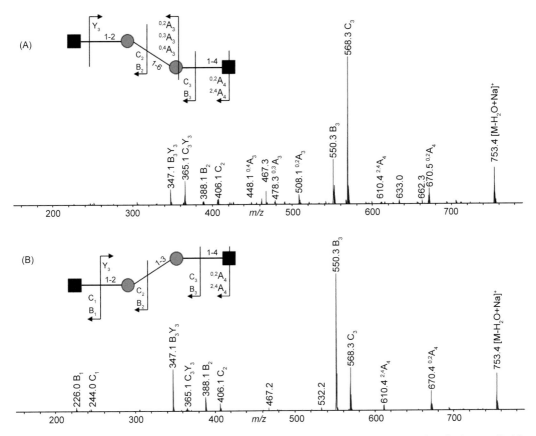

Figure 7. Positive-ion fragmentation mass spectra of two isomeric sodiated tetrasaccharide from urine of a G_{M2}-gangliosisis patient with precursor ion *m/z* 771.5 A and B from Fig. 6. Reprinted with permission (Bruggink et al. 2012).

Materials and Methods

Materials

To prepare the eluents analytical reagent grade sodium hydroxide (50 percentage w/w), sodium acetate were obtained from J.T. Baker (Deventer, The Netherlands). Sulfuric acid (AR) used for the desalter regenerant and the makeup solution sodium chloride (AR) came from J.T. Baker. The acetonitrile was from Biosolve (Valkenswaard, The Netherlands). Water from a Milli-Q synthesis system from Millipore BV (Amsterdam, The Netherlands) was used throughout. Details on urine samples are given in Table 9.

Sample Preparation

To isolate oligosaccharides from biological samples, SPE graphitized carbon cartridges were used, as previous described (Packer et al. 1998). A 200 µL sample was diluted with 1800 µL water and loaded on a Carbograph SPE (210142) from Alltech Associates Inc. (Deerfield, IL). To desalt the urine sample the cartridge was washed with 6 mL of water. The isolated oligosaccharides were eluted from the column with 3 mL of 25 percent acetonitrile containing 0.05 percent trifluoroacetic acid. The eluate was evaporated under a nitrogen stream at room temperature until the volume was decreased by 50 percent. The remaining solution was lyophilized and reconstituted with 200 µL water and was then ready for injection on the chromatography system.

Table 8. Disease related glycans of sialidosis. Modified from Bruggink et al. 2012 and reprinted with permission.

Composition	m/z	Charge	Ret. time (min)	Fragment ions
HNS	697.6/719.5	$[M+Na]^+/[M-H+2Na]^+$	21.3	516.2 HS; 498.2 HS-18; 406.1 HN; 388.1 HN-18; 354.0 S; 336.1 S-18; 318.0 S-2x18; 226.0 N-18
H_3N_2S	1224.5/1246.8 624.1/635.1	$[M+Na]^+/[M-H+2Na]^+$ $[M+2Na]^{2+}/[M-H+3Na]^{2+}$	21.8	1043.4/533.3 H_3NS-18; 1025.4/524.3 H_3NS-18; 933.4/477.9 H_3N_2; 915.4 H_3N_2-18; 881.5/452.3 H_2NS; 863.3/443.0 H_2NS-18; 771.4 H_2N; 753.5 H_2N-18; 730.4 H_3N; 712.5 H_3N-18; 719.4 HNS; 701.4 HNS-18; 568.4 H_2N; 550.2 H_2N-18; 516.3 HS; 498.3 HS-18; 406.1 HN; 388.1 HN-18; 365.0 H_2; 347.3 H_2-18; 354.0 S; 336.0 S-18; 243.9 N; 226.0 N-18; 208.0 N-2x18; 203.1 H; 185.0 H-18
H_5N_3S	887.6/898.3	$[M+2Na]^{2+}/[M-H+3Na]^{2+}$	23.7	1460.5 H_5N_3; 1442.6 H_5N_3-18; 1408.6 H_4N_2S; 1390.3 H_4N_2S-18; 1257.6 H_5N_2; 1095.5 H_4N_2-18; 1077.6 H_4N_2-18; 1025.2 H_3NS-18; 915.4 H_3N_2-18; 892.2 H_4N; 881.3 H_2NS; 797.4 H_4N_3S-9; 796.9 H_5N_2S; 771.5 H_2N; 694.5 H_3N-2x18; 640.5 H_5N; 605.0 H_4NS-9; 568.2 H_2N; 541.0 H_4N_2-2x9; 388.2 HN-18; 336.1/314.0 S-18
$H_5N_3S_2$	1033.1/1044.1/1055.1	$[M+2Na]^{2+}/[M-H+3Na]^{2+}/[M-2H+4Na]^{2+}$	29.1	1773.4/898.5 H_5N_3S; 1733.1/1755.3/889.4 H_5N_3S-18; 1571.4/797.5 H_4N_3S-18; 1570.5 H_5N_3S; 1460.2/741.9 H_5N_2; 1408.4 H_4N_2S; 1368.8 H_4N_3S-18; 1095.5 H_4N_2; 953.4 H_5N_2; 915.5 H_3N_2-18; 892.1 H_4N; 701.2 HNS-18; 694.4 H_3N-2x18; 605.3 H_4NS-9; 596.1 H_4NS-2x9; 313.9 S
$H_6N_4S_2$	1237.4	$[M-2H+4Na]^{2+}$	28.8	
$H_3SO_3N_2S$	1304.3/1348.2 664.0/674.5/685.8	$[M+Na]^+/[M-2H+3Na]^+$ $[M+2Na]^{2+}/[M-H+3Na]^{2+}/[M-2H+4Na]^{2+}$	21.8	933.5 $H_3(SO_3)N_2$; 701.4 H(SO_3)NS-18; 645.6/634.9 H_3N_2S; 634.5 $H_2(SO_3)N$; 516.3 H(SO_3)S; 196.0 HN
$H_5SO_3N_3S$	1854.3/1876.3/ 927.2/938.3/949.4	$[M-H+2Na]^+/[M-2H+3Na]^+/$ $[M+2Na]^{2+}/[M-H+3Na]^{2+}/[M-2H+4Na]^{2+}$	22.0	
$H_5SO_3N_3S_2$	2166.6/1083.8	$[M-2H+3Na]^+/[M-H+3Na]^{2+}$	33.8	

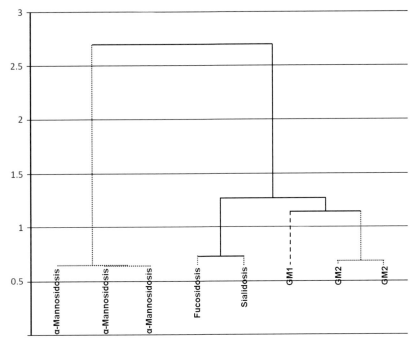

Figure 8. Dendrogram of hierarchical cluster analysis of lysosomal storage diseases α-mannosidosis, fucosidosis, G_{M1}-gangliosidosis, G_{M2}-gangliosidosis, and sialidosis.

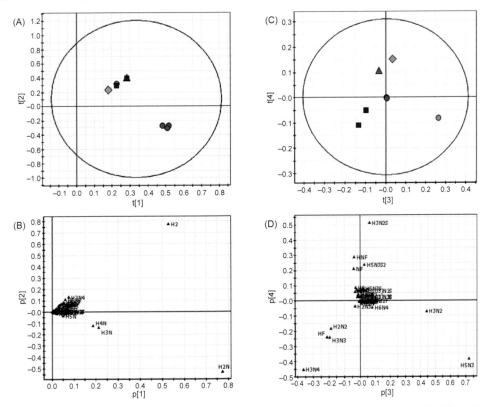

Figure 9. Loading plots based on PC1 and PC2 (A and B). Loading plots based on PC3 and PC4 (C and D). Black triangle fucosidosis, dark circle is α-mannosidosis, light gray circle is G_{M1}-gangliosidosis, dark square is G_{M2}-gangliosidosis, and diamond is sialidosis.

Table 9. Sample information. Reprinted with permission (Bruggink et al. 2012).

Sample code	Disorder	Creatinine (mmol/L)
U1	Fucosidosis	2.22
U2	G_{M1}-gangliosidosis	1.04
U3	G_{M2}-gangliosidosis	5.37
U4	G_{M2}-gangliosidosis	1.04
U5	α-Mannosidosis	18.86
U6	α-Mannosidosis	8.46
U7	α-Mannosidosis	14.52
U8	Sialidosis	Not determined

Capillary HPAEC

A modified Dionex BioLC system from Thermo Fisher Scientific (Sunnyvale, CA, USA) was converted into a capillary chromatographic system comprising a microbore GP40 quaternary gradient pump, a Famos micro autosampler with a full PEEK (polyether ether ketone) injector equipped with a 1 µL loop and an ED40 electrochemical detector. BioLC control, data acquisition from the ED40 detector and, signal integration was supported by Dionex Chromeleon V6.8 software (Thermo Fisher Scientific). This modified system has been described in detail before (Bruggink et al. 2005), for the system layout see Fig. 1. A prototype capillary column (250 x 0.4 mm I.D.) packed with CarboPac PA200 resin was manufactured by Thermo Fisher Scientific. To make the GP40 pump suitable for delivering a eluent flow rate of 10 µL·min⁻¹ a splitter out of PEEK tubing and a TEE-piece was made. The pump was provided with water (eluent A), 500 mM sodium hydroxide (eluent B), and 500 mM sodium acetate (eluent C). All separations were performed at room temperature. The following ternary gradient was used for separating oligosaccharides of fucosidosis, G_{M2}-gangliosidosis, and sialidosis: an isocratic part of 76% A + 24% B (–20 to –14 min) to wash the column with sodium hydroxide, followed by the column equilibration with 88% A + 12% B (–14 to 0 min), continued with a linear sodium acetate gradient (0–55 min) to 25.5% A + 12% B + 62.5% C for the separation. For separating oligosaccharides of α-mannosidosis and G_{M1}-gangliosidosis the following ternary gradient was used: isocratic column wash with sodium hydroxide 76% A + 24% B (–20 to –14 min), followed by column equilibration with 88% A + 12% B (–14 to 0 min), continued by a linear sodium hydroxide gradient (0 to 9.1 min) to 60% A + 40% B; 60% A + 40% B, was kept isocratic for a period of 9.1 to 12.5 min, than a linear sodium acetate gradient (12.5 to 21.6 min) to 85.2% A + 12% B + 2.8% C, followed by a second linear sodium acetate gradient (21.6 to 104 min) to 60.5% A + 12% B + 27.5% C. Injection of the sample takes place at time 0.0 min.

The ED40 detector applies the following waveform to the gold working electrode: E_1 = 0.1 V (t_d = 0.00–0.20 s, t_1 = 0.20–0.40 s), E_2 = –2.0 V (t_2 = 0.41–0.42 s), E_3 = 0.6 V (t_3 = 0.43 s), E_4 = –0.1 V (t_4 = 0.44–0.50 s) versus an Ag/AgCl reference electrode (Rocklin et al. 1998). A 1 mm gold work electrode and a 25 µm gasket were installed.

Mass Spectrometry

An Esquire 3000 ion trap mass spectrometer from Bruker Daltonics (Bremen, Germany), equipped with an electrospray ionization (ESI) source was coupled to the capillary chromatographic system. The eluent flows through an inline prototype desalter (Thermo Fisher Scientific) to convert the eluent into an ESI compatible fluid. The desalter is continually regenerated with dilute sulfuric acid to exchange sodium ions in the eluent with hydronium ions. This delivers volatile acetic acid and water in the direction of the ion trap MS. To obtain efficient ionization a microbore AGP-1 (Thermo Fisher Scientific) was modified as an auxiliary pump to pump the makeup solution (0.6 mM NaCl in 50 percent acetonitrile). The makeup solution was pumped into the eluent flow via a MicroTEE (P-775 Upchurch Scientific, Oak Harbor, WA, USA) at a flow rate of 4.6 µL·min^{-1}. The ion-trap MS operated in the positive mode at the following conditions: dry temperature 325ºC, nebulizer 103 kPa, dry gas 7 l·min^{-1}, capillary voltage –3500 V, target mass m/z 850, scan speed 13000 m/z per s in MS and MS/MS mode. For tandem MS automatic selection of three precursors was applied.

Data Analysis

Data Analysis (version 3.3, Bruker Daltonics) was used to manually interpret MS as well as MS/MS spectra. To determine the peak area of the individual oligosaccharides, extracted ion chromatograms (EIC) were produced from the MS spectra. Signals of all detected charge states and isomers corresponding to the same compound were summed followed by normalizing the peak areas to the sum of all glycan peak areas of one sample. Subsequently, data matrices were analyzed by PCA using SIMCA-P+ (version 12.0, Umetrics, Sweden) software package.

Keywords: Anion-exchange chromatography, Fucosidosis, Glycans, G$_{M1}$-Gangliosidosis, G$_{M2}$-Gangliosidosis, HPAE, Integrated pulsed amperometric detection, Mannosidosis, Mass spectrometry, Oligosaccharides, Ring fragmentation, Sialidosis, Pulsed amperometric detection

References

Achyuthan, K. E. and A. M. Achyuthan. 2001. Comparative enzymology, biochemistry and pathophysiology of human exo-alpha-sialidases (neuraminidases). Comp Biochem Physiol B Biochem Mol Biol 129: 29–64.

An, Y., S. P. Young, S. L. Hillman, J. L. Van Hove, Y. T. Chen and D. S. Millington. 2000. Liquid chromatographic assay for a glucose tetrasaccharide, a putative biomarker for the diagnosis of Pompe disease. Anal Biochem 287: 136–143.

Aronson, N. N., Jr. and M. J. Kuranda. 1989. Lysosomal degradation of Asn-linked glycoproteins. FASEB J 3: 2615–2622.

Bruggink, C., M. Wuhrer, C. A. M. Koeleman, V. Barreto, Y. Liu, C. Pohl et al. 2005. Oligosaccharide analysis by capillary-scale high-pH anion-exchange chromatography with on-line ion-trap mass spectrometry. J Chromatogr B Analyt Technol Biomed Life Sci 829: 136–143.

Bruggink, C., B. J. Poorthuis, M. Piraud, R. Froissart, A. M. Deelder and M. Wuhrer. 2010. Glycan profiling of urine, amniotic fluid and ascitic fluid from galactosialidosis patients reveals novel oligosaccharides with reducing end hexose and aldohexonic acid residues. FEBS J 277: 2970–2986.

Bruggink, C. 2012. Oligosaccharide analysis by high-performance anion-exchange chromatography hyphenated to integrated pulsed amperometric detection and on-line ion-trap mass spectrometry. pp. 379–391. In: Bhattacharyya, L. and J. S. Rohrer (eds.). Applications of Ion Chromatography in the Analysis of Pharmaceutical and Biological Products. John Wiley and Sons Inc., Hoboken, New Jersey.

Bruggink, C., B. J. Poorthuis, A. M. Deelder and M. Wuhrer. 2012. Analysis of urinary oligosaccharides in lysosomal storage disorders by capillary high-performance anion-exchange chromatography-mass spectrometry. Anal Bioanal Chem 403: 1671–1683.

Cantz, M., J. Gehler and J. Spranger. 1977. Mucolipidosis I: Increased sialic acid content and deficiency of an alpha-N-acetylneuraminidase in cultured fibroblasts. Biochem Biophys Res Commun 74: 732–738.

Cantz, M. and B. Ulrich-Bott. 1990. Disorders of glycoprotein degradation. J Inherit Metab Dis 13: 523–537.

Dean, J. A. 1999. Lange's Handbook of Chemistry, 15th edn. McGraw-Hill, Inc., New York.

Domon, B. and C. E. Costello. 1988. A systematic nomenclature for carbohydrate fragmentations in FAB-MS/MS spectra of glycoconjugates. J Glycoconj 5: 397–409.

Ferreira, J. A., M. R. Domingues, A. Reis, M. A. Monteiro and M. A. Coimbra. 2009. Differentiation of isomeric Lewis blood groups by positive ion electrospray tandem mass spectrometry. Anal Biochem 397: 186–196.

Hardy, M. R. and R. R. Townsend. 1988. Separation of positional isomers of oligosaccharides and glycopeptides by high-performance anion-exchange chromatography with pulsed amperometric detection. Proc Natl Acad Sci USA 85: 3289–3293.

Harvey, D. J. 2000. Electrospray mass spectrometry and fragmentation of N-linked carbohydrates derivatized at the reducing terminus. J Am Soc Mass Spectrom 11: 900–915.

Hoffman, L. M., D. Amsterdam, S. E. Brooks and L. Schneck. 1977. Glycosphingolipids in fetal Tay-Sachs disease brain and lung cultures. J Neurochem 29: 551–559.

Hou, Y., R. Tse and D. J. Mahuran. 1996. Direct determination of the substrate specificity of the alpha-active site in heterodimeric beta-hexosaminidase A. Biochemistry (Mosc) 35: 3963–3969.

Kin, N. M. 1987. Comparison of the urinary glycoconjugates excreted by patients with type I and type II fucosidosis. Clin Chem 33: 44–47.

Kolter, T. and K. Sandhoff. 2006. Sphingolipid metabolism diseases. Biochim Biophys Acta 1758: 2057–2079.

Landing, B. H., F. N. Silverman, D. L. Chadwick, M. E. Lahey, M. D. Jacoby and J. M. Raig. 1964. Familial neurovisceral lipidosis. An analysis of eight cases of a syndrome previously reported as "Hurler-variant," "Pseudo-Hurler," and "Tay-Sachs disease with visceral involvement". Am J Dis Child 108: 503–522.

Lee, Y. C. 1990. High-performance anion-exchange chromatography for carbohydrate analysis. Anal Biochem 189: 151–162.

Lundblad, A., J. Lundsten, N. E. Nordén, S. Sjöblad, S. Svensson, P. A. Öckerman et al. 1978. Urinary abnormalities in fucosidosis. Eur J Biochem 83: 513–521.

Mahuran, D. J. 1999. Biochemical consequences of mutations causing the G_{M2} gangliosidoses. Biochim Biophys Acta 1455: 105–138.

Mechref, Y., M. V. Novotny and C. Krishnan. 2003. Structural characterization of oligosaccharides using MALDI-TOF/TOF tandem mass spectrometry. Anal Chem 75: 4895–4903.

Michalski, J. C. and A. Klein. 1999. Glycoprotein lysosomal storage disorders: alpha- and beta-mannosidosis, fucosidosis and alpha-N-acetylgalactosaminidase deficiency. Biochim Biophys Acta 1455: 69–84.

Mohr, M. D., K. O. Bornsen and H. M. Widmer. 1995. Matrix-assisted laser desorption/ionization mass spectrometry: improved matrix for oligosaccharides. Rapid Commun Mass Spectrom 9: 809–814.

Neville, D. C., R. A. Dwek and T. D. Butters. 2009. Development of a single column method for the separation of lipid- and protein-derived oligosaccharides. J Proteome Res 8: 681–687.

Ockerman, P. A. 1969. Diseases of glycoprotein storage. Lancet 1: 734.

Ockerman, P. A., S. Autio and N. E. Norden. 1973. Diagnosis of mannosidosis. Lancet 1: 207–208.

Packer, N. H., M. A. Lawson, D. R. Jardine and J. W. Redmond. 1998. A general approach to desalting oligosaccharides released from glycoproteins. Glycoconj J 15: 737–747.

Peelen, G. O., J. G. de Jong and R. A. Wevers. 1994. HPLC analysis of oligosaccharides in urine from oligosaccharidosis patients. Clin Chem 40: 914–921.

Penn, S. G., M. T. Cancilla and C. B. Lebrilla. 1996. Collision-induced dissociation of branched oligosaccharide ions with analysis and calculation of relative dissociation thresholds. Anal Chem 68: 2331–2339.

Rabin, S., J. R. Stillian, V. Barreto, K. Friedman and M. Toofan. 1993. New membrane-based electrolytic suppressor device for suppressed conductivity detection in ion chromatography. J Chromatogr 640: 97–109.

Rocklin, R. D., A. P. Clarke and M. Weitzhandler. 1998. Improved long-term reproducibility for pulsed amperometric detection of carbohydrates via a new quadruple-potential waveform. Anal Chem 70: 1496–1501.

Rubin, M., G. Karpati, L. S. Wolfe, S. Carpenter, M. H. Klavins and D. J. Mahuran. 1988. Adult onset motor neuronopathy in the juvenile type of hexosaminidase A and B deficiency. J Neurol Sci 87: 103–119.

Schindler, D., T. Kanzaki and R. J. Desnick. 1990. A method for the rapid detection of urinary glycopeptides in alpha-N-acetylgalactosaminidase deficiency and other lysosomal storage diseases. Clin Chim Acta 190: 81–91.

Sewell, A. C. 1979. An improved thin-layer chromatographic method for urinary oligosaccharide screening. Clin Chim Acta 92: 411–414.

Spina, E., L. Sturiale, D. Romeo, G. Impallomeni, D. Garozzo, D. Waidelich et al. 2004. New fragmentation mechanisms in matrix-assisted laser desorption/ionization time-of-flight/time-of-flight tandem mass spectrometry of carbohydrates. Rapid Commun Mass Spectrom 18: 392–398.

Strecker, G., M. C. Herlant-Peers, B. Fournet and J. Montreul. 1977. Structure of seven oligosaccharides excreted in the urine of a patient with Sandhoff's disease (G_{M2} gangliosidosis-variant O). Eur J Biochem 81: 165–171.

Takahashi, Y. and T. Orii. 1989. Severity of G_{M1} gangliosidosis and urinary oligosaccharide excretion. Clin Chim Acta 179: 153–162.

Thayer, J. R., J. S. Rohrer, N. Avdalovic and R. P. Gearing. 1998. Improvements to in-line desalting of oligosaccharides separated by high-pH anion exchange chromatography with pulsed amperometric detection. Anal Biochem 256: 207–216.

Townsend, R. R., M. R. Hardy, O. Hindsgaul and Y. C. Lee. 1988. High-performance anion-exchange chromatography of oligosaccharides using pellicular resins and pulsed amperometric detection. Anal Biochem 174: 459–470.

Townsend, R. R., M. R. Hardy, D. A. Cumming, J. P. Carver and B. Bendiak. 1989. Separation of branched sialylated oligosaccharides using high-pH anion-exchange chromatography with pulsed amperometric detection. Anal Biochem 182: 1–8.

van Pelt, J., J. P. Kamerling, H. D. Bakker and J. F. Vliegenthart. 1991. A comparative study of sialyloligosaccharides isolated from sialidosis and galactosialidosis urine. J Inherit Metab Dis 14: 730–740.

Vellodi, A. 2005. Lysosomal storage disorders. Br J Haematol 128: 413–431.

Warner, T. G., R. D. De Kremer, D. Applegarth and A. K. Mock. 1986. Diagnosis and characterization of G_{M2} gangliosidosis type II (Sandhoff disease) by analysis of the accumulating N-acetyl-glucosaminyl oligosaccharides with high performance liquid chromatography. Clin Chim Acta 154: 151–164.

Weiskopf, A. S., P. Vouros and D. J. Harvey. 1998. Electrospray ionization-ion trap mass spectrometry for structural analysis of complex N-linked glycoprotein oligosaccharides. Anal Chem 70: 4441–4447.

Weiss, J. 2004. Handbook of Ion Chromatography. Third, Completely Revised and Updated Edition, 3 edn. Wiley-VCH Verlag GmbH & Co. KGaA, Weinheim.

Winchester, B. 2005. Lysosomal metabolism of glycoproteins. Glycobiology 15: 1R–15R.

Wuhrer, M., A. M. Deelder and Y. E. van der Burgt. 2011. Mass spectrometric glycan rearrangements. Mass Spectrom Rev 30: 664–680.

Wuhrer, M. 2013. Glycomics using mass spectrometry. Glycoconj J 30: 11–22.

CHAPTER 4

Glycosaminoglycan Binding by the Lyme Disease Spirochete is a Determinant of Tissue Tropism and Disease

Yi-Pin Lin,[1,a] *Marcia S. Osburne,*[1,b] *Michael J. Pereira,*[2] *Jenifer Coburn*[3] *and John M. Leong*[1,*]

Introduction

Upon transmission to humans by a vector tick bite, the Lyme disease bacterium, *Borrelia burgdorferi* sensu lato, can establish a local skin infection and may then disseminate further to multiple tissues, including the joints, heart, skin, and nervous system (Steere 2001). Clinical manifestations of infection in humans are quite variable and have been associated with genotypic differences in infecting strains. Interactions with mammalian cells and extracellular matrix (ECM) are critical for colonization of diverse sites in the mouse model of infection and many *B. burgdorferi* cell- or ECM-binding surface-localized attachment factors (adhesins) have been identified. Adhesins, which are likely to promote chronic multisystem disease and contribute to human disease diversity, often target host glycosaminoglycans (GAGs). An understanding of this infectious process is complicated by the multiplicities of target tissues and adhesins, many of which exhibit multiple attachment functions and vary in sequence. Detailed analysis of DbpA and BBK32, two adhesins that recognize dermatan sulfate GAG, indicate that (a) GAG-recognition by *B. burgdorferi* promotes colonization in a tissue-specific manner; and (b) sequence variation in adhesins influences the spectrum of tissues colonized. Recently, the *B. burgdorferi*-encoded OspF-related protein family, which

[1] Department of Molecular Biology and Microbiology, Tufts University School of Medicine, 136 Harrison Ave., Boston, MA 02111.

[a] E-mail: Yi-Pin.Lin@tufts.edu

[b] E-mail: Marcia.Osburne@tufts.edu

[2] Department of Molecular Biology and Microbiology, Tufts University School of Medicine, Sackler School of Graduate Biomedical Sciences, 136 Harrison Ave., Boston, MA 02111.
E-mail: Michael.Pereira@tufts.edu

[3] Division of Infectious Disease, and Center for Infectious Disease Research, Medical College of Wisconsin, 8701 Watertown Plank Rd., Milwaukee, WI 53226.
E-mail: jcoburn@mcw.edu

* Corresponding author: John.Leong@tufts.edu

encompasses more than seven paralogs, has been shown to recognize heparan sulfate GAG, suggesting that the complex and diverse manifestations of Lyme disease are influenced by strain-specific allelic variation of adhesins and differences in the repertoire of GAG-binding activities.

Clinical Importance and Biology of Lyme Disease Spirochetes

Lyme disease has become one of the most prevalent vector borne diseases in the United States, totaling approximately 30,000 confirmed cases in 2013. Although spreading, the disease is concentrated in the New England area—95% of all US cases occur in Connecticut, Maine, Massachusetts, New Hampshire, Rhode Island, and Vermont—with an average incidence of 75.1 (42.2–107.6) confirmed cases per 100,000 population per year. Recent data suggest that the current annual economic impact of Lyme disease in the US is approximately $1.3 billion, further emphasizing the need for the development of more effective treatment and prevention strategies (Adrion et al. 2015).

B. burgdorferi sensu lato, the causative agent of Lyme disease (Burgdorfer et al. 1982), encompasses several species of spirochetal (spiral-shaped) bacteria, but the three major human pathogens are *B. burgdorferi* sensu stricto, *B. afzelii*, and *B. garinii*. *B. burgdorferi* is the sole known agent of Lyme disease in the United States, whereas the latter two species are the prevalent agents in Eurasia (Chao and Shih 2002). The genome of Lyme disease spirochetes is highly complex, consisting of a single linear chromosome and a variety of endogenous linear and circular plasmids. Some of these plasmids, and the products they encode, are required for *in vitro* cultivation, for infection of laboratory mice, and/or for survival in the tick vector (see below) (Chung et al. 2002); other extrachromosomal elements seem to be required only for colonization of certain tissue sites (Liveris et al. 1996). The particular plasmid profile can differ among Lyme disease strains.

The Lyme spirochete is transmitted to the mammalian or avian host through the bite of certain members of the *Ixodes* genus of ticks, and the ability to readily transmit between the tick and animal hosts, typically rodents, is fundamental in the life cycle of the Lyme spirochete (Kornblatt et al. 1984, Piesman et al. 1987, Philipp and Johnson 1994). The *B. burgdorferi* life cycle is complex and dependent upon both tick and higher animal hosts for its propagation and transmission (Lane et al. 1991, Shih et al. 2002, Tilly et al. 2008). In order to be stably propagated in the enzootic cycle, a spirochete inoculated into a host animal must establish a persistent skin infection so as to be efficiently transmitted into the subsequent generation of (uninfected) ticks, which typically feed on the animal months or even a year later. This long-term persistence in the mammalian host implies that the Lyme spirochete has evolved to spread within that host and to evade immunity.

Lyme Disease Spirochetes Differ in Specific Tissues They Colonize and in Clinical Manifestations They Cause

The manifestations of human Lyme disease reflect the spirochetes' ability to cause chronic systemic infection in its natural mammalian hosts. Following the tick bite, spirochetes multiply and produce an outwardly spreading skin infection at the site of the bite, leading to the formation of the expanding pathognomonic erythema migrans rash that appears in approximately 70–80% of patients (Aguero-Rosenfeld et al. 2005), and can sometimes take on a "bulls-eye" appearance (Fig. 1). *B. burgdorferi*, like many other pathogenic spirochetes such as *Leptospira interrogans* and *Treponema pallidum*, can also disseminate via the bloodstream to colonize multiple tissues, including the heart, joints, or nervous system, producing symptoms such as arthritis, carditis, and neurologic conditions (Shapiro et al. 2014) that may persist, particularly if not treated promptly (Auwaerter et al. 2004).

Adding to the inherent complexity of this process is the observation that tissue tropism and disease manifestations appear to differ significantly among Lyme disease spirochetes. For example, *B. burgdorferi* is associated with arthritis, whereas *B. afzelii* is more commonly associated with skin manifestations such as acrodermatitis, and *B. garinii* is associated with neurological manifestations (van Dam et al. 1993, Anthonissen et al. 1994, Wang et al. 1999, Behera et al. 2008, Moriarty et al. 2008). In addition, even within

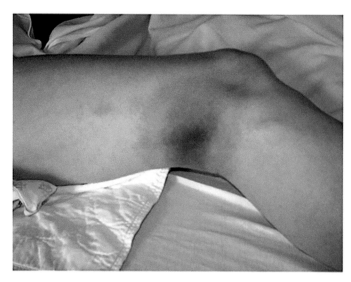

Figure 1. Erythema migrans, a characteristic skin lesion of Lyme disease. This migrating rash at the site of the bite of an infected tick reflects a spreading dermal infection. Photo courtesy of Lucas Wolf.

a Lyme spirochete species, there appears to be marked strain-dependent differences in tissue tropism—*B. burgdorferi* strains that are differentiated on the basis of genetic markers often differ in their ability to cause disseminated infection (Liveris et al. 1996, Seinost et al. 1999, Wang et al. 2001, Dolan et al. 2004).

Interactions of *B. burgdorferi* with Mammalian Components are Mediated by Multiple Surface Adhesive Proteins that Promote Tissue Colonization

The capacity of microbial pathogens to colonize distant tissue depends on their ability to establish an infectious niche at these sites. Thus, attachment to mammalian cells or extracellular matrix (ECM) is a common activity of pathogenic microbes, and it has been long established that *B. burgdorferi* is capable of binding to cultured mammalian cells (Fig. 2). Indeed, the process of dissemination through the vasculature can be visualized by intravital microscopy of fluorescent *B. burgdorferi* in living mice (Fig. 3) (Moriarty et al. 2008, Norman et al. 2008). Detailed analyses of these events reveal dissemination to be a multi-stage process initiated by attachment to the endothelial wall, followed by extravasation and then colonization (Moriarty et al. 2008) (Fig. 4). The endothelial attachment step can be further subdivided into: (1) tethering, defined as traversing 100 μm of the vessel wall in less than one second; (2) dragging, i.e., traversing 100 μm in one to 20 seconds; (3) stationary adherence, i.e., fixed attachment for > 20 seconds; and (4) extravasation (Fig. 4) (Moriarty et al. 2008).

Given the complexity of interactions between the Lyme spirochete and host tissues, including multistep interactions with vessel wall and differing tissue tropisms among strains, it is not surprising that *B. burgdorferi* sensu lato utilizes multiple attachment pathways to localize to specific tissues. Most pathogenic bacteria produce adhesins, i.e., surface proteins that mediate attachment to host components, to promote tissue localization and colonization (Finlay and Falkow 1997, Coburn et al. 2013). Lyme disease spirochetes in particular produce a large number of documented or putative adhesins (Coburn et al. 2013, Brissette and Gaultney 2014). Some of these adhesins are chromosomally encoded, but several are encoded by extrachromosomal plasmids, which, as mentioned above, may not be precisely conserved among all Lyme disease strains.

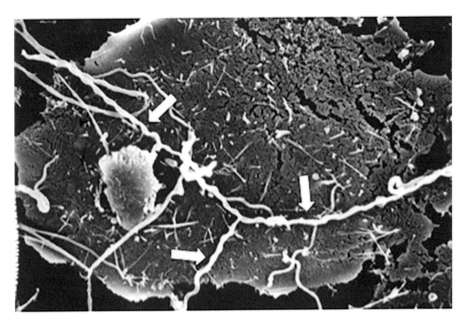

Figure 2. The Lyme disease spirochete attaches to cultured mammalian cells. *B. burgdorferi* strain G39/40 was added to cultured monolayers of Hep-2 human epithelial cells and subjected to scanning electron microscopy. Arrows indicate *B. burgdorferi* spirochetes bound to the surface of the cell. Photo provided by Judith Reichler.

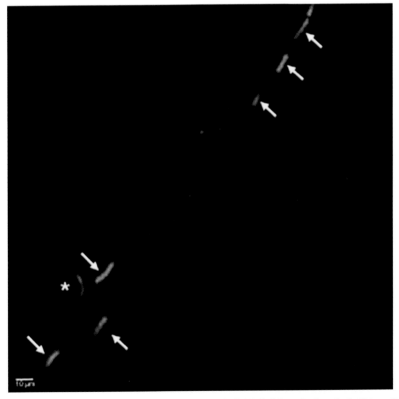

Figure 3. Vascular interactions by the Lyme disease spirochete. GFP-labeled *Borrelia burgdorferi* interacting with a post capillary venule of a mouse knee joint, visualized by intravital microscopy (IVM). Endothelial cells were labeled by Alexa 555-conjugated antibody against PECAM-1 (Red). The scale bar is 10 μm. Spirochetes attaching to endothelium and invading tissues are indicated by arrows and an asterisk, respectively. Photo courtesy of Devender Kumar.

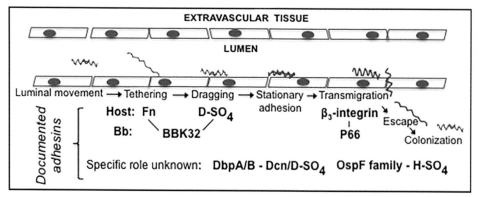

Figure 4. *B. burgdorferi* adhesins, several of which bind GAGs, promote tissue colonization. Invasion across the vessel wall can be described as occurring in multiple steps: (a) tethering, i.e., interactions where the spirochete traverses 100 μm along the vessel in less than one second; (b) dragging, i.e., spirochetes traverse 100 μm in 1–20 seconds; (c) stationary adhesion, i.e., spirochetes remain at a single site for 20 seconds or longer; and (d) transmigration, i.e., spirochetes migrate through the vessel wall. The Fn-binding and dermatan sulfate-binding (D-SO4) activities of BBK32 have been implicated in tethering and dragging, respectively. The integrin-binding activity of another adhesin, P66, has been implicated in transmigration. The specific roles of other documented adhesins, such as DbpA and DbpB, which bind decorin (Dcn) and D-SO$_4$, or OspF family members, which bind heparan sulfate (H-SO4), are unknown. (For clarity, many documented or candidate adhesins have been omitted.)

Glycosaminoglycans are Common Targets of *Borrelia* Adhesins

Although targets of Lyme disease adhesins include integrins, glycolipids and ECM proteins such as collagen or fibronectin (Fn) (Coburn et al. 2013, Brissette and Gaultney 2014), glycosaminoglycans (GAGs) are particularly common receptors for *B. burgdorferi* adhesins (Isaacs 1994, Leong et al. 1995, Parveen and Leong 2000, Parveen et al. 2003, Fischer et al. 2006, Lin et al. 2015a,b). GAGs are long, linear repeating disaccharides that can be divided into different classes depending upon the sugar composition, the glycosidic linkage between each monosaccharide, and the degrees and types of sulfation (Aquino et al. 2010). GAGs are widely and differentially expressed on the surface and in the ECM of many mammalian cell types (Kjellen and Lindhal 1991) and include heparin, heparan sulfate, chondroitin-4-sulfate, chondroitin-6-sulfate, dermatan sulfate, and keratan sulfate. Binding of *B. burgdorferi* to many different cell types, including those of endothelial and neural origin, was shown to be mediated by GAGs, but the specific class of GAGs that was most important for promoting bacterial binding differed among cell types (Isaacs 1994, Leong et al. 1995, 1998). *B. burgdorferi* strains collectively recognize a wide variety of GAGs, including dermatan sulfate, heparin and heparan sulfate (Isaacs 1994, Leong et al. 1995). Importantly, however, specific Lyme disease spirochete strains recognized different subsets of GAGs (Leong et al. 1995, 1998, Parveen et al. 1999).

GAG-binding Activity Promotes *B. burgdorferi* Colonization and May Contribute to Observed Species- and Strain-specific Differences in Tissue Tropism

Infectious strains of Lyme disease spirochetes were consistently found to display GAG-binding activity, whereas some (highly passaged in the laboratory) noninfectious strains, which may lack one or more endogenous plasmids, appeared to lose binding activity (Leong et al. 1995). This observation raised the possibility that GAG binding was an essential property of infectious strains, perhaps serving to establish an infectious niche by promoting bacterial localization in tissues. A first step in testing this hypothesis was the identification of GAG-binding adhesins. In fact, *B. burgdorferi* produces several outer surface proteins that recognize GAGs (Parveen and Leong 2000, Parveen et al. 2003, Fischer et al. 2006, Lin et al. 2015a,b). Here we will focus on two GAG-binding adhesins in particular, BBK32 and DbpA.

The Dermatan Sulfate-binding Activity of the *B. burgdorferi* Adhesin BBK32 Promotes Joint Colonization

BBK32 is a surface lipoprotein of *B. burgdorferi* that was first identified on the basis of its ability to bind to the ECM protein fibronectin (Probert and Johnson 1998), and subsequently shown to harbor a separate GAG-binding activity that promoted mammalian cell attachment (Fischer et al. 2006). A *B. burgdorferi* mutant defective for BBK32 displayed a defect in skin and joint colonization during the first seven days of infection (Seshu et al. 2006, Hyde et al. 2011), indicating that this surface adhesin was indeed a colonization factor. BBK32 produced in a high passage, noninfectious and otherwise poorly adherent strains not only conferred the ability to bind purified GAGs and cultured mammalian cells, but also promoted bacterial localization to the joint after intravenous (i.v.) inoculation (Lin et al. 2015b). Intravital microscopy analysis of a high passage strain producing BBK32 showed that this adhesin promotes transient adhesion (i.e., tethering and dragging) to the vasculature of living mice (Norman et al. 2008). Further, compared to wild type infectious *B. burgdorferi*, a *bbk32*-deficient mutant showed significantly reduced transient adhesion at the joint vasculature after intravenous inoculation of mice, indicating that BBK32 contributes to transient vascular interaction (Moriarty et al. 2008, Lin et al. 2015b).

These data indicated that BBK32 was an adhesive colonization factor, but left unanswered the question of whether GAG- or Fn-binding, or both, were critical for colonization. The fibronectin-binding region of BBK32 included residues 158 to 182 (Probert et al. 2001), and a BBK32 mutant (BBK32Δ158–182) lacking these residues was incapable of promoting binding of *B. burgdorferi* to fibronectin (Lin et al. 2015b). The dermatan sulfate GAG-binding region of BBK32 was mapped to a separate region, residues 45 to 68, and a BBK32 mutant (BBK32Δ45–68) lacking this region was defective in binding to dermatan sulfate, as well as to some mammalian cell types (Lin et al. 2015b). Interestingly, both BBK32Δ158–182 and BBK32Δ45–68 displayed defects in binding cultured mammalian cells, but differed in which cell lines they were incapable of binding (Lin et al. 2015b).

The observations above raised the possibility that the GAG- and Fn-binding activities of BBK32 might promote distinct aspects of colonization during mammalian infection. In fact, after i.v. inoculation, a *B. burgdorferi* mutant that produced the Fn-binding-defective BBK32Δ158–182 colonized all tissues assayed, whereas a mutant producing the GAG-binding-defective BBK32Δ45–68 was diminished for localization to joints (Lin et al. 2015b). Compared to wild type BBK32 or the Fn-binding-defective BBK32Δ158–182, the GAG-binding-defective BBK32Δ45–68 exhibited diminished dragging interaction in the microvasculature (Moriarty et al. 2012). Thus, the dermatan sulfate-binding activity of the BBK32 adhesin mediates a specific bacterial interaction with the vasculature, thus promoting spirochetal localization and ultimately colonization of the joint.

The Decorin- and Dermatan Sulfate-binding Activity of the *B. burgdorferi* Adhesin DbpA Promotes Tissue Colonization in an Allele-specific Manner

Lyme disease spirochetes produce the decorin- and dermatan-sulfate binding surface lipoprotein DbpA (Guo et al. 1998, Parveen et al. 2003), that mediates bacterial attachment to several cultured mammalian cells (Fischer et al. 2006, Benoit et al. 2011, Salo et al. 2011). Lyme disease spirochetes also produce the co-regulated DbpB, a paralog that binds decorin and dermatan sulfate and has partially overlapping function during mammalian infection (Blevins et al. 2008, Shi et al. 2008, Weening et al. 2008, Imai et al. 2013). While DbpB is highly conserved, DbpA is highly allelically variable, with sequence similarities as low as 58% between variants encoded by different strains and species (Roberts et al. 1998). The affinity of this adhesin for decorin and dermatan sulfate (Lin et al. 2014), as well as its ability to promote attachment to mammalian cells (Benoit et al. 2011), varies with the allele. The ability to bind to decorin and dermatan sulfate is critical for the colonization function of DbpA, as mutants that specifically abrogate this binding activity are incapable of promoting tissue colonization (Fortune et al. 2014, Lin et al. 2014). Given that *B. burgdorferi* strains differ in their ability to cause disseminated infections and that human infections by *B. burgdorferi*, *B. garinii* and *B. afzelii* are associated with distinct chronic manifestations, an obvious hypothesis is that the sequence variation of adhesins such as DbpA may contribute to strain-specific differences in tissue tropism.

To test whether allelic variation of DbpA might influence tissue tropism, groups of mice were infected with a set of isogenic *B. burgdorferi* strains that differ only in the DbpA allele produced. In fact, variation in DbpA sequence was associated with differences in the efficiency of colonization of the inoculation site, heart, and joint, with concomitant differences in disease severity (Lin et al. 2014). Interestingly, the DbpA derived from strain N40, a *B. burgdorferi* sensu stricto isolate, promoted more robust colonization of the joint than DbpA variants derived from *B. garinii* or *B. afzelii* strains, a finding that correlates with the noted rheumatological manifestations of human *B. burgdorferi* infection (van Dam et al. 1993, Anthonissen et al. 1994, Wang et al. 2002). These findings suggest that strain-specific variations of *Borrelia* surface adhesins may influence tissue tropism.

A *Borrelia* Paralogous Family of Heparan Sulfate-binding Adhesins May Contribute to Tissue Colonization

To identify candidate *B. burgdorferi* adhesins, a surface display phage library of *B. burgdorferi* proteins was injected en masse i.v. into mice, and phage specifically enriched in different tissues were identified. Several members of the OspF family were isolated from joints, heart and bladder, suggesting a potential adhesive function (Antonara et al. 2007). The OspF-related proteins comprise a distinct subclass of the so-called "Erp" proteins (Akins et al. 1999, Caimano et al. 2000). *B. burgdorferi* sensu lato carries 6 to 10 homologous copies of a 32-kb circular plasmid (cp32) encoding Erp surface lipoproteins (Akins et al. 1995, Marconi et al. 1996, Stevenson et al. 1996, Akins et al. 1999, Brissette et al. 2008). The repertoire of Erp proteins varies from strain to strain (Brissette et al. 2008). Each of these OspF-related proteins tested was subsequently shown to bind to heparan sulfate. One family member, ErpG, was shown to promote spirochetal binding to heparan sulfate and was further tested for the ability to mediate bacterial binding to cultured cells (Lin et al. 2015a). Interestingly, ErpG promoted binding to glial cells, but not to SW982 synovial, SVEC endothelial, A549 epithelial, or CHO-K1 cells, suggesting that this adhesin might, like BBK32 and DbpA, promote tissue-specific colonization. *B. burgdorferi* strains containing transposon insertions into genes encoding two OspF-related proteins (i.e., ErpK or OspF) showed significantly reduced colonization of murine joints, heart, and skin, providing evidence that these proteins may contribute to tissue colonization (Lin et al. 2012). Further analysis of the infection phenotypes of OspF family protein mutants is required to clarify their roles in tissue colonization, but given the strain-specific differences in the OspF family protein repertoire, it is tempting to speculate that the expression profile of paralogous adhesins might be another contributing factor in the tissue tropism variation observed among Lyme disease spirochete strains.

Concluding Remarks and Future Studies

Colonization by bacterial pathogens is a complex multistep process involving a multitude of distinct interactions between microbe and host components. The Lyme disease spirochete, by virtue of its enzootic cycle, is highly adapted for systemic infection of its mammalian or avian host, a property reflected in the multisystemic nature of human Lyme disease. Tissue colonization by Lyme disease *Borrelia* is promoted by the production of surface adhesins, typically lipoproteins, that promote bacterial localization in, and subsequent colonization of, diverse tissues. GAGs, which are ubiquitously produced in all tissues, are common targets of Lyme disease *Borrelia* adhesins, and GAG binding has been rigorously demonstrated, in the case of BBK32 and DbpA, to promote colonization by these spirochetes.

Given the noted apparent variation in tissue tropism among Lyme disease spirochetes, an important finding is that different strains display different GAG-binding profiles. Differences in the spectrum of GAGs targeted by different *Borrelia* strains may be a manifestation of allelic variation of key GAG-binding adhesins, such a DbpA, as well as differences in the expression profiles of a multitude of GAG-binding adhesins, such as the OspF family of surface lipoproteins. An attractive hypothesis, illustrated in Fig. 5,

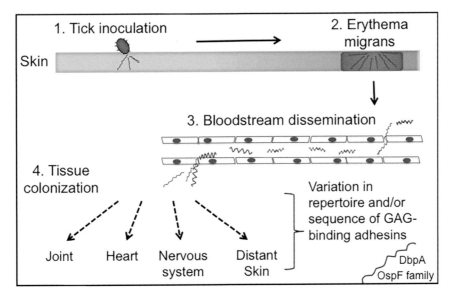

Figure 5. Potential role of adhesins in tissue tropism. *B. burgdorferi* establishes a skin infection, erythema migrans, after tick inoculation, and then disseminates via the blood. The specific set of tissues subsequently colonized may be influenced by the adhesive properties of the infecting spirochete.

is that the GAG-binding profile of a specific Lyme disease strain is an important determinant of tissue tropism, and, potentially, subsequent disease in humans.

Initial evidence for this hypothesis has been developed for one adhesin, DbpA, but further investigation is clearly required to test this model and to gain a detailed understanding of the events leading to stable colonization. For example, although subclasses of GAGs are found relatively enriched in distinct subsets of mammalian tissues, generally GAGs are ubiquitously expressed in a variety of tissues (Couchman and Ljubimov 1989, Scott et al. 1997, Iozzo 1998). Hence, how does dermatan sulfate binding (e.g., by BBK32) promote colonization of a specific tissue (e.g., joint)? In addition, several GAG-binding adhesins have been identified, but whether other GAG-binding adhesins are yet to be characterized is not yet known. In addition to OspF-related proteins, *in vivo* phage display selection identified other *Borrelia* surface proteins that may promote spirochetal binding to mammalian tissues (Antonara et al. 2007). One of these, OspC, is produced and required specifically during the establishment of mammalian infection (Grimm et al. 2004, Tilly et al. 2006). Another, Lmp1, plays a role in the establishment of persistent infection (Yang et al. 2009). Finally, other pathogenic spirochetes that efficiently cause systemic disease with high frequency are also known to produce GAG-binding surface proteins [*Leptospira*: see (Breiner et al. 2009, Andrade and Brown 2012, Ching et al. 2012, Robbins et al. 2015), *Treponema pallidum*: see (Fitzgerald et al. 1985, Fitzgerald and Repesh 1987), *Treponema denticola*: see (Haapasalo et al. 1996)], but their roles in tissue colonization and tropism are relatively unexplored. Our hope is that a detailed analysis of the role of GAG recognition by the Lyme disease spirochete, a pathogen highly adapted to colonize diverse tissues, will reveal general principles in tissue colonization that can be extrapolated to other pathogenic microbes.

Acknowledgements

Supported by R01AI093104 (to J.C. and J.M.L.). We thank Lucas Wolf and Linden Hu for the photograph of erythema migrans, and Devender Kumar and George Chaconas for the photograph of spirochetes in the vasculature. The authors declare no competing financial interests.

Keywords: glycosaminoglycans, Lyme disease, infection, tissue tropism, adhesin, *Borrelia burgdorferi*, colonization

References

Adrion, E. R., J. Aucott, K. W. Lemke and J. P. Weiner. 2015. Health care costs, utilization and patterns of care following Lyme disease. PLoS One 10: e0116767.

Aguero-Rosenfeld, M. E., G. Wang, I. Schwartz and G. P. Wormser. 2005. Diagnosis of lyme borreliosis. Clin Microbiol Rev 18: 484–509.

Akins, D. R., S. F. Porcella, T. G. Popova, D. Shevchenko, S. I. Baker, M. Li et al. 1995. Evidence for *in vivo* but not *in vitro* expression of a *Borrelia burgdorferi* outer surface protein F (OspF) homologue. Mol Microbiol 18: 507–520.

Akins, D. R., M. J. Caimano, X. Yang, F. Cerna, M. V. Norgard and J. D. Radolf. 1999. Molecular and evolutionary analysis of *Borrelia burgdorferi* 297 circular plasmid-encoded lipoproteins with OspE- and OspF-like leader peptides. Infect Immun 67: 1526–1532.

Andrade, G. I. and P. D. Brown. 2012. A comparative analysis of the attachment of *Leptospira interrogans* and *L. borgpetersenii* to mammalian cells. FEMS Immunol Med Microbiol 65: 105–115.

Anthonissen, F. M., M. De Kesel, P. P. Hoet and G. H. Bigaignon. 1994. Evidence for the involvement of different genospecies of *Borrelia* in the clinical outcome of Lyme disease in Belgium. Res Microbiol 145: 327–331.

Antonara, S., R. M. Chafel, M. LaFrance and J. Coburn. 2007. *Borrelia burgdorferi* adhesins identified using *in vivo* phage display. Mol Microbiol 66: 262–276.

Aquino, R. S., E. S. Lee and P. W. Park. 2010. Diverse functions of glycosaminoglycans in infectious diseases. Prog Mol Biol Transl Sci 93: 373–394.

Auwaerter, P. G., J. Aucott and J. S. Dumler. 2004. Lyme borreliosis (Lyme disease): Molecular and cellular pathobiology and prospects for prevention, diagnosis and treatment. Expert Rev Mol Med 6: 1–22.

Behera, A. K., E. Durand, C. Cugini, S. Antonara, L. Bourassa, E. Hildebrand et al. 2008. *Borrelia burgdorferi* BBB07 interaction with integrin alpha3beta1 stimulates production of pro-inflammatory mediators in primary human chondrocytes. Cell Microbiol 10: 320–331.

Benoit, V. M., J. R. Fischer, Y. P. Lin, N. Parveen and J. M. Leong. 2011. Allelic variation of the Lyme disease spirochete adhesin DbpA influences spirochetal binding to decorin, dermatan sulfate, and mammalian cells. Infect Immun 79: 3501–3509.

Blevins, J. S., K. E. Hagman and M. V. Norgard. 2008. Assessment of decorin-binding protein A to the infectivity of *Borrelia burgdorferi* in the murine models of needle and tick infection. BMC Microbiol 8: 82.

Breiner, D. D., M. Fahey, R. Salvador, J. Novakova and J. Coburn. 2009. *Leptospira interrogans* binds to human cell surface receptors including proteoglycans. Infect Immun 77: 5528–5536.

Brissette, C. A., A. E. Cooley, L. H. Burns, S. P. Riley, A. Verma, M. E. Woodman et al. 2008. Lyme borreliosis spirochete Erp proteins, their known host ligands, and potential roles in mammalian infection. Int J Med Microbiol 298 Suppl 1: 257–267.

Brissette, C. A. and R. A. Gaultney. 2014. That's my story, and I'm sticking to it—an update on *B. burgdorferi* adhesins. Front Cell Infect Microbiol 4: 41.

Burgdorfer, W., A. G. Barbour, S. F. Hayes, J. L. Benach, E. Grunwaldt and J. P. Davis. 1982. Lyme disease-a tick-borne spirochetosis? Science 216: 1317–1319.

Caimano, M. J., X. Yang, T. G. Popova, M. L. Clawson, D. R. Akins, M. V. Norgard et al. 2000. Molecular and evolutionary characterization of the cp32/18 family of supercoiled plasmids in *Borrelia burgdorferi* 297. Infect Immun 68: 1574–1586.

Chao, L. L. and C. M. Shih. 2002. Molecular characterization of Lyme disease spirochetes (*Borrelia burgdorferi* sensu lato) isolated in Taiwan by restriction fragment length polymorphism analysis of 5S(rrf)-23S(rrl) intergenic spacer amplicons. Am J Trop Med Hyg 67: 504–510.

Ching, A. T., R. D. Favaro, S. S. Lima, A. Chaves Ade, M. A. de Lima, H. B. Nader et al. 2012. *Leptospira interrogans* shotgun phage display identified LigB as a heparin-binding protein. Biochem Biophys Res Commun 427: 774–779.

Chung, Y. C., H. Y. Tsai, C. M. Shih, L. L. Chao and R. Y. Lin. 2002. Lyme disease in childhood: Report of one case. Acta Paediatr Taiwan 43: 162–165.

Coburn, J., J. Leong and G. Chaconas. 2013. Illuminating the roles of the *Borrelia burgdorferi* adhesins. Trends Microbiol 21: 372–379.

Couchman, J. R. and A. V. Ljubimov. 1989. Mammalian tissue distribution of a large heparan sulfate proteoglycan detected by monoclonal antibodies. Matrix 9: 311–321.

Dolan, M. C., J. Piesman, B. S. Schneider, M. Schriefer, K. Brandt and N. S. Zeidner. 2004. Comparison of disseminated and nondisseminated strains of *Borrelia burgdorferi* sensu stricto in mice naturally infected by tick bite. Infect Immun 72: 5262–5266.

Finlay, B. B. and S. Falkow. 1997. Common themes in microbial pathogenicity revisited. Microbiol Mol Biol Rev 61: 136–169.

Fischer, J. R., K. T. LeBlanc and J. M. Leong. 2006. Fibronectin binding protein BBK32 of the Lyme disease spirochete promotes bacterial attachment to glycosaminoglycans. Infect Immun 74: 435–441.

Fitzgerald, T. J., J. N. Miller, L. A. Repesh, M. Rice and A. Urquhart. 1985. Binding of glycosaminoglycans to the surface of *Treponema pallidum* and subsequent effects on complement interactions between antigen and antibody. Genitourin Med 61: 13–20.

Fitzgerald, T. J. and L. A. Repesh. 1987. The hyaluronidase associated with *Treponema pallidum* facilitates treponemal dissemination. Infect Immun 55: 1023–1028.

Fortune, D. E., Y. P. Lin, R. K. Deka, A. M. Groshong, B. P. Moore, K. E. Hagman et al. 2014. Identification of lysine residues in the *Borrelia burgdorferi* DbpA adhesin required for murine infection. Infect Immun 82: 3186–3198.

Grimm, D., C. H. Eggers, M. J. Caimano, K. Tilly, P. E. Stewart, A. F. Elias et al. 2004. Experimental assessment of the roles of linear plasmids lp25 and lp28-1 of *Borrelia burgdorferi* throughout the infectious cycle. Infect Immun 72: 5938–5946.

Guo, B. P., E. L. Brown, D. W. Dorward, L. C. Rosenberg and M. Hook. 1998. Decorin-binding adhesins from *Borrelia burgdorferi*. Mol Microbiol 30: 711–723.

Haapasalo, M., P. Hannam, B. C. McBride and V. J. Uitto. 1996. Hyaluronan, a possible ligand mediating *Treponema denticola* binding to periodontal tissue. Oral Microbiol Immunol 11: 156–160.

Hyde, J. A., E. H. Weening, M. Chang, J. P. Trzeciakowski, M. Hook, J. D. Cirillo et al. 2011. Bioluminescent imaging of *Borrelia burgdorferi in vivo* demonstrates that the fibronectin-binding protein BBK32 is required for optimal infectivity. Mol Microbiol 82: 99–113.

Imai, D. M., D. S. Samuels, S. Feng, E. Hodzic, K. Olsen and S. W. Barthold. 2013. The early dissemination defect attributed to disruption of decorin-binding proteins is abolished in chronic murine Lyme borreliosis. Infect Immun 81: 1663–1673.

Iozzo, R. V. 1998. Matrix proteoglycans: from molecular design to cellular function. Annu Rev Biochem 67: 609–652.

Isaacs, R. D. 1994. *Borrelia burgdorferi* bind to epithelial cell proteoglycans. J Clin Invest 93: 809–819.

Kjellen, L. and U. Lindahl. 1991. Proteoglycans: Structures and interactions. Annu Rev Biochem 60: 443–475.

Kornblatt, A. N., A. C. Steere and D. G. Brownstein. 1984. Experimental Lyme disease in rabbits: Spirochetes found in erythema migrans and blood. Infect Immun 46: 220–223.

Lane, R. S., J. Piesman and W. Burgdorfer. 1991. Lyme borreliosis: relation of its causative agent to its vectors and hosts in North America and Europe. Annu Rev Entomol 36: 587–609.

Leong, J. M., P. E. Morrissey, E. Ortega-Barria, M. E. Pereira and J. Coburn. 1995. Hemagglutination and proteoglycan binding by the Lyme disease spirochete, *Borrelia burgdorferi*. Infect Immun 63: 874–883.

Leong, J. M., H. Wang, L. Magoun, J. A. Field, P. E. Morrissey, D. Robbins et al. 1998. Different classes of proteoglycans contribute to the attachment of *Borrelia burgdorferi* to cultured endothelial and brain cells. Infect Immun 66: 994–999.

Lin, T., L. Gao, C. Zhang, E. Odeh, M. B. Jacobs, L. Coutte et al. 2012. Analysis of an ordered, comprehensive STM mutant library in infectious *Borrelia burgdorferi*: insights into the genes required for mouse infectivity. PLoS One 7: e47532.

Lin, Y. P., V. Benoit, X. Yang, R. Martinez-Herranz, U. Pal and J. M. Leong. 2014. Strain-specific variation of the decorin-binding adhesin DbpA influences the tissue tropism of the lyme disease spirochete. PLoS Pathog 10: e1004238.

Lin, Y. P., R. Bhowmick, J. Coburn and J. M. Leong. 2015a. Host cell heparan sulfate glycosaminoglycans are ligands for OspF-related proteins of the Lyme disease spirochete. Cell Microbiol (in press).

Lin, Y. P., Q. Chen, J. A. Ritchie, N. P. Dufour, J. R. Fischer, J. Coburn et al. 2015b. Glycosaminoglycan binding by *Borrelia burgdorferi* adhesin BBK32 specifically and uniquely promotes joint colonization. Cell Microbiol 17: 860–875.

Liveris, D., G. P. Wormser, J. Nowakowski, R. Nadelman, S. Bittker, D. Cooper et al. 1996. Molecular typing of *Borrelia burgdorferi* from Lyme disease patients by PCR-restriction fragment length polymorphism analysis. J Clin Microbiol 34: 1306–1309.

Marconi, R. T., S. Y. Sung, C. A. Hughes and J. A. Carlyon. 1996. Molecular and evolutionary analyses of a variable series of genes in *Borrelia burgdorferi* that are related to *ospE* and *ospF*, constitute a gene family, and share a common upstream homology box. J Bacteriol 178: 5615–5626.

Moriarty, T. J., M. U. Norman, P. Colarusso, T. Bankhead, P. Kubes and G. Chaconas. 2008. Real-time high resolution 3D imaging of the lyme disease spirochete adhering to and escaping from the vasculature of a living host. PLoS Pathog 4: e1000090.

Moriarty, T. J., M. Shi, Y. P. Lin, R. Ebady, H. Zhou, T. Odisho et al. 2012. Vascular binding of a pathogen under shear force through mechanistically distinct sequential interactions with host macromolecules. Mol Microbiol 86: 1116–1131.

Norman, M. U., T. J. Moriarty, A. R. Dresser, B. Millen, P. Kubes and G. Chaconas. 2008. Molecular mechanisms involved in vascular interactions of the Lyme disease pathogen in a living host. PLoS Pathog 4: e1000169.

Parveen, N., D. Robbins and J. M. Leong. 1999. Strain variation in glycosaminoglycan recognition influences cell-type-specific binding by lyme disease spirochetes. Infect Immun 67: 1743–1749.

Parveen, N. and J. M. Leong. 2000. Identification of a candidate glycosaminoglycan-binding adhesin of the Lyme disease spirochete *Borrelia burgdorferi*. Mol Microbiol 35: 1220–1234.

Parveen, N., M. Caimano, J. D. Radolf and J. M. Leong. 2003. Adaptation of the Lyme disease spirochaete to the mammalian host environment results in enhanced glycosaminoglycan and host cell binding. Mol Microbiol 47: 1433–1444.

Philipp, M. T. and B. J. Johnson. 1994. Animal models of Lyme disease: Pathogenesis and immunoprophylaxis. Trends Microbiol 2: 431–437.

Piesman, J., T. N. Mather, R. J. Sinsky and A. Spielman. 1987. Duration of tick attachment and *Borrelia burgdorferi* transmission. J Clin Microbiol 25: 557–558.

Probert, W. S. and B. J. Johnson. 1998. Identification of a 47 kDa fibronectin-binding protein expressed by *Borrelia burgdorferi* isolate B31. Mol Microbiol 30: 1003–1015.

Probert, W. S., J. H. Kim, M. Hook and B. J. Johnson. 2001. Mapping the ligand-binding region of *Borrelia burgdorferi* fibronectin-binding protein BBK32. Infect Immun 69: 4129–4133.

Robbins, G. T., B. L. Hahn, K. V. Evangelista, L. Padmore, P. S. Aranda and J. Coburn. 2015. Evaluation of cell binding activities of *Leptospira* ECM adhesins. PLoS Negl Trop Dis 9: e0003712.

Roberts, W. C., B. A. Mullikin, R. Lathigra and M. S. Hanson. 1998. Molecular analysis of sequence heterogeneity among genes encoding decorin binding proteins A and B of *Borrelia burgdorferi* sensu lato. Infect Immun 66: 5275–5285.

Salo, J., V. Loimaranta, P. Lahdenne, M. K. Viljanen and J. Hytonen. 2011. Decorin binding by DbpA and B of *Borrelia garinii*, *Borrelia afzelii*, and *Borrelia burgdorferi* sensu stricto. J Infect Dis 204: 65–73.

Scott, P. G., T. Nakano and C. M. Dodd. 1997. Isolation and characterization of small proteoglycans from different zones of the porcine knee meniscus. Biochim Biophys Acta 1336: 254–262.

Seinost, G., D. E. Dykhuizen, R. J. Dattwyler, W. T. Golde, J. J. Dunn, I. N. Wang et al. 1999. Four clones of *Borrelia burgdorferi* sensu stricto cause invasive infection in humans. Infect Immun 67: 3518–3524.

Seshu, J., M. D. Esteve-Gassent, M. Labandeira-Rey, J. H. Kim, J. P. Trzeciakowski, M. Hook et al. 2006. Inactivation of the fibronectin-binding adhesin gene bbk32 significantly attenuates the infectivity potential of *Borrelia burgdorferi*. Mol Microbiol 59: 1591–1601.

Shapiro, L., P. Whelan and C. Magro. 2014. Case 18-2014: A man with a rash, myalgia, and weakness. N Engl J Med 371: 1361.

Shi, Y., Q. Xu, K. McShan and F. T. Liang. 2008. Both decorin-binding proteins A and B are critical for the overall virulence of *Borrelia burgdorferi*. Infect Immun 76: 1239–1246.

Shih, C. M., L. L. Chao and C. P. Yu. 2002. Chemotactic migration of the Lyme disease spirochete (*Borrelia burgdorferi*) to salivary gland extracts of vector ticks. Am J Trop Med Hyg 66: 616–621.

Steere, A. C. 2001. Lyme disease. N Engl J Med 345: 115–125.

Stevenson, B., K. Tilly and P. A. Rosa. 1996. A family of genes located on four separate 32-kilobase circular plasmids in *Borrelia burgdorferi* B31. J Bacteriol 178: 3508–3516.

Tilly, K., J. G. Krum, A. Bestor, M. W. Jewett, D. Grimm, D. Bueschel et al. 2006. *Borrelia burgdorferi* OspC protein required exclusively in a crucial early stage of mammalian infection. Infect Immun 74: 3554–3564.

Tilly, K., P. A. Rosa and P. E. Stewart. 2008. Biology of infection with *Borrelia burgdorferi*. Infect Dis Clin North Am 22: 217–234.

van Dam, A. P., H. Kuiper, K. Vos, A. Widjojokusumo, B. M. de Jongh, L. Spanjaard et al. 1993. Different genospecies of *Borrelia burgdorferi* are associated with distinct clinical manifestations of Lyme borreliosis. Clin Infect Dis 17: 708–717.

Wang, G., A. P. van Dam, I. Schwartz and J. Dankert. 1999. Molecular typing of *Borrelia burgdorferi* sensu lato: Taxonomic, epidemiological, and clinical implications. Clin Microbiol Rev 12: 633–653.

Wang, G., C. Ojaimi, R. Iyer, V. Saksenberg, S. A. McClain, G. P. Wormser et al. 2001. Impact of genotypic variation of *Borrelia burgdorferi* sensu stricto on kinetics of dissemination and severity of disease in C3H/HeJ mice. Infect Immun 69: 4303–4312.

Wang, G., C. Ojaimi, H. Wu, V. Saksenberg, R. Iyer, D. Liveris et al. 2002. Disease severity in a murine model of lyme borreliosis is associated with the genotype of the infecting *Borrelia burgdorferi* sensu stricto strain. J Infect Dis 186: 782–791.

Weening, E. H., N. Parveen, J. P. Trzeciakowski, J. M. Leong, M. Hook and J. T. Skare. 2008. *Borrelia burgdorferi* lacking DbpBA exhibits an early survival defect during experimental infection. Infect Immun 76: 5694–5705.

Yang, X., A. S. Coleman, J. Anguita and U. Pal. 2009. A chromosomally encoded virulence factor protects the Lyme disease pathogen against host-adaptive immunity. PLoS Pathog 5: e1000326.

CHAPTER 5

The Role of Viral Envelope Protein Glycosylation in Pathogenesis of Influenza A Virus

Kevan L. Hartshorn

Introduction

Influenza A virus (IAV) presents an ongoing major threat to human health and there is much yet to be learned about the role of innate immunity during IAV infection (Tripathi et al. 2015). Although IAV elicits strong adaptive immune responses, it is prone to rapid genomic variation either through small incremental mutations or major changes resulting from exchange of genome segments with those of animal strains (reassortment). These genomic changes allow IAV to escape immune responses generated against prior strains. Generally the small incremental changes lead to seasonal epidemics, whereas reassortment leads to pandemics. The presence of animal reservoirs allows introduction of avian or pig strains (or genes from these strains) into humans resulting in pandemics, as in 2009 (Dawood et al. 2009). Seasonal epidemics of influenza virus still contribute tremendous morbidity and mortality including annual mortality in the USA of ~40,000 (Morens 2003). Certain groups of individuals are more susceptible to severe outcomes of seasonal IAV: those at extremes of age, smokers, individuals with chronic obstructive pulmonary disease (COPD), cystic fibrosis or asthma, diabetes mellitus, cardiovascular disease, or immune compromise. Some otherwise healthy young people die during seasonal epidemics, sometimes due to bacterial super-infection (e.g., note recent association of IAV with MRSA pneumonia) (Hartshorn 2010). Pandemics cause more indiscriminate mortality in young healthy adults than seasonal IAV (Hartshorn 2013). There is a period of 5–7 days prior to arrival of CD8+ T cells in the lung after exposure to a new IAV strain and innate defense is critical at this time. The innate immune response to IAV is highly complex and this chapter will focus on the initial phase of the response in respiratory tract.

The Role of Soluble Inhibitors in Airway Lining Fluid in the Initial Defense Against IAV

Our research has focused on soluble inhibitors in the respiratory lining fluids which provide the first barrier to infection. This initial inhibition reduces infection of the respiratory epithelium with minimal inflammation and reduced potential for viral spread to the lung. Key soluble inhibitors include surfactant protein D

Boston University School of Medicine, 650 Albany Street, Boston, MA 02465.
  E-mail: khartsho@bu.edu

(SP-D), surfactant protein A (SP-A), H-ficolin and LL-37 and other anti-microbial peptides. SP-A and SP-D are members of the "collectin" family of host defense lectins which includes also mannose binding lectin (MBL) and several other collectins found in bovines or other species. The collectins generally have a multimeric structure composed of collagenous arms which have trimeric globular neck and carbohydrate recognition domains (NCRDs) at the C-terminus. A cysteine rich N-terminal domain enables the formation of multimeric assemblies of trimers. In the case of SP-D, from 4 to up to 32 trimers can be assembled in a single molecule (see Fig. 1 for electron micrograph of a typical 4 armed or dodecameric molecule of SP-D).

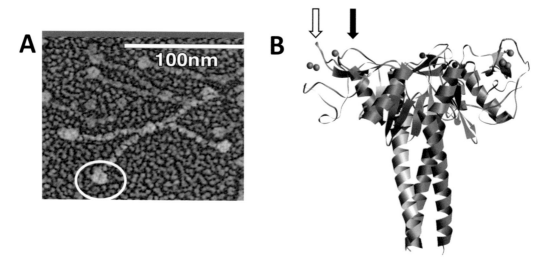

Figure 1. **Electron micrograph of dodecameric, intact SP-D molecule (A) and ribbon diagram of the trimeric neck and carbohydrate recognition domains (NCRD) of SP-D (B).** The white circle in panel A is included to highlight the globular NCRD component of the molecule. In panel B the white and black arrows indicate ridges surrounding the lectin binding site of the NCRD. The ridge indicated by the white arrow is formed by the D325 residue and that shown by the dark arrow is formed by R343.

SP-A and MBL have shorter collagen domains and instead of forming a cross-like structure they appear as a bunch of tulips with up to six arms. Our earlier *in vitro* and mouse studies demonstrated that SP-D and SP-A play key roles in the initial defense response to infection with seasonal IAV strains (Hartshorn et al. 1994, LeVine et al. 2001). These findings have been confirmed by several other groups (Reading et al. 1997, Li et al. 2002, Hawgood et al. 2004, Vigerust et al. 2007). We also showed that SP-D contributes most of the innate inhibitory activity of human bronchoalveolar lavage fluid (BALF) to these strains (Hartshorn et al. 1994, White et al. 2007) and that binding to the Influenza virus A hemagglutinin (HA) and HA-associated glycans is key for neutralization by SP-D (Hartshorn et al. 2000a). We recently showed that H-ficolin (Hakata Antigen) is present in BALF of healthy volunteer donors and that removal of H-ficolin from human BALF or serum reduces antiviral activity for IAV (Verma et al. 2012). Of interest, although SP-A and H-ficolin function as lectins they appear to cause IAV neutralization by a different mechanism which involves presenting decoy sialylated ligands to the viral HA (Hartshorn et al. 1997, Verma et al. 2012).

Understanding potential defects in the initial soluble barrier to infection can explain why some subjects or some viral strains are associated with more severe infection. We recently showed that unlike seasonal IAV, pandemic IAV strains from 1918 (H1N1), 1957 (H2N2), 1968 (H3N2) and 2009 (H1N1) and avian H5N1 are not inhibited by SP-D (Qi et al. 2011). A common feature of pandemic human IAV as well as avian and some porcine strains (and most mouse adapted strains) is relative lack of glycosylation on the globular head domain of the HA (Vigerust et al. 2007, Hartshorn et al. 2008, Job et al. 2010, Tate et al. 2011). As H1 and H3 HAs evolved over time in humans they acquired more glycosylation (likely in part to shield key parts of the HA from antibody recognition) and became more sensitive to inhibition by SP-D or MBL which acts through the same mechanism as SP-D (Hartshorn et al. 1993). In contrast, H-ficolin does inhibit H1N1pdm (Verma et al. 2012). Overall our recent findings suggest that one of the reasons for the high level of infectivity and pathogenicity associated with pandemic IAV is an ability to bypass key components of the initial soluble barrier to infection. It is also likely that deficiencies in SP-D levels or activity could account for the susceptibility of specific vulnerable populations to seasonal IAV. For instance, diabetic mice are more susceptible to IAV in part due to inhibition of SP-D by glucose (Reading et al. 1998). Smokers and individuals with COPD or cystic fibrosis have reduced levels of SP-D and SP-A (Honda et al. 1996, Lomas et al. 2009, Sims et al. 2008). In many inflammatory states multimerization and function of SP-D are altered. Furthermore there are polymorphic forms of SP-D and SP-A, some of which have reduced activity against IAV *in vitro* and are associated with respiratory infections (Leth-Larsen et al. 2005, Mikerov et al. 2008, Thomas et al. 2009).

If an IAV strain can bypass or overwhelm the soluble barriers to infection additional layers of defense are deployed. The key initial cellular defenders include respiratory epithelial cells, neutrophils and alveolar macrophages. There are extensive data showing that each of these cell types respond to IAV and contribute importantly to clearance as we recently reviewed (Tripathi et al. 2015). Infected respiratory epithelial cells play a key role in the innate response both by generating interferons and other innate inhibitors, and by sending out danger signals to recruit inflammatory cells. Resident alveolar macrophages and dendritic cells play critical roles in mounting the immune response as well. Neutrophils, activated monocytes, natural killer cells and innate and adaptive lymphocytes are recruited by signals released by the resident cells. The ideal outcome at this point is to restrict inflammation to the upper airway until adaptive immune cells can arrive. The soluble inhibitors still play key roles at this level by modulating epithelial and phagocytes responses. For example, SP-D, SP-A, H-ficolin and various antimicrobial peptides increase phagocyte uptake of IAV (Tecle et al. 2007, White et al. 2014). We recently showed that IAV stimulates neutrophil extracellular trap (NET) formation and this response is greatly potentiated by LL-37 (Tripathi et al. 2014).

With more extensive infection, in particular infection of the lung, more serious illness ensues with complications of viral pneumonia of bacterial super-infection (Hartshorn 2010). At this level both innate and adaptive responses are critical for recovery, but both can also cause harmful inflammation that can cause morbidity or even mortality (Tripathi et al. 2015). H5N1 and some pandemic strains are associated with more profound inflammatory responses and illness in humans and animal models (Hartshorn 2013). An important finding from *in vitro* and murine studies is that SP-D, SP-A and LL-37 inhibit inflammatory responses to IAV infection (LeVine et al. 2001, Hawgood et al. 2004). For SP-D this effect parallels reduction in viral load but SP-A can inhibit inflammation independent of effects on viral load (Li et al. 2002).

Carbohydrate Based Inhibition of IAV

The findings described above made it a high priority to understand the mechanism of inhibition of IAV by SP-D, since it plays key roles in different aspects of the initial defense barrier against seasonal strains of IAV. It was first established by Dr. E. Margot Anders and her collaborators at the University of Melbourne, Australia, that mammalian serum β-inhibitors of IAV are calcium dependent lectins and that inhibition of H3N2 and H1N1 seasonal strains of IAV depends on the presence of high mannose glycans on the viral HA of these strains (Anders et al. 1990, Hartley et al. 1992, Reading et al. 1997). The antiviral activity of these proteins was eliminated by carrying out incubation in EDTA or addition of mannan. Repeated propagation of viral strains in the presence of bovine serum caused outgrowth of β-inhibitor resistant strains which were found to have lost specific oligosaccharide attachment sites on the head region of their HA. They showed that the inhibitors were conglutinin (in the case of bovine serum) or MBL in other mammalian sera. In collaboration with Dr. Anders and others we confirmed that purified human MBL and bovine conglutinin are strong calcium-dependent inhibitors of seasonal IAV strains, but not of the highly mouse adapted PR-8 H1N1 strain which lacks glycosylation on the head region of its HA (Hartshorn et al. 1993). SP-A and SP-D were discovered to be members of the collectin family present at highest concentration in respiratory lining fluids (Haagsman et al. 1987, Wright et al. 1987, Persson et al. 1990, Rust et al. 1991). SP-A and SP-D were also shown to be present in mucosal secretions including those of the gastrointestinal and genitourinary tracts and other epithelia (Madsen et al. 2000). In collaboration with Dr. Erika Crouch (Washington University, St. Louis), the discoverer of SP-D, we demonstrated that

SP-D has strong influenza viral neutralizing activity and that it can induce viral aggregation and promote viral uptake by neutrophils (Hartshorn et al. 1994). Subsequent studies confirmed that deletion of SP-D in mice results in higher viral loads and markedly increased inflammatory responses upon infection with seasonal strains of IAV (LeVine et al. 2001, Hawgood et al. 2004).

Another group of serum inhibitors which have been called γ-inhibitors have been shown to act in a calcium independent manner which is abrogated by treating the inhibitor with neuraminidase. Classic serum γ-inhibitors include α2-macroglobulin and serum amyloid and pentraxin proteins (Ryan-Poirier and Kawaoka 1993, Job et al. 2013a). These are highly sialylated proteins and their ability to inhibit IAV depends upon having sialic acids in the appropriate linkage for recognition by the viral HA. Avian and mouse adapted HA molecules recognize sialic acids in a α(2-3)-linkage, while human strains recognize preferentially those in an α(2-6) linkage characteristic of sialylation found in the human respiratory tract. SP-A (Iwaarden et al. 1993, Hartshorn et al. 1997) and the related collagenous lectin H-ficolin inhibit IAV in this manner (Verma et al. 2012). β-inhibition appears to provide a stronger method of viral neutralization for seasonal IAV based murine studies and studies of human BAL fluid, in which SP-D is the most important inhibitory factor (Hartshorn et al. 1994). γ-Inhibitors can be undermined by the ability of the viral neuraminidase to remove sialic acids from the inhibitor thus freeing up the virus to escape and succeed in infecting their target respiratory epithelial cells. This is most obvious with airway mucins which cause only transient inhibition or viral aggregation. Inhibition by mucin can be strongly potentiated by addition of a neuraminidase inhibitor (e.g., oseltamivir—an important antiviral drug used to treat IAV) (White et al. 2005, 2009). In contrast, inhibitors have the potential to inhibit strains resistant to of β-inhibitors, since they do not depend on glycosylation of the viral HA and in some cases have increased activity against IAV strains lacking HA glycosylation (Hartshorn et al. 1997).

Analyzing the Molecular Mechanism of Inhibition of Infectivity of IAV by SP-D

Based on these various findings it became very important to try to understand at a molecular level how SP-D (and presumably related β-inhibitors) inhibit IAV infection and by extension why they cannot inhibit pandemic IAV strains. For SP-D, binding affinity for glycans is greatly potentiated by the formation of multimers with 4 or more trimeric arms (as compared to single trimeric arms of the molecule) (Brown-Augsburger et al. 1996, Hartshorn et al. 1996). To generate the fully oligomerized molecule in recombinant form it is necessary to use mammalian expression systems (Hartshorn et al. 1996). Our initial studies with conglutinin and MBL suggested that the NCRDs of these proteins might have greater intrinsic antiviral activity than that of SP-D. The challenge was to find a way to compare the activity of these NCRDs while accounting for effects of their differing N-terminal and collagen domains. To address this problem we produced chimeric molecules having the N-terminal and collagen domains of SP-D and the NCRD of SP-D. These chimeric molecules have significantly increased antiviral activity than either parent molecule (SP-D, conglutinin or MBL) (Hartshorn et al. 2000b, White et al. 2000, Zhang et al. 2002), supporting the concept that the intrinsic activity of the serum collectin NCRDs is greater than that of SP-D. Additional bovine collectins, CL-43 and CL-46, were discovered by Uffe Holmskov and his laboratory (University of Odense, Denmark) (Rothmann et al. 1997, Hansen et al. 2002). In collaboration with Holmskov we found evidence that these collectins had increased antiviral activity compared to SP-D, likely based on differences in glycan binding properties (Hartshorn et al. 2002).

The NCRD of SP-D was shown to be expressed in high concentrations in bacteria with the neck region guiding trimerization of the molecule (Lim et al. 1994, Kishore et al. 1996). This opened up the possibility to directly compare antiviral activities among isolated NCRDs which would eliminate potential confounding effects of the N-terminal and collagen domains. Indeed, the trimeric NCRD of CL-43 and CL-45 were found to have strong antiviral activity (Crouch et al. 2005, Hartshorn et al. 2010a). Unfortunately, the wild type human NCRD was found to have greatly reduced ability to bind IAV, and no measurable neutralizing activity for IAV (Crouch et al. 2005). Of note, the CL-43 and CL-45 trimers were able to cause viral aggregation despite lacking the multimeric structure of a full length collectin (Hartshorn et al. 2010b).

An important step in carrying this research forward was the determination of the crystal structure of the NCRD of SP-D (Hakansson et al. 1999, Shrive et al. 2003). It was known that specific residues (in human SP-D the glutamic acid, proline, and asparagine or EPN sequence at residues 321-3) were involved in chelating calcium in the lectin site and determining the monosaccharide specificity of the molecule. Changing the EPN sequence to glutamine, proline and aspartic acid (QPD) was shown to alter monosaccharide preference from mannose and glucose to galactose, and replacing the glutamic acid with a lysine was shown to eliminate lectin activity altogether (Ogasawara and Voelker 1995, Hartshorn et al. 2000b).

In collaborative studies involving site directed mutagenesis, functional assays (saccharide binding and antiviral activity) and structural analysis involving Drs. Crouch (Washington University School of Medicine), Seaton and Head (Boston University School of Medicine) and our laboratory, we were able to characterize the contributions of specific NCRD residues with antiviral activity and to progressively increase antiviral activities of NCRDs. Key features of the crystal structure of the SP-D CRD include ridges on either side of the monosaccharide binding pocket formed by the D325 and R343 residues (see Fig. 1B). We noted various changes in these residues in serum collectins. Most notably, arginine 343 (R343) is replaced by a hydrophobic residue in the serum collectins (MBL, conglutinin, CL-43 and CL-46). Variations in the aspartic acid 325 (D325) residue were also found in various collectins. For instance, in rat and mouse SP-D there are asparagines instead of aspartic acids at residue 324 and 325 (i.e., D324N and D325N) substitutions as compared to human SP-D. Substituting the N for D in these two positions in human SP-D resulted in a subtle shift in binding site structure, saccharide binding specificity, and viral binding ability (Crouch et al. 2006).

Substituting a hydrophobic residue (alanine, isoleucine, or valine) for R343 caused a shift toward increased binding affinity for GlcNAc (Crouch et al. 2009), resulting from a different orientation of the monosaccharide in the binding pocket. Although ability to bind mannose monosaccharide was not altered, the ability to bind elongated mannose chains or mannan polymer was greatly increased. The structural basis for this was shown to be a different orientation of dimannose or longer chains in the binding pocket. Instead of the terminal mannose residue attaching to the calcium in the binding site, the penultimate mannose bound resulting in a different orientation of the saccharide across the surface of the CRD. Importantly, the R343 substitutions resulted in a marked increase in antiviral activity for IAV (Crouch et al. 2009). The R343V substitution had the greatest effect with significantly more antiviral activity than when alanine was substituted for R343. Of further interest the R343V substituted molecule also caused viral aggregation, an unexpected effect given lack of a multimeric structure (Hartshorn et al. 2010b).

Further steps included substituting D325 of human SP-D with an alanine, and creating a double mutant NCRD with both D325A and R343V mutations (Crouch et al. 2011). This molecule had a further increase in antiviral activity compared to R343V, including greater neutralizing activity for seasonal strains, marked viral aggregating activity, and ability to inhibit pandemic strains including the 2009 H1N1 strains which were fully resistant to full length SP-D multimers (Nikolaidis et al. 2014). Dr. Seaton and her group were able to obtain crystal structures of wild type and mutant SP-D NCRDs alone or co-crystallized with small saccharide chains (refs needed? I can send them to you but you said you were having problems with your refs. So let me know what you want to do.).

We found that the optimal initial model for determining the molecular basis for IAV inhibition by SP-D involved the Aichi68 H3N2 viral strain which is representative of the pandemic strains of 1968. This strain was not inhibited by wild type NCRD but strongly inhibited by the D325A+R343V mutant (Goh et al. 2013). The D325A+R343V mutant also strongly aggregated Aichi68 viral particles while wild type NCRD did not. The Aichi68 strain has the glycan at 165 which has been shown to be important in inhibition of H3N2 strains of IAV by collectins and the structure of its HA was already published (Sauter et al. 1992). Native full length SP-D has some ability to inhibit Aichi68 but greatly reduced compared to inhibition of more recent, seasonal H3N2 strains and reduced compared to the D325A+R343V trimer. The main pre-requisites for determining the molecular basis for IAV neutralization by SP-D included determination of the structure on man9 as present at site 165 on the Aichi68 HA and determination of structures of wild type and mutant versions of the human SP-D NCRD in the presence and absence of man9 and also Mass Spectrometry studies of purified H3N2 HA to characterize glycans actually present on the HA.

Dr. Seaton and Dr. Rynkiewicz (Boston University School of Medicine, Physiology and Biophysics) were able to determine the crystal structures of the NCRDs in presence and absence of man9 (Crouch et al. 2011, Goh et al. 2013). Dr. Joseph Zaia (Boston University School of Medicine, Biochemistry) and his laboratory were able to take bromelain solubilized HA from IAV strains and determine the glycan structures on present, including confirmation that the glycan at 165 on H3N2 strains is, in fact, occupied and predominantly high mannose (Crouch et al. 2011). Determining the three dimensional structure of man9 as it exists at site 165 on the HA was challenging since crystallographic images only reveal the first 2 or 3 monosaccharides of the chain. However, using available crystal structures of HA, SP-D, and man9, it was possible to construct starting models of SP-D bound to HA at site 165. Having these structures it was then possible for Dr. Boon Goh and Klaus Schulten (University of Illinois, Urbana-Champaign, Physics) to determine the most energetically favorable structures of NCRDs with the glycosylated HA using molecular modeling and molecular dynamics (Goh et al. 2013). There were several key findings in this study. First it was determined that both with type NCRD and D325A+R343V can overlie and obstruct the sialic acid binding site of the HA after attachment to man9 at 165 accounting for ability inhibit hemagglutination activity and infectivity (Fig. 2).

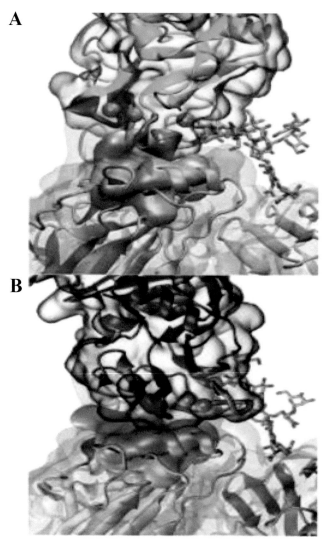

Figure 2. Inhibition of the HA sialic acid binding site. The binding site, located on HA, is shown as a pink surface; the remainder of HA is shown in cartoon and transparent surface representation in cyan; the Man-9 chain linked to HA is shown in licorice representation in red-orange. (A) HA bound to wild type NCRD, the latter shown in cartoon and transparent surface representation in green. (B) HA bound to D325A+R343V, the latter shown in cartoon and transparent surface representation in purple. Two loop regions of both wild type and D325A+R343V, colored in tan and blue, are seen to cover and thereby inhibit the sialic acid binding site (Figure reprinted with permission from Goh et al. 2013).

The D325A+R343V complex with HA was found to be more stable due both to additional hydrogen bonds and added hydrophobic protein-protein interaction HA residues and Ala325 and Pro319 of D325A+R343V, accounting in part for the increased neutralizing activity of this mutant NCRD. As noted, the R343V change results in a different mechanism of binding to dimannose or man9, in which the penultimate mannose, rather the terminal mannose, binds to the lectin site calcium (Crouch et al. 2009, 2011, Goh et al. 2013). This change results in a different orientation of the whole D325A+R343V trimer compared to wild type NCRD. In the orientation favored by D325A+R343V the other heads of the trimer extend outward in such a way that they are positioned to interact with other HA molecules (Fig. 3).

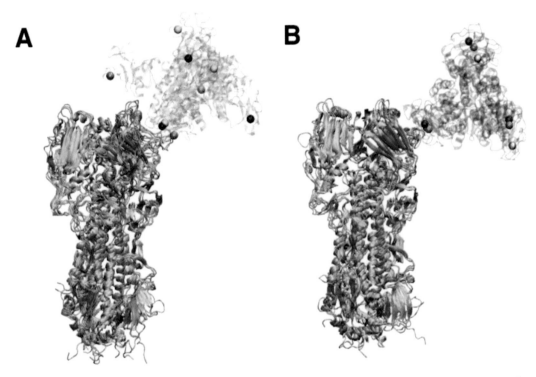

Figure 3. Differences in orientation in HA complexes with WT (A) or D325A+R343V (B)—The figure represents the endpoints of three repeated simulations. Calcium ions are represented in orange, red and white; WT and D325A+R343V are in transparent cartoon representation in green and purple, respectively; HA is shown in cartoon representation in cyan (Figure reprinted with permission from Goh et al. 2013).

By extension this latter finding explains the ability of D325A+R343V and related NCRDs to cause viral aggregation despite lacking the multimeric structure of the full length molecule. These studies provided for the first time an atomic-level molecular view of the interaction of a host defense lectin with a viral glycoprotein target.

Future Directions and Caveats

An important next step in these studies will be determination of the mechanism through which D325A+R343V (or a related mutant D325S+R343V which has similar activity to D325A+R343V) inhibits pandemic H1N1 strains, like those of 1918 and 2009 (Nikolaidis et al. 2014). Key to this study will be determination of the true glycan structures on the HA of these strains by the glycomic studies being pioneered by Dr. Joseph Zaia (Boston University School of Medicine). The crystal structures of both the 1918 and 2009 H1 HA have been published and molecular modeling and molecular dynamics studies will follow.

As noted above the key glycan for collectin attachment on H1N1 strains appears to be that at position 104. This position differs in being lower down on the HA head than 165 of H3N2 strains, so the binding orientation of NCRDs may be quite different as well. The 2009 H1N1 pandemic strains have already evolved such that their seasonal descendants have additional potential N-linked glycan attachment sites. Future studies of these strains, including potential increased sensitivity to SP-D will be important. Such studies can be greatly facilitated by reverse genetics which allows production of recombinant strains of IAV with deliberate addition or subtraction of N-linked glycan attachment sequences (Neumann et al. 2013).

Studies of porcine surfactant protein D led by Martin van Eijk and Henk Haagsman (University of Utrecht, Netherlands) have shown that this version of SP-D has distinctive NCRD properties leading to increased anti-influenza activity (van Eijk et al. 2003, Hillaire et al. 2012). These include presence of an N-linked, sialylated glycan attachment on the NCRD itself (not present on any other version of SP-D) and distinctive features of the lectin site itself. The presence of the N-linked sugar allows porcine SP-D to act as both a B and γ-inhibitor and inhibit IAV strains not inhibited by human SP-D (including porcine, avian and pandemic strains). In collaboration with Drs. Seaton and Rynkiewicz, the crystal structure of the porcine SP-D NCRD was obtained showing a distinctive additional loop adjacent to the lectin site which stabilizes the interaction with man9 (van Eijk et al. 2012). The porcine SP-D NCRD was found to have greater intrinsic neutralizing activity even in the absence of its N-linked glycan, presumably due to these changes adjacent to the lectin site. Hence, further molecular studies of porcine SP-D are another important direction for research.

Another important avenue for future is determination of other potential impacts of HA glycans on viral pathogenesis including shield regions of the HA from antibody recognition (Wei et al. 2010, Wanzeck et al. 2011, Job et al. 2013b), modulation of binding affinity or even specificity of the HA (Tsuchiya et al. 2002), and interactions with other host defense lectins like the macrophage mannose receptor, DC-SIGN, or galectins all of which play roles in host defense against IAV (Londrigan et al. 2011, Tate et al. 2011, Yang et al. 2011). It should be noted that such lectin interactions can also be hijacked by the virus to promote infection (Spear et al. 2003, Londrigan et al. 2011).

It will be important as well to study interaction of mutant NCRDs with additional avian strains. There is a vast reservoir of avian strains (with 16 HA types) and although only H1-H3 have successfully become established in the human population, the potential is there for novel pandemics with other HA types. There is a high level of concern regarding especially the H5, H7 and H9 subtypes that have infected humans with relatively high mortality rates. Fortunately none of these viral subtypes have adapted for efficient transmission among humans thus far. A recent study by Qi et al. evaluated recombinant strains containing the HA of avian strains (H1 through H16) combined with other genes segments taken from a low pathogenicity, SP-D-sensitive human H1N1 strain (Qi et al. 2014). All of these recombinant strains were resistant to SP-D, presumably due to minimal glycosylation on their HA head regions. All of these strains were resistant to SP-D; however, only a subset of them strains (H1, H3, H5, H9, H11 and H13) were highly pathogenic in mice and cytopathic in human bronchial epithelial cells. Hence, although the HA of the avian strains is critical for interactions with SP-D and pathogenicity, other properties of the HA besides lack of inhibition by SP-D must contribute to pathogenicity. The case for SP-D resistance as an important contributory factor for increased pathogenicity of human pandemic H1 and H3 strains remains strong in any case, since simple addition of additional glycans to the HA of these strains does reduce pathogenicity in mice (Vigerust et al. 2007, Tate et al. 2012).

Conclusions

Influenza A viruses (IAVs) are a major ongoing public health problem due to their ability to undergo continuous mutation of viral surface proteins. Lectin interactions are central to infectivity of IAV and many other viruses. For IAV cell binding and the initial steps of the viral life cycle in the cell are determined by the viral hemagglutinin (HA) through its ability to bind to specific sialic acid conjugates on the surface of respiratory epithelial cells or immune cells. Lectin interactions also play a key role in the innate response to IAV. IAV is a prime example of the importance of innate immunity in early host protection against infection. Our research has focused on the role of soluble lectin inhibitors in lung fluids that provide an initial barrier to IAV infection and also modulate host inflammatory responses to the virus. In this review we describe in detail the role of the pulmonary surfactant collectin, surfactant protein D (SP-D), in host defense against IAV. SP-D appears to play a particularly important role in defense against seasonal IAV strains. In contrast, pandemic IAV strains are not inhibited by human SP-D due to relative lack of glycosylation of the IAV head or cell binding portion of their HA. In addition, avian strains of IAV generally have limited HA glycosylation and are not inhibited by SP-D. We have generated mutant versions of SP-D with increased affinity for mannose rich glycans and these mutants have increased ability to neutralize seasonal IAV, as well as being able to inhibit pandemic IAV *in vitro* and *in vivo*. Through crystallography, molecular modeling, and molecular dynamics we have determined the molecular mechanism of binding of SP-D to the IAV HA and established the basis for increased inhibitory activity of mutant versions of SP-D. These studies provide the first detailed molecular mechanism for viral inhibition by an innate lectin inhibitor. The studies were highly collaborative requiring shared expertise in virology, structural biology, protein chemistry, and glycomics.

Acknowledgements

Dr. Hartshorn's work was supported by NIH grants AI-83222 and HL-069031. The author gratefully acknowledge the contribution to this work by Drs. Erika Crouch (Washington University School of Medicine, USA), Uffe Holmskov (University of Odense, Denmark), Barbara Seaton (Boston University School of Medicine, USA), Martin van Eijk (University of Utrecht, Netherlands) and Joseph Zaia (Boston University School of Medicine, USA) and Boon Chong Goh (University of Illinois, Urbana-Champaign, USA). The author also thankful to other colleagues noted in the text for their impact in the presented study. In particular, the author appreciates Dr. Barbara Seaton (Boston University School of Medicine, USA) for her careful review of the manuscript.

Keywords: surfactant protein D, collectin, innate immunity, hemagglutinin, molecular dynamics

References

Anders, E. M., C. A. Hartley and D. C. Jackson. 1990. Bovine and mouse serum beta inhibitors of influenza A viruses are mannose-binding lectins. Proc Natl Acad Sci USA 87: 4485–9.

Brown-Augsburger, P., K. L. Hartshorn, D. Chang, K. Rust, C. Fliszar, H. G. Welgus et al. 1996. Site directed mutagenesis of Cys15 and Cys20 of pulmonary surfactant protein D: Expression of a trimeric protein with altered anti-viral properties. J Biol Chem 271: 13724–13730.

Crouch, E., Y. Tu, D. Briner, B. McDonald, K. Smith, U. Holmskov et al. 2005. Ligand specificity of human surfactant protein D: expression of a mutant trimeric collectin that shows enhanced interactions with influenza A virus. J Biol Chem 280: 17046–56.

Crouch, E. C., K. Smith, B. McDonald, D. Briner, B. Linders, J. McDonald et al. 2006. Species differences in the carbohydrate binding preferences of surfactant protein D. Am J Respir Cell Mol Biol 35: 84–94.

Crouch, E., K. Hartshorn, T. Horlacher, B. McDonald, K. Smith, T. Cafarella et al. 2009. Recognition of mannosylated ligands and influenza A virus by human surfactant protein D: contributions of an extended site and residue 343. Biochemistry 48: 3335–45.

Crouch, E., N. Nikolaidis, F. X. McCormack, B. McDonald, K. Allen, M. J. Rynkiewicz et al. 2011. Mutagenesis of surfactant protein D informed by evolution and x-ray crystallography enhances defenses against influenza A virus *in vivo*. J Biol Chem 286: 40681–92.

Dawood, F. S., S. Jain, L. Finelli, M. W. Shaw, S. Lindstrom, R. J. Garten et al. 2009. Emergence of a novel swine-origin influenza A (H1N1) virus in humans. N Engl J Med 360: 2605–15.

Goh, B. C., M. J. Rynkiewicz, T. R. Cafarella, M. R. White, K. L. Hartshorn, K. Allen et al. 2013. Molecular mechanisms of inhibition of influenza by surfactant protein D revealed by large-scale molecular dynamics simulation. Biochemistry 52: 8527–8538.

Haagsman, H. P., S. Hawgood, T. Sargeant, D. Buckley, R. T. White, K. Drickamer et al. 1987. The major lung surfactant protein, SP 28-36, is a calcium-dependant, carbohydrate-binding protein. J Biol Chem 262: 13877–13880.

Hakansson, K., N. K. Lim, H. J. Hoppe and K. B. M. Reid. 1999. Crystal structure of the trimeric alpha helical coiled-coil and the three lectin domains of human lung surfactant protein D. Structure 24: 255–264.

Hansen, Soren, Dorte Holm, Vivi Moeller, Lars Vitved, Christian Bendixen, Kenneth B.M. Reid et al. 2002. CL-46, a novel collectin highly expressed in bovine thymus and liver. J Immunol 169: 5726–5734.

Hartley, C. A., D. C. Jackson and E. M. Anders. 1992. Two distinct serum mannose-binding lectins function as beta inhibitors of influenza virus: Identification of bovine serum beta inhibitor as conglutinin. J Virol 66: 4358–63.

Hartshorn, K. L., K. Sastry, M. R. White, E. M. Anders, M. Super, R. A. Ezekowitz et al. 1993. Human mannose-binding protein functions as an opsonin for influenza A viruses. J Clin Invest 91: 1414–20.

Hartshorn, K. L., E. C. Crouch, M. R. White, P. Eggleton, A. I. Tauber, D. Chang et al. 1994. Evidence for a protective role of pulmonary surfactant protein D (SP-D) against influenza A viruses. J Clin Invest 94: 311–319.

Hartshorn, K., D. Chang, K. Rust, M. White, J. Heuser and E. Crouch. 1996. Interactions of recombinant human pulmonary surfactant protein D and SP-D multimers with influenza A. Am J Physiol 271: L753–62.

Hartshorn, K. L., M. R. White, V. Shepherd, K. Reid, J. C. Jensenius and E. C. Crouch. 1997. Mechanisms of anti-influenza activity of surfactant proteins A and D: Comparison with serum collectins. Am J Physiol 273: L1156–66.

Hartshorn, K. L., M. R. White, D. R. Voelker, J. Coburn, K. Zaner and E. C. Crouch. 2000a. Mechanism of binding of surfactant protein D to influenza A viruses: Importance of binding to haemagglutinin to antiviral activity. Biochem J 351 Pt 2: 449–58.

Hartshorn, K. L., K. N. Sastry, D. Chang, M. R. White and E. C. Crouch. 2000b. Enhanced anti-influenza activity of a surfactant protein D and serum conglutinin fusion protein. Am J Physiol Lung Cell Mol Physiol 278: L90–8.

Hartshorn, K. L., U. Holmskov, S. Hansen, P. Zhang, T. Meschi, T. Mogues et al. 2002. Distinctive anti-influenza properties of recombinant collectin 43. Biochem J 366: 87–96.

Hartshorn, K. L., R. Webby, M. R. White, T. Tecle, C. Pan, S. Boucher et al. 2008. Role of viral hemagglutinin glycosylation in anti-influenza activities of recombinant surfactant protein D. Respir Res 9: 65.

Hartshorn, K. L. 2010. New look at an old problem. Bacterial superinfection after influenza. Am J Pathol 176: 536–539.

Hartshorn, K., M. White, K. Smith, G. Sorensen, Y. Kuroki, U. Holmskov et al. 2010a. Increasing antiviral activity of surfactant protein d trimers by introducing residues from bovine serum collectins: dissociation of mannan-binding and antiviral activity. Scand J Immunol 72: 22–30.

Hartshorn, K. L., M. R. White, T. Tecle, G. L. Sorensen, U. Holmskov and E. C. Crouch. 2010b. Viral aggregating and opsonizing activity in collectin trimers. Am J Physiol Lung Cell Mol Physiol 298: L79–88.

Hartshorn, K. L. 2013. Why does pandemic influenza virus kill? Am J Pathol 183: 1125–7.

Hawgood, S., C. Brown, J. Edmondson, A. Stumbaugh, L. Allen, J. Goerke et al. 2004. Pulmonary collectins modulate strain-specific influenza a virus infection and host responses. J Virol 78: 8565–72.

Hillaire, M. L., M. van Eijk, N. J. Nieuwkoop, S. E. Vogelzang-van Trierum, R. A. Fouchier, A. D. Osterhaus et al. 2012. The number and position of N-linked glycosylation sites in the hemagglutinin determine differential recognition of seasonal and 2009 pandemic H1N1 influenza virus by porcine surfactant protein D. Virus Res 169: 301–5.

Honda, Y., H. Takahashi, Y. Kuroki, T. Akino and S. Abe. 1996. Decreased contents of surfactant proteins A and D in BAL fluids of Healthy smokers. Chest 109: 1006–9.

Iwaarden, J. F. van, C. A. Benne, J. A. G. van Strijp, J. Verhoef, L. M. G. van Golde and C. A. Kraaijeveld. 1993. Surfactant protein A (SP-A) prevents infection of cells by influenza A virus. Am Rev Resp Dis 148: A146.

Job, E. R., Y. M. Deng, M. D. Tate, B. Bottazzi, E. C. Crouch, M. M. Dean et al. 2010. Pandemic H1N1 influenza A viruses are resistant to the antiviral activities of innate immune proteins of the collectin and pentraxin superfamilies. J Immunol 185: 4284–91.

Job, E. R., B. Bottazzi, B. Gilbertson, K. M. Edenborough, L. E. Brown, A. Mantovani et al. 2013a. Serum amyloid P is a sialylated glycoprotein inhibitor of influenza A viruses. PLoS One 8: e59623.

Job, E. R., Y. M. Deng, K. K. Barfod, M. D. Tate, N. Caldwell, S. Reddiex et al. 2013b. Addition of glycosylation to influenza A virus hemagglutinin modulates antibody-mediated recognition of H1N1 2009 pandemic viruses. J Immunol 190: 2169–77.

Kishore, U., J. Wang, H. Hoppe and K. B. M. Reid. 1996. The alpha helical neck region of human lung SP-D is essential for binding of the carbohydrate recognition domains to lipopolysaccharides and phospholipids. Biochem J 318: 505–511.

Leth-Larsen, R., P. Garred, H. Jensenius, J. Meschi, K. Hartshorn, J. Madsen et al. 2005. A common polymorphism in the SFTPD gene influences assembly, function, and concentration of surfactant protein D. J Immunol 174: 1532–8.

LeVine, A. M., J. A. Whitsett, K. L. Hartshorn, E. C. Crouch and T. R. Korfhagen. 2001. Surfactant protein D enhances clearance of influenza A virus from the lung *in vivo*. J Immunol 167: 5868–73.

Li, G., J. Siddiqui, M. Hendry, J. Akiyama, J. Edmondson, C. Brown et al. 2002. Surfactant protein-A—deficient mice display an exaggerated early inflammatory response to a beta-resistant strain of influenza A virus. Am J Respir Cell Mol Biol 26: 277–82.

Lim, B., J. Wang, U. Holmskov, S. Thiel, J. C. Jensenius, H. J. Hoppe et al. 1994. Expression of the carbohydrate recognition domain of lung surfactant protein D and demonstration of its binding to lipopolysaccharides of gram-negative bacteria. Biochem Biophis Res Comm 202: 1674–1680.

Lomas, D. A., E. K. Silverman, L. D. Edwards, N. W. Locantore, B. E. Miller, D. H. Horstman et al. 2009. Serum surfactant protein D is steroid sensitive and associated with exacerbations of COPD. Eur Respir J 34: 95–102.

Londrigan, S. L., S. G. Turville, M. D. Tate, Y. M. Deng, A. G. Brooks and P. C. Reading. 2011. N-linked glycosylation facilitates sialic acid-independent attachment and entry of influenza A viruses into cells expressing DC-SIGN or L-SIGN. J Virol 85: 2990–3000.

Madsen, J., A. Kliem, I. Tornoe, K. Skjodt, C. Koch and U. Holmskov. 2000. Localization of lung surfactant protein D on mucosal surfaces in human tissues. J Immunol 164: 5866–70.

Mikerov, A. N., M. White, K. Hartshorn, G. Wang and J. Floros. 2008. Inhibition of hemagglutination activity of influenza A viruses by SP-A1 and SP-A2 variants expressed in CHO cells. Med Microbiol Immunol 197: 9–12.

Morens, D. M. 2003. Influenza-related mortality: Considerations for practice and public health. JAMA 289: 227–9.

Neumann, G., M. Ozawa and Y. Kawaoka. 2013. Reverse genetics of influenza viruses. Methods Mol Biol 865: 193–206.

Nikolaidis, N. M., M. R. White, K. Allen, S. Tripathi, L. Qi, B. McDonald et al. 2014. Mutations flanking the carbohydrate binding site of surfactant protein D confer antiviral activity for pandemic influenza A viruses. Am J Physiol Lung Cell Mol Physiol 306: L1036–44.

Ogasawara, Y. and D. R. Voelker. 1995. Altered carbohydrate recognition specificity engineered into surfactant protein D reveals different binding mechanisms for phosphatidylinositol and glucosylceramide. J Biol Chem 270: 14725–14732.

Persson, A., D. Chang and E. Crouch. 1990. Surfactant protein D is a divalent cation-dependent carbohydrate-binding protein. J Biol Chem 265: 5755–5760.

Qi, L., J. C. Kash, V. G. Dugan, B. W. Jagger, Y. F. Lau, Z. M. Sheng et al. 2011. The ability of pandemic influenza virus hemagglutinins to induce lower respiratory pathology is associated with decreased surfactant protein D binding. Virology 412: 426–34.

Qi, L., L. M. Pujanauski, A. S. Davis, L. M. Schwartzman, D. S. Chertow, D. Baxter et al. 2014. Contemporary avian influenza a virus subtype h1, h6, h7, h10, and h15 hemagglutinin genes encode a Mammalian virulence factor similar to the 1918 pandemic virus h1 hemagglutinin. MBio 5: e02116–14.

Reading, P. C., L. S. Morey, E. C. Crouch and E. M. Anders. 1997. Collectin-mediated antiviral host defense of the lung: Evidence from influenza virus infection of mice. J Virol 71: 8204–12.

Reading, P. C., J. Allison, E. C. Crouch and E. M. Anders. 1998. Increased susceptibility of diabetic mice to influenza virus infection: Compromise of collectin-mediated host defense of the lung by glucose. J Virol 72: 6884–6887.

Rothmann, A. B., H. D. Mortensen, U. Holmskov and P. Hojrup. 1997. Structural characterization of bovine collectin-43. Eur J Biochem 243: 630–635.

Rust, K., L. Grosso, V. Zhang, D. Chang, A. Persson, W. Longmore et al. 1991. Human surfactant protein D: SP-D contains a C-type lectin carbohydrate recognition domain. Ar Biochem and Biophys 290: 116–126.

Ryan-Poirier, K. A. and Y. Kawaoka. 1993. Alpha 2-macroglobulin is the major neutralizing inhibitor of influenza A virus in pig serum. Virology 193: 974–6.

Sauter, N. K., J. E. Hanson, G. D. Glick, J. H. Brown, R. L. Crowther, S. J. Park et al. 1992. Binding of influenza virus hemagglutinin to analogs of its cell-surface receptor, sialic acid: analysis by proton nuclear magnetic resonance spectroscopy and X-ray crystallography. Biochemistry 31: 9609–21.

Shrive, A. K., H. A. Tharia, P. Strong, U. Kishore, I. Burns, P. J. Rizkallah et al. 2003. High-resolution structural insights into ligand binding and immune cell recognition by human lung surfactant protein D. J Mol Biol 331: 509–23.

Sims, M. W., R. M. Tal-Singer, S. Kierstein, A. I. Musani, M. F. Beers, R. A. Panettieri et al. 2008. Chronic obstructive pulmonary disease and inhaled steroids alter surfactant protein D (SP-D) levels: A cross-sectional study. Respir Res 9: 13.

Spear, G. T., M. R. Zariffard, J. Xin and M. Saifuddin. 2003. Inhibition of DC-SIGN-mediated trans infection of T cells by mannose-binding lectin. Immunology 110: 80–5.

Tate, M. D., E. R. Job, A. G. Brooks and P. C. Reading. 2011. Glycosylation of the hemagglutinin modulates the sensitivity of H3N2 influenza viruses to innate proteins in airway secretions and virulence in mice. Virology 413: 84–92.

Tate, M. D., A. G. Brooks and P. C. Reading. 2012. Specific sites of N-linked glycosylation on the hemagglutinin of H1N1 subtype influenza A virus determine sensitivity to inhibitors of the innate immune system and virulence in mice. J Immunol 187: 1884–94.

Tecle, T., M. R. White, D. Gantz, E. C. Crouch and K. L. Hartshorn. 2007. Human neutrophil defensins increase neutrophil uptake of influenza A virus and bacteria and modify virus-induced respiratory burst responses. J Immunol 178: 8046–52.

Thomas, N. J., S. Diangelo, J. C. Hess, R. Fan, M. W. Ball, J. M. Geskey et al. 2009. Transmission of surfactant protein variants and haplotypes in children hospitalized with respiratory syncytial virus. Pediatr Res 66: 70–73.

Tripathi, S., M. R. White, G. Wang and K. Hartshorn. 2014. LL-37 modulates human phagocyte responses to influenza A virus. J Leukoc Biol 96: 931–938.

Tripathi, S., M. R. White and K. L. Hartshorn. 2015. The amazing innate immune response to influenza A virus infection. Innate Immun 21: 73–98.

Tsuchiya, E., K. Sugawara, S. Hongo, Y. Matsuzaki, Y. Muraki, Z. N. Li et al. 2002. Effect of addition of new oligosaccharide chains to the globular head of influenza A/H2N2 virus haemagglutinin on the intracellular transport and biological activities of the molecule. J Gen Virol 83: 1137–46.

van Eijk, M., M. R. White, E. C. Crouch, J. J. Batenburg, A. B. Vaandrager, L. M. Van Golde et al. 2003. Porcine pulmonary collectins show distinct interactions with influenza A viruses: Role of the N-linked oligosaccharides in the carbohydrate recognition domain. J Immunol 171: 1431–40.

van Eijk, M., M. J. Rynkiewicz, M. R. White, K. L. Hartshorn, X. Zou, K. Schulten et al. 2012. A unique sugar-binding site mediates the distinct anti-influenza activity of pig surfactant protein D. J Biol Chem 287: 26666–77.

Verma, A., M. White, V. Vathipadiekal, S. Tripathi, J. Mbianda, M. Ieong et al. 2012. Human H-ficolin inhibits replication of seasonal and pandemic influenza A viruses. J Immunol 189: 2478–87.

Vigerust, D. J., K. B. Ulett, K. L. Boyd, J. Madsen, S. Hawgood and J. A. McCullers. 2007. N-linked glycosylation attenuates H3N2 influenza viruses. J Virol 81: 8593–600.

Wanzeck, K., K. L. Boyd and J. A. McCullers. 2011. Glycan shielding of the influenza virus hemagglutinin contributes to immunopathology in mice. Am J Respir Crit Care Med 183: 776–773.

Wei, C. J., J. C. Boyington, K. Dai, K. V. Houser, M. B. Pearce, W. P. Kong et al. 2010. Cross-neutralization of 1918 and 2009 influenza viruses: Role of glycans in viral evolution and vaccine design. Sci Transl Med 2: 24ra21.

White, M. R., E. Crouch, D. Chang, K. Sastry, N. Guo, G. Engelich et al. 2000. Enhanced antiviral and opsonic activity of a human mannose-binding lectin and surfactant protein D chimera. J Immunol 165: 2108–15.

White, M. R., E. Crouch, M. van Eijk, M. Hartshorn, L. Pemberton, I. Tornoe et al. 2005. Cooperative anti-influenza activities of respiratory innate immune proteins and neuraminidase inhibitor. Am J Physiol Lung Cell Mol Physiol 288: L831–40.

White, M. R., T. Tecle, E. C. Crouch and K. L. Hartshorn. 2007. Impact of neutrophils on antiviral activity of human bronchoalveolar lavage fluid. Am J Physiol Lung Cell Mol Physiol 293: L1293–9.

White, M. R., E. J. Helmerhorst, A. Ligtenberg, M. Karpel, T. Tecle, W. L. Siqueira et al. 2009. Multiple components contribute to ability of saliva to inhibit influenza viruses. Oral Microbiol Immunol 24: 18–24.

White, M. R., R. Kandel, S. Tripathi, D. Condon, L. Qi, J. Taubenberger et al. 2014. Alzheimer's associated beta amyloid protein inhibits influenza A virus and modulates viral interactions with phagocytes. PLOS ONe 9: e101364.

Wright, J. R., R. E. Wager, S. Hawgood, L. Dobbs and J. A. Clements. 1987. Surfactant apoprotein Mr = 26,000–36,000 enhances uptake of liposomes by type II cells. J Biol Chem 262: 2888–2894.

Yang, M. L., Y. H. Chen, S. W. Wang, Y. J. Huang, C. H. Leu, N. C. Yeh et al. 2011. Galectin-1 binds to influenza virus and ameliorates influenza virus pathogenesis. J Virol 85: 10010–20.

Zhang, L., K. L. Hartshorn, E. C. Crouch, M. Ikegami and J. A. Whitsett. 2002. Complementation of pulmonary abnormalities in SP-D(–/–) mice with an SP-D/conglutinin fusion protein. J Biol Chem 277: 22453–9.

CHAPTER 6

Application of Lectin Histochemistry for the Diagnosis of Lysosomal Storage Diseases

Joseph Alroy,[1,]* *Min Fang,*[2,a] *Andrew G. Plaut*[3] and *Gary Sahagian*[2,b]

Introduction

Lectins (from the Latin word legere, to select), are sugar-binding proteins or glycoproteins that agglutinate cells and/or precipitate glycoconjugates that have saccharides of appropriate complementarity (Table 1 and Alroy et al. 1984a). The interaction of lectins with particular carbohydrates can be as specific as the interaction between antigens and antibodies (Ghazarian et al. 2011). When lectins are conjugated directly or indirectly to a "visualant" so they can be detected on tissues, they are useful as probes for identifying the presence of specific carbohydrate residues in histological sections. A recent review highlighted the usefulness of both glycan-binding antibodies and lectins in the characterization of tissue glycoconjugates (Tang et al. 2015). This illustrated the difference in the expression of glycoconjugates in normal glomerulus and glomerulus of a patient with I cell disease, as shown in Figs. 1 and 2 (Castagnaro et al. 1987).

Different mammalian species may have similar terminal residues on glycoproteins, an example being mammalian Brunner's glands (Fig. 3, Skutelskey et al. 1989).

However, glycoconjugate expression may differ among mammalian species, an example being the vascular endothelium (Alroy et al. 1987). Only human endothelial cells are stained with UEA-1, while most other species are stained with GS-1. Similarly, different lectins show diversity in staining and distribution of carbohydrate residues in normal skin (Schaumburg-Lever et al. 1984a), in proliferative lesions (Schaumburg-Lever et al. 1986), and in psoriasis (Schaumburg-Lever et al. 1984b). Lectins have been used to characterize the carbohydrate distribution in the optical cornea (Panjwani et al. 1986b).

[1] Department of Integrated Pathophysiology and Pathobiology, Tufts University School of Medicine, 136 Harrison Avenue, Boston, Massachusetts, 02111.
[2] Department of Developmental, Molecular and Chemical Biology, Tufts University School of Medicine, 136 Harrison Avenue, Boston, Massachusetts, 02111.
[a] E-mail: min.fang@tufts.edu
[b] E-mail: gary.sahagian@tufts.edu
[3] Department of Medicine, Division of Gastroenterology, Tufts University School of Medicine and Tufts Medical Center, 800 Washington Street, Boston, Massachusetts, 02111.
   E-mail: aplaut@tuftsmedicalcenter.org
* Corresponding author: joealroy@gmail.com

Table 1. Lectins used in laboratory for identifying carbohydrate units.

Lectin origin	Common name	Acronym	Concentration (mg/ml)	Major Sugar Specificity	Binding Inhibitor
Arachishypogea	Peanut	PNA	20	β-D-Galp-(1→3)-D-Gal	Lactose
Concanavalia ensiformis	Jack bean	ConA	10	*a*-D-Glc, *a*-D-Man	*a*-D-Man*p*OMc
Datura stramonium	Jimsonweed	DSA	10	[β-D-Galp-(1→4)-b-D-Glc*p*NAc-(1→3)]$_n$	(β-D-Glc*p*NAc)$_{2-3}$
Dolichos biflorus	Horse gran	DBA	10	*a*-D-GalNAc	*a*-D-GalNAc
Glycine max	Soybean	SBA	10	*a*-D-GalNAc, *a*-D-Gal	*a*-D-GalNAc
Griffonia simplicifolia	Bandeirea	GS-I	50	*a*-D-Gal	Lactose
Lens culinaris	Common lentil	LCA	10	*a*-D-Gal, *a*-D-Man	*a*-D-Man*p*OMc
Ulex europaeus	Gorse	UEA-I	10	α-L-fucose	α-L-fucose

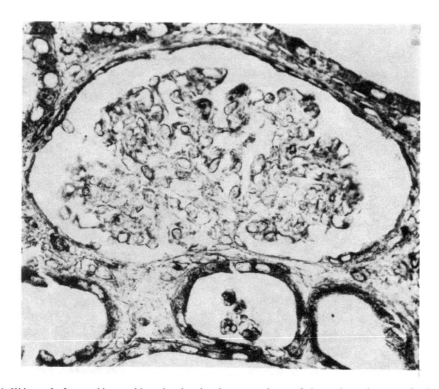

Figure 1. Kidney of a 2 year old normal boy showing the plasma membrane of glomerular podocytes stained with ConA (*Concanavalia ensiformis*).

Alterations in lectin staining have also been observed in macular dystrophy (Panjwani et al. 1986a), and retinoblastoma (Brandenstein et al. 1987). Lectins have also been used to demonstrate the modulation of carbohydrate residues in regenerative nodules of pancreatic acini and pancreatic acinar carcinoma (Skutelskey et al. 1987), and in breast lesions (Fig. 4, Skutelskey et al. 1988).

A study of lectin histochemistry of the intestinal epithelium of domestic fowl (Gallus domesticus) has shown that enterocytes in different segments of the intestine bear glycoconjugates that may play a significant role in host-parasite interaction (Alroy et al. 1989). A study of 3 different *Eimeria* sporozoites (the infectious stage) species have shown that their surface lectins differ in specificity to enterocytes glycoconjugates. These lectins appear likely to play a role in determining the site of infection (Strout et al. 1994). Lectin histochemistry has also been used to identify the surface glycoconjugates of *Giardialamblia*

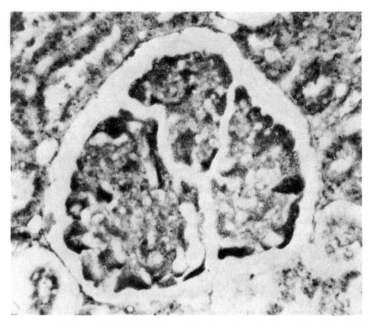

Figure 2. Kidney of 9 ½-year old boy who has I Cell Disease showing enlarged podocytes heavily stained with ConA.

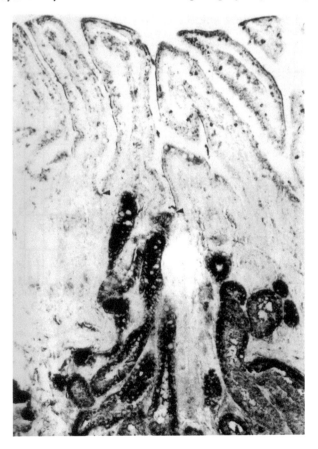

Figure 3. Histologic section through normal human duodenum illustrating intense staining of Brunner's glands and their ducts with WGA.

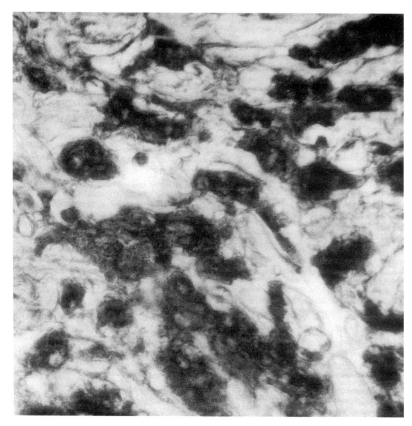

Figure 4. High magnification photomicrograph of an infiltrating ductal carcinoma of the breast showing ConA staining is restricted to the cytoplasm and plasma membrane of the neoplastic cells.

trophozoites (Ward et al. 1988). Lectins have been used to show that terminal residues of glycolipids and glycoproteins consisting of lipofuscin, an aging pigment in neurons and myocytes, change with age (Monserrat et al. 1995). Differences have been reported in glycoconjugates of enterocytes between colitis and cancer-prone tamarins when compared to enterocytes from resistant primates (Moore et al. 1988a). Glycoconjugate changes in inflamed and neoplastic epithelium and in colitis and cancer-prone tamarins have been observed (Moore et al. 1988b). Lectin histochemistry has been used to characterize nephrogenic adenomas and embryonic tubules (Devine et al. 1984). It has also been used for predicting behavior of non-neoplastic urothelium in human urinary bladder (Alroy et al. 1982). There also is a difference in lectin staining of seminal vesicle as well as between central and peripheral prostatic zones. In intraductal breast dysplasia there is markedly reduced staining compared to normal tissue, consistent with impaired differentiation (McNeal et al. 1988). In mucinous prostate adenocarcinoma there is a correlation between the degree of differentiation and the patterns of lectin staining (McNeal et al. 1991). A recent review focused on the role of carbohydrates and lectins in cancer therapeutics (Ghazarian et al. 2011).

In this review, we address the role of lectins in the diagnosis and the identification of terminal residues in glycoproteins and in glycolipids stored in lysosomal storage diseases.

Lysosomes as Subcellular Organelles

Lysosomes are catabolic organelles that digest and recycle many cellular and extracellular materials including glycoproteins, glycosaminoglycans, sphingolipids, glycogen and proteins. These membrane-bound organelles are present in all nucleated cells and were first described in 1955 by Christian de Duve (Boyd 1963); they are the primary disposal and recycling centers of the cell. They have approximately

25 membrane proteins including the vacuolar proton pump (v-ATPase) and they contain more than 50 known hydrolytic enzymes that participate with associated accessory proteins in turnover of intracellular and extracellular macromolecules (Saftig and Klumperman 2009). These enzymes include glycosidases, lipases, nucleases, phosphatases, proteases, and sulfatases that are active at acidic pH in the range of pH 4.5 to 5. The enzymes are synthesized in the rough endoplasmic reticulum (RER) and reach their final destination in the lysosome following a series of posttranslational lysosomal targeting modifications involving protein and carbohydrate recognition signals. Most details of these modifications and transport pathways are known. The hydrophobic amino-terminal signal peptide on the nascent enzyme protein directs its transport into the lumen of the RER where it undergoes glycosylation of selected asparagine residues. The protein signal peptide is then cleaved and oligosaccharides are processed by removal of 3 glucose residues and 1 mannose residue. The modified hydrolases are then transported to the Golgi apparatus where they acquire mannose-6-phosphate residues on their oligosaccharide side chains by the action of two enzymes, UPD-*N*-acetylglucosamine-1-phosphate transferase and GlcNAc-phosphoglycosidase. Hydrolases that contain mannose-6-phosphate are recognized and bound by mannose-6-phosphate receptors (MPRs), transmembrane proteins that transport the hydrolases to endosomes for subsequent delivery to lysosomes. Upon arrival into endosomes the hydrolases are dissociated from the receptors, and the free receptors are then recycled back to the Golgi apparatus and reutilized. Deficiency of the Golgi enzyme N-acetylglucosamine-1-phosphotransferase results in a deficiency of multiple lysosomal enzymes because they are not correctly targeted. This enzyme is encoded by 3 different genes whose mutations lead to multiple enzyme deficiency states such as mucolipidosis II and III (ML-II and ML-III, respectively). A few lysosomal enzymes are transmitted to lysosomes via the membrane protein sortilin (Libin and Morales 2009). It is noteworthy that all lysosomal hydrolases are soluble proteins, with the exception of glucocerebrosidase and acid phosphatase. These lysosomal membrane proteins reach the lysosome independent of the mannose 6-phosphate and sortilin targeting pathways.

Lysosomal membrane proteins are classified into several different functional groups. For example, ion transporter proteins such as the proton/chloride transporter *ClC-7* and *Ostm1* result in osteopetrosis with neuronal storage (Pangrazio et al. 2010) and a transient receptor potential (TRP) defect in the mucolipin 1 (ML-1) protein, which is an ion channel, leads to mucolipidosis IV (ML-IV). Cystinosin (Bendavid et al. 2004), sialin (Aula et al. 2002) are export proteins that participate in efflux of cystamine and free sialic acid from the lysosome to the cytosol, respectively. A hybrid enzyme/transporter protein complex with 4 different transmembrane enzymes is deficient in mucopolysaccharidosis III (MPSIII) resulting in abnormal storage of heparin sulfate. Other transporter proteins include Niemann-Pick C-1 (NPC-1) and NPC-2 that are membrane proteins that have a role in cholesterol transport from late endosomes and lysosomes into the cytosol (Fernandez-Valero et al. 2005), and the lysosomal-associated membrane proteins (LAMPs), LAMP-1 (Huynh et al. 2007) and LAMP-2 (Zeevi et al. 2007).

Lysosomal Storage Diseases

Lysosomal storage diseases (LSDs) are a large group of genetically determined or acquired heterogeneous metabolic disorders. Currently there are 56 known such inherited disorders (Table 2, Alroy et al. 2014) and these include four newly identified forms of abnormal lysosomal storage of ceroid lipofuscinosis (NCL-11, NCL-12, NCL-13, and NCL 14) in human patients (reviewed Cotman et al. 2013, Boustany 2013, Table 2) and forty spontaneous diseases that have been described in animals (Alroy and Lyons 2014). LSDs are diverse disorders usually resulting from the deficiency of one or more hydrolytic enzymes that participate in turnover of cellular and extracellular macromolecules but in some cases, result from deficiencies of nonenzymatic proteins or proteins that are involved in lysosomal biogenesis, targeting, degradation or product export. LSDs can affect different cell types, tissues and organs, and the accumulation in a particular cell type depends on cell function, metabolism and life span. Brain lesions comprise two-thirds of all LSDs and are particularly prevalent. The amount of substrate to be catabolized is influenced by the composition of the cell membrane, rate of membrane recycling, rate of cellular catabolism, life span of the cells, phagocytic ability of the affected cells and nature of the phagocytosed substrates. The catabolism in lysosomes of many macromolecules such as glycosaminoglycans is known to involve a cascading, linear

Table 2. Lysosomal storage diseases.

Disease	Deficient Hydrolases	Primary Storage Products	Major Organ Involvement
Mucopolysaccharidoses (MPS)			
MPS-I Hurler, Scheie syndrome	α-L-Iduronidase	Dermatan sulfate, Heparan sulfate	CNS, connective tissue, heart, skeleton, cornea
MPS-II Hunter syndrome	Iduronate sulfatase	Dermatan sulfate, Heparan sulfate	CNS, connective tissue, heart, skeleton
MPS-III Sanfilippo syndrome			
Subtype A	Sulfaminidase	Heparan sulfate	CNS
Subtype B	α-N-Acetylglucosaminidase	Heparan sulfate	CNS
Subtype C	Acetyl CoA α-glucosaminidae acetyltransferase	Heparan sulfate	CNS
Subtype D	N-acetylglucosaminidase 6-sulfatase	Heparan sulfate	CNS
MPS-IV Morquio syndrome			
Type A	Galactose 6-sulfatase	Chondroitin-4 sulfate, Keratan sulfate	Cartilage, skeleton, cornea, heart
Type B	β-Galactosidase	Keratan sulfate	Cartilage, skeleton, cornea
MPS-VI Maroteaux-Lamy syndrome	Arylsulfatase β-N-acetylglucosamine 4-sulfatase	Dermatan sulfate	Skeleton, cornea, heart
MPS-VII Sly syndrome	β-Glucuronidase	Dermatan sulfate, Heparan sulfate, Chondroitin 4-6sulfate	CNS, connective tissue, skeleton, heart
MPS-IX hyaluronidase deficiency	Hyaluronidase	Hyaluronan	Periarticular soft tissue
Sphingolipidoses (lipid storage disease)			
Glucocerebrosidosis (Gaucher disease)	β-Glucocerebrosidase	Glucosylceramide	
Infantile type 2			CNS, spleen, liver, bone marrow
Juvenile type 3			CNS, spleen, liver, bone marrow
Adult type I			spleen, liver, bone marrow
Fabry disease	α-Galactosidase	Trihexosylceramide	Blood vessels of skin, kidney, brain

Disease	Enzyme/protein defect	Stored material	Tissue distribution
Schindler disease	α-N-acetylgalactosaminidase	Sialylated and asialopeptides and oligosaccharides	CNS, PNS
Metachromatic leukodystrophy	Arylsulfatase A	Galactosylsulfatide	CNS, liver, kidney, gallbladder
Multiple sulfatase deficiency	At least 7 lysosomal sulfatase and a microsomal sulfatase		CNS, visceral organs and skeleton
Niemann-Pick A and B	Sphingomyelinase	Sphingomyelin	CNS, liver, spleen, bone marrow
Niemann-Pick Type C (NPC-1 and NPC-2)	Proteins required for lipid transport through late endosome	Unesterified cholesterol and sphingolipids	CNS, liver, spleen
G_{M1}-gangliosidosis	β-Galactosidase	G_{M1}-ganglioside, Oligosaccharides Keratan sulfate	CNS, skeleton, viscera
G_{M2}-gangliosidosis			
Tay-Sachs disease, A variant	β-Hexosaminidase A	G_{M2}-ganglioside	CNS
Sandhoff disease	β-Hexosaminidases A and B	G_{M2}-ganglioside, oligosaccharides	CNS
AB variant	Deficiency of G_{M2}-activator protein	G_{M2}-ganglioside	CNS
Galactosialidosis	Protective protein/Cathepsin A, resulting in Deficiency of β-hexosaminidase and α-neuraminidase	Glycolipids and oligosaccharides	CNS, spleen, liver, skeleton
Globoid cell leukodystrophy (Krabbe's disease)	Galactocerebroside β-galactosidase	Galactosylsphingosine	CNS
Farber granulomatosis	Ceramidase	Ceramide	Subcutaneous nodules, joints, larynx, liver, lung, heart
Wolman disease	Acid lipase/cholesterol esterase	Triglycerides, cholesterol Esters	Liver, spleen, adrenal
Disorders of glycoprotein degradation			
Aspartylglucosaminuria	Aspartylglucosaminidase	Fragments of glycoprotein, aspartyl-2-deoxy-2-ceramide glucosamine, N-linked oligosaccharides	CNS, connective tissue, bone marrow
α-Mannosidosis	α-Mannosidase	N-linked oligosaccharides	CNS, skeleton, liver, spleen

Table 2. contd....

Table 2. contd....

Disease	Deficient Hydrolases	Primary Storage Products	Major Organ Involvement
β-Mannosidosis	β-Mannosidase	N-linked oligosaccharides	CNS, skeleton, liver, spleen
Fucosidosis	α-Fucosidase	Oligosaccharides and glycolipids	CNS, spleen, liver
Sialidosis (Mucolipidosis-I) ML-I	Neuraminidase	Fragments of glycoprotein	CNS, spleen, liver, skeleton
Neuronal ceroid lipofuscinoses (NCL)			
Infantile NCL (CLN-1)	Palmitoyl protein thioesterase	Protein, saposins A and D	CNS, heart, endothelial cells, retina
Classic late infantile NCL (CLN-2)	Pepstatin-sensitive protease, tripeptidylpeptidase	Mitochondrial subunit C of ATPase synthase	CNS, retina
Classic juvenile NCL (CLN-3)	(Battenin) lysosomal transmembrane protein	Mitochondrial subunit C of ATPase synthase	CNS, heart, endothelial cells, retina
Adult NCL (CLN-4)	Unknown	Mitochondrial subunit C of ATPase synthase	CNS, heart, endothelial cells
Late infantile (Finnish variant) NCL (CLN-5)	Transmembrane protein	Mitochondrial subunit C of ATPase synthase	CNS, heart, endothelial cells
Late infantile (Indian variant) NCL (CLN-6)	Endoplasmic reticulum transmembrane protein	Mitochondrial subunit C of ATPase synthase	CNS, heart, endothelial cells
Late infantile (Turkish variant) NCL (CLN-7)	Protein	Mitochondrial subunit C of ATPase synthase	CNS
Progressive epilepsy with mental retardation, Northern epilepsy NCL (CLN-8)	Transmembrane protein	Mitochondrial subunit C of ATPase synthase	CNS
Glycogen storage disease Pompe disease type II	α-Glucosidase (acid maltase)	Glycogen	CNS, muscle, heart
Abnormal lysosomal membrane transport			
Mucolipidosis-II (I-cell disease)	N-acetylglucosaminyl-phosphotransferase, resulting in multiple enzyme deficiencies	Mucopolysaccharides, glycolipids, glycoproteins	CNS, connective tissue, skeleton, heart, kidney
Mucolipidosis-III (pseudo-Hurler polydystrophy)	N-acetylglucosaminyl-phosphotransferase, resulting in multiple enzyme deficiencies	Mucopolysaccharides, glycolipids, glycoproteins	Joint and connective tissue predominantly
Mucolipidosis IV	TRPML-I	Glycolipids	CNS, connective tissue

Danon's disease	Deficiency of LAMP-2, lysosomal associated membrane protein	Glycogen	CNS, muscle, heart
Infantile osteopetrosis and neuronal storage	OSTMI Chloride Channel 7	Glycoproteins and glycolipids	CNS, skeleton
Disorders of lysosomal efflux			
Cystinosis	Cysteine efflux mediator	Cysteine	Kidney
Salla disease	Sialic acid efflux mediator	Free sialic acid	CNS
Infantile sialuria	Sialic acid efflux mediator	Free sialic acid	CNS, kidney, liver
Other			
Acid phosphatases	Acid phosphatase		CNS, skeleton

sequence of reactions in which the product of one reaction becomes the substrate for the next. Therefore, the concentration of any substrate in normal or abnormal amounts can be determined by the influx rate of the substrate, the kinetic parameters of the degrading enzyme, or by the rate of export of the degraded material.

The major classification of LSDs is based on the type of material that is stored which gives these illnesses descriptive terms such as glycoprotein storage diseases, mucolipidosis, mucopolysaccharidoses, neuronal ceroid-lipofucinosis and sphingolipidosis (Alroy et al. 1991). The nature of the material actually stored in lysosomes of such patients in abnormal amounts is readily accomplished using lectin histochemistry (Alroy et al. 1988a,b,c). This identification of storage material in specimens from a wide range of lysosomal storage diseases allows the identification of which tissues and cells are affected, and provides a way to analyze the stored material (Alroy et al. 1984a).

A good example of the usefulness of lectin histochemistry was illustrated by the ability to diagnosis α-mannosidosis from sections of paraffin embedded tissues studied ten years after autopsy (Alroy et al. 1984a). However, care must be taken in interpreting results because identification may be influenced by whether or not the tissue was "fixed", how it was fixed, and whether or not materials such as glycolipids were extracted from the tissue during embedding in paraffin. Whereas glycoproteins and oligosaccharides can be readily identified in stored paraffin sections (Alroy et al. 1986b), frozen sections are required for identification of stored glycolipids. In practice, fluorescently tagged lectins are used for lectin histochemistry, and such tags used as visualants have high sensitivity and ease of use. However, some stored lipids are autofluorescent and this is a drawback that can interfere with accurate interpretation of specific staining and with tissue morphology (Alroy et al. 1984a). This drawback can be readily addressed by examination of control non-stained sections. Furthermore, since the strength of lectin binding depends on the concentration of both the lectin and its carbohydrate target as well as the time of incubation, it is important to carefully optimize and standardize the conditions of staining (Alroy and Lyons 2014).

In many lysosomal storage diseases there is variation in staining depending on the cells and tissue that one is examining (see Table 2), and among patients with the same storage disease, lectin staining of tissues can differ in appearance. This indicates that multiple factors influence the degradation of stored material, and this can differ among patients, or even tissues from the same patient. A clear example of this is found in tissues who have accumulation of glycolipids in mucopolysaccharidosis storage diseases (Alroy et al. 2013). When examined by electron microscopy, tissue samples from mucopolysaccharidoses display lamellated membrane structure accumulation (i.e., glycolipids) in addition to the primary storage of fine fibrillar material (i.e., glycosaminoglycans) in the same lysosome (Alroy et al. 2013). This heterogeneous appearance can occur because of a general loss of lysosomal function caused by the altered lysosomal microenvironment (Avila and Convit et al. 1975). In I-cell disease functional loss of *N*-acetylglucosamine 1-phosphotransferase, the enzyme that initiates construction of mannose-6-phosphate on newly synthesized lysosomal hydrolases (Castagnaro et al. 1987a), results in deficiency of many lysosomal hydrolases and accumulation of a wide range of lysosomal degradation products. In fact, there is only one known storage disease in which only a single type of carbohydrate is stored, that being the free sialic acid stored as a result of the lysosomal sialic acid transport protein (Pueschel et al. 1988). In some lysosomal storage diseases the terminal residue catabolized by the deficient hydrolase is present both in glycolipids and glycoproteins (Alroy et al. 1986b). The diagnosis of such diseases may require the use of several lectins that differ in specificity so that the nature of residues other than those at the terminal end of the oligosaccharide can be identified (Castagnaro et al. 1987b). For example, some diseases such as G_{M1}-gangliosidosis (Alroy and Lyons 2014), Gaucher's disease (Figs. 5 and 6, DeGasperi et al. 1990), fucosidosis (Alroy et al. 1986b) and Niemann-Pick C and D (Weintraub et al. 1992) the deficient hydrolase cleaves similar terminal residue of glycolipids and glycoproteins.

Glycoprotein-storage Diseases

These disorders from an inborn deficiency of one or more lysosomal hydrolases that degrade O- or N-linked glycans (Alroy et al. 1984).

α-Mannosidosis is due to deficiency of lysosomal α-mannosidase (Thomas 2001) leading to accumulation of oligosaccharides containing α-D-mannosyl groups and one or two 2-acetamido-2-

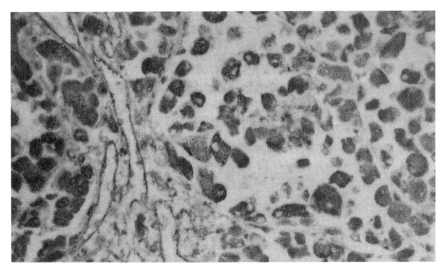

Figure 5. Frozen section of a spleen from a child with type I Gaucher's disease showing strong staining of the cytoplasm of enlarged cells with ConA.

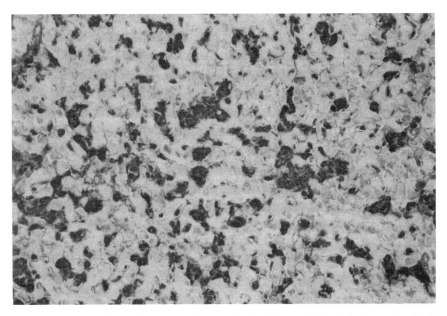

Figure 6. Liver tissue (imbedded in paraffin) from an 11 year old girl with type III Gaucher's disease showing Kupfer cells stained with Lens culinaris agglutinin.

deoxy-β-D-glucose residues at the reducing end (Alroy and Lyons 2014). Cells in paraffin sections from patients and animals with *a*-mannosidosis can be stained with *Concanavalia ensiformis* agglutinin (ConA), succinylated wheat germ agglutinin (S-WGA as shown in Fig. 7 and in Alroy et al. 1984b), or wheat germ agglutinin (WGA). In contrast, tissues from such patients do not stain with *Ulex europaeus* agglutinin-I (UEA-I) (Fig. 7).

Currently there is no known lectin that recognizes β-mannosides. Lectin staining can highlight the storage of undegraded oligosaccharides that have terminal α-mannosyl and β-N-acetyl glucosaminyl residues in cats, cattle and goats intoxicated by eating plants that contain swainsonine (Alroy et al. 1985).

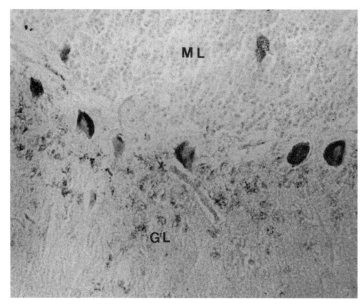

Figure 7. Photomicrograph of brain tissue from a 2-year-old patient deficient in α-mannosidase showing intense staining of the neuronal cytoplasm with ConA.

Fucosidosis occurs through a deficiency of the enzyme α-fucosidase (Thomas 2001) resulting in storage of oligosaccharides and sphingolipids that have terminal α-L-fucosyl residues. Accumulation of cells that accumulate molecules with α-L-fucosyl residues can be stained with UEA-I (Fig. 8, Alroy et al. 1985).

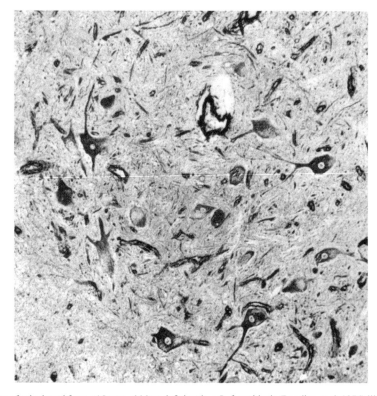

Figure 8. Section of spinal cord from a 15 year-old-boy deficient in α-L-fucosidosis (Landing et al. 1976) illustrating neurons with enlarged cytoplasm are intensely stained with UEA-I.

The storage of oligosaccharides with α-L-fucosyl residues can be demonstrated on paraffin sections, while the sphingolipid with terminal α-L-fucosyl residues can be seen only with frozen sections.

Mucolipidoses

Mucolipidosis II (I-Cell Disease) is characterized by deficient activity of *N*-acetylglucosamine phosphotransferase, resulting in the absence of D-mannose-6-phosphate units, which are required for delivery of newly synthesized lysosomal hydrolase to the lysosome. Mutations of the gene result in multiple enzyme deficiency (Kornfeld and Sly 2001). Paraffin sections of kidney from patients affected with I-cell disease show staining with ConA, WGA and S-WGA suggesting storage of sialylated, N-linked oligosaccharides (Castagnaro et al. 1987b).

Mucolipidosis IV is a rare neurodegenerative lysosomal storage disease due to mutation of MCOLN1 that encodes the transient receptor mucolipin (TRPML1), which is lysosomal ion channel permeable to cations (Coblentz et al. 2014). Lectin histochemistry of paraffin section showed only light staining of neuronswith ConA. In contrast, frozen sections of brain, liver and kidney stained positively with several lectins including ConA, RCA-I, LCA, WGA and PNA (Fig. 9, Folkerth et al. 1995).

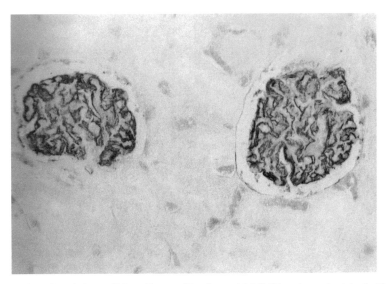

Figure 9. Frozen section of renal glomeruli from 21-year-old patients with ML IV are intensely stained with PNA, whereas tubular, endothelial and blood cells are not.

Sphingolipidoses

These disorders are also known as glycolipid storage diseases. In this group of diseases, deficient enzyme activity or deficient activator protein activity results in aberrant sphingolipid catabolism which result in lysosomal storage of lipids, glycolipids, glycoproteins and oligosaccharides. The cellular storage of oligosaccharides in tissues that were embedded in paraffin sections can be demonstrated in patients with fucosidosis (Fig. 8). Oligosaccharides can also be demonstrated both on frozen and paraffin sections as seen in spleen of a child with type I Gaucher's disease (Figs. 6 and 7, DeGasperi et al. 1990). Different cell types in mucolipidosis IV are stained differently in frozen sections and paraffin sections. In G_{M1} gangliosidosis there is deficient activity of β-galactosidase which catalyze terminal β-galactosyl residues from glycolipids, glycoproteins and oligosaccharides (Suzuki et al. 2001). In G_{M1} gangliosidosis, paraffin sections from brain of different species stained with different lectins including *Griffonia simplicifolia* agglutinin-I (GS-I) (Fig. 10, Alroy et al. 1988a).

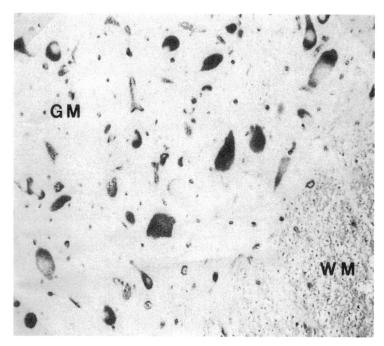

Figure 10. Paraffin section of cerebrum from a dog with G$_{M1}$ gangliosidosis revealing gray matter (GM) and white matter (WM). The neurons and the endothelial cells are strongly stained with *Griffonia simplicifolia* agglutinin GS-I.

G$_{M2}$ gangliosidosis is a group of 3 different lysosomal storage diseases. Tay-Sachs disease is due to deficient activity of the α-subunit of β-hexosaminidase (Hex A), Sandhoff disease is due to deficient activity of the β-subunit (Hex A+B) and Prosaposin Deficiency Disease is a deficiency of saposin A activity which is a G$_{M2}$ activator protein (Gravel et al. 2001). In Tay-Sachs disease, frozen and paraffin sections of brain stain with different lectins including peanut agglutinin PNA (Fig. 11, Alroy et al. 1988b).

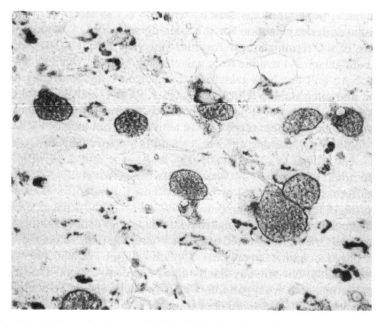

Figure 11. Section of cerebral cortex from 2-year-old child with Tay-Sachs disease showing meganeurons stained with peanut agglutinin (PNA).

Similar frozen and paraffin sections of brain from patient with Sandhoff disease stain strongly with ConA and UEA-I while visceral cells, astrocytes and macrophages are stained with S-WGA (Fig. 12, Alroy et al. 1988).

In Krabbe's disease there is storage of galactosylceramide which is the major constituent of myelin and it affects the white matter (Wenger et al. 2001). Morphologically it is characterized by demyelination and the presence of globoid cells around blood vessels. Lectin staining of paraffin sections of brain from human, cats, dogs, and twitcher mice revealed that only S-WGA stains positively in all these species (Figs. 13 and 14, Alroy et al. 1986a) but some lectins like PNA could stain in other species.

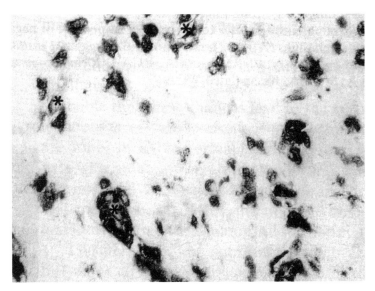

Figure 12. Paraffin section of cerebral cortex from 2 and 1/2-year-old boy with Sandhoff disease revealing macrophages, microglial and endothelial cells stained with succinylated-WGA (S-WGA).

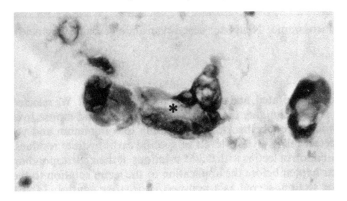

Figure 13. Paraffin section of the white matter of 18-month-old girl with Krabbe's Disease showing perivascular (asterisk) infiltration of macrophages positively stained with succinylated-WGA (S-WGA).

Fabry disease is caused by deficient activity of α-galactosidase, which results in lysosomal storage of glycosphingolipids with terminal a-galactosyl residues (Desnick et al. 2001). Lectin histochemistry of unfixed frozen sections of kidney stain with RCA-I and BS-I, but corresponding paraffin sections are negative (Faraggiana et al. 1981) indicating storage of glycosphingolipid. Epon embedded sections of the eccrine glands from skin biopsy stain with RCA-I and GS-I indicating the storage of glycosphingolipids with terminal α-galactosyl and β-galactosyl residues (Kanda et al. 2000). Storage of free sialic acid is

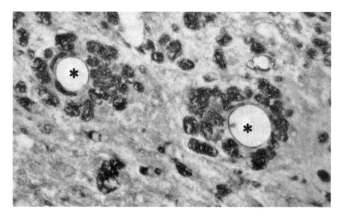

Figure 14. Paraffin section of brain from 39-week-old dog with Krabbe's disease. White matter is infiltrated with macrophages which form perivascular (asterisk) packets of cells. The cytoplasm of the macrophages is stained with succinylated-WGA (S-WGA).

due to malfunction of the lysosomal transporter membrane protein, sialin, which exports free sialic acid from lysosomes (Kleta et al. 2003). Storage of free sialic acid was demonstrated with WGA (Fig. 15, Pueschel et al. 1988).

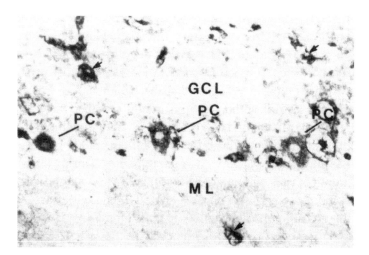

Figure 15. Paraffin section of the cerebellum from a child with infantile sialic acid storage disease illustrating a granular cell layer (GCL) and a molecular cell layer (MCL). The Purkinje cells (PC) and the vascular endothelium (arrows) are slightly enlarged and are intensely stained with wheat germ agglutinin (WGA).

Neuronal Ceroid Lipofuscinosis (NCL)

This is a group of 13 different diseases (Cotman et al. 2013). The hallmark of NCL is the histopathologic finding of lysosomal autofluorescent lipopigments "aging pigment" in brain and other tissues (Hofmann and Peltonen 2001). The neurons in patients with infantile lysosomal storage disease that is associated with osteopetrosisis characterized by storage of both carbohydrate and lipids in neurons. Lectin histochemistry highlight the accumulation of oligosaccharides containing β- and α-galactosyl residues (Fig. 16, Alroy et al. 1995).

Infantile lysosomal storage disease associated with osteopetrosis is a very rare disease. It is due to mutations in CLCN7 (Pangrazio et al. 2010). Paraffin sections of brains stained with luxol fast blue revealed the storage of glycolipid presence, and staining with lectins including *Griffonia simplicifolia*-I (GS-I) (Fig. 17, Alroy et al. 1994) revealed storage of oligosaccharides.

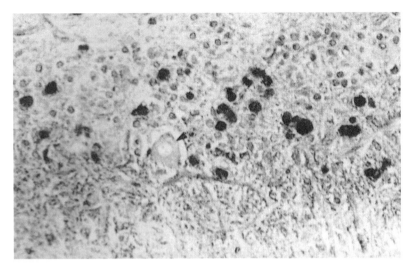

Figure 16. Paraffin section of atrophic cerebellum of dog with neuronal ceroid lipofuscinosis stained with *Dolichos biflorus* agglutinin (DBA). The glial cells are DBA-positive, but Purkinje cells and glial cells are unstained.

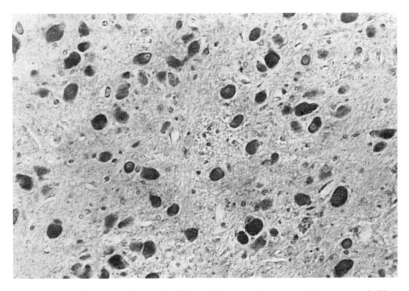

Figure 17. Photomicrograph of brain from 2-month-old boy with neuronal storage with osteopetrosis illustrating neuronal staining with *Griffonia simplicifolia*-I (GS-I).

Conclusions

As indicated in this review, lectins are useful in characterizing glycoconjugates such as glycolipids in frozen sections and glycoproteins in paraffin sections in the cells and tissues of mammals with storage diseases. During epithelial cell differentiation, proliferation and malignant transformation, the structure and composition of their cellular glycoconjugates are known to vary. Using the described methodology, one is able to follow such changes histologically. In addition, the role that glycoconjugates may play at sites of protozoan parasite infection can also be followed by lectin histochemistry. The use of lectins as probes have an especially important role in the diagnosis of lysosomal storage diseases and in understanding of the clinical manifestations of these disorders such as cloudy cornea, skeletal abnormalities and dysmyelogenesis that can result from the faulty recycling of glycoconjugates.

Keywords: Lectin Glycoconjugate, Lectin histochemistry, Lysosomal storage diseases

References

Alroy, J., F. C. Zoaka, J. A. Heaney and A. A. Ucci. 1982. Lectins as a probe for carbohydrate residues in non-neoplastic urothelium of urinary bladder. J Urol 128: 1889–193.

Alroy, J., A. A. Ucci and M. E. A. Periera. 1984a. Lectins: histochemical probes for specific carbohydrate residues. pp. 67–88. *In*: DeLellis, R. A. (ed.). Advance in Immunohistochemistry. Masson Inc., New York.

Alroy, J., U. Orgad, A. A. Ucci and M. E. A. Pereira. 1984b. Identification of glycoprotein storage disease by lectins. A new diagnostic method. J Histochem Cytochem 32: 1280–1294.

Alroy, J., U. Orgad, A. A. Ucci and V. E. Gavris. 1985. Swainsonine toxicosis mimics lectin histochemistry of mannosidosis. Vet Path 22: 311–316.

Alroy, J., A. A. Ucci, V. Goyal and A. Aurilio. 1986a. Histochemical similarities between human and animal globoid cells in Krabbe's disease: Lectin study. Acta Neuropathol 71: 26–31.

Alroy, J., A. A. Ucci, V. Goyal and W. Woods. 1986b. Lectin histochemistry of glycolipid storage diseases on frozen and paraffin-embedded tissue sections. J Histochem Cytochem 34: 501–505.

Alroy, J., V. Goyal and F. Skutelsky. 1987. Lectin histochemistry of mammalian endothelium. Histochemistry 86: 603–607.

Alroy, J., V. Goyal and C. D. Warren. 1988a. Lectin histochemistry of gangliosidosis. I. Neural tissue in four mammalian species. Acta Neuropathol 76: 109–114.

Alroy, J., L. S. Adelman and C. D. Warren. 1988b. Lectin histochemistry of gangliosidosis II. Neurovisceral tissues from patients with Sandhoff's disease. Acta Neuropathol 76: 359–365.

Alroy, J., A. A. Ucci and M. E. A. Periera. 1988c. Lectin histochemistry. pp. 93–131. *In*: DeLellis, R. A. (ed.). An Update Advance in Immunohistochemistry. Raven Press, New York.

Alroy, J., V. Goyal, N. W. L. Lukacs, R. L. Taylor, R. G. Strout, H. D. Ward et al. 1989. Glycoconjugates of the intestinal epithelium of the domestic fowl (Gallus domesticus): A lectin histochemistry study. Histochemical J 21: 187–193.

Alroy, J., R. De Gasperi and C. D. Warren. 1991. Application of lectin histochemistry and carbohydrate analysis to the characterization of lysosomal storage diseases. Carbohydrate Res 213: 229–250.

Alroy, J., M. Castagnaro, E. Skutelsky and I. Lomakina. 1994. Lectin histochemistry of infantile lysosomal storage associated with osteopetrosis. Acta Neuropathol 87: 594–597.

Alroy, J., M. Castagnaro, J. P. McCoy, D. Brum, A. Sisson, P. F. Daniel et al. 1995. Neuronal ceroid lipofuscinoses disease in Australian Blue Heelers: clinical, morphological and histochemical studies. Eur J Vet Pathol 1: 61–68.

Alroy, J., R. Pfannl and A. A. Ucci. 2013. Electron microscopy as a useful tool in the diagnosis of lysosomal storage diseases. pp. 237–267. *In*: Stirling, J. W., A. Curry and B. Eyden (eds.). Diagnostic Electron Microscopy: A Practical Guide to Interpretation and Technique. A John Wiley & Sons Ltd.

Alroy, J. and J. A. Lyons. 2014. Lysosomal storage diseases. Inborn Errors of Metabolism & Screening 1–20.

Alroy, J., C. Garganta and G. Wiederschain. 2014. Secondary biochemical and morphological consequences in lysosomal storage diseases. Biochemistry (Moscow) 79: 782–801.

Aula, N., A. Jalanko, P. Aula and L. Peltonen. 2002. Unraveling the molecular pathogenesis of free sialic acid storage disorders: Altered targeting of mutant sialin. Molecular Genetics and Metabolism 77: 99–107.

Avila, J. L. and J. Convit. 1975. Inhibition of leucocytic lysosomal enzymes by glycosaminoglycan *in vitro*. The Biochemical Journal 152: 57–64.

Bendavid, C., R. Kleta, R. Long, M. Ouspenskaia, M. Muenk, B. R. Haddad et al. 2004. Fish diagnosis of the common 57-kb deletion in CTNS causing cystinosis. Hum Genet 115: 510–514.

Boustany, R. M. N. 2013. Lysosomal storage diseases-the horizon expands. Nat Rev Neurol 9: 583–598.

Boyd, W. C. 1963. The lectin: The present status. Vox Sang 8: 1–32.

Brandenstein, D. S., M. M. Rodrigues, J. Alroy and S. Brownstein. 1987. Lectin binding in retinoblastoma. Current Eye Research 6: 1141–1150.

Castagnaro, M., J. Alroy, A. A. Ucci and R. H. Glew. 1987a. Lectin histochemistry of feline kidneys from six different storage diseases. Virchows Arch B 54: 16–26.

Castagnaro, M., J. Alroy, A. A. Ucci and R. Jaffe. 1987b. Lectin histochemistry and ultrastructure of kidneys from patients with I-cell disease. Arch Pathol Lab Med 111: 285–290.

Coblentz, J., C. S. T. Croix and K. Kiselvov. 2014. Loss of TRPML1 promotes production of reactive oxygen species: Is oxidative damage a factor in mucolipidosis IV? Biochem J 457: 361–368.

Cotman, S. L., A. Karaa, J. F. Staropoli and K. B. Sims. 2013. Neuronal ceroid lipofucinosis: Impact of recent genetic advances and expansion of the clinicopathologic spectrum. Curr Neurol Neurosci Rep. 13(8): 366.

DeGasperi, R., J. Alroy, R. Richard, V. Goyal, U. Orgad, R. E. Lee et al. 1990. Glycoprotein storage in Gaucher's disease: Lectin histochemistry and biochemical studies. Lab Invest 63: 385–393.

Desnick, R. J., A. Y. Ioannou and C. M. Eng. 2001. α-Galactosidase A deficiency: Fabry disease. pp. 3733–3774. *In*: Scriver, C. R., A. L. Beaudet, W. S. Sly, D. Valle, B. Childs, K. W. Kinzler et al. (eds.). The Metabolic and Molecular Basis of Inherited Diseases. Vol. 3, 8th edition, McGraw-Hill, New York.

De Duve, C. 1955. The lysosome turns fifty. Nature Cell Biol 7: 847–849.

Devine, P., A. A. Ucci, H. Krain, V. E. Gravis, J. A. Bhaganvan, J. A. Heaney et al. 1984. Nephrogenic adenoma and embryonic kidney tubules share PNA receptor sites. Am J Clin Path Lab Med 81: 728–732.

Faraggiana, T., J. Churg, E. Grishman, L. Strauss, A. Prado, D. F. Bishop et al. 1981. Light and electron microscopic histochemistry of Fabry's disease. Am J Pathol 103: 247–262.

Fernandez-Valero, E. M., A. Ballart, C. Iturriaga, M. Lluch, J. Macias, M. T. Vanier et al. 2005. Identification of 25 new mutations unrelated Spanish Niemann-Pick C patients genotype-phenotype correlations. Clin Genet 68: 245–254.

Folkerth, R. D., J. Alroy, I. Lomakina, E. Skutelskyy, S. S. Raghavan and E. H. Kolodny. 1995. Mucolipidosis IV: Morphology and histochemistry of an autopsy case. J Neuropathol Exp Neurol l54: 154–164.

Ghazarian, H., B. Idoni and S. B. Oppenheimer. 2011. A glycobiology review: Carbohydrates, lectins and implications in cancer therapeutics. Acta Histochemica 113: 236–247.

Gravel, R. A., M. M. Kaback, R. L. Proid, K. Sandhoff, K. Suzuki and K. Suzuki. 2001. The GM2 gangliosidosis. pp. 3827–3876. *In*: Scriver, C. R., A. L. Beaudet, W. S. Sly, D. Valle, B. Childs, K. W. Kinzler et al. (eds.). The Metabolic & Molecular Bases of Inherited Disease, Vol. 3, 8th edition. McGraw-Hill.

Hofmann, S. L. and L. Peltonen. 2001. The neuronal ceroid lipofuscinosis. pp. 3877–3894. *In*: Scriver, C. R., A. L. Beaudet, W. S. Sly, D. Valle, B. Childs, K. W. Kinzler et al. (eds.). The Metabolic & Molecular Bases of Inherited Disease, Vol. 3, 8 edition. McGraw-Hill, New York.

Huynh, K. K., E. -L. Eskelinen, C. C. Scott, A. Malevanets, P. Saftig and S. Grinstein. 2007. LAMP proteins are required for fusion of lysosomes and phagosomes. EMBO J 28: 313–324.

Kanda, K., S. Nakao, S. Tsuyama, F. Murata and T. Kanzaki. 2000. Fabry disease: Ultrastructural lectin histochemical analysis of lysosomal deposits. Virchows Arch 436: 36–42.

Kleta, R., D. J. Aughton, M. J. Rivkin, M. Huizing, E. Strovel, Y. Anikster et al. 2003. Biochemical and molecular analyses of infantile free sialic acid storage in North American children. Am J Med Genet 120A: 28–33.

Kornfeld, S. and W. S. Sly. 2001. I-cell disease and pseudo-Hurler polydystrophy: Disorders of lysosomal enzyme phosphorylation and localization. pp. 3507–3572. *In*: Scriver, C. R., A. L. Beaudet, W. S. Sly, D. Valle, B. Childs, K. W. Kinzler et al. (eds.). The Metabolic & Molecular Bases of Inherited Disease, Vol. 3, 8th edition. McGrawHill, New York.

Libin, C. M. and C. R. Morales. 2009. The interactomic of sertolin: An ancient lysosomal receptor evolving new functions. Histol Histopathol 24: 481–492.

McNeal, J. E., I. Leav, J. Alroy and E. Skutelsky. 1988. Differential lectin staining of central and peripheral zones of the prostate and alterations in dysplasia. Am J Clin Pathol 89: 41–48.

McNeal, J. E., J. Alroy, A. Villers, E. A. Redwine, F. S. Freiha and T. A. Stamey. 1991. Mucinous differentiation in prostatic adenocarcinoma. Hum Pathol 22: 979–988.

Monserrat, A. J., S. H. Benavides, A. Berra, S. Farina, S. C. Vicario and E. A. Porta. 1995. Lectin histochemistry of lipofuscin and certain ceroid pigments. Histochemistry 103: 435–445.

Moore, R., N. King and J. Alroy. 1988a. Characterization of colonic cellular glycoconjugates in colitis and cancer-prone Tamarins versus colitis and cancer resistant primates. Am J Pathol 131: 477–483.

Moore, R., N. King J. Alroy. 1988b. Modulation of cellular glycoconjugates in quiescent, inflamed and neoplastic colonic epithelium of colitis and cancer-prone Tamarins. Am J Pathol 131: 484–489.

Pangrazio, A., M. Pusch, L. L. Kurland, E. Frattini, E. Lamino, P. M. Tamhankar et al. 2010. Molecular and clinical heterogeneity in CLCN7-dependent osteopetrosis: report of 20 novel mutations. Human Mutation 32: E1071–E1080.

Panjwani, N., M. M. Rodrigues, J. Alroy, D. Albert and J. Baum. 1986a. Alterations in stromal glycoconjugates in macular corneal dystrophy. Invest Ophthalmol Vis Sci 27: 1211–1216.

Panjwani, N., P. Moulton, J. Alroy and J. Baum. 1986b. Localization of lectin binding sites in human, cat and rabbit corneas. Invest Ophthalmol Vis Sci 27: 1280–1284.

Pueschel, S. M., P. A. O'Shea, J. Alroy, M. Ambler, F. Dangond, P. Daniel et al. 1988. Infantile sialic acid storage disease associated with renal disease. Pediat Neurol 4: 207–212.

Saftig, P. and J. Klumperman. 2009. Lysosomal biogenesis and lysosomal membrane proteins: trafficking meets function. Nat Rev Mol Cell Biol 10: 623–635.

Schaumburg-Lever, G., J. Alroy, A. A. Ucci and W. F. Lever. 1984a. Distribution of carbohydrate residues in normal skin. Arch Dermatol Res 276: 216–233.

Schaumburg-Lever, G., J. Alroy, A. A. Ucci, W. F. Lever and C. F. Orfanos, C.E. 1984b. Cell surface carbohydrates in psoriasis. Defective cytoplasmic transport by glycoconjugates carrying fucose residues suggested by lectin staining. J Am Acad Dermatol 11: 1087–1094.

Schaumburg-Lever, G., J. Alroy, A. A. Ucci and W. F. Lever. 1986. Cell surface carbohydrates in proliferative epidermal lesions. II. Masking of peanut agglutinin (PNA) binding sites in solar keratosis, Bowen's disease, and squamous cell carcinoma by neuraminic acid. J Cutaneous Pathology 13: 163–171.

Skutelskey, E., J. Alroy, A. A. Ucci, J. L. Carpenter and F. M. Moore. 1987. Modulation of carbohydrate residues in regenerative nodules and neoplasms of canine and feline pancreas. Am J Pathol 126: 25–32.

Skutelskey, E., S. Hoenig, B. Griffel and J. Alroy. 1988. The distribution of lectin receptor sites in human breast lesions. Path Res and Pract 183: 469–476.

Skutelskey, E., R. P. Moore and J. Alroy. 1989. Lectin histochemistry of mammalian Brunner's glands. Histochemistry 90: 383–390.

Strout, R. G., J. Alroy, N. W. Likacs, H. D. Ward and M. E. A. Pereira. 1994. Developmental regulated lectins in Eimeria species and their role in avian coccidiosis. J Parasitol 80: 946–951.

Suzuki, Y., O. Oshima and E. Nanba. 2001. β-Galactosidase deficiency (β-galactosidosis): GM1 galactosidosis and Morquio B Disease. pp. 3775–3826. *In*: Scriver, C. R., A. L. Beaudet, W. S. Sly, D. Valle, B. Childs, K. W. Kinzler et al. (eds.). The Metabolic & Molecular Bases of Inherited Disease, 8th edition, McGrawHill, New York.

Tang, H., P. Hsueh, D. Kletter, M. Bern and B. Haab. 2015. The detection and discovery of glycan motifs in biological samples using lectins and antibodies: new methods and opportunities 126: 167–202.

Thomas, G. H. 2001. Disorders of glycoprotein degradation: α-mannosidosis, β-mannosidosis, fucosidosis, and sialidosis. pp. 3507–3572. *In*: Scriver, C. R., A. L. Beaudet, W. S. Sly, D. Valle, B. Childs, K. W. Kinzler et al. (eds.). The Metabolic & Molecular Bases of Inherited Disease, Vol. 3, 8th edition. McGrawHill, New York.

Ward, H. D., J. Alroy, B. I. Lev, G. T. Keusch and M. E. A. Pereira. 1988. Biology of Giardia Lamblia: Detection of N-Acetyl-D-Glucosamine as the only surface saccharide moiety and identification of two distinct subsets of trophozoites by lectin binding. J Exp Med 167: 73–88.

Weintraub, H., J. Alroy, R. DeGasperi, V. Goyal, E. Skutelskey, P. G. Pentchev et al. 1992. Storage of glycoprotein in NCTR-Balb/C mouse: Lectin histochemistry, and biochemical studies. Virchows Archiv B Cell Pathol 62: 347–352.

Wenger, D. A., K. Suzuki, Y. Suzuki and K. Suzuki. 2001. Galactoceramide lipidosis: Globoid cell leukodystrophy (Krabbe disease). pp. 3669–3694. *In*: Scriver, C. R., A. L. Beaudet, W. S. Sly, D. Valle, B. Childs, K. W. Kinzler et al. (eds.). The Metabolic & Molecular Bases of Inherited Disease, Vol. 3, 8th edition. McGrawHill, New York.

Zeevi, D. A., A. Frunkin and G. Bach. 2007. TRPML and lysosomal function. Biochimica et Biophysica Acta 1772: 851–858.

CHAPTER 7

Computational Approaches for Studying Carbohydrate-Lectin Interactions in Infection

Tamir Dingjan,[1,a] Elizabeth Yuriev[1,b],* and Paul A. Ramsland[2],*

Introduction

Bacterial infection typically begins by the pathogen adhering to host tissue through the action of one or more cell-surface molecules called adhesins (Ofek and Doyle 1994). Adhesion permits the bacterium to withstand tissue cleansing processes, enhances access to local nutrients, and allows wandering pathogens to begin colonization. Bacterial adhesins recognize a variety of host tissues through interactions with different cell-surface targets. One important group of targets for bacterial adhesins are saccharides (glycans) that are displayed on a wide range of host glycoproteins and glycolipids. Carbohydrate-binding adhesins are often referred to as lectins as they contain one or more carbohydrate-binding (or lectin type) domains. Among the many carbohydrate tissue determinants, human blood group and related saccharides are known targets for bacterial adhesion of important human bacterial pathogens (examples of bacterial pathogens that recognize blood group related glycans are *Helicobacter pylori* (Lindén et al. 2008, Ishijima et al. 2011), *Escherichia coli* (Lund et al. 1987, Hung et al. 2002), and *Pseudomonas aeruginosa* (Gilboagarber et al. 1994, Chemani et al. 2009)). The role of carbohydrate binding by bacterial lectins in respiratory infection is illustrated in Fig. 1.

The A, B and H/O blood group determinants are expressed not only on red blood cells, but also on many epithelial surfaces in the body including the respiratory, urinary and gastrointestinal tracts (Ravn and Dabelsteen 2000). Similarly, the Lewis blood and tissue group carbohydrates (Le^a, Le^b, Le^x, and Le^y) are expressed in several healthy tissues, which are important sites of bacterial colonization and infection (Sakamoto et al. 1986). With respect to bacterial lectin recognition, the blood group related glycans are normally displayed at the ends of longer carbohydrate chains attached to glycoproteins or glycolipids, but are defined by saccharide molecular structures or determinants (Fig. 2), which can be selectively recognised by antibodies and lectins (Dingjan et al. 2015).

[1] Monash Institute of Pharmaceutical Sciences, Monash University, Parkville, VIC 3052, Australia.
[a] E-mail: tamir.dingjan@monash.edu
[b] E-mail: elizabeth.yuriev@monash.edu
[2] Centre for Biomedical Research, Burnet Institute, Melbourne, VIC 3004, Australia.
  E-mail: pramsland@burnet.edu.au
* Corresponding authors

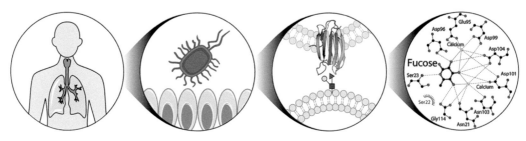

Figure 1. Schematic diagram of carbohydrate-lectin interactions in respiratory infection.

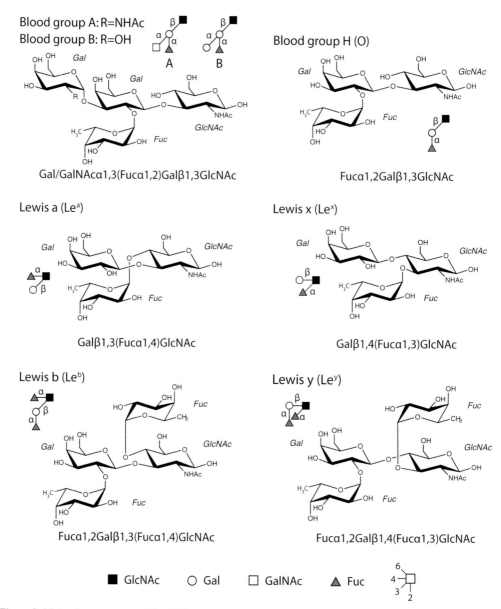

Figure 2. Molecular structures of the ABO and Lewis blood group determinants, shown with linear and schematic representations. The cartoon represents the monosaccharides of each blood group determinant with glycosidic attachment positions shown by the line angle according to the key. Anomeric configurations are labelled α or β.

Structural and biophysical characterization of bacterial lectin binding interactions with host carbohydrates is often used to rationalize the observed patterns of infectivity, and can be useful for the structure-based development of anti-adhesive molecules as potential anti-infectives. For defining the three-dimensional structures of protein-carbohydrate complexes, the main experimental techniques are X-ray crystallography and NMR spectroscopy (Poveda and Jimenez-Barbero 1998, Kogelberg et al. 2003, Roldos et al. 2011, del Carmen Fernandez-Alonso et al. 2012, Koharudin and Gronenborn 2012). More recently, glycan array profiling has also emerged as a valuable tool to determine the structural features of carbohydrate determinants that are critical for bacterial lectin binding to host glycans (Taylor and Drickamer 2009, Campbell and Gildersleeve 2011, Van Damme et al. 2011, Song et al. 2012, Hirabayashi et al. 2013, Kletter et al. 2013). However, carbohydrates remain challenging targets to characterize using only experimental methods. For example, the conformational flexibility and repeating structures of oligosaccharides can confound NMR analysis, a technique which depends on averaging of conformational states (DeMarco and Woods 2008). Crystallization of carbohydrate-protein complexes and glycoproteins remains a hurdle for X-ray crystallography, but through improvements in methods for crystallization, protein expression and carbohydrate synthesis, progress is still being made (Jeffries et al. 2012). However, perhaps due to the lack of integration between state-of-the-art computational methods and crystallographic structure refinement approaches, there remain significant issues (Agirre et al. 2015) with many of the saccharide structures of carbohydrate-protein crystal structures deposited in the Protein Data Bank (PDB) (Berman et al. 2000). Isolation and synthesis of carbohydrates is another challenge to experimental characterization of carbohydrate-protein complexes, but has been an area of significant progress in recent years (Bertozzi and Kiessling 2001, Boltje et al. 2009, Zulueta et al. 2015). With the advent of glycan-based microarrays, it has been possible to generate significantly more information regarding the specificity and cross-reactivity of carbohydrate-binding proteins (Song et al. 2012). However, interpreting the results of glycan array screens is not without difficulties and factors such as glycan density, effects of spacers, and proximity of the solid support (e.g., glass slides) can all impact on the structure-activity information derived from these binding techniques (Liang and Wu 2009, Taylor and Drickamer 2009, Rillahan and Paulson 2011).

Computational methods provide an alternative approach for the structural characterization of carbohydrate-protein interactions by both complementing and augmenting experimentally determined data (Fig. 3). Computational simulation can illuminate the atomic scale processes that mediate biological behaviour, from the shape of a given carbohydrate in solution to the structural features underlying lectin selectivity and specificity (Woods and Tessier 2010). This information is then directly applicable to the design of lectin-binding molecules. In this chapter, we present a brief explanation of some general features of carbohydrate-protein binding interactions and conformational properties that are relevant to structural predictions by *in silico*, or computational, approaches. We also discuss two complementary computational

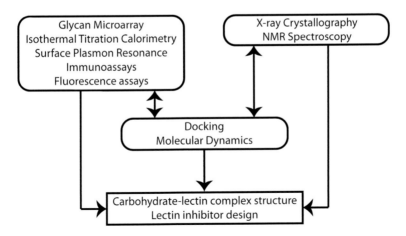

Figure 3. Combining experimental and computational approaches for the characterization of carbohydrate-lectin complexes and the design of lectin inhibitors.

techniques, docking and molecular dynamics (MD) that are frequently used to explore structure-activity relationships of carbohydrate-binding proteins such as bacterial lectins. Finally, we present some key examples illustrating how integrated experimental and computational approaches may be used to dissect the structural basis of bacterial lectin specificity for blood group and related glycans. Such information is critical for understanding the mechanisms of colonization and infection of humans.

For further information on how computational techniques can be used to study carbohydrates and carbohydrate-binding proteins we refer readers to some excellent reviews and book chapters (DeMarco and Woods 2008, Fadda and Woods 2010, Agostino et al. 2012, Sousa et al. 2013, Pérez and Tvaroška 2014, Johnson et al. 2015).

Carbohydrate Binding Interactions

Carbohydrate-protein complexes are held together by multiple intermolecular interactions. Unlike in protein-protein interactions or interactions between proteins and small chemical entities (e.g., traditional drugs and drug-like molecules), hydrogen bonding contributes the majority of the stabilizing forces between a carbohydrate ligand and a lectin. Hydrogen bonds are established either directly between the carbohydrate and the protein or via water-mediation. Hydrophobic CH-π interactions, metal ion coordination, and solvent reordering are also critical factors involved in carbohydrate-lectin interactions. These binding interactions are briefly outlined below as they are important considerations for the prediction of carbohydrate-protein complexes by computational approaches.

Carbohydrates feature many hydroxyl moieties, allowing them to participate in multiple simultaneous hydrogen-bonding interactions. Each hydroxyl group is capable of donating a hydrogen bond via the attached hydrogen atom, while simultaneously receiving one or two hydrogen bonds via the oxygen atom. Hydrogen bonds, donated by lectin residues, usually involve main-chain amide protons, with less frequent participation by side-chain amides (i.e., asparagine and glutamine) (Weis and Drickamer 1996, Dam and Brewer 2007). Binding site acceptors of hydrogen bond interactions are frequently acidic side-chains (i.e., aspartic and glutamic acids). These acidic moieties are planar, allowing them to accept two hydrogen bonds from adjacent carbohydrate hydroxyls simultaneously. Amino acid hydroxyl groups (i.e., tyrosine, serine, and threonine side-chains) are not frequently involved in hydrogen bond interactions, suggesting that the entropic cost to restrict their motion outweighs the stabilization value of the hydrogen bond (Weis and Drickamer 1996, Dam and Brewer 2007).

The balancing act between entropic and enthalpic contributions to binding is relevant to the role of structured water molecules. Before formation of the complex, both saccharide and binding site are coated in a layer of structured water molecules, held in position by hydrogen bonds (Lemieux 1996, Hummer 2010). Upon carbohydrate binding, these water molecules are either displaced by the incoming ligand or incorporated into the binding interactions as hydrogen bond mediators. The fate of bound water molecules depends on the balance between the entropic benefit that accompanies their removal to bulk solvent, and the enthalpic cost to dislodge them from the binding site (Michel et al. 2009).

As discussed, the extensive hydrogen bonding interactions found in carbohydrate-protein complexes are accomplished by the many polar hydroxyl groups which commonly adorn saccharides. However, the orientations of these polar moieties also create hydrophobic zones on carbohydrates, allowing non-polar interactions with protein residues. These often take the form of hydrophobic stacking between the apolar face of a monosaccharide unit and an aromatic amino acid side-chain (e.g., tryptophan, phenylalanine, and tyrosine) in the lectin binding site (Dam and Brewer 2007). Interactions with aliphatic side-chains are rarely seen, indicating that most hydrophobic interactions are of the CH-π type, in which the slightly electropositive saccharide aliphatic protons closely associate with the electronegative delocalized π-electrons (Gabius 1998).

The glycosidic bonds linking saccharides are an important and unique structural feature of carbohydrates. The high degree of variability in glycosidic linkages (anomeric state, dihedral angle, and attachment position) increases the density with which biological signals can be encoded. Branched glycan structures far surpass the complexity obtained with linear biological oligomers such as proteins and DNA (Gabius 2008). In addition to the branching and attachment positions within oligosaccharide structures, the conformations around glycosidic linkages are an important feature. The dihedral angles occupied by glycosidic linkages are influenced by the anomeric and exoanomeric electronic effects. The anomeric effect refers to the preference observed for electronegative anomeric substituents to occupy an axial position, rather than the sterically preferred equatorial geometry (Miljkovic 2010). The prevailing explanation for this effect is that of hyperconjugation between the C1-O5 and C1-O1 (Vila and Mosquera 2007). The exoanomeric effect similarly arises from interactions between the glycosidic linkage ether oxygen (O1) and the ring oxygen (O5), resulting in preferences for certain torsion angles around the O5-C1-O1-C_x dihedral (Miljkovic 2010) (also termed the φ-angle). Lastly, the gauche effect controls the orientation around the O5-C5-C6-O6 dihedral. Electrostatic and solvent interactions cause a preference for a gauche orientation of O6 and O5 (Kirschner and Woods 2001). Thus, carbohydrates are complex biological molecules with unique properties that are important to consider when making predictions about their structure. The handling of glycosidic dihedral angles by modelling approaches is a key requirement for accuracy (Nivedha et al. 2014).

Computational Modelling of Carbohydrate-Lectin Complexes

Carbohydrate-lectin modelling is used to predict how saccharides are bound by lectins and to investigate the binding forces operating in the complexes. These insights can suggest structural mechanisms that explain observed binding properties. For example, the thermodynamic aspects of carbohydrate-lectin binding, which can be determined by calorimetry, can be structurally rationalized as the combination of intermolecular interactions (including water-mediated hydrogen bonding networks) and the hydrophobic effect caused by the expulsion of water molecules from the binding site during binding. Lectin selectivity measured by glycan arrays can potentially be explained based on computational predictions of favourable binding interactions between the lectin and each saccharide in the array. Importantly, when experimental observations are effectively combined with modelling insights, the resultant understanding of carbohydrate recognition can guide the structure-based design of lectin inhibitors.

To allow the modelling of carbohydrate-lectin complexes, the binding interactions and conformational properties outlined above (section "Carbohydrate binding interactions") are represented as mathematical functions termed molecular mechanics force fields. Both modelling methods described in this chapter, docking and molecular dynamics, make use of force fields to simulate carbohydrate-lectin complexes. Both docking and MD can be used to examine the structural and dynamic aspects of carbohydrate-lectin recognition (section "Molecular modelling of bacterial lectin-carbohydrate complexes").

Molecular Mechanics Force Fields

In a carbohydrate-lectin complex, intermolecular interactions and structural geometries of the binding partners contribute to the total potential energy of the complex. The combined set of mathematical functions describing the energy of a system (the force field) is integral to most modelling methods. The general form of a force field, accompanied by the relevant carbohydrate-protein structural features, is shown in Fig. 4.

Force fields use the coordinates, distances and angles of a system's atomic structures with parameters derived experimentally or by quantum calculation to give the potential energy of the system. In the general force field form shown in Fig. 4, the first three terms describe the potential energy related to the positions of bonded atoms, and the final two terms define the potential energy derived from the positions of non-bonded atoms which interact through space. The bond and angle terms describe the energy of the system's bond lengths l_i and bond angles θ_i as they deviate from equilibrium values l_{i0} and θ_{i0}. The torsional term represents potential energy of rotation around bonds (dihedral angle ω_j) as a periodic function with periodicity n and phase γ_i. The non-bonded terms describe interactions between atoms i and j, separated by distance r_{ij}. The van der Waals interactions are represented as a Lennard-Jones potential with σ_{ij} and ε denoting the ideal distance and the depth of the potential well, respectively. The Coulomb term describes charge-based interactions between the atoms with charges represented by q_i and q_j. Selected energetic terms are tuned or scaled by force constants (a_i, b_i, c_i, and k).

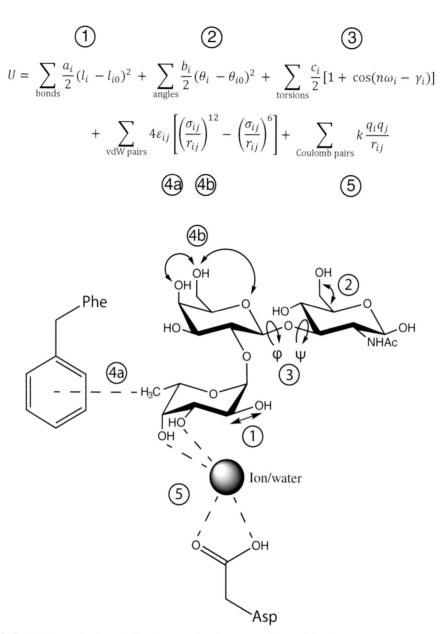

$$U = \sum_{\text{bonds}} \frac{a_i}{2}(l_i - l_{i0})^2 + \sum_{\text{angles}} \frac{b_i}{2}(\theta_i - \theta_{i0})^2 + \sum_{\text{torsions}} \frac{c_i}{2}[1 + \cos(n\omega_i - \gamma_i)]$$

$$+ \sum_{\text{vdW pairs}} 4\varepsilon_{ij}\left[\left(\frac{\sigma_{ij}}{r_{ij}}\right)^{12} - \left(\frac{\sigma_{ij}}{r_{ij}}\right)^6\right] + \sum_{\text{Coulomb pairs}} k\frac{q_i q_j}{r_{ij}}$$

Figure 4. General form of a force field with examples of corresponding carbohydrate structural features. 1. Bond stretching; 2. Angle fluctuation; 3. Torsional rotation around bonds, with specific glycosidic torsions labelled (φ – O5-C1-O1-C$_x$; ψ – C1-O1-C$_x$-C$_{x-1}$); 4a. van der Waals interactions in CH-π bonds; 4b. van der Waals interactions between neighbouring atoms; 5. Charge-mediated attraction forces, here exemplified by ion- or water-mediated interactions.

Due to unique interaction patterns, carbohydrates are challenging to model. The high number of chiral centres, flexibility inherent to glycosidic linkages and ring conformations, and subtle electronic features all add to the complexity of carbohydrate simulation. Nevertheless, force fields accurately describing the atomic behaviour and properties of carbohydrates have been developed. For more in-depth comparisons, see (Xiong et al. 2015) and (Fadda and Woods 2010).

The most commonly used force fields specifically developed for carbohydrates (OPLS-AA-SEI, GROMOS 53A6$_{\text{GLYC}}$, CHARMM36 and GLYCAM06) aim to accurately represent carbohydrates in complex with proteins and other biomolecules (Foley et al. 2012). These four force fields are similarly accurate in their descriptions of saccharide conformations and properties and differ mostly by the range of modifications or alternate sugars they can describe (Hemmingsen et al. 2004, Stortz et al. 2009). The OPLS-AA-SEI parameter set accurately reproduces calculated relative energies for gluco-, manno-, and galactopyranose, but has not yet been applied to the wider assortment of saccharides (Kony et al. 2002). The GROMOS53A6$_{GLYC}$ force field carbohydrate parameters currently describe unbranched hexopyranoses of mono- to oligosaccharide size (Pol-Fachin et al. 2012), and has been extended to include glycoprotein torsional parameters (Pol-Fachin et al. 2014). However, amino sugars, sialic acids, and other sugar derivatives are not included (Hansen and Hünenberger 2011). CHARMM36 includes the main pyranoses and furanoses in both anomeric states with all glycosidic linkages, but only supports D enantiomers (Guvench et al. 2011). Parameters for carbohydrates linked to phosphate and sulfate functional groups are also included (Mallajosyula et al. 2012). A recent addition to the CHARMM force field includes Drude polarization, allowing bonds to be represented as dynamic dipoles rather than partial charges (Patel et al. 2015). Application to the simulation of carbohydrates showed increased accuracy for the calculation of conformational energies and the reproduction of crystallographic structures (Vanommeslaeghe and MacKerell 2015). GLYCAM06 presents the most widely applicable parameter set, allowing the description of most saccharides in α or β anomers, D or L enantiomers and all possible glycosidic linkage positions and torsions (Kirschner et al. 2008). Usability is enhanced by an online interface (Woods 2005) for the construction of carbohydrate molecules. For the simulation of protein-carbohydrate complexes, GLYCAM06 paired with AMBER99SB is a frequently used combination (Fadda and Woods 2010, Sapay et al. 2013).

Force fields for other aspects of carbohydrate simulation are also available. The MM3 force field (Allinger et al. 1989) is commonly used to determine conformational energies of glycosidic linkages (Mendonca et al. 2002, Stortz and French 2008). The Martini coarse-grained force field has been extended to include carbohydrates, and is suitable for the simulation of phase behaviour in lipid-aqueous systems (Lopez et al. 2009). A coarse-grained force field specifically for long glycosaminoglycans has also been recently reported (Samsonov et al. 2015). However, these approximations are not suitable for studying atomic-level details in carbohydrate-protein complexes.

Docking

Docking is an efficient modelling method used to predict bound protein-ligand complex structures. To do this, different ligand conformations are explored and placed in the protein binding site, resulting in docked "poses". The binding energy of each of these associations is evaluated using an appropriate "scoring" function, and the complexes are ranked accordingly. In this way, docking predicts valuable information: the conformations and relative orientations of the protein and ligand and an estimation of the energetic favourability of multiple arrangements (Yuriev et al. 2011). Docking programs abound, although the majority of published docking experiments are performed by three programs: AutoDock, GOLD and Glide (Yuriev and Ramsland 2013).

The main strength of docking methods is their speed; many thousands of docked poses can be produced in a single day using readily available computational resources. This speed in predicting ligand-protein complexes makes docking the method of choice for rapidly evaluating vast libraries of potential ligands (Lionta et al. 2014, Yuriev et al. 2015). However, this speed results from a number of approximations in the representation of proteins and ligands, mainly relating to the choice of method used to handle flexibility and scoring. Until recently, proteins have been typically treated rigidly in docking, without exploring the motion of binding site amino acid side-chains or larger motions of the backbone. While including protein flexibility can benefit docking accuracy in multiple scenarios (Sotriffer 2011, Lill 2011), no clear suggestions for best practice have yet been established (Yuriev et al. 2015). Similarly, the calculation of the potential energy of docked poses (i.e., scoring) is also a recognized challenge. While docking programs can generally produce correct geometries, they are not as capable when ranking or comparing poses on energetic terms (Warren et al. 2006, Plewczynski et al. 2011). Scoring functions can be based on force fields, but they must also be able to deal with solvation and entropic effects in a manner applicable to a wide range of systems (Yuriev and Ramsland 2013). Scoring functions are constrained by the overarching requirement for high speed calculation, imposing simplifications that can limit accuracy (Sousa et al. 2013).

Recent developments incorporating empirical data or higher levels of quantum theory continue to address and improve docking scoring functions (Yuriev et al. 2015).

Similar to described above, carbohydrate docking is faced with several unique challenges. Specifically, predicting carbohydrate ring conformations is difficult. Many hexopyranoses prefer $^4C_1$ chair conformations, but selected monosaccharides such as fucose and mannose occupy a $^1C_4$ conformation. The CH-π interactions formed between aromatic amino acids and aliphatic carbohydrate protons are poorly modelled, despite contributing significantly to binding. The involvement of bound water molecules in mediating binding interactions is not handled well or is often ignored by docking procedures. The high degree of flexibility inherent to oligosaccharide molecules (multiple rotatable hydroxyl groups and glycosidic torsions) presents barriers to thorough conformational sampling. Finally, the subtle electronic effects that influence carbohydrate conformation around glycosidic bonds (the anomeric, exoanomeric, and gauche effects) are generally not considered, to the detriment of docking accuracy.

Current developments in carbohydrate docking are beginning to answer these challenges. Energy gains or losses associated with carbohydrate stereoelectronic effects can be applied to docked poses (Nivedha et al. 2014). By filtering for inappropriate glycosidic torsion angles, unrealistic docked poses can be rejected and higher docking accuracy attained. In more simple approaches, appropriate torsion angles can be selected post-docking. Vetting of docked carbohydrate glycosidic torsion angles can be done by comparison to established favourable values (Yuriev et al. 2008, Agostino et al. 2010, Nurisso et al. 2010, Topin et al. 2013).

While the involvement of water molecules in carbohydrate-lectin binding is best investigated using MD simulation in explicit solvent environments, docking methods can also factor in some of the effects of solvation. In a study of *Escherichia coli* heat-labile enterotoxin (a galactoside-binding protein containing multiple lectin domains), Minke et al. (1999) reported increased docking accuracy when including high-occupancy crystallographic waters and GRID-predicted waters in the protein structure. Samsonov et al. (2011) extended this method to glycosaminoglycan-protein complexes, demonstrating slight improvements to docking performance across multiple docking programs. A different approach by Gauto et al. (2013) involved modification of the AutoDock scoring function to represent regions of high water density at the protein surface, rather than specify explicit water molecules. Similar modifications to the DOCK scoring function account for the displacement of water molecules by carbohydrates in docking (Sun et al. 2014). Finally, prediction of carbohydrate hydroxyl oxygen positions based on binding site solvent structure in the unliganded state has also been shown to improve the quality of docking predictions (Modenutti et al. 2015). While these adjustments to docking methods do not fully incorporate a solvent environment, docking procedures have shown a promising capacity to at minimum handle the structural contributions of solvation in carbohydrate-protein interactions.

An important consideration for docking is the validation of the method against known structures to determine the potential quality of predictions of unknown ligand-protein systems. Docking validation studies cover a range of research questions. Several investigations have addressed database-spanning multi-program analyses (Warren et al. 2006, Hartshorn et al. 2007, Cross et al. 2009, Plewczynski et al. 2011). Further, docking programs have been applied to and validated for specific ligand-protein complex types such as carbohydrate-antibody (Yuriev et al. 2008, Agostino et al. 2009, 2011a) and carbohydrate-lectin (Nurisso et al. 2008, Agostino et al. 2011b). Other studies have focussed on individual proteins, for example, glycogen phosphorylase (Alexacou et al. 2008), *Ralstonia solanacearum* lectin (Mishra et al. 2012), and *Escherichia coli* FimH (Sperling et al. 2006). Validation is typically accomplished by comparing docked pose output to crystallographic structures, using the numerical geometric root-mean-square-distance (RMSD) measure. However, RMSD alone can reject correct poses that differ geometrically from the crystallographic structure; considering binding site interactions as a co-measure of docking accuracy is therefore recommended (Kroemer et al. 2004, Agostino et al. 2009).

Carbohydrate-protein docking can be accurately performed using generally applicable docking software. GLIDE (Friesner et al. 2004, Halgren et al. 2004, Friesner et al. 2006) consistently ranks highly in docking validation studies (Nurisso et al. 2008, Agostino et al. 2009, 2011b), closely followed by AutoDock (Morris et al. 2009). Carbohydrate docking validation studies have revealed that the highest scored pose is frequently not the most accurate. The "scoring problem" is one of the most persistent challenges to docking methods, and multiple strategies have been proposed to overcome it (Yuriev et al. 2015). One such method is to tune the scoring function to perform accurately on a specific target, and software designed specifically for carbohydrate-protein docking in this way does exist. SLICK (Sugar-Lectin Interactions and Docking) (Kerzmann et al. 2006) is a scoring function including a carbohydrate-specific CH-π term. Implemented in the Biochemical Algorithms Library as BALLDock/SLICK, the program has been shown to accurately generate and score carbohydrate-lectin complexes (Kerzmann et al. 2008, Hildebrandt et al. 2010).

Molecular Dynamics

Molecular Dynamics is a simulation method that applies Newton's laws of motion to atoms to calculate their motion over time. MD allows the study of dynamic molecular events, including protein conformational motions, ligand recognition, and ion transport (Dror et al. 2012).

MD simulations begin with the coordinates of an atomic system, such as may be obtained experimentally from X-ray crystallography and NMR spectroscopy or theoretically from template-based (homology) modelling, fold recognition, docking, and other modelling approaches. These coordinates are then placed in an explicit solvent environment and prepared for simulation by a series of minimization and equilibration calculations. At the start of the MD simulation, the initial forces and accelerations of each atom are calculated using a force field. By specifying a temperature and pressure, the initial velocities can be assigned, and the system's motion simulated for a short time, typically at the single femtosecond scale. After this time period, the velocities are recalculated for the updated positions; simulation then iterates until reaching the specified total duration. The length of the timestep is enforced by the need to capture the fastest motion in the system, usually the vibration of C-H bonds (Leach 2001).

Simulations must be long enough to include the behaviour under investigation in statistically relevant frequencies; this can be achieved by combining lengthy durations with replicate simulations. For this reason, classical MD is computationally intensive and is acutely limited by available computational resources. Current typical hardware can feasibly achieve simulation durations up to a microsecond for an average carbohydrate-protein complex. More advanced forms of MD, such as simulated annealing (Yi et al. 1991), replica exchange (Zhang et al. 2005), and metadynamics (Sutto et al. 2012) explore the energetics of the system more thoroughly, reducing the duration required for comprehensive sampling.

MD simulations usually employ an explicit solvent environment of atomistic water, allowing investigation into the dynamic role of water in carbohydrate-protein complexes. The displacement of water molecules from protein binding sites contributes significantly to ligand affinity (Michel et al. 2009, Hummer 2010), especially for carbohydrate-lectin complexes (Modenutti et al. 2015), which frequently exchange bound water molecules for carbohydrate hydroxyl groups at the same locations (Gauto et al. 2013). By identifying regions of water binding, probable locations for carbohydrate hydroxyl groups in the bound complex can be predicted. MD is well-suited for the identification of water sites due to the presence of explicit solvent molecules and has been successfully applied to the task (Li and Lazaridis 2005, Gauto et al. 2009, 2011). The role of water as an interaction mediator in carbohydrate-protein complexes can also be effectively analysed using MD simulation, and is mostly achieved by using radial pair distributions to determine proximity to carbohydrate hydroxyls (Andersson and Balling Engelsen 1999, Corzana et al. 2004, Reynolds et al. 2008, Sauter and Grafmuller 2015). More complex analyses consider additional factors, such as the lifetimes of water-mediated hydrogen bonds (Jana and Bandyopadhyay 2012). The presence of an atomistic, explicit solvent body in MD simulations allows detailed analysis of the role of water, both as an interaction mediator and displaced molecule.

Molecular Modelling of Bacterial Lectin-Carbohydrate Complexes

As mentioned above, bacterial lectins often bind to human blood group carbohydrates during infection. The binding interactions can be studied using a variety of biophysical assay methods (e.g., glycan arrays, isothermal titration calorimetry, STD-NMR, fluorescence spectroscopy) and structural techniques (X-ray crystallography, NMR spectroscopy). The information gained from these experiments characterizes the binding behaviour and static structure of the bound complex. Subsequent investigation into the structural basis for the observed binding calls for computational modelling using the methods presented above. In this section, a number of modelling studies are discussed, which illustrate the application of these methods to lectin-blood group carbohydrate complexes for three bacterial lectins: *P. aeruginosa* lectins LecA (PA-IL) and LecB (PA-IIL), and *Burkholderia ambifaria* lectin BambL (Table 1). These lectins bind fucosylated human blood group antigens, facilitating bacterial adhesion to human respiratory epithelia. Blood group selectivity has been determined for these lectins using a combination of biophysical assays, and crystallographic structures have been solved in complex with multiple human blood group saccharides. Modelling studies investigating various aspects of blood group binding are shown in Table 1.

Table 1. Binding and computational characterization of selected bacterial lectins.

Research purpose	Computational method	Reference
Burkholderia ambifaria BambL (blood groups: H, Le^y)		(Audfray et al. 2012)
to investigate recognition of fucosylated blood group saccharides	Docking (Glide)	(Topin et al. 2013)
Pseudomonas aeruginosa PA-IL/LecA (blood groups: B, Pk, P1)		(Gilboagarber et al. 1994)
to rationalize binding selectivity	Docking (AutoDock 3.05, Sybyl 7.3), MD (AMBER 8)	(Blanchard et al. 2008)
to rationalize binding thermodynamics	Docking (AutoDock 3, Sybyl), MD (AMBER 8)	(Nurisso et al. 2010)
to rationalize blood group binding affinities	Docking	(Mitchell et al. 2002)
to rationalize observed multivalency effects	MD	(Kadam et al. 2011)
to investigate dendrimer binding	MD	(Johansson et al. 2008)
to investigate glycocluster cross-linking	Modelling (Sybyl)	(Marotte et al. 2007a)
to design high affinity glycopeptide inhibitors	Docking (Glide)	(Kadam et al. 2013a)
Pseudomonas aeruginosa PA-IIL/LecB (blood groups: sLe^a > Le^a, H type 2 > Le^b, Le^y, Le^x, A tri)		(Perret et al. 2005, Topin et al. 2013)
to investigate recognition of fucosylated blood group saccharides	Docking (Glide)	(Topin et al. 2013)
to rationalize fucose binding affinity	MD (AMBER 8)	(Mishra et al. 2008)
to interrogate energetics of monosaccharide binding	MD (AMBER 8)	(Mishra et al. 2010)
to quantify effect of mutations on affinity	Docking (AutoDock 3.1), MD (AMBER)	(Kriz et al. 2014)

Programs and version numbers are shown if reported.

Pseudomonas aeruginosa Lectins, PA-IL and PA-IIL (LecA and LecB)

Binding Specificity

The opportunistic respiratory pathogen *P. aeruginosa* is responsible for the majority of mortality associated with cystic fibrosis (Govan and Deretic 1996). Two of its many lectins, PA-IL and PA-IIL (also termed LecA and LecB), are toxic to respiratory endothelial cells (Bajoletlaudinat et al. 1994) and inhibit their ciliary beating (Adam et al. 1997), respectively. Both lectins facilitate adhesion to lung tissue by binding to epithelial cell surfaces (Kirkeby et al. 2007). LecA and LecB reside within the bacterial cytoplasm, in the periplasm and on both the cytoplasmic and outer membranes (Glick and Garber 1983, Tielker et al. 2005, Funken et al. 2012).

The binding specificities and affinities of LecA and LecB have been thoroughly investigated for a range of glycans. LecA is selective for galactose (K$_d$ of 87.5 ± 3.5 μM) (Kadam et al. 2011), and also binds to *N*-acetyl-D-galactosamine (Garber et al. 1992). Hydrophobic substituents at the anomeric position increase binding affinity (Garber et al. 1992, Chen et al. 1998), as for *p*-nitrophenyl-β-D-galactoside (K_d of 14.1 ± 0.2 µM) (Kadam et al. 2011) and napthyl-β-D-galactoside (K_d of 6.3 ± 0.4 µM) (Rodrigue et al. 2013). Disaccharides containing terminal α-D-galactose at the non-reducing end are also bound (e.g., Galα1,2/3/4Galβ1OMe, K_d of 37/132/115 µM) (Nurisso et al. 2010), though only melibiose (Galα1,6Glc) is bound more strongly than monosaccharide-size glycans (Lanne et al. 1994, Chen et al. 1998). Among blood group determinants, LecA binds to A, B, H, P, Pk, and P1 glycans, with a preference for B, Pk and P1 which feature a Galα1,3/4 non-reducing terminal (Gilboagarber et al. 1994). Thus, the Galα1,3/4 saccharide is the binding epitope of LecA.

The second *P. aeruginosa* lectin, LecB, is selective for fucose-containing saccharides, with an uncommonly high binding affinity for the monosaccharide (fucose K_d of 0.6 µM) (Garber et al. 1987). Other monosaccharides (L-fucosamine, L-galactose, mannose and fructose) are bound with lower affinity (Sabin et al. 2006). Analogues containing hydrophobic groups are also bound more potently, with *p*-nitrophenyl-α-L-fucose displaying twice the inhibitory activity of L-fucose. Disaccharides containing the Fucα1,4GlcNAc moiety are bound strongly (Marotte et al. 2007b). Binding to a range of human blood group determinants identified Le[a] as the strongest-bound glycan (K_d of 0.2 µM), followed by H type 2 and Le[x] (K_d of 3.4 µM) (Mitchell et al. 2002, Perret et al. 2005, Wu et al. 2006, Topin et al. 2013).

Crystal Structures

Both *P. aeruginosa* lectins are composed of β-sandwich folds of eight antiparallel β-strands arranged in two sheets and oligomerize to form tetramers (Imberty et al. 2004). The first crystal structures of LecA were reported by Karaveg et al. (2003) and Cioci et al. (2003) (PDB IDs: 1L7L, 1OKO, 1UOJ), determined in the unliganded state and in complex with galactose. Complexes with longer di- and tri-galactosides were also determined (Blanchard et al. 2008, Nurisso et al. 2010) (PDB IDs: 2VXJ, 2WYF). As inhibitor development progressed, complexes featuring galactosyl-conjugated glycopeptide dendrimers (Kadam et al. 2011, 2013a) (PDB IDs: 3ZYB, 3ZYH, 3ZYF, 4LKF, 4LKD, 4LKE) and aromatic glycosides (Rodrigue et al. 2013, Kadam et al. 2013b) (PDB IDs: 4A6S, 4LJH, 4LK6, 4LK7) were determined. Recently, a second glucose-binding site was identified in complex with melibiose (Blanchard et al. 2014) (PDB ID: 4AL9). Complexes with highly potent anti-adhesive galactoside conjugates have also been recently reported (Novoa et al. 2014) (PDB IDs: 4CP9, 4CPB).

The crystallographic structure of LecB was first reported by (Mitchell et al. 2002) in complex with fucose (PDB ID: 1GZT). Complexes with fructose and mannose monosaccharides soon followed (Loris et al. 2003) (PDB IDs: 1OXC, 1OUR, 1OVP, 1OVS), including an especially high-resolution structure bound to fucose (Mitchell et al. 2005) (PDB ID: 1UZV). Complexes with human milk saccharides (Perret et al. 2005) (PDB IDs: 1W8F, 1W8H), methyl-β-D-arabinose and L-arabinose (Sabin et al. 2006) (PDB IDs: 2BOJ, 2BP6) have also been determined. A mutagenesis study of the specificity-determining loop region of the LecB binding site revealed the role of specific amino acids in complex with fucose and mannose (Adam et al. 2007) (PDB IDs: 2JDM, 2JDN, 2JDP, 2JDU, 2JDY). Several complexes bound to glycomimetics have been structurally characterized (Marotte et al. 2007b, Hauck et al. 2013) (PDB IDs: 2JDH, 2JDK, 2VUC, 2VUD, 3ZDV). Finally, a structure featuring a perdeuterated version of LecB has been recently released (PDB ID: 4CE8).

Docking

Docking has been used in several studies to elucidate the interactions that cause glycan selectivity in binding assays. Using docking to simulate LecA complexed with Galα1,4Gal produced a pose similar to the crystallized complex with Galα1,3Gal (Blanchard et al. 2008). However, when lipid chains were modelled attached to the docked carbohydrates, only Galα1,4Gal orientation allowed for parallel placement of lipid tails as found in membranes *in vivo*, suggesting that the higher affinity for the Galα1,4Gal epitope is due to the cell surface presentation. An early study docking Le[x] into LecB revealed a steric clash between the *N*-acetyl methyl group and multiple binding site residues, explaining the weaker observed affinity for Le[x] (Mitchell et al. 2002). More recently, a panel of blood group carbohydrates (Le[a], sialyl Le[a], Le[x], sialyl Le[x], H type 1, H type 2 and A) were docked to LecB by Topin et al. (2013), revealing the role of hydrogen bonding interactions in determining binding affinity. Le[x] made no hydrogen bonds, whereas Le[a] and sialyl Le[a] formed one hydrogen bond between GlcNAc-O6 and Asp96 and between the glycerol group and Glu86, respectively. The higher binding affinities for Le[a] and sialyl Le[a] were therefore proposed to depend on hydrogen bonding interactions. The A trisaccharide, the lowest affinity carbohydrate, also made multiple hydrogen bonding interactions when docked, but with conformational strain around the Fucα1,2Gal glycosidic linkage, suggesting that carbohydrate binding conformation has a greater impact on LecB binding than the formation of hydrogen bonds. The only hydrogen bonds seen in the H type 1 docked poses involved the GlcNAc anomeric oxygen and the best H type 2 pose showed no hydrogen bonds. Since H type 2 is strongly bound by LecB, the paucity of hydrogen bonding interactions suggests that hydrophobic interactions may also be a high priority for LecB binding.

Molecular Dynamics

MD simulations of the *P. aeruginosa* lectins were carried out to analyse thermodynamic and multivalent aspects of binding. Simulation of LecB in complex with a range of monosaccharides revealed the greatest involvement of water molecules when fucose was bound, suggesting a source for the high enthalpic binding component for the LecB-fucose interaction (Mishra et al. 2008). A thermodynamic and computational study of the binding of Galα1,2Gal, Galα1,3Gal and Galα1,4Gal by LecA revealed more frequent hydrogen bond interactions and greater stability within the binding site in the Galα1,2Gal complex compared to the other digalactosides (Nurisso et al. 2010). These findings were suggested to explain the thermodynamic observations, both the larger enthalpic component of Galα1,2Gal binding (due to stronger hydrogen bonding interactions) and the higher entropic penalty (less motion within the bound complex reflecting greater conformational restraint).

Where binding site interactions require conformational motion of the binding site residues or carbohydrate hydroxyl groups, MD can prove a valuable analysis method. The formation of hydrophobic saccharide surface areas created by the arrangement of hydroxyl groups around monosaccharides has been studied by MD for LecB bound to multiple monosaccharides (Mishra et al. 2010). The individual roles of LecB binding site residues within the selectivity-determining loop region (residues 22–24) have been determined using a combination of docking, MD simulation, and free-energy calculation (Kriz et al. 2014). By comparing docked poses featuring a series of LecB mutants with wild-type crystallographic complexes, the binding contributions of each position were elucidated. In this investigation, mutants were generated *in silico* and docking was used to predict bound complexes with fucose and mannose monosaccharides. Owing to the orientation of residues at position 24 away from the binding site, the role of mutants at this position was not fully elucidated by static docking methods. MD simulation was employed to allow dynamic motion, giving the full range of motion available to position 24, and suggesting a role for hydrophobic stacking interactions involving that area of the binding site (Kriz et al. 2014).

The multivalent arrangement of LecA and LecB has prompted the exploration of multivalent inhibitors (Mammen et al. 1998, Pieters 2009), recently reviewed by (Cecioni et al. 2015). A class of multivalent ligands, glycodendrimers display carbohydrate epitopes extended towards multiple lectin binding sites by extended linker structures (Deguise et al. 2007, Chabre and Roy 2008, Pera et al. 2010). A key aim for glycodendrimer inhibitor design is the simultaneous binding or bridging of multiple lectin sites. In this area, modelling methods can assist with distance measurements on the atomic scale and analysis of conformational behaviour of glycodendrimers. MD has been used to assess the bridging capabilities of glycosylated dendrimers for glycopeptidic LecA inhibitors (Johansson et al. 2008, Kadam et al. 2011). Marotte et al. (2007a) used modelling to assess the conformations and distances exhibited by various non-peptide linkers. Docking has been applied to screen for single point mutations in galactosylated tripeptides to select LecA binders for further development (Kadam et al. 2013a). These examples demonstrate the utility of computational methods for guiding and informing the design of multivalent bacterial lectin inhibitors.

Burkholderia ambifaria **Lectin, BambL**

Binding Specificity

Burkholderia ambifaria is an opportunistic human respiratory pathogen, able to infect immune- and lung function-compromised individuals, such as cystic fibrosis patients (Coenye et al. 2001). *B. ambifaria* has been reported to recognize a range of fucosylated human blood group determinants to accomplish tissue adhesion (Audfray et al. 2012). The recently characterized *B. ambifaria* lectin (BambL) has a micromolar affinity for fucose, and similar affinities for terminally fucosylated blood group determinants. The H type 2 and Le^y determinants are the most strongly bound, followed by the A trisaccharide, the B trisaccharide, and the type 1 Lewis glycans (Le^a and Le^b) (Audfray et al. 2012, 2013).

Crystal Structures

BambL has been crystallized in complex with multiple human blood group oligosaccharides (Audfray et al. 2012, Topin et al. 2013) (saccharide and PDB IDs: apo, 3ZW0; Le^x, 3ZW1; H type 1, 3ZW2; B, 3ZWE; H type 2, 3ZZV). The crystallographic structure of BambL showed that this lectin adopts a 6-fold β-propeller architecture composed of three monomers. Each BambL monomer contains a carbohydrate-binding site and additional carbohydrate-binding sites are formed as clefts involving neighbouring BambL monomers in the hexameric β-propeller assembly.

Docking

Report by Topin et al. (2013) presents docking of multiple blood group saccharides to BambL and identifies the role of saccharide conformation in determining binding selectivity. In the predicted docked poses, H type 1 and 2 saccharides were both heavily involved in hydrogen bonding interactions in the binding site, and both occupied lowest energy conformers of the Fucα1,2Gal linkage, but the type 1 and type 2 poses differed with respect to the Galβ1,4GlcNAc linkage: the best H type 2 pose was bound in the lowest energy conformer, but H type 1 featured a higher energy distorted form. This structural observation matches the observed higher potency of BambL for H type 2 and demonstrates the influence of conformational distortions upon binding (Topin et al. 2013). Conformational distortions were also observed for Le^a and Le^x saccharides, as the internally-stacked galactose and fucose saccharides are disrupted by binding site residues. The docked poses suggest that binding is accompanied by a shift in the carbohydrate conformation from the lowest energy "closed" conformation to higher energy open forms (Topin et al. 2013).

Conclusions

Bacterial infection of human hosts involves interactions between bacterial proteins and human blood group and related saccharides. Experimental methods have been used to probe binding specificities and affinities for carbohydrate-lectin complexes, but these methods are not well able to integrate the large amount of glycan-protein interaction data now available. Thus, computational modelling approaches are often used to study the structural basis for observed behaviours such as binding selectivity, multivalency, and thermodynamic profiles of a wide range of carbohydrate-lectin systems. A number of case studies illustrate the value of docking and MD as useful computational tools for the detailed analysis of carbohydrate-protein interactions and the design of anti-infective bacterial lectin inhibitors.

Acknowledgements

TD is supported by an Australian Postgraduate Award. The authors gratefully acknowledge the contribution toward this study from the Victorian Operational Infrastructure Support Program received by the Burnet Institute.

Keywords: Bacterial lectin, carbohydrate binding interactions, carbohydrate-lectin binding, computational modelling, docking, force field, molecular dynamics

References

Adam, E. C., B. S. Mitchell, D. U. Schumacher, G. Grant and U. Schumacher. 1997. *Pseudomonas aeruginosa* II lectin stops human ciliary beating: Therapeutic implications of fucose. Am J Respir Crit Care Med 155: 2102–2104.

Adam, J., M. Pokorna, C. Sabin, E. P. Mitchell, A. Imberty and M. Wimmerova. 2007. Engineering of PA-IIL lectin from *Pseudomonas aeruginosa*—Unravelling the role of the specificity loop for sugar preference. BMC Struct Biol 7: 36.

Agirre, J., G. Davies, K. Wilson and K. Cowtan. 2015. Carbohydrate anomalies in the PDB. Nat Chem Biol 11: 303–303.

Agostino, M., C. Jene, T. Boyle, P. A. Ramsland and E. Yuriev. 2009. Molecular docking of carbohydrate ligands to antibodies: Structural validation against crystal structures. J Chem Inf Model 49: 2749–2760.

Agostino, M., M. S. Sandrin, P. E. Thompson, E. Yuriev and P. A. Ramsland. 2010. Identification of preferred carbohydrate binding modes in xenoreactive antibodies by combining conformational filters and binding site maps. Glycobiology 20: 724–735.

Agostino, M., M. S. Sandrin, P. E. Thompson, P. A. Ramsland and E. Yuriev. 2011a. Peptide inhibitors of xenoreactive antibodies mimic the interaction profile of the native carbohydrate antigens. Biopolymers 96: 193–206.

Agostino, M., E. Yuriev and P. A. Ramsland. 2011b. A computational approach for exploring carbohydrate recognition by lectins in innate immunity. Front Immunol 2: 23.

Agostino, M., P. A. Ramsland and E. Yuriev. 2012. Docking of carbohydrates into protein binding sites. pp. 111–138. *In*: Yuriev, E. and P. A. Ramsland (eds.). Structural Glycobiology. CRC Press, Boca Raton, FL, USA.

Alexacou, K. M., J. M. Hayes, C. Tiraidis, S. E. Zographos, D. D. Leonidas, E. D. Chrysina et al. 2008. Crystallographic and computational studies on 4-phenyl-N-(beta-D-glucopyranosyl)-1H-1,2, 3-triazole-1-acetamide, an inhibitor of glycogen phosphorylase: Comparison with alpha-D-glucose, N-acetyl-beta-D-glucopyranosylamine and N-benzoyl-N '-beta-D-glucopyranosyl urea binding. Proteins: Struct, Funct, Bioinf 71: 1307–1323.

Allinger, N. L., Y. H. Yuh and J. H. Lii. 1989. Molecular mechanics. The MM3 force field for hydrocarbons. 1. J Am Chem Soc 111: 8551–8566.

Andersson, C. and S. Balling Engelsen. 1999. The mean hydration of carbohydrates as studied by normalized two-dimensional radial pair distributions. J Mol Graphics Model 17: 101–105.

Audfray, A., J. Claudinon, S. Abounit, N. Ruvoen-Clouet, G. Larson, D. F. Smith et al. 2012. Fucose-binding lectin from opportunistic pathogen Burkholderia ambifaria binds to both plant and human oligosaccharidic epitopes. J Biol Chem 287: 4335–4347.

Audfray, A., A. Varrot and A. Imberty. 2013. Bacteria love our sugars: Interaction between soluble lectins and human fucosylated glycans, structures, thermodynamics and design of competing glycocompounds. C R Chim 16: 482–490.

Bajoletlaudinat, O., S. Giroddebentzmann, J. M. Tournier, C. Madoulet, M. C. Plotkowski, C. Chippaux et al. 1994. Cytotoxicity of Pseudomonas-aeruginosa internal lectin PA-I to respiratory epithelial-cells in primary culture. Infect Immun 62: 4481–4487.

Berman, H. M., J. Westbrook, Z. Feng, G. Gilliland, T. N. Bhat, H. Weissig et al. 2000. The protein data bank. Nucleic Acids Res 28: 235–242.

Bertozzi, C. R. and L. L. Kiessling. 2001. Chemical glycobiology. Science 291: 2357–2364.

Blanchard, B., A. Nurisso, E. Hollville, C. Tetaud, J. Wiels, M. Pokorna et al. 2008. Structural basis of the preferential binding for globo-series glycosphingolipids displayed by *Pseudomonas aeruginosa* lectin I. J Mol Biol 383: 837–853.

Blanchard, B., A. Imberty and A. Varrot. 2014. Secondary sugar binding site identified for LecA lectin from *Pseudomonas aeruginosa*. Proteins: Struct, Funct, Bioinf 82: 1060–1065.

Boltje, T. J., T. Buskas and G. -J. Boons. 2009. Opportunities and challenges in synthetic oligosaccharide and glycoconjugate research. Nat Chem 1: 611–622.

Campbell, C. and J. Gildersleeve. 2011. Tools for glycomics: Glycan and lectin microarrays. pp. 205–227. *In*: Wang, B. and G. -J. Boons (eds.). Carbohydrate Recognition. John Wiley & Sons, Inc., Hoboken, NJ, USA.

Cecioni, S., A. Imberty and S. Vidal. 2015. Glycomimetics versus multivalent glycoconjugates for the design of high affinity lectin ligands. Chem Rev 115: 525–561.

Chabre, Y. M. and R. Roy. 2008. Recent trends in glycodendrimer syntheses and applications. Curr Top Med Chem 8: 1237–1285.

Chemani, C., A. Imberty, S. de Bentzmann, M. Pierre, M. Wimmerova, B. P. Guery et al. 2009. Role of LecA and LecB lectins in *Pseudomonas aeruginosa*-induced lung injury and effect of carbohydrate ligands. Infect Immun 77: 2065–2075.

Chen, C. P., S. C. Song, N. Gilboa-Garber, K. S. S. Chang and A. M. Wu. 1998. Studies on the binding site of the galactose-specific agglutinin PA-IL from *Pseudomonas aeruginosa*. Glycobiology 8: 7–16.

Cioci, G., E. P. Mitchell, C. Gautier, M. Wimmerova, D. Sudakevitz, S. Perez et al. 2003. Structural basis of calcium and galactose recognition by the lectin PA-IL of *Pseudomonas aeruginosa*. FEBS Lett 555: 297–301.

Coenye, T., E. Mahenthiralingam, D. Henry, J. J. LiPuma, S. Laevens, M. Gillis et al. 2001. Burkholderia ambifaria sp. nov., a novel member of the Burkholderia cepacia complex including biocontrol and cystic fibrosis-related isolates. Int J Syst Evol Microbiol 51: 1481–1490.

Corzana, F., M. S. Motawia, C. H. Du Penhoat, S. Perez, S. M. Tschampel, R. J. Woods et al. 2004. A hydration study of (1→4) and (1→6) linked α-glucans by comparative 10 ns molecular dynamics simulations and 500-MHz NMR. J Comput Chem 25: 573–586.

Cross, J. B., D. C. Thompson, B. K. Rai, J. C. Baber, K. Y. Fan, Y. Hu et al. 2009. Comparison of several molecular docking programs: Pose prediction and virtual screening accuracy. J Chem Inf Model 49: 1455–1474.

Dam, T. K. and C. F. Brewer. 2007. 3.21—Fundamentals of lectin–carbohydrate interactions. pp. 397–452. *In*: Kamerling, H. (ed.). Comprehensive Glycoscience. Elsevier, Oxford, UK.

Deguise, I., D. Lagnoux and R. Roy. 2007. Synthesis of glycodendrimers containing both fucoside and galactoside residues and their binding properties to PA-IL and PA-IIL lectins from *Pseudomonas aeruginosa*. New J Chem 31: 1321–1331.

del Carmen Fernandez-Alonso, M., D. Diaz, M. Alvaro Berbis, F. Marcelo, J. Canada and J. Jimenez-Barbero. 2012. Protein-carbohydrate interactions studied by NMR: From molecular recognition to drug Design. Curr Protein Pept Sci 13: 816–830.

DeMarco, M. L. and R. J. Woods. 2008. Structural glycobiology: A game of snakes and ladders. Glycobiology 18: 426–440.

Dingjan, T., I. Spendlove, L. G. Durrant, A. M. Scott, E. Yuriev and P. A. Ramsland. 2015. Structural biology of antibody recognition of carbohydrate epitopes and potential uses for targeted cancer immunotherapies. Mol Immunol (in press). doi: 10.1016/j.molimm.2015.02.028.

Dror, R. O., R. M. Dirks, J. P. Grossman, H. F. Xu and D. E. Shaw. 2012. Biomolecular simulation: A computational microscope for molecular biology. Annu Rev Biophys 41: 429–452.

Fadda, E. and R. J. Woods. 2010. Molecular simulations of carbohydrates and protein–carbohydrate interactions: motivation, issues and prospects. Drug Discov Today 15: 596–609.

Foley, B. L., M. B. Tessier and R. J. Woods. 2012. Carbohydrate force fields. Wiley Interdiscip Rev: Comput Mol Sci 2: 652–697.

Friesner, R. A., J. L. Banks, R. B. Murphy, T. A. Halgren, J. J. Klicic, D. T. Mainz et al. 2004. Glide: A new approach for rapid, accurate docking and scoring. 1. Method and assessment of docking accuracy. J Med Chem 47: 1739–1749.

Friesner, R. A., R. B. Murphy, M. P. Repasky, L. L. Frye, J. R. Greenwood, T. A. Halgren et al. 2006. Extra precision glide: Docking and scoring incorporating a model of hydrophobic enclosure for protein−ligand complexes. J Med Chem 49: 6177–6196.

Funken, H., K. -M. Bartels, S. Wilhelm, M. Brocker, M. Bott, M. Bains et al. 2012. Specific association of lectin LecB with the surface of *Pseudomonas aeruginosa*: Role of outer membrane protein OprF. PLoS One 7: e46857.

Gabius, H. J. 1998. The how and why of protein-carbohydrate interaction: A primer to the theoretical concept and a guide to application in drug design. Pharm Res 15: 23–30.

Gabius, H. J. 2008. Glycans: Bioactive signals decoded by lectins. Biochem Soc Trans 36: 1491–1496.

Garber, N., U. Guempel, N. Gilboagarber and R. J. Doyle. 1987. Specificity of the fucose-binding lectin of Pseudomonas-aeruginosa. FEMS Microbiol Lett 48: 331–334.

Garber, N., U. Guempel, A. Belz, N. Gilboagarber and R. J. Doyle. 1992. On the specificity of the d-galactose-binding lectin (PA-I) of Pseudomonas-aeruginosa and its strong binding to hydrophobic derivatives of D-galactose and thiogalactose. Biochim Biophys Acta 1116: 331–333.

Gauto, D. F., S. Di Lella, C. M. A. Guardia, D. A. Estrin and M. A. Marti. 2009. Carbohydrate-binding proteins: Dissecting ligand structures through solvent environment occupancy. J Phys Chem B 113: 8717–8724.

Gauto, D. F., S. Di Lella, D. A. Estrin, H. L. Monaco and M. A. Marti. 2011. Structural basis for ligand recognition in a mushroom lectin: solvent structure as specificity predictor. Carbohydr Res 346: 939–948.

Gauto, D. F., A. A. Petruk, C. P. Modenutti, J. I. Blanco, S. Di Lella and M. A. Marti. 2013. Solvent structure improves docking prediction in lectin-carbohydrate complexes. Glycobiology 23: 241–258.

Gilboagarber, N., D. Sudakevitz, M. Sheffi, R. Sela and C. Levene. 1994. PA-I and PA-II lectin interactions with the Abo(H)-blood and P-blood group glycosphingolipid antigens may contribute to the broad-spectrum adherence of Pseudomonas-aeruginosa to human tissues in secondary infections. Glycoconjugate J 11: 414–417.

Glick, J. and N. Garber. 1983. The intracellular-localization of Pseudomonas-aeruginosa lectins. J Gen Microbiol 129: 3085–3090.

Govan, J. R. W. and V. Deretic. 1996. Microbial pathogenesis in cystic fibrosis: Mucoid *Pseudomonas aeruginosa* and Burkholderia cepacia. Microbiol Rev 60: 539–574.

Guvench, O., S. S. Mallajosyula, E. P. Raman, E. Hatcher, K. Vanommeslaeghe, T. J. Foster et al. 2011. CHARMM additive all-atom force field for carbohydrate derivatives and its utility in polysaccharide and carbohydrate–protein modeling. J Chem Theory Comput 7: 3162–3180.

Halgren, T. A., R. B. Murphy, R. A. Friesner, H. S. Beard, L. L. Frye, W. T. Pollard et al. 2004. Glide: A new approach for rapid, accurate docking and scoring. 2. Enrichment factors in database screening. J Med Chem 47: 1750–1759.

Hansen, H. S. and P. H. Hünenberger. 2011. A reoptimized GROMOS force field for hexopyranose-based carbohydrates accounting for the relative free energies of ring conformers, anomers, epimers, hydroxymethyl rotamers, and glycosidic linkage conformers. J Comput Chem 32: 998–1032.

Hartshorn, M. J., M. L. Verdonk, G. Chessari, S. C. Brewerton, W. T. M. Mooij, P. N. Mortenson et al. 2007. Diverse, high-quality test set for the validation of protein-ligand docking performance. J Med Chem 50: 726–741.

Hauck, D., I. Joachim, B. Frommeyer, A. Varrot, B. Philipp, H. M. Moller et al. 2013. Discovery of two classes of potent glycomimetic inhibitors of *Pseudomonas aeruginosa* LecB with distinct binding modes. ACS Chem Biol 8: 1775–1784.

Hemmingsen, L., D. E. Madsen, A. L. Esbensen, L. Olsen and S. B. Engelsen. 2004. Evaluation of carbohydrate molecular mechanical force fields by quantum mechanical calculations. Carbohydr Res 339: 937–948.

Hildebrandt, A., A. K. Dehof, A. Rurainski, A. Bertsch, M. Schumann, N. C. Toussaint et al. 2010. BALL—biochemical algorithms library 1.3. BMC Bioinf 11: 5.

Hirabayashi, J., M. Yamada, A. Kuno and H. Tateno. 2013. Lectin microarrays: Concept, principle and applications. Chem Soc Rev 42: 4443–4458.

Hummer, G. 2010. Molecular binding under water's influence. Nat Chem 2: 906–907.

Hung, C. S., J. Bouckaert, D. Hung, J. Pinkner, C. Widberg, A. DeFusco et al. 2002. Structural basis of tropism of *Escherichia coli* to the bladder during urinary tract infection. Mol Microbiol 44: 903–915.

Imberty, A., M. Wimmerova, E. P. Mitchell and N. Gilboa-Garber. 2004. Structures of the lectins from *Pseudomonas aeruginosa*: insights into the molecular basis for host glycan recognition. Microbes Infect 6: 221–228.

Ishijima, N., M. Suzuki, H. Ashida, Y. Ichikawa, Y. Kanegae, I. Saito et al. 2011. BabA-mediated adherence is a potentiator of the Helicobacter pylori type IV secretion system activity. J Biol Chem 286: 25256–25264.

Jana, M. and S. Bandyopadhyay. 2012. Restricted dynamics of water around a protein-carbohydrate complex: Computer simulation studies. J Chem Phys 137: 055102.

Jeffries, C. M., W. Farrugia and P. A. Ramsland. 2012. Crystallography and small-angle scattering of carbohydrate-protein complexes and glycoproteins. pp. 3–28. *In*: Yuriev, E. and P. A. Ramsland (eds.). Structural Glycobiology. CRC Press, Boca Raton, FL, USA.

Johansson, E. M., S. A. Crusz, E. Kolomiets, L. Buts, R. U. Kadam, M. Cacciarini et al. 2008. Inhibition and dispersion of *Pseudomonas aeruginosa* biofilms by glycopeptide dendrimers targeting the fucose-specific lectin LecB. Chem Biol 15: 1249–1257.

Johnson, Q., R. Lindsay, L. Petridis and T. Shen. 2015. Investigation of carbohydrate recognition via computer simulation. Molecules 20: 7700–7718.

Kadam, R. U., M. Bergmann, M. Hurley, D. Garg, M. Cacciarini, M. A. Swiderska et al. 2011. A Glycopeptide dendrimer inhibitor of the galactose-specific lectin LecA and of *Pseudomonas aeruginosa* biofilms. Angew Chem, Int Ed 50: 10631–10635.

Kadam, R. U., M. Bergmann, D. Garg, G. Gabrieli, A. Stocker, T. Darbre et al. 2013a. Structure-based optimization of the terminal tripeptide in glycopeptide dendrimer inhibitors of *Pseudomonas aeruginosa* biofilms targeting LecA. Chem -Eur J 19: 17054–17063.

Kadam, R. U., D. Garg, J. Schwartz, R. Visini, M. Sattler, A. Stocker et al. 2013b. CH-pi "T-shape" interaction with histidine explains binding of aromatic galactosides to *Pseudomonas aeruginosa* lectin LecA. ACS Chem Biol 8: 1925–1930.

Karaveg, K., Z. J. Liu, W. Tempel, R. J. Doyle, J. P. Rose and B. C. Wang. 2003. Crystallization and preliminary X-ray diffraction analysis of lectin-1 from *Pseudomonas aeruginosa*. Acta Crystallogr, Sect D: Biol Crystallogr 59: 1241–1242.

Kerzmann, A., D. Neumann and O. Kohlbacher. 2006. SLICK—Scoring and energy functions for protein-carbohydrate interactions. J Chem Inf Model 46: 1635–1642.

Kerzmann, A., J. Fuhrmann, O. Kohlbacher and D. Neumann. 2008. BALLDock/SLICK: A new method for protein-carbohydrate docking. J Chem Inf Model 48: 1616–1625.

Kirkeby, S., M. Wimmerova, D. Moe and A. K. Hansen. 2007. The mink as an animal model for *Pseudomonas aeruginosa* adhesion: Binding of the bacterial lectins (PA-IL and PA-IIL) to neoglycoproteins and to sections of pancreas and lung tissues from healthy mink. Microbes Infect 9: 566–573.

Kirschner, K. N. and R. J. Woods. 2001. Solvent interactions determine carbohydrate conformation. Proc Natl Acad Sci USA 98: 10541–10545.

Kirschner, K. N., A. B. Yongye, S. M. Tschampel, J. González-Outeiriño, C. R. Daniels, B. L. Foley et al. 2008. GLYCAM06: A generalizable biomolecular force field. Carbohydrates J Comput Chem 29: 622–655.

Kletter, D., S. Singh, M. Bern and B. B. Haab. 2013. Global comparisons of lectin–glycan interactions using a database of analyzed glycan array data. Mol Cell Proteomics 12: 1026–1035.

Kogelberg, H., D. Solis and J. Jimenez-Barbero. 2003. New structural insights into carbohydrate-protein interactions from NMR spectroscopy. Curr Opin Struct Biol 13: 646–653.

Koharudin, L. M. I. and A. M. Gronenborn. 2012. Nuclear magnetic resonance studies of carbohydrate-protein interactions. pp. 29–46. *In*: Yuriev, E. and P. A. Ramsland (eds.). Structural Glycobiology. CRC Press, Boca Raton, FL, USA.

Kony, D., W. Damm, S. Stoll and W. F. Van Gunsteren. 2002. An improved OPLS-AA force field for carbohydrates. J Comput Chem 23: 1416–1429.

Kriz, Z., J. Adam, J. Mrazkova, P. Zotos, T. Chatzipavlou, M. Wimmerova et al. 2014. Engineering the *Pseudomonas aeruginosa* II lectin: Designing mutants with changed affinity and specificity. J Comput-Aided Mol Des 28: 951–960.

Kroemer, R. T., A. Vulpetti, J. J. McDonald, D. C. Rohrer, J. Y. Trosset, F. Giordanetto et al. 2004. Assessment of docking poses: Interactions-based accuracy classification (IBAC) versus crystal structure deviations. J Chem Inf Comput Sci 44: 871–881.

Lanne, B., J. Ciopraga, J. Bergstrom, C. Motas and K. A. Karlsson. 1994. Binding of the galactose-specific Pseudomonas-aeruginosa lectin, PA-I, to glycosphingolipids and other glycoconjugates. Glycoconjugate J 11: 292–298.

Leach, A. 2001. Molecular Modelling: Principles and Applications. Prentice Hall, Upper Saddle River, NJ, USA.

Lemieux, R. U. 1996. How water provides the impetus for molecular recognition in aqueous solution. Acc Chem Res 29: 373–380.

Li, Z. and T. Lazaridis. 2005. The effect of water displacement on binding thermodynamics: Concanavalin A. J Phys Chem B 109: 662–670.

Liang, C. -H. and C. -Y. Wu. 2009. Glycan array: A powerful tool for glycomics studies. Expert Rev Proteomics 6: 631–645.

Lill, M. A. 2011. Efficient incorporation of protein flexibility and dynamics into molecular docking simulations. Biochemistry 50: 6157–6169.

Lindén, S., J. Mahdavi, C. Semino-Mora, C. Olsen, I. Carlstedt, T. Borén et al. 2008. Role of ABO secretor status in mucosal innate immunity and H. pylori Infection. PLoS Pathog 4: e2.

Lionta, E., G. Spyrou, D. K. Vassilatis and Z. Cournia. 2014. Structure-based virtual screening for drug discovery: Principles, applications and recent advances. Curr Top Med Chem 14: 1923–1938.

Lopez, C. A., A. J. Rzepiela, A. H. de Vries, L. Dijkhuizen, P. H. Hunenberger and S. J. Marrink. 2009. Martini coarse-grained force field: Extension to carbohydrates. J Chem Theory Comput 5: 3195–3210.

Loris, R., D. Tielker, K. E. Jaeger and L. Wyns. 2003. Structural basis of carbohydrate recognition by the lectin LecB from *Pseudomonas aeruginosa*. J Mol Biol 331: 861–870.

Lund, B., F. Lindberg, B. I. Marklund and S. Normark. 1987. The PapG protein is the alpha-D-galactopyranosyl-(1-4)-beta-D-galactopyranose-binding adhesin of uropathogenic *Escherichia-coli*. Proc Natl Acad Sci USA 84: 5898–5902.

Mallajosyula, S. S., O. Guvench, E. Hatcher and A. D. MacKerell. 2012. CHARMM additive all-atom force field for phosphate and sulfate linked to carbohydrates. J Chem Theory Comput 8: 759–776.

Mammen, M., S. K. Choi and G. M. Whitesides. 1998. Polyvalent interactions in biological systems: Implications for design and use of multivalent ligands and inhibitors. Angew Chem, Int Ed 37: 2755–2794.

Marotte, K., C. P. Eville, C. Sabin, M. M. Pymbock, A. Imberty and R. Roy. 2007a. Synthesis and binding properties of divalent and trivalent clusters of the Lewis a disaccharide moiety to *Pseudomonas aeruginosa* lectin PA-IIL. Org Biomol Chem 5: 2953–2961.

Marotte, K., C. Sabin, C. Preville, M. Moume-Pymbock, M. Wimmerova, E. P. Mitchell et al. 2007b. X-ray structures and thermodynamics of the interaction of PA-IIL from *Pseudomonas aeruginosa* with disaccharide derivatives. ChemMedChem 2: 1328–1338.

Mendonca, S., G. P. Johnson, A. D. French and R. A. Laine. 2002. Conformational analyses of native and permethylated disaccharides. J Phys Chem A 106: 4115–4124.

Michel, J., J. Tirado-Rives and W. L. Jorgensen. 2009. Energetics of displacing water molecules from protein binding sites: Consequences for ligand optimization. J Am Chem Soc 131: 15403–15411.

Miljkovic, M. 2010. Carbohydrate: Synthesis, Mechanisms, and Stereoelectric Effects. Springer, New York, NY, USA.

Minke, W. E., D. J. Diller, W. G. J. Hol and C. Verlinde. 1999. The role of waters in docking strategies with incremental flexibility for carbohydrate derivatives: Heat-labile enterotoxin, a multivalent test case. J Med Chem 42: 1778–1788.

Mishra, N. K., P. Kulhánek, L. Šnajdrová, M. Petřek, A. Imberty and J. Koča. 2008. Molecular dynamics study of *Pseudomonas aeruginosa* lectin-II complexed with monosaccharides. Proteins: Struct, Funct, Genet 72: 382–392.

Mishra, N. K., Z. Křiž, M. Wimmerová and J. Koča. 2010. Recognition of selected monosaccharides by *Pseudomonas aeruginosa* Lectin II analyzed by molecular dynamics and free energy calculations. Carbohydr Res 345: 1432–1441.

Mishra, S. K., J. Adam, M. Wimmerova and J. Koca. 2012. *In silico* mutagenesis and docking study of ralstonia solanacearum RSL lectin: Performance of docking software to predict saccharide binding. J Chem Inf Model 52: 1250–1261.

Mitchell, E., C. Houles, D. Sudakevitz, M. Wimmerova, C. Gautier, S. Perez et al. 2002. Structural basis for oligosaccharide-mediated adhesion of *Pseudomonas aeruginosa* in the lungs of cystic fibrosis patients. Nat Struct Biol 9: 918–921.

Mitchell, E. P., C. Sabin, L. Snajdrova, M. Pokorna, S. Perret, C. Gautier et al. 2005. High affinity fucose binding of *Pseudomonas aeruginosa* lectin PA-IIL: 1.0 A resolution crystal structure of the complex combined with thermodynamics and computational chemistry approaches. Proteins 58: 735–746.

Modenutti, C., D. Gauto, L. Radusky, J. Blanco, Á. Turjanski, S. Hajos et al. 2015. Using crystallographic water properties for the analysis and prediction of lectin-carbohydrate complex structures. Glycobiology 25: 181–196.

Morris, G. M., R. Huey, W. Lindstrom, M. F. Sanner, R. K. Belew, D. S. Goodsell et al. 2009. AutoDock4 and AutoDockTools4: Automated docking with selective receptor flexibility. J Comput Chem 30: 2785–2791.

Nivedha, A. K., S. Makeneni, B. L. Foley, M. B. Tessier and R. J. Woods. 2014. Importance of ligand conformational energies in carbohydrate docking: Sorting the wheat from the chaff. J Comput Chem 35: 526–539.

Novoa, A., T. Eierhoff, J. Topin, A. Varrot, S. Barluenga, A. Imberty et al. 2014. A LecA ligand identified from a galactoside-conjugate array inhibits host cell invasion by *Pseudomonas aeruginosa*. Angew Chem, Int Ed 53: 8885–8889.

Nurisso, A., S. Kozmon and A. Imberty. 2008. Comparison of docking methods for carbohydrate binding in calcium-dependent lectins and prediction of the carbohydrate binding mode to sea cucumber lectin CEL-III. Mol Simul 34: 469–479.

Nurisso, A., B. Blanchard, A. Audfray, L. Rydner, S. Oscarson, A. Varrot et al. 2010. Role of water molecules in structure and energetics of *Pseudomonas aeruginosa* lectin I interacting with disaccharides. J Biol Chem 285: 20316–20327.

Ofek, I. and R. Doyle. 1994. Principles of bacterial adhesion. pp. 1–15. *In*: Ofek, I. and R. Doyle (eds.). Bacterial Adhesion to Cells and Tissues. Springer US, New York, NY, USA.

Patel, D. S., X. He and A. D. MacKerell. 2015. Polarizable empirical force field for hexopyranose monosaccharides based on the classical drude oscillator. J Phys Chem B 119: 637–652.

Pera, N. P., H. M. Branderhorst, R. Kooij, C. Maierhofer, M. van der Kaaden, R. M. J. Liskamp et al. 2010. Rapid screening of lectins for multivalency effects with a glycodendrimer microarray. ChemBioChem 11: 1896–1904.

Pérez, S. and I. Tvaroška. 2014. Carbohydrate–protein interactions: Molecular modeling insights. pp. 9–136. *In*: Derek, H. (ed.). Advances in Carbohydrate Chemistry and Biochemistry. Academic Press, San Diego, CA, USA.

Perret, S., C. Sabin, C. Dumon, M. Pokorna, C. Gautier, O. Galanina et al. 2005. Structural basis for the interaction between human milk oligosaccharides and the bacterial lectin PA-IIL of *Pseudomonas aeruginosa*. Biochem J 389: 325–332.

Pieters, R. J. 2009. Maximising multivalency effects in protein-carbohydrate interactions. Org Biomol Chem 7: 2013–2025.

Plewczynski, D., M. Lazniewski, R. Augustyniak and K. Ginalski. 2011. Can we trust docking results? Evaluation of seven commonly used programs on PDBbind database. J Comput Chem 32: 742–755.

Pol-Fachin, L., V. H. Rusu, H. Verli and R. D. Lins. 2012. GROMOS 53A6GLYC, an improved GROMOS force field for hexopyranose-based carbohydrates. J Chem Theory Comput 8: 4681–4690.

Pol-Fachin, L., H. Verli and R. D. Lins. 2014. Extension and validation of the GROMOS 53A6(GLYC) parameter set for glycoproteins. J Comput Chem 35: 2087–2095.

Poveda, A. and J. Jimenez-Barbero. 1998. NMR studies of carbohydrate-protein interactions in solution. Chem Soc Rev 27: 133–143.

Ravn, V. and E. Dabelsteen. 2000. Tissue distribution of histo-blood group antigens. APMIS 108: 1–28.

Reynolds, M., A. Fuchs, T. K. Lindhorst and S. Perez. 2008. The hydration features of carbohydrate determinants of Lewis antigens. Mol Simul 34: 447–460.

Rillahan, C. D. and J. C. Paulson. 2011. Glycan microarrays for decoding the glycome. Annu Rev Biochem 80: 797–823.

Rodrigue, J., G. Ganne, B. Blanchard, C. Saucier, D. Giguere, T. C. Shiao et al. 2013. Aromatic thioglycoside inhibitors against the virulence factor LecA from *Pseudomonas aeruginosa*. Org Biomol Chem 11: 6906–6918.

Roldos, V., F. Javier Canada and J. Jimenez-Barbero. 2011. Carbohydrate-protein interactions: A 3D view by NMR. ChemBioChem 12: 990–1005.

Sabin, C., E. P. Mitchell, M. Pokorna, C. Gautier, J. P. Utille, M. Wimmerova et al. 2006. Binding of different monosaccharides by lectin PA-IIL from *Pseudomonas aeruginosa*: Thermodynamics data correlated with X-ray structures. FEBS Lett 580: 982–987.

Sakamoto, J., K. Furukawa, C. Cordon-Cardo, B. W. T. Yin, W. J. Rettig, H. F. Oettgen et al. 1986. Expression of Lewisa, Lewisb, X, and Y blood group antigens in human colonic tumors and normal tissue and in human tumor-derived cell lines. Cancer Res 46: 1553–1561.

Samsonov, S. A., J. Teyra and M. T. Pisabarro. 2011. Docking glycosaminoglycans to proteins: analysis of solvent inclusion. J Comput-Aided Mol Des 25: 477–489.

Samsonov, S. A., L. Bichmann and M. T. Pisabarro. 2015. Coarse-grained model of glycosaminoglycans. J Chem Inf Model 55: 114–124.

Sapay, N., A. Nurisso and A. Imberty. 2013. Simulation of carbohydrates, from molecular docking to dynamics in water. Methods Mol Biol 924: 469–483.

Sauter, J. and A. Grafmuller. 2015. Solution properties of hemicellulose polysaccharides with four common carbohydrate force fields. J Chem Theory Comput 11: 1765–1774.

Song, X., D. F. Smith and R. D. Cummings. 2012. Glycan-based arrays for determining specificity of carbohydrate-binding proteins. pp. 163–174. *In*: Yuriev, E. and P. A. Ramsland (eds.). Structural Glycobiology. CRC Press, Boca Raton, FL, USA.

Sotriffer, C. A. 2011. Accounting for induced-fit effects in docking: What is possible and what is not? Curr Top Med Chem 11: 179–191.

Sousa, S. F., A. J. M. Ribeiro, J. T. S. Coimbra, R. P. P. Neves, S. A. Martins, N. S. H. N. Moorthy et al. 2013. Protein-ligand docking in the new millennium—A retrospective of 10 years in the field. Curr Med Chem 20: 2296–2314.

Sperling, O., A. Fuchs and T. K. Lindhorst. 2006. Evaluation of the carbohydrate recognition domain of the bacterial adhesin FimH: Design, synthesis and binding properties of mannoside ligands. Org Biomol Chem 4: 3913–3922.

Stortz, C. A. and A. D. French. 2008. Disaccharide conformational maps: Adiabaticity in analogues with variable ring shapes. Mol Simul 34: 373–389.

Stortz, C. A., G. P. Johnson, A. D. French and G. I. Csonka. 2009. Comparison of different force fields for the study of disaccharides. Carbohydr Res 344: 2217–2228.

Sun, H., L. Zhao, S. Peng and N. Huang. 2014. Incorporating replacement free energy of binding-site waters in molecular docking. Proteins: Struct, Funct, Bioinf 82: 1765–1776.

Sutto, L., S. Marsili and F. L. Gervasio. 2012. New advances in metadynamics. Wiley Interdiscip Rev: Comput Mol Sci 2: 771–779.

Taylor, M. E. and K. Drickamer. 2009. Structural insights into what glycan arrays tell us about how glycan-binding proteins interact with their ligands. Glycobiology 19: 1155–1162.

Tielker, D., S. Hacker, R. Loris, M. Strathmann, J. Wingender, S. Wilhelm et al. 2005. *Pseudomonas aeruginosa* lectin LecB is located in the outer membrane and is involved in biofilm formation. Microbiology 151: 1313–1323.

Topin, J., J. Arnaud, A. Sarkar, A. Audfray, E. Gillon, S. Perez et al. 2013. Deciphering the glycan preference of bacterial lectins by glycan array and molecular docking with validation by microcalorimetry and crystallography. PLoS One 8: e71149.

Van Damme, E. M., D. Smith, R. Cummings and W. Peumans. 2011. Glycan arrays to decipher the specificity of plant lectins. pp. 757–767. *In*: Wu, A. M. (ed.). The Molecular Immunology of Complex Carbohydrates-3. Springer US, New York, NY, USA.

Vanommeslaeghe, K. and A. D. MacKerell. 2015. CHARMM additive and polarizable force fields for biophysics and computer-aided drug design. Biochim Biophys Acta 1850: 861–871.

Vila, A. and R. A. Mosquera. 2007. Atoms in molecules interpretation of the anomeric effect in the O-C-O unit. J Comput Chem 28: 1516–1530.

Warren, G. L., C. W. Andrews, A. -M. Capelli, B. Clarke, J. LaLonde, M. H. Lambert et al. 2006. A critical assessment of docking programs and scoring functions. J Med Chem 49: 5912–5931.

Weis, W. I. and K. Drickamer. 1996. Structural basis of lectin-carbohydrate recognition. Annu Rev Biochem 65: 441–473.

Woods, R. J. 2005. GLYCAM Web. Complex Carbohydrate Research Center, University of Georgia, Athens, GA. Retrieved June 1, 2015, from http://www.glycam.com.

Woods, R. J. and M. B. Tessier. 2010. Computational glycoscience: Characterizing the spatial and temporal properties of glycans and glycan-protein complexes. Curr Opin Struct Biol 20: 575–583.

Wu, A. M., J. H. Wu, T. Singh, J. H. Liu, M. S. Tsai and N. Gilboa-Garber. 2006. Interactions of the fucose-specific *Pseudomonas aeruginosa* lectin, PA-IIL, with mammalian glycoconjugates bearing polyvalent Lewis(a) and ABH blood group glycotopes. Biochimie 88: 1479–1492.

Xiong, X., Z. Chen, B. P. Cossins, Z. Xu, Q. Shao, K. Ding et al. 2015. Force fields and scoring functions for carbohydrate simulation. Carbohydr Res 401: 73–81.

Yi, J. -Y., J. Bernholc and P. Salamon. 1991. Simulated annealing strategies for molecular dynamics. Comput Phys Commun 66: 177–180.

Yuriev, E., M. S. Sandrin and P. A. Ramsland. 2008. Antibody-ligand docking: Insights into peptide-carbohydrate mimicry. Mol Simul 34: 461–468.

Yuriev, E., M. Agostino and P. A. Ramsland. 2011. Challenges and advances in computational docking: 2009 in review. J Mol Recognit 24: 149–164.

Yuriev, E. and P. A. Ramsland. 2013. Latest developments in molecular docking: 2010–2011 in review. J Mol Recognit 26: 215–239.

Yuriev, E., J. Holien and P. A. Ramsland. 2015. Improvements, trends, and new ideas in molecular docking: 2012–2013 in review. J Mol Recognit (in press). doi: 10.1002/jmr.2471.

Zhang, W., C. Wu and Y. Duan. 2005. Convergence of replica exchange molecular dynamics. J Chem Phys 123: 154105.

Zulueta, M. M. L., D. Janreddy and S. -C. Hung. 2015. One-pot methods for the protection and assembly of sugars. Isr J Chem 55: 347–359.

CHAPTER 8

Altered Sialylation of Glycoproteins and Its Impact on Disease Pathogenesis

Ida Annunziata[a] and *Alessandra d'Azzo**

Introduction

Sialic acids comprise a large family of derivatives of the sugar neuraminic acid (Varki 2008). Their structural diversity and ubiquitous distribution in nature reflect the broad range of biological functions that these sugars control. Because of their terminal position on the glycan chains of glycoproteins and glycolipids and their negative charge, sialic acids are potent modulators of the structure and biochemical properties of soluble and membrane glycoconjugates, and play a critical role in fundamental processes ranging from tissue development and differentiation, to innate immunity, inflammation, and response to pathogens (Varki and Schauer 2009).

In mammalian cells, homeostatic control of the sialic acid content in glycoproteins and glycoconjugates is achieved by the concerted and opposite actions of synthetic and degradative enzymes. The cycle of biosynthesis, transfer, removal and recycling of sialic acids is a complex cascade involving multiple steps that occur in different cell compartments (Varki and Schauer 2009). Considering the many events that modulate the extent and composition of bound sialic acids, one would predict that there would be numerous, naturally occurring genetic lesions that might ultimately result in altered sialylation. However, only a hand full of genetic defects affecting either the synthesis or the degradation of sialic acids bound to glycoproteins and glycoconjugates have been identified, suggesting that mutations interfering with any steps of sialic acid biogenesis might be incompatible with life. In this review we give a brief account of what has been reported to date on the pathogenic effects of altered sialylation of specific glycoconjugates in genetic diseases affecting the synthesis or the degradation of this sugar moiety.

Sialic Acid Biosynthesis and Function

Sialic acids are cyclic, 9-carbon amino sugars found in virtually all eukaryotic cells and in some prokaryotes (Warren and Felsenfeld 1962, Tanner 2005, Severi et al. 2007). Their strategic position at the non-reducing terminal end of glycan chains and their unusual structural diversity account for the numerous vital roles assigned to this sugar moiety. Because of their bulky, acidic, and negatively charged nature, sialic acids

Department of Genetics, St. Jude Children's Research Hospital, 262 Danny Thomas Pl., Memphis TN 38105, USA.
[a] E-mail: ida.annunziata@stjude.org
* Corresponding author: Sandra.dazzo@stjude.org

can drastically alter the biochemical properties and half-life of glycoproteins in circulation, as well as the stability and trafficking of intracellular glycoconjugates (Fukuda et al. 1989, Yogalingam et al. 2008, Bork et al. 2009). As the exposed residues of plasma membrane glycoproteins and glycosphingolipids, sialic acids function as recognition sites or receptors in a plethora of physiological processes and signaling cascades, regulating, among others, neuroplasticity, glomerular filtration, fertilization, cell differentiation and blood cells removal from circulation (Aminoff et al. 1977, Andrews 1979, Traving and Schauer 1998, Topfer-Petersen 1999, Varki 2008, Varki and Schauer 2009, Ravindran et al. 2013, Sondermann et al. 2013, Schnaar et al. 2014). Sialic acids are also critical components of innate immunity in vertebrates, a role exerted via their ability to bind in *cis* to specific I-type or C-type lectins, siglecs (sialic acid-binding immunoglobulin-type lectins) and selectins, at the cell surface, thereby masking the underneath glycan chain and preventing recognition by pathogens (Crocker et al. 1998, Varki 2007, Schauer 2009, Varki and Gagneux 2012). On the other hand, sialic acids serve as receptors or ligands for viruses and bacteria, and therefore take a direct part in the infection process (Sharon and Lis 1993, Karlsson 1995, Schauer 2000, Hidari et al. 2007, Schauer 2009).

The core structure of all sialic acid derivatives is neuraminic acid, and N-acetyl-neuraminic acid (Neu5Ac) is the structure more commonly present. Chemical modifications and substitutions at different carbon positions of Neu5Ac expand the diversity of the underlying glycan chain and specify the unique makeup of the glycocalix in outer and inner membranes of different cell types. In vertebrates, the biosynthesis of the Neu5Ac occurs primarily in the cytosol and starts with the production of ManNAc-6-P (N-acetyl-mannosamine 6-phosphate) from UDP-GlcNAc (Uridine diphosphate N-acetylglucosamine) (Fig. 1). This reaction is a rate-limiting step and is catalyzed by the bifunctional, two-domain enzyme, glucosamine

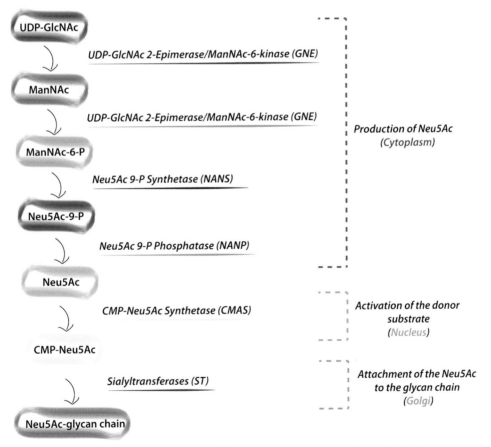

Figure 1. Biosynthesis of Neu5Ac. Schematic of the different reactions and enzymes that synthesize N-acetylneuraminic acid (Neu5Ac).

(UDP-N-acetyl)-2-epimerase/N-acetylmannosamine kinase (GNE). As epimerase GNE first converts UDP-GlcNAc to ManNAc (N-acetylmannosamine) by the removal of the UDP and epimerization of the sugar; using its kinase activity GNE then gives rise to ManNAc-6-P by adding a phosphate group to ManNAc (Hinderlich et al. 1997, Stasche et al. 1997). Condensation of ManNAc-6-P with phosphoenolpyruvate generates the phosphorylated sialic acid precursor Neu5Ac-9-P (N-acetyl-neuraminic acid-9-phosphate) that is then de-phosphorylated in Neu5Ac. In order to be transferred to an oligosaccharide chain, Neu5Ac requires to be activated into a nucleotide donor substrate. This reaction that occurs in the nucleus promotes the attachment of Neu5Ac to cytidine 5'-triphosphate (CTP) to produce the CMP-Neu5Ac. This intermediate is then transferred back to the cytosol and imported into the Golgi where it is used as substrate acceptor for the sialyltransferases (Fig. 1).

Sialyltransferases

Sialyltransferases are a large family of more than 20 enzymes, which catalyze the transfer of Neu5Ac to the newly synthesized oligosaccharide chain of glycoconjugates. They generate specific carbohydrate linkages for sialic acid (α2→3, α2→6, α2→8) and show a strict preference for the acceptor sugar residue. Based on the glycosidic linkage they generate, sialyltransferases are classified in four families: α2→3 and α2→6 β-galactoside; α2→6 and α2→8 GalNAc (*N*-Acetylgalactosamine). Several sialyltransferase genes share their genomic architecture and encode for enzymes that have similar functions. The existence of sialyltransferases that apparently act on the same linkage reflect the need for a tight regulation of the expression and abundance of sialylated glycoconjugates. Given their high number, cell distribution and substrate selectivity, it is no surprise that sialyltransferases have been implicated in human diseases, particularly in cancer (Blomme et al. 2009, Bos et al. 2009, Audry et al. 2011, Falconer et al. 2012, Lu et al. 2014). Increased expression of sialyltransferases has been reported in several types of neoplasia and in plasma of cancer patients (Kessel and Allen 1975, Schultz et al. 2012, Bull et al. 2014, Glavey et al. 2014). In tumor cells, upregulation of sialyltransferases results in hypersialylation of glycoconjugates at surface membranes, affecting cell-cell and cell-ECM interaction, cell migration/adhesion, intracellular signaling and metastatic potential (Bull et al. 2014). For example, the sialyltransferase ST6GalNAc-I [(α-N-acetyl-neuraminyl-2,3-β-galactosyl-1,3)-N-acetylgalactosaminide α-2,6-sialyltransferase-I] is thought to contribute to the generation of the mucin-associated sialyl-Tn antigen, a marker of metastatic carcinoma (Marcos et al. 2010, Heimburg-Molinaro et al. 2011), and ST6GalNAc-V, imparts metastatic potential to breast cancer (Bos et al. 2009). Thus, deregulated expression of these enzymes positively correlates with cancer progression, metastasis and poor prognosis. However, to date no genetic or somatic mutations in any of the sialyltransferase genes have been linked to disease conditions, including cancer. For a comprehensive review on this topic see for example Dall'Olio et al. 2014 and Bull et al. 2014 (Bull et al. 2014, Dall'Olio et al. 2014).

Sialidases

At some point in their life cycle, the sialic acids attached to glycoproteins and glycoconjugates must be removed to initiate the degradation of the glycan chain and the recycling of the sugar residues. In eukaryotes, this occurs by the regulated action of only 4 enzymes known as sialidases or neuraminidases (NEUs), a family of exoglycosidases. Reflecting the role of their target sialic acid substrates (Varki and Schauer 2009), sialidases have been implicated in basic biological processes, ranging from cell proliferation/differentiation and cell adhesion, to receptor recognition, signal transduction, degradation of gangliosides and glycoproteins, immune response and vesicular trafficking (Monti et al. 2010, Giacopuzzi et al. 2012, Miyagi and Yamaguchi 2012, Smutova et al. 2014). Based on their subcellular localization, these enzymes are classified as lysosomal (NEU1), cytosolic (NEU2), plasma-membrane (NEU3), and mitochondrial/lysosomal/intracellular membranes (NEU4). The 4 mammalian sialidases have a unique tissue distribution, pH optimum, biochemical properties, and preference for sialic acid linkages (Monti et al. 2010). NEU1 shows a high degree of conservation among all the mammals (for example, mouse and human NEU1 are 90% identical) and its primary structure is more homologous to bacterial neuraminidases than to other vertebrate NEUs. NEU2, NEU3 and NEU4 instead are more similar to each other than to NEU1, suggesting that their genes have appeared after recent gene duplication in vertebrates (Monti et al. 2010, Giacopuzzi et al. 2012).

All NEUs have a common active site and similar sequence motifs (Gaskell et al. 1995, Taylor 1996). A highly conserved domain (F/Y) RIP, located at the N terminus includes the arginine (Arg) residue that is part of the neuraminidase catalytic triad (Rothe et al. 1991, Vimr 1994). A second characteristic of sialidases is a short conserved sequence of 8 amino acids, Ser/Thr-X-Asp-X-Gly-X-Thr-Trp/Phe, which is repeated 2 to 5 times in each of the proteins. This motif was designated the "Asp box," because all of the aspartic acid residues are conserved among members of this family of enzymes (Roggentin et al. 1993). Although the function of the Asp-boxes remains unknown, this motif has been implicated in substrate recognition and binding (Rothe et al. 1991). Structural models of all mammalian NEUs were first generated by molecular replacement using the 3D structure of viral and bacterial neuraminidases (Fig. 2) (Colman 1994, Bonten et al. 2009). However, in 2005 the high resolution x-ray structure of human NEU2 was solved in its apo form or bound to its competitive inhibitor Neu5Ac2en(2-deoxy-2,3-dehydro-N-acetylneuraminic acid, DANA) (Chavas et al. 2005). The 3D structure revealed that the enzyme shares a common fold with viral and bacterial sialidases, referred as super-barrel or six-bladed β-propeller (Chavas et al. 2005).

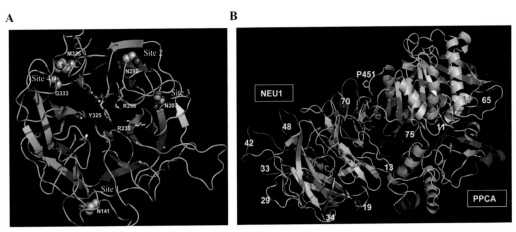

Figure 2. Structural model of NEU1 and NEU1-PPCA heterodimer. (A) Molecular replacement model of NEU1 based on the crystal structure of *M. Viridifaciences* sialidase. (B) structural model of NEU1-PPCA heterodimer; NEU1 peptides 13 (red) and 70 (blue) interact with PPCA peptide 74 (red) and PPCA residue Pro-451. Adapted from (Bonten et al. 2009).

Even though the 4 mammalian sialidases are likely to share structural characteristics, these enzymes are differentially expressed during development and in adult tissues and organs, which indicates that they are under a strict spatio-temporal regulation and have a distinct role in controlling the turnover or processing of sialoglycoconjugates (Hasegawa et al. 2001). Of the 4 mammalian sialidases NEU1 is the most abundant and ubiquitously expressed. The enzyme is present in virtually all tissues and cells, but its expression levels vary greatly, likely reflecting variations in the metabolic/catabolic needs and substrate availability among different cell types (d'Azzo and Bonten 2010, Monti et al. 2010). In addition, another feature that distinguishes NEU1 from the other NEUs is its strict dependency on association with the serine carboxypeptidase protective protein/cathepsin A (PPCA) for correct compartmentalization, catalytic activation and stability in lysosomes (Fig. 2). NEU1 is in fact part of a high molecular weight, multiprotein complex containing PPCA and the glycosidase β-galactosidase (β-GAL). In complex with PPCA, NEU1 and β-GAL are "protected", i.e., they are stable and active in the lysosomal compartment, hence the name protective protein. Within the complex, PPCA functions as an essential chaperone which targets/transfer NEU1 to the lysosomes.

Genetic Diseases Linked to Hyposialylation of Glycoproteins

Hereditary Inclusion Body Myopathy

Hereditary inclusion body myopathy (HIBM) is a rare autosomal recessive disease that presents in adulthood and affects primarily the long muscles (Yunis and Samaha 1971, Nonaka et al. 1981). The disorder is linked to mutations in the *GNE* gene that causes loss of function of either the epimerase or the kinase activity of the protein, depending on their positions within the primary structure of GNE (Eisenberg et al. 1999, 2001). After diagnosis the disease progresses slowly over a period of 2–3 decades and manifests with increasing weakness of mainly leg muscles, albeit with an unusually selective pathology that spares the quadriceps. In addition, GNE deficiency does not affect the ocular, pharyngeal and respiratory muscles. At the end stage of the disease, patients are bound to a wheelchair. Histopathologically, the affected muscle shows red rimmed vacuoles with Gomori's trichrome stain, autophagic vacuoles containing β-amyloid, tau, and presenilin (Griggs et al. 1995). Electron micrographs of the affected muscle reveal cytoplasmic and nuclear inclusion bodies containing cellular products and membrane remnants, a hallmark of the disease. HIBM occurs worldwide, but is especially common among Persian Jews. It is allelic with Nonaka myopathy, an autosomal recessive distal myopathy, identified in Japanese patients (Nonaka et al. 1981).

The *GNE* gene produces at least 6 spliced transcripts; the major transcript consists of 13 exons and encodes for a protein that is ubiquitously expressed with the highest levels found in the liver. The protein has a multidomain architecture: the N-terminal portion embeds the epimerase activity while the C-terminal portion comprises the kinase catalytic activity (Hinderlich et al. 1997). Over 70 mutations have been identified in the *GNE* gene; these occur in various combinations in both the epimerase and the kinase domains, with the most common missense mutation, p.M712T, identified in the Persian-Jewish population, affecting the kinase domain (Eisenberg et al. 2003). Other two common mutations have been identified and are the p.V572L, and p.D176V, both occurring in patients of Japanese origin.

The effects of *GNE* mutations on either the epimerase, the kinase or both activities of the enzyme have been tested in patients' muscle biopsies, and in culture fibroblasts, myoblasts and lymphoblasts (Noguchi et al. 2004, Nonaka et al. 2005, Salama et al. 2005, Sparks et al. 2005, Savelkoul et al. 2006, Huizing and Krasnewich 2009). In most cases, both functions of the enzyme were reduced but not completely abolished. Furthermore, mutations affecting one of the catalytic domains of the enzyme often resulted in perturbation of the other catalytic domain. These features have made it difficult to dissect the causative effects of specific mutation(s), and link them to the observed pathogenesis. To further complicate this issue some investigators have hypothesized that the activity of other enzymes involved in the sialic acid biosynthetic pathway may influence the effect(s) of any given *GNE* mutations on enzyme functions and penetrance of disease phenotypes (Krause et al. 2005). Thus, until now no cellular and molecular mechanisms have been identified, which link GNE deficiency to the formation of the muscle inclusion bodies characteristic of the disease.

For differential diagnosis of HIBM patients, analysis of total sialic acid in plasma has demonstrated a measurable reduction in total protein sialylation. However, *in vitro* assays using several cell types have shown only a modest reduction in enzymatic activity, likely due to the presence of sialylated factors in the medium of cultured cells (see below). The other possible explanation is that some cells may be less sensitive to deficiency of GNE than others for the *de novo* synthesis of sialic acids. Nevertheless, HIBM remains to date a conundrum and more studies in faithful models of the disease may be needed to shed light on the mechanisms underlying this disease pathogenesis.

Sialuria

Sialuria, previously known as French type Sialuria, is a rare disease characterized by cytoplasmic accumulation and excessive excretion of free NeuAc in the urine (Montreuil et al. 1968, Enns et al. 2001). This disease is also associated with *GNE* mutation occurring in the allosteric site of the enzyme, which responds to levels of CMP-Neu5Ac in a negative feedback loop. Remarkably, HIBM patients do not show sialuria. Clinical features of the disease include mild developmental delay, slightly prolonged neonatal jaundice, coarse facies, hepatomegaly and frequent infections of the respiratory tract (Seppala et al. 1999). Analysis of patients' fibroblasts has revealed a clear overproduction of CMP-NeuAc (Wopereis et al. 2006). HPLC of patients' serum proteins demonstrated hypersialylation of α2,6-linked NeuAc in core 1 O-glycans while N-glycans were only marginally affected (Wopereis et al. 2006). Also for this rare disease the underlying molecular pathways responsible for pathogenesis are currently unknown.

GNE Animal Models

Mouse

The initial attempt to generate a mouse model of GNE deficiency using classic gene targeting of the chromosomal locus failed, because mice homozygous for the null allele were embryonic lethal between E8.5 and E9.5 (Schwarzkopf et al. 2002). Analysis of ES cell lines, homozygous for the null allele, showed absence of mRNA and protein, and no detectable GNE enzymatic activity. Under culturing conditions with low sialylated proteins in the medium, these deficient ES cells had more than 75% reduction in the levels of PM sialic acids compared to wild type ES cells (Schwarzkopf et al. 2002). This feature could be in part corrected by culturing the null cells in serum containing medium. Interestingly, in the KO ES cells NCAM did not carry any polysialic acids, and polysialylation of this moiety could not be restored by the sialic acids recycled from degradation of sialylated glycoproteins present in the culture medium. However, feeding KO cells with the precursor of sialic acids ManAc restored polysialylation of NCAM (Schwarzkopf et al. 2002). These results demonstrated that sialic acids can be synthesized *in vitro* from ManAc without the need for the GNE epimerase activity, which is instead essential *in vivo*. In contrast, the phosphorylation of ManAc can be catalyzed also by other kinases, making the kinase activity of GNE partially redundant (Schwarzkopf et al. 2002).

Because *GNE*-null mice were embryonic lethal, investigators have generated two additional mouse models using different targeting strategies (Galeano et al. 2007, Malicdan et al. 2007, Sela et al. 2013). Transgenic mouse lines carrying either the D176V or the M712T mutation found in HIBM patients were crossed into the GNE deficient background. The first model, GNE^{-/-}hGNED176V-Tg mice (Malicdan et al. 2007), develop a clinical phenotype that closely resembles the human disease; the mice present with muscle weakness and muscle pathology around 30 weeks of age, marked hyposialylation of serum and muscle glycoproteins, and formation of amyloid bodies in the affected myofibers. Interestingly, muscle weakness is antecedent to the appearance of rimmed vacuoles, the hallmark of the disease. In order to identify, potential therapeutics for GNE myopathy, a screening of several synthetic sugar compounds was carried out and tested in the GNE^{-/-}hGNED176V-Tg mice (Malicdan et al. 2012). This study identified peracetylated ManAc as a compound that efficiently rescues the muscle phenotype in a dose dependent manner (Malicdan et al. 2012). Unfortunately, this compound also raised cellular sialic acids levels in different tissues. Even tough, the excess sialic acids was quickly excreted into the urine, this issue raised concerns and prompted a quest for additional compounds. Searching for alternative synthetic sugars, the molecule sialyllactose was found to improve muscle phenotype, rescue locomotion activity, halt disease progression and increase total sialylation (Yonekawa et al. 2014).

The *GNE*^{-/-}hGNEM712T-Tg (Galeano et al. 2007), which carry the most common mutation found in HIBM patients, do not develop a myopathy and die few days after birth. These mice present with a severe hematuria and proteinuria as a result of abnormalities in the glomerular basement membrane. Podocalyxin, the major sialoprotein in foot podocytes of the kidney, was found to be hyposialylated. Administration of ManNAc to the mutant pups rescues in part the perinatal mortality and increases sialylation of podocalyxin. A possible explanation for these results is that two Gne splice variants are present in mice, which are the orthologs of two human isoforms, GNE1 and GNE2 (Yardeni et al. 2013). The mGne1 seems to be the most ubiquitously expressed, while mGne2 is differentially expressed in mouse tissues with liver, heart and brain showing undetectable or low expression of the protein (Yardeni et al. 2013). The GNE^{-/-}hGNEM712T-Tg mice showed no difference in the levels of expression of the two murine splice variants, but treatment of mice with ManAc increased preferentially the levels of the tissue-specific variant mGne2, which resulted in significantly elevated GNE enzymatic activity (Yardeni et al. 2013).

Zebrafish

Since the GNE gene and protein show high degree of conservation between zebrafish and human, a zebrafish model was recently generated (Daya et al. 2014). Characterization of the spatio-temporal expression of Gne in zebrafish revealed a maternal expression of the gene in one-cell stage embryos, which diminished with time, and differential pattern of expression of the gene in different tissues. Muscle expression of Gne was observed in the first 3 days post fertilization and decreased after this initial stage. Knocking down the zebrafish *Gne* gene with antisense morpholino caused overt developmental abnormalities and high mortality rate. Morphants present with a plethora of phenotypic variants, ranging from marginally reduced length to severely shortened trunk length. Characterization of the antisense morpholino mutants showed impairment in loco motoractivity and muscle development. Specifically, slow and fast muscle morphology and structure were severely affected. Overall these data point to an essential function of Gne in myofibers development and organization; hence, this zebrafish mutant could represent a faithful model of the disease (Daya et al. 2014).

Genetic Diseases Linked to Hypersialylation of Glycoproteins

Sialidosis

The fundamental role of the NEU1 in maintaining cell and tissue homeostasis is documented by the systemic, clinical manifestations associated with defective or deficient enzyme activity. Deficiency of NEU1 gives rise to two neurosomatic glycoprotein storages diseases: sialidosis due to primary genetic lesions in the *NEU1* gene, and galactosialidosis (GS) due to a primary genetic defect of PPCA and secondary deficiency of NEU1 (d'Azzo et al. 2013, Thomas 2013).

Patients with sialidosis and those with GS have similar clinical and biochemical features, and both are characterized by multiple phenotypes that are classified according to the age of onset and severity of the symptoms. Type I (normomorphic) sialidosis, a mild non-neuropathic form of the disease, is associated with cherry-red spot myoclonus syndrome, onset in the second decade of life, and progressively impaired vision. Type II (dysmorphic) sialidosis, the severe, neuropathic form, comprises 3 subtypes based on the age at onset: congenital or hydropic (in utero onset), infantile (0–12 months), and juvenile (2–20 years). All patients with Type II sialidosis eventually demonstrate a progressive mucopolysaccharidosis-like phenotype, including cherry-red spot myoclonus, coarse facies, visceromegaly, dysostosis multiplex, and severe mental retardation (d'Azzo et al. 2015). Patients with congenital Type II sialidosis present with hydrops fetalis, neonatal ascites, or both; these infants are either stillborn or die shortly after birth (Thomas 2013, d'Azzo et al. 2015). Chemical and NMR-spectroscopic analyses of the storage products in patients' urine and fibroblasts demonstrated increased levels of linear and branched sialyloligosaccharides (Kuriyama et al. 1981, van Pelt et al. 1988, Takahashi et al. 1991, van Pelt et al. 1991). We and others have identified a number of mutations in patients with either Type I or II sialidosis (d'Azzo et al. 2015). The penetrance and degree of severity of the symptoms in these patients correlate closely with the type of NEU1 mutations involved and, in turn, the levels of residual enzyme activity.

Galactosialidosis

Although Galactosialidosis (GS) is not genetically linked to NEU1 it is briefly mentioned here given that a the disease is associated with severely reduced or deficient NEU1 activity, secondary to a primary defect in PPCA (d'Azzo and Bonten 2010, d'Azzo et al. 2013, Bonten et al. 2014). In fact patients with sialidosis and those with GS share many clinical and biochemical features that are attributed at least in part to the loss of NEU1 function in both diseases. As observed in sialidosis, patients with GS are clinically heterogeneous and differ widely in severity and age of onset of the symptoms. The early onset forms of the disease develop a very severe systemic condition associated with fetal hydrops, skeletal dysplasia, visceromegaly, renal and cardiac failure, variable neurological involvement and early death. It has similarity to the early onset congenital forms of sialidosis, although GS infants have Mucopolysaccharidosis-like features with course facial features and severe bone abnormalities while those this sialidosis lack an overt dysmorphic phenotype.

NEU1 Mouse Models

Neu1$^{-/-}$ Mouse: A Model of Type II Sialidosis

Neu1$^{-/-}$ mice develop a systemic and CNS disease that closely recapitulates the early onset, type II form of sialidosis and have a reduced life span (de Geest et al. 2002). Mutant mice present signs of the disease at birth, with progressive urinary excretion of sialylated oligosaccharides and expansion of the lysosomal system in cells of virtually all systemic organs and the nervous system, as well as tissues of mesenchymal origin (Fig. 3).

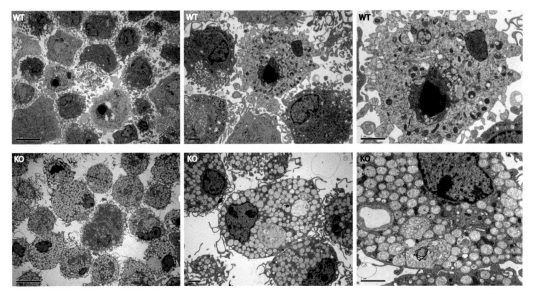

Figure 3. Lysosomal expansion in sialidosis. Expansion of the lysosomal system in macrophages isolated from *Neu1$^{-/-}$* mice.

The cells that are mostly targeted are epithelia, reticulo-endothelia and histiocytes. *Neu1* null mice also present with growth retardation, hepatosplenomegaly, edema, kyphosis of the lumbar spine, lordosis of the cervical and thoracic spine, neurological impairment and muscle hypotonia and atrophia. Ultimately *Neu1$^{-/-}$* mice suffer from dyspnea, severe loss of weight, diffuse edema, gait abnormalities and tremor (de Geest et al. 2002).

Several pathological signs documented in the sialidosis patients are phenocopied in the *Neu1$^{-/-}$* mice. They include: progressive splenomegaly, which is accompanied by extramedullary hematopoiesis (EMH); kidney dysfunction, which is associated with extensive and progressive lysosomal vacuolization of the renal tubular epithelium, leading to widespread edema; muscle atrophy and hypotonia, which is linked to abnormal expansion of the connective tissue that infiltrates the muscle bed and results in myofibers degeneration (de Geest et al. 2002, Zanoteli et al. 2010). In the brain, the most affected cells are those of the epithelium of the choroid plexus and the endothelium of the ependymal layer (de Geest et al. 2002, Annunziata et al. 2013). In addition, lysosomal expansion and ballooning is observed in affected microglia and perivascular macrophages, which are commonly juxtaposed to degenerating neurons, eliciting an extensive microgliosis. All the pathogenic signs identified so far in the *Neu1$^{-/-}$* mouse model can be, at least in part, attributed to the activation of a common pathogenic pathway, excessive lysosomal exocytosis, discussed in details below. The downstream effects of excessive lysosomal exocytosis on tissue homeostasis vary depending on the biological and functional characteristics of the various organs, and on the spectrum of tissue-specific sialylated substrates that are the target of the enzyme *in vivo*.

Neu1⁻/⁻; NEU1^{V54M} Mouse: A Model of Type I Sialidosis

The *Neu1*$^{-/-}$; *NEU1*^{V54M}, a transgenic mouse model of type I sialidosis carries the amino acid substitution V54M, previously identified in a non-neuropathic adult patient (Bonten et al. 2000). This mouse model was created by crossing a *NEU1*^{V54M} transgenic mice into the *Neu1*$^{-/-}$ background (Bonten et al. 2013). These mice are fertile and viable and appear to have no early signs of disease and have measurable Neu1 enzymatic activity. The mice have no CNS condition and a normal lifespan. Later in life, mutant mice develop edema, enlargement of the kidneys and prominent oligosacchariduria (Bonten et al. 2013). Neu1 activity is reduced in all the organs tested, although residual levels vary greatly and range from 30% to 80% of control values. Histopathological and biochemical characterization of these mice makes them an exploitable model for experiment with therapeutic interventions possibly amenable for patients with type I sialidosis.

Mechanism of Pathogenesis Linked to Altered sialylation of Glycoproteins

GNE Role in Muscle Development and Homeostasis

Hyposialylation of cellular proteins appear to be the major cause of the muscle phenotype observed in patients with HIBM. In fact, administration of sialic acid or the biosynthetic precursor ManAc rescues or stop muscle pathology in the GNE myopathy models. However, it is still unclear how deficiency of GNE leads to the human disease and it is speculated that additional mechanisms may contribute to pathogenesis. Using GNE deficient ES cells it was indeed shown that the enzyme might also play a role in cell differentiation and proliferation (Weidemann et al. 2010). In fact, *Gne*$^{-/-}$ cells proliferate at a faster rate compared to wild-type cells and their growth rate appears to directly correlate to the levels of available GNE protein. Furthermore, growth related genes that may be involved in this proliferative phenotype were shown to be differentially expressed in Gne deficient ES cells. Comparison of the developmental profile of cultured ES cells, mimicking embryogenesis *in vitro*, has confirmed a role for GNE in the early development of skeletal and cardiac muscle (Milman Krentsis et al. 2011). Using several differentiation protocols, it was observed that Gne deficient ES cells rarely differentiated in culture and, if they did, their differentiation state was only partial. It was also shown that wild-type and *Gne* KO ES cells acquired a cardiac fate at the same time, but the KO cardiomyocytes had a shorter lifespan in culture than the wild-type cardiomyocytes, and also beat abnormally. Differentiation markers like Pax7 and MyoD were almost completely absent in the *Gne* KO cardiac cells, confirming their inability to fully differentiate (Milman Krentsis et al. 2011). These data imply that GNE may have additional functions on heart development and may explain the observed embryonic lethality.

NEU1 as Negative Regulator of Lysosomal Exocytosis

Studies directed to the understanding of the molecular bases of splenomegaly, which is recurrent in sialidosis patients and in the mouse model of the disease, brought to the identification of an unexpected function of NEU1, that of negative regulator of lysosomal exocytosis (Yogalingam et al. 2008). The latter is a Ca^{2+} regulated process present in both secretory and non-secretory cells and delegated to pivotal cellular functions, like the repair or replenishment of damaged plasma membrane (PM), the release of specialized proteins, the removal of pathogenic bacteria or the release of human immunodeficiency virus from infected cells (Rodriguez et al. 1997, Yogalingam et al. 2008, Griffiths et al. 2010, Samie and Xu 2014) (Fig. 4). During lysosomal exocytosis a selected pool of lysosomes are recruited to the cytoskeletal network and docked at the PM. A spike in intracellular Ca^{2+} promotes the fusion of docked lysosomes with the PM, and

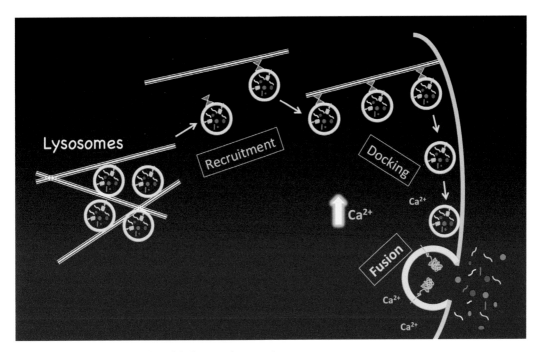

Figure 4. Schematic representation of the lysosomal exocytosis process.

the release of lysosomal contents extracellularly (Andrews 2000, Yogalingam et al. 2008). Thus, lysosomal exocytosis is an intrinsic physiological process that cells use for the homeostatic control of PM integrity and ECM replenishment or remodeling (Fig. 4).

The intracellular movement of exocytic lysosomes and their docking at the PM involve the lysosomal integral membrane protein LAMP1 (Yogalingam et al. 2008). LAMP1 is an important structural component of lysosomes, localized abundantly in the limiting membrane of the organelles and sparsely at the PM, unless cells undergo exocytosis. Its primary structure consists of a single transmembrane domain, a small, C-terminal cytoplasmic tail of 12-amino-acids and a highly glycosylated and sialylated *N*-terminal portion facing the lumen of the lysosomes (Yogalingam et al. 2008, Schwake et al. 2013). LAMP1 is a natural target of NEU1 activity; hence, NEU1 loss of function leaves the protein' sialic acids unprocessed or partially processed, and LAMP1 accumulates in an hypersialylated state at the lysosomal membrane, a feature that renders these lysosomes particularly prone to dock at the PM ready to engage in lysosomal exocytosis. The end result is excessive exocytosis of lysosomal contents into the extracellular space with deleterious consequences for PM and ECM integrity (Yogalingam et al. 2008). Thus, NEU1 is the first and so-far only negative-regulator of lysosomal exocytosis, and LAMP-1 is an active component of this process (Yogalingam et al. 2008).

Several genetic diseases have been described that are associated with impaired exocytosis of lysosomes, and share common clinical features of auto-immunodeficiency, albinism and bleeding disorders (Huynh et al. 2004, Stinchcombe et al. 2004). Characterization of these genetic defects has allowed the identification of basic components required for the movement of lysosomes along the cytoskeletal network and for their fusion with the PM (Holt et al. 2006, Luzio et al. 2014). Now there is compelling evidence that LAMP1 is indeed a key player in this process and that LAMP1 sialic acid content dictates the extent of lysosomal exocytosis. Considering the variety of physiological processes that are influenced by lysosomal exocytosis, it is predictable that its extent in any cell type would significantly affect the characteristic and composition of the PM and the surrounding ECM and would contribute to disease pathogenesis (Yogalingam et al. 2008, Wu et al. 2010, Zanoteli et al. 2010, Annunziata et al. 2013). Thus, the Neu1 deficient mice provide an ideal model to dissect the downstream effects of excessive rather than impaired lysosomal exocytosis on tissue homeostasis (Yogalingam et al. 2008, Schwake et al. 2013).

Extramedullary Hematopoiesis and Splenomegaly

The initial characterization of the *Neu1⁻/⁻* mice identified a progressive and time dependent enlargement of the spleen, which was accompanied by progressive increase in total cell count. This was paralleled by increased number of erythroid precursors and megakaryocytes. Further analyses revealed an increased number of hematopoietic progenitors in the peripheral blood, which was accompanied by a lower number of progenitors in the bone marrow (BM). All these pathological characteristics were suggestive of extramedullary hematopoiesis (EMH) (de Geest et al. 2002). Moreover, an attempt to treat *Neu1⁻/⁻* mice with transplantation of genetically engineered BM cells expressing NEU1 failed because long term engraftment was unsuccessful (Yogalingam et al. 2008). In search of mechanisms that would elucidate the lack of BM engraftment in *Neu1⁻/⁻* mice and the progressive EMH, it was discovered that NEU1 negatively regulates lysosomal exocytosis.

Excessive exocytosis of lysosomal contents into the bone niche by the KO BM cells changes dramatically the characteristics of the bone marrow microenvironment. The sequence of events that ensue can be summarized as follows: increased levels of active proteases, such as neutrophil elastase and cathepsin G, exocytosed by *Neu1⁻/⁻* BM neutrophils and macrophages into the BM extracellular fluid (BMEF) lead to inactivation of the serine protease inhibitors, serpina1 and serpina3, and premature degradation of the vascular cell adhesion molecule 1 (VCAM-1) at the surface of the BM stromal cells, a key molecule for the retention of hematopoietic progenitor cells (HPC) in the bone niche. Loss of retention of HCP in the bone niche pushes hematopoiesis to a peripheral organ, like the spleen, a phenomenon that explains the increased mobilization of HPC in the peripheral blood and the time dependent spleen enlargement observed in the mutant mice (Yogalingam et al. 2008). This study showed for the first time that excessive lysosomal exocytosis can trigger a pathogenic cascade that strictly depends on the level of sialylation of LAMP-1 controlled by NEU1, and underscored the importance of this enzyme in lysosomal biogenesis during the occurrence of BM hematopoiesis (Fig. 5).

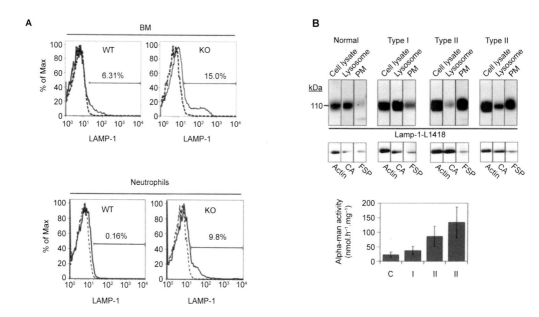

Figure 5. Excessive lysosomal exocytosis in sialidosis. (A) FACS analysis of total BM cells from 3-month-old WT and KO littermates with FITC-conjugated anti-LAMP-1 showed increased levels of Lamp1 at the PM of BM cells and neutrophils; (B) top, PM and lysosomal preparations purified from normal fibroblasts, type I (mild), and type II (severe) sialidosis fibroblasts were analyzed on immunoblots with anti-LAMP-1, bottom, increased α-man activity was assayed in the medium of type II sialidosis fibroblasts as a measure of lysosomal exocytosis; excessive lysosomal exocytosis correlates with the levels of residual activity measure in the different sialidosis patients. Adapted from (Yogalingam et al. 2008).

Myopathy

Osteoskeletal deformities and muscle hypotonia have been described in patients with sialidosis and are recapitulated in the *Neu1*[−/−] mice. Pathological analysis of the skeletal muscle in Neu1 deficient mice revealed apro found expansion of the epimysial and perimysial connective tissue, characterized by hyper-proliferation of myo-fibroblasts, upregulation and massive deposition of collagens and other ECM components, and activation of matrix metalloproteinases and their cognate inhibitors (Zanoteli et al. 2010, Neves et al. 2015). Together these features are reminiscent of incipient fibrosis (Zanoteli et al. 2010). Similarly to BM cells, *Neu1*[−/−] myo-fibroblasts cultured *in vitro* showed increased levels of oversialylated Lamp1 and, in turn, excessive exocytosis of lysosomal hydrolases, including cathepsin B and cathepsin L (Zanoteli et al. 2010). Muscle fibers located adjacent to the expanded connective tissue displayed widespread invagination of their sarcolemma. Histopathological and immunohistochemical examination of the affected areas of the muscle confirmed the presence of increased levels of Lamp1, lysosomal cathepsins, metalloproteinases and other hydrolytic enzymes. Thus, the progressive loss of muscle mass and muscle atrophy characteristic of the *Neu1*[−/−] mice as well as of patients with sialidosis can be explained at least in part by the abnormal lysosomal exocytosis of active proteases and hydrolases by connective tissue myo-fibroblasts, which increasingly affects the integrity of the basement membranes of muscle cells and provokes the progressive infiltration/invasion of the muscle bed by the ever-expanding connective tissue. Interestingly, the myopathy in *Neu1*[−/−] mice, as it is the case in IBM2, is not associated with necrosis or inflammation.

Anacusis

Another phenotype that is commonly found in sialidosis patients and in *Neu1*[−/−] mice is anacusis, or hearing loss which is evident in all the anatomical part of the ear (Wu et al. 2010, Thomas 2013). Light and electron microscopic studies of the ear unveiled thickening of the cerumen in the external auditory canal and severe otitis media; infiltration of connective tissue in the middle ear ossicles with signs of persistent inflammation; extensive vacuolization consistent with ballooning of the lysosomal system was also observed in several cells of the cochlea and was most commonly found in the marginal cells of the stria vascularis. Many of these changes are likely the end result of excessive lysosomal exocytosis into the endolymph. Actually, numerous lysosomes docking at the apical surface of the marginal cells were positive for Lamp1 and Lamp2 (Wu et al. 2010). Increased levels of lysosomal content into the endolymphatic liquid maybe accountable for changes in endolymphatic potential, defective sound transduction in the sensory cells and ultimately be the cause of progressive hearing loss (Wu et al. 2010).

Neurodegeneration, a Link to Alzheimer's Disease

Through studies of mouse models of LSDs, it is becoming increasingly apparent that these pediatric conditions develop pathological signs, especially in the CNS, which resemble adult neurodegenerative diseases, like Alzheimer's disease (AD) and Parkinson disease (Ohmi et al. 2009, 2011, Keilani et al. 2012, Sidransky and Lopez 2012, Martins et al. 2015). As observed in other LSD models, the *Neu1*[−/−] mice exhibit early in life a brain phenotype with signs of early aging. However, what makes the *Neu1*[−/−] mouse model unique compared to other LSD models is the presence of amyloid deposits resembling the plaques characteristic of AD (Annunziata et al. 2013). Histopathological analyses of the *Neu1*[−/−] brain identified numerous multifocal, eosinophilic deposits, heterogeneous in size and shape, especially in the CA3 region of the hippocampus. These deposits contain proteinaceous material that stained positive with the Congo red/Chrysamine-G derivative Methoxy-X04, a compound with high affinity for amyloid. At the ultrastructural level, the same region of the *Neu1*[−/−] brain showed many dystrophic neurites, filled with electron dense vacuoles, likely representing autophagosomes or autophagolysosomes. These phenotypic changes can be directly linked to Neu1 loss of function for the following reasons: (1) in absence of Neu1, the amyloid precursor protein (APP) is oversialylated and accumulates in lysosomal fractions isolated from the hippocampus of *Neu1*[−/−] mice. These results identified APP as a natural substrate of NEU1; (2) accumulated APP is proteolytically processed to generate toxic Aβ peptides which are detected in purified lysosomes from hippocampal extracts and in the amyloid deposits; (3) combined accumulation of APP and Aβ peptides promotes the formation of the toxic amyloid peptide Aβ42; (4) the levels of secreted Aβ42 are higher in *Neu1*[−/−] cerebrospinal fluid and in the medium of *Neu1*[−/−] hippocampal neurosphere cultures than in the corresponding control samples (Annunziata et al. 2013). Finally, the demonstration that in absence of Neu1 Aβ is released via lysosomal exocytosis identifies this process as a novel mechanism for the extracellular deposition of this toxic peptide. Indeed, deletion of Neu1 in a transgenic mouse model of AD accelerates APP accumulation and plaque formation. On the other hand, exogenous expression of Neu1 in the brain of these AD mice largely reduced plaque occurrence. Combined these observations clearly link Neu1 loss of function to the occurrence of an AD-like phenotype in the sialidosis mice, and identify NEU1 enzyme activity as a risk factor for the development of this disease (Annunziata et al. 2013).

Conclusions

It is increasingly recognized that the spatiotemporal composition of sialic acids on glycoproteins and glycoconjugates plays a pivotal role in a myriad of fundamental cellular processes that control development/differentiation of cells and tissues, intracellular trafficking and signalling, cell-cell and cell-ECM cross-talks, cell survival and cell death. This review touches upon the pathogenic effects associated with hyposialylation or hypersialylation of specific glycoproteins as the result of genetic defects in enzymes that control either the early steps of sialic acid biosynthesis or the processing and degradation of bound sialic acids. We highlight how changes in sialic acid content affect the properties and functions of glycoproteins and impact on the physiological pathways they regulate, ultimately leading to loss of cell and tissue homeostasis and disease pathogenesis.

Acknowledgements

We apologize for not being able to cite all the outstanding contributions by other investigators in this field of research due to space constraints. We thank Dr. Gerard Grosveld for critical reading of this manuscript. A. D'Azzo holds the Jewelers for Children Endowed Chair in Genetics and Gene Therapy. This work was funded in part by NIH grants GM60905 and DK52025, the Assisi Foundation of Memphis, the American Lebanese Syrian Associated Charities (ALSAC) and the National Tay-Sachs & Allied Disease Association (NTSAD). A. D'Azzo and I. Annunziata are named as co-inventors on the patent application "Methods and compositions to detect the level of lysosomal exocytosis activity and methods of use", number PCT/US2012/052629 based, in part, on the research reported herein.

Keywords: sialic acids, neuraminidases, NEU1, GNE, sialidosis, galactosialidosis, inclusion body myopathy, lysosomal exocytosis

References

Aminoff, D., W. F. Bruegge, W. C. Bell, K. Sarpolis and R. Williams. 1977. Role of sialic acid in survival of erythrocytes in the circulation: Interaction of neuraminidase-treated and untreated erythrocytes with spleen and liver at the cellular level. Proc Natl Acad Sci USA 74: 1521–1524.

Andrews, N. W. 2000. Regulated secretion of conventional lysosomes. Trends Cell Biol 10: 316–321.

Andrews, P. M. 1979. Glomerular epithelial alterations resulting from sialic acid surface coat removal. Kidney Int 15: 376–385.

Annunziata, I., A. Patterson, D. Helton, H. Hu, S. Moshiach, E. Gomero et al. 2013. Lysosomal NEU1 deficiency affects amyloid precursor protein levels and amyloid-beta secretion via deregulated lysosomal exocytosis. Nat Commun 4: 2734.

Audry, M., C. Jeanneau, A. Imberty, A. Harduin-Lepers, P. Delannoy and C. Breton. 2011. Current trends in the structure-activity relationships of sialyltransferases. Glycobiology 21: 716–726.

Blomme, B., C. Van Steenkiste, N. Callewaert and H. Van Vlierberghe. 2009. Alteration of protein glycosylation in liver diseases. J Hepatol 50: 592–603.

Bonten, E. J., W. F. Arts, M. Beck, A. Covanis, M. A. Donati, R. Parini et al. 2000. Novel mutations in lysosomal neuraminidase identify functional domains and determine clinical severity in sialidosis. Hum Mol Genet 9: 2715–2725.

Bonten, E. J., Y. Campos, V. Zaitsev, A. Nourse, B. Waddell, W. Lewis et al. 2009. Heterodimerization of the sialidase NEU1 with the chaperone protective protein/cathepsin A prevents its premature oligomerization. J Biol Chem 284: 28430–28441.

Bonten, E. J., G. Yogalingam, H. Hu, E. Gomero, D. van de Vlekkert and A. d'Azzo. 2013. Chaperone-mediated gene therapy with recombinant AAV-PPCA in a new mouse model of type I sialidosis. Biochim Biophys Acta 1832: 1784–1792.

Bonten, E. J., I. Annunziata and A. d'Azzo. 2014. Lysosomal multienzyme complex: Pros and cons of working together. Cell Mol Life Sci 71: 2017–2032.

Bork, K., R. Horstkorte and W. Weidemann. 2009. Increasing the sialylation of therapeutic glycoproteins: The potential of the sialic acid biosynthetic pathway. J Pharm Sci 98: 3499–34508.

Bos, P. D., X. H. Zhang, C. Nadal, W. Shu, R. R. Gomis, D. X. Nguyen et al. 2009. Genes that mediate breast cancer metastasis to the brain. Nature 459: 1005–1009.

Bull, C., M. A. Stoel, M. H. den Brok and G. J. Adema. 2014. Sialic acids sweeten a tumor's Life. Cancer Res 74: 3199–3204.

Chavas, L. M., C. Tringali, P. Fusi, B. Venerando, G. Tettamanti, R. Kato et al. 2005. Crystal structure of the human cytosolic sialidase Neu2. Evidence for the dynamic nature of substrate recognition. J Biol Chem 280: 469–475.

Colman, P. M. 1994. Influenza virus neuraminidase: Structure, antibodies, and inhibitors. Protein Sci 3: 1687–1696.

Crocker, P. R., E. A. Clark, M. Filbin, S. Gordon, Y. Jones, J. H. Kehrl et al. 1998. Siglecs: A family of sialic-acid binding lectins. Glycobiology 8, 2 v.

d'Azzo, A. and E. Bonten. 2010. Molecular mechanisms of pathogenesis in a glycosphingolipid and a glycoprotein storage disease. Biochem Soc Trans 38: 1453–1457.

d'Azzo, A., G. Andria, E. Bonten and I. Annunziata. 2013. The Online Metabolic & Molecular Bases of Inherited Diseases. McGraw-Hill Publishing Co., New York.

d'Azzo, A., E. Machado and I. Annunziata. 2015. Pathogenesis, emerging therapeutic targets and treatment in sialidosis. Expert Opin Orphan Drugs 3: 491–504.

Dall'Olio, F., N. Malagolini, M. Trinchera and M. Chiricolo. 2014. Sialosignaling: Sialyltransferases as engines of self-fueling loops in cancer progression. Biochim Biophys Acta 1840: 2752–2764.

Daya, A., G. D. Vatine, M. Becker-Cohen, T. Tal-Goldberg, A. Friedmann, Y. Gothilf et al. 2014. Gne depletion during zebrafish development impairs skeletal muscle structure and function. Hum Mol Genet 23: 3349–3361.

de Geest, N., E. Bonten, L. Mann, J. de Sousa-Hitzler, C. Hahn and A. d'Azzo. 2002. Systemic and neurologic abnormalities distinguish the lysosomal disorders sialidosis and galactosialidosis in mice. Hum Mol Genet 11: 1455–1464.

Eisenberg, I., C. Thiel, T. Levi, E. Tiram, Z. Argov, M. Sadeh et al. 1999. Fine-structure mapping of the hereditary inclusion body myopathy locus. Genomics 55: 43–48.

Eisenberg, I., N. Avidan, T. Potikha, H. Hochner, M. Chen, T. Olender et al. 2001. The UDP-N-acetylglucosamine 2-epimerase/N-acetylmannosamine kinase gene is mutated in recessive hereditary inclusion body myopathy. Nat Genet 29: 83–87.

Eisenberg, I., G. Grabov-Nardini, H. Hochner, M. Korner, M. Sadeh, T. Bertorini et al. 2003. Mutations spectrum of GNE in hereditary inclusion body myopathy sparing the quadriceps. Hum Mutat 21: 99.

Enns, G. M., R. Seppala, T. J. Musci, K. Weisiger, L. D. Ferrell, D. A. Wenger et al. 2001. Clinical course and biochemistry of sialuria. J Inherit Metab Dis 24: 328–336.

Falconer, R. A., R. J. Errington, S. D. Shnyder, P. J. Smith and L. H. Patterson. 2012. Polysialyltransferase: A new target in metastatic cancer. Curr Cancer Drug Targets 12: 925–939.

Fukuda, M. N., H. Sasaki, L. Lopez and M. Fukuda. 1989. Survival of recombinant erythropoietin in the circulation: The role of carbohydrates. Blood 73: 84–89.

Galeano, B., R. Klootwijk, I. Manoli, M. Sun, C. Ciccone, D. Darvish et al. 2007. Mutation in the key enzyme of sialic acid biosynthesis causes severe glomerular proteinuria and is rescued by N-acetylmannosamine. J Clin Invest 117: 1585–1594.

Gaskell, A., S. Crennell and G. Taylor. 1995. The three domains of a bacterial sialidase: A β-propeller, an immunoglobulin module and a galactose-binding jelly-roll. Structure 3: 1197–1205.

Giacopuzzi, E., R. Bresciani, R. Schauer, E. Monti and G. Borsani. 2012. New insights on the sialidase protein family revealed by a phylogenetic analysis in metazoa. PLoS One 7: e44193.

Glavey, S. V., S. Manier, A. Natoni, A. Sacco, M. Moschetta, M. R. Reagan et al. 2014. The sialyltransferase ST3GAL6 influences homing and survival in multiple myeloma. Blood 124: 1765–1776.

Griffiths, G. M., A. Tsun and J. C. Stinchcombe. 2010. The immunological synapse: A focal point for endocytosis and exocytosis. J Cell Biol 189: 399–406.

Griggs, R. C., V. Askanas, S. DiMauro, A. Engel, G. Karpati, J. R. Mendell et al. 1995. Inclusion body myositis and myopathies. Ann Neurol 38: 705–713.

Hasegawa, T., C. Feijoo Carnero, T. Wada, Y. Itoyama and T. Miyagi. 2001. Differential expression of three sialidase genes in rat development. Biochem Biophys Res Commun 280: 726–732.

Heimburg-Molinaro, J., M. Lum, G. Vijay, M. T. Jain, A. Almogren and K. Rittenhouse-Olson. 2011. Cancer vaccines and carbohydrate epitopes. Vaccine 29: 8802–8826.

Hidari, K. I., S. Shimada, Y. Suzuki and T. Suzuki. 2007. Binding kinetics of influenza viruses to sialic acid-containing carbohydrates. Glycoconj J 24: 583–590.

Hinderlich, S., R. Stasche, R. Zeitler and W. Reutter. 1997. A bifunctional enzyme catalyzes the first two steps in N-acetylneuraminic acid biosynthesis of rat liver. Purification and characterization of UDP-N-acetylglucosamine 2-epimerase/N-acetylmannosamine kinase. J Biol Chem 272: 24313–24318.

Holt, O. J., F. Gallo and G. M. Griffiths. 2006. Regulating secretory lysosomes. J Biochem 140: 7–12.

Huizing, M. and D. M. Krasnewich. 2009. Hereditary inclusion body myopathy: A decade of progress. Biochim Biophys Acta 1792: 881–887.

Huynh, C., D. Roth, D. M. Ward, J. Kaplan and N. W. Andrews. 2004. Defective lysosomal exocytosis and plasma membrane repair in Chediak-Higashi/beige cells. Proc Natl Acad Sci USA 101: 16795–16800.

Karlsson, K. A. 1995. Microbial recognition of target-cell glycoconjugates. Curr Opin Struct Biol 5: 622–635.

Keilani, S., Y. Lun, A. C. Stevens, H. N. Williams, E. R. Sjoberg, R. Khanna et al. 2012. Lysosomal dysfunction in a mouse model of Sandhoff disease leads to accumulation of ganglioside-bound amyloid-beta peptide. J Neurosci 32: 5223–5236.

Kessel, D. and J. Allen. 1975. Elevated plasma sialyltransferase in cancer patient. Cancer Res 35: 670–672.

Krause, S., S. Hinderlich, S. Amsili, R. Horstkorte, H. Wiendl, Z. Argov et al. 2005. Localization of UDP-GlcNAc 2-epimerase/ManAc kinase (GNE) in the Golgi complex and the nucleus of mammalian cells. Exp Cell Res 304: 365–379.

Kuriyama, M., T. Ariga, S. Ando, M. Suzuki, T. Yamada and T. Miyatake. 1981. Four positional isomers of sialyloligosaccharides isolated from the urine of a patient with sialidosis. J Biol Chem 256: 12316.

Lu, J., T. Isaji, S. Im, T. Fukuda, N. Hashii, D. Takakura et al. 2014. beta-Galactoside alpha2,6-sialyltranferase 1 promotes transforming growth factor-beta-mediated epithelial-mesenchymal transition. J Biol Chem 289: 34627–34641.

Luzio, J. P., Y. Hackmann, N. M. Dieckmann and G. M. Griffiths. 2014. The biogenesis of lysosomes and lysosome-related organelles. Cold Spring Harb Perspect Biol 6: a016840.

Malicdan, M. C., S. Noguchi, I. Nonaka, Y. K. Hayashi and I. Nishino. 2007. A Gne knockout mouse expressing human GNE D176V mutation develops features similar to distal myopathy with rimmed vacuoles or hereditary inclusion body myopathy. Hum Mol Genet 16: 2669–2682.

Malicdan, M. C., S. Noguchi, T. Tokutomi, Y. Goto, I. Nonaka, Y. K. Hayashi et al. 2012. Peracetylated N-acetylmannosamine, a synthetic sugar molecule, efficiently rescues muscle phenotype and biochemical defects in mouse model of sialic acid-deficient myopathy. J Biol Chem 287: 2689–2705.

Marcos, N., E. Bennett, J. Gomes, A. Magalhaes, C. Gomes, L. David et al. 2010. Expression of sialyltransferase ST6GalNAc-I and sialyl-Tn antigen in human gastrointestinal tissues. Glycobiology 20: 1499–1500.

Martins, C., H. Hulkova, L. Dridi, V. Dormoy-Raclet, L. Grigoryeva, Y. Choi et al. 2015. Neuroinflammation, mitochondrial defects and neurodegeneration in mucopolysaccharidosis III type C mouse model. Brain 138: 336–355.

Milman Krentsis, I., I. Sela, R. Eiges, V. Blanchard, M. Berger, M. Becker Cohen et al. 2011. GNE is involved in the early development of skeletal and cardiac muscle. PLoS One 6: e21389.

Miyagi, T. and K. Yamaguchi. 2012. Mammalian sialidases: Physiological and pathological roles in cellular functions. Glycobiology 22: 880–896.

Monti, E., E. Bonten, A. D'Azzo, R. Bresciani, B. Venerando, G. Borsani et al. 2010. Sialidases in vertebrates: A family of enzymes tailored for several cell functions. Adv Carbohydr Chem Biochem 64: 403–479.

Montreuil, J., G. Biserte, G. Strecker, G. Spik, G. Fontaine and J. P. Farriaux. 1968. Description of a new type of melituria, called sialuria. Clin Chim Acta 21: 61–69.

Neves, J. C., V. R. Rizzato, A. Fappi, M. M. Garcia, G. Chadi, D. van de Vlekkert et al. 2015. Neuraminidase-1 mediates skeletal muscle regeneration. Biochim Biophys Acta 1852: 1755–1764.

Noguchi, S., Y. Keira, K. Murayama, M. Ogawa, M. Fujita, G. Kawahara et al. 2004. Reduction of UDP-N-acetylglucosamine 2-epimerase/N-acetylmannosamine kinase activity and sialylation in distal myopathy with rimmed vacuoles. J Biol Chem 279: 11402–11407.

Nonaka, I., N. Sunohara, S. Ishiura and E. Satoyoshi. 1981. Familial distal myopathy with rimmed vacuole and lamellar (myeloid) body formation. J Neurol Sci 51: 141–155.

Nonaka, I., S. Noguchi and I. Nishino. 2005. Distal myopathy with rimmed vacuoles and hereditary inclusion body myopathy. Curr Neurol Neurosci Rep 5: 61–65.

Ohmi, K., L. C. Kudo, S. Ryazantsev, H. Z. Zhao, S. L. Karsten and E. F. Neufeld. 2009. Sanfilippo syndrome type B, a lysosomal storage disease, is also a tauopathy. Proc Natl Acad Sci USA 106: 8332–8337.

Ohmi, K., H. Z. Zhao and E. F. Neufeld. 2011. Defects in the medial entorhinal cortex and dentate gyrus in the mouse model of Sanfilippo syndrome type B. PLoS One 6: e27461.

Ravindran, M. S., L. B. Tanner and M. R. Wenk. 2013. Sialic acid linkage in glycosphingolipids is a molecular correlate for trafficking and delivery of extracellular cargo. Traffic 14: 1182–1191.

Rodriguez, A., P. Webster, J. Ortego and N. W. Andrews. 1997. Lysosomes behave as Ca2+-regulated exocytic vesicles in fibroblasts and epithelial cells. J Cell Biol 137: 93–104.

Roggentin, P., R. Schauer, L. Hoyer and E. Vimr. 1993. MicroReview: The sialidase superfamily and its spread by horizontal gene transfer. Mol Microbiol 9: 915–921.

Rothe, B., B. Rothe, P. Roggentin and R. Schauer. 1991. The sialidase gene from Clostridium septicum: Cloning, sequencing, expression in *Escherichia coli* and identification of conserved sequences in sialidases and other proteins. Mol Gen Genet 226: 190–197.

Salama, I., S. Hinderlich, Z. Shlomai, I. Eisenberg, S. Krause, K. Yarema et al. 2005. No overall hyposialylation in hereditary inclusion body myopathy myoblasts carrying the homozygous M712T GNE mutation. Biochem Biophys Res Commun 328: 221–226.

Samie, M. A. and H. Xu. 2014. Lysosomal exocytosis and lipid storage disorders. J Lipid Res 55: 995–1009.

Savelkoul, P. J., I. Manoli, S. E. Sparks, C. Ciccone, W. A. Gahl, D. M. Krasnewich et al. 2006. Normal sialylation of serum N-linked and O-GalNAc-linked glycans in hereditary inclusion-body myopathy. Mol Genet Metab 88: 389–390.

Schauer, R. 2000. Achievements and challenges of sialic acid research. Glycoconj J 17: 485–499.

Schauer, R. 2009. Sialic acids as regulators of molecular and cellular interactions. Curr Opin Struct Biol 19: 507–514.

Schnaar, R. L., R. Gerardy-Schahn and H. Hildebrandt. 2014. Sialic acids in the brain: gangliosides and polysialic acid in nervous system development, stability, disease, and regeneration. Physiol Rev 94: 461–518.

Schultz, M. J., A. F. Swindall and S. L. Bellis. 2012. Regulation of the metastatic cell phenotype by sialylated glycans. Cancer and Metastasis Reviews 31: 501–518.

Schwake, M., B. Schroder and P. Saftig. 2013. Lysosomal membrane proteins and their central role in physiology. Traffic 14: 739–748.

Schwarzkopf, M., K. P. Knobeloch, E. Rohde, S. Hinderlich, N. Wiechens, L. Lucka et al. 2002. Sialylation is essential for early development in mice. Proc Natl Acad Sci USA 99: 5267–5270.

Sela, I., L. Yakovlev, M. Becker Cohen, M. Elbaz, N. Yanay, U. Ben Shlomo et al. 2013. Variable phenotypes of knockin mice carrying the M712T Gne mutation. Neuromolecular Med 15: 180–191.

Seppala, R., V. P. Lehto and W. A. Gahl. 1999. Mutations in the human UDP-N-acetylglucosamine 2-epimerase gene define the disease sialuria and the allosteric site of the enzyme. Am J Hum Genet 64: 1563–1569.

Severi, E., D. W. Hood and G. H. Thomas. 2007. Sialic acid utilization by bacterial pathogens. Microbiology 153: 2817–2822.

Sharon, N. and H. Lis. 1993. Carbohydrates in cell recognition. Sci Am 268: 82–89.

Sidransky, E. and G. Lopez. 2012. The link between the GBA gene and parkinsonism. Lancet Neurol 11: 986–998.

Smutova, V., A. Albohy, X. Pan, E. Korchagina, T. Miyagi, N. Bovin et al. 2014. Structural basis for substrate specificity of mammalian neuraminidases. PLoS One 9: e106320.

Sondermann, P., A. Pincetic, J. Maamary, K. Lammens and J. V. Ravetch. 2013. General mechanism for modulating immunoglobulin effector function. Proc Natl Acad Sci USA 110: 9868–9872.

Sparks, S. E., C. Ciccone, M. Lalor, E. Orvisky, R. Klootwijk, P. J. Savelkoul et al. 2005. Use of a cell-free system to determine UDP-N-acetylglucosamine 2-epimerase and N-acetylmannosamine kinase activities in human hereditary inclusion body myopathy. Glycobiology 15: 1102–1110.

Stasche, R., S. Hinderlich, C. Weise, K. Effertz, L. Lucka, P. Moormann et al. 1997. A bifunctional enzyme catalyzes the first two steps in N-acetylneuraminic acid biosynthesis of rat liver. Molecular cloning and functional expression of UDP-N-acetyl-glucosamine 2-epimerase/N-acetylmannosamine kinase. J Biol Chem 272: 24319–24324.

Stinchcombe, J., G. Bossi and G. M. Griffiths. 2004. Linking albinism and immunity: the secrets of secretory lysosomes. Science 305: 55–59.

Takahashi, K., Y. Tamanoue, M. Yanagida, Y. Sakurai, T. Takahashi and K. Sutoh. 1991. Specific cleavages of arginyl peptide bonds at basic amino acid pairs by a serine proteinase from the microsomal membranes of rat liver. Biochem Biophys Res Commun 175: 1152–1158.

Tanner, M. E. 2005. The enzymes of sialic acid biosynthesis. Bioorg Chem 33: 216–228.

Taylor, G. 1996. Sialidases: Structures, biological significance and therapeutic potential. Curr Opin Struct Biol 6: 830–837.

Thomas, G. 2013. The Online Metabolic & Molecular Bases of Inherited Diseases. McGraw-Hill Publishing Co., New York.

Topfer-Petersen, E. 1999. Carbohydrate-based interactions on the route of a spermatozoon to fertilization. Hum Reprod Update 5: 314–329.

Traving, C. and R. Schauer. 1998. Structure, function and metabolism of sialic acids. Cell Mol Life Sci 54: 1330–1349.

van Pelt, J., D. G. van Bilsen, J. P. Kamerling and J. F. Vliegenthart. 1988. Structural analysis of O-glycosidic type of sialyloligosaccharide-alditols derived from urinary glycopeptides of a sialidosis patient. Eur J Biol Chem 174: 183–187.

van Pelt, J., H. Bakker, J. P. Kamerling and J. F. Vliegenthart. 1991. A comparative study of sialyloligosaccharides isolated from sialidosis and galactosialidosis urine. J Inherit Metab Dis 14: 730.

Varki, A. 2007. Glycan-based interactions involving vertebrate sialic-acid-recognizing proteins. Nature 446: 1023–1029.

Varki, A. 2008. Sialic acids in human health and disease. Trends Mol Med 14: 351–360.

Varki, A. and R. Schauer. 2009. Sialic acids. *In*: Varki, A., R. D. Cummings, J. D. Esko, H. H. Freeze, P. Stanley, C. R. Bertozzi et al. (eds.). Essentials of Glycobiology. Cold Spring Harbor (NY).

Varki, A. and P. Gagneux. 2012. Multifarious roles of sialic acids in immunity. Ann N Y Acad Sci 1253: 16–36.

Vimr, E. 1994. Microbial sialidases: Does bigger always mean better? Trends in Microbiology 2: 271–277.

Warren, L. and H. Felsenfeld. 1962. The biosynthesis of sialic acids. J Biol Chem 237: 1421–1431.

Weidemann, W., C. Klukas, A. Klein, A. Simm, F. Schreiber and R. Horstkorte. 2010. Lessons from GNE-deficient embryonic stem cells: Sialic acid biosynthesis is involved in proliferation and gene expression. Glycobiology 20: 107–117.

Wopereis, S., U. M. Abd Hamid, A. Critchley, L. Royle, R. A. Dwek, E. Morava et al. 2006. Abnormal glycosylation with hypersialylated O-glycans in patients with sialuria. Biochim Biophys Acta 1762: 598–607.

Wu, X., K. A. Steigelman, E. Bonten, H. Hu, W. He, T. Ren et al. 2010. Vacuolization and alterations of lysosomal membrane proteins in cochlear marginal cells contribute to hearing loss in neuraminidase 1-deficient mice. Biochim Biophys Acta 1802: 259–268.

Yardeni, T., K. Jacobs, T. K. Niethamer, C. Ciccone, Y. Anikster, N. Kurochkina et al. 2013. Murine isoforms of UDP-GlcNAc 2-epimerase/ManNAc kinase: Secondary structures, expression profiles, and response to ManNAc therapy. Glycoconj J 30: 609–618.

Yogalingam, G., E. J. Bonten, D. van de Vlekkert, H. Hu, S. Moshiach, S. A. Connell et al. 2008. Neuraminidase 1 is a negative regulator of lysosomal exocytosis. Dev Cell 15: 74–86.

Yonekawa, T., M. C. Malicdan, A. Cho, Y. K. Hayashi, I. Nonaka, T. Mine et al. 2014. Sialyllactose ameliorates myopathic phenotypes in symptomatic GNE myopathy model mice. Brain 137: 2670–2679.

Yunis, E. J. and F. J. Samaha. 1971. Inclusion body myositis. Lab Invest 25: 240–248.

Zanoteli, E., D. van de Vlekkert, E. J. Bonten, H. Hu, L. Mann, E. M. Gomero et al. 2010. Muscle degeneration in neuraminidase 1-deficient mice results from infiltration of the muscle fibers by expanded connective tissue. Biochim Biophys Acta 1802: 659–672.

CHAPTER 9

Role of Glycosylation in TOLL-like Receptor Activation and Pro-inflammatory Responses

Schammim Ray Amith,[1] Samar Abdulkhalek[2] and Myron R. Szewczuk[3],*

Introduction

Infectious and inflammatory diseases caused by microbial pathogens, once highly prevalent only in the developing world, are now cause for global concern. The mammalian Toll-like receptors (TLRs) are one of the families of sensor receptors that recognize pathogen-associated molecular patterns (PAMPs). Not only are TLRs crucial sensors of microbial (e.g., viral, bacterial and parasitic) infections in innate immune cells, they also play important roles in the pathophysiology of infectious, inflammatory and autoimmune diseases. Thus, the intensity and duration of TLR responses against invading microbial pathogens and endogenous danger signals must be tightly controlled. It follows that studies on the structural integrity of TLRs, their ligand interactions and signaling components may provide important information essential to our understanding of TLR-dependent immunological protection and disease intervention. Although the signaling pathways of TLR sensors are well characterized, the parameters controlling interactions between these receptors and their ligands still remain poorly defined. Here, we summarize the current understanding of TLR structure, function and signaling, and highlight the role of glycosylation and sialylation in TLR activation. The key interactions that induce TLR activation are identified in a novel TLR-signaling platform. A mammalian neuraminidase-1 (Neu1 sialidase) and matrix metalloproteinase 9 (MMP9) cross-talk in alliance with the G-protein coupled receptor (GPCR) neuromedin B is uncovered which is essential for TLR-induced receptor activation, cellular signaling and pro-inflammatory responses.

[1] Department of Biochemistry, University of Alberta, Edmonton, AB, T6G 2H7, Canada.
  E-mail: amith@ualberta.ca
[2] General Requirement Unit, Fatima College of Health Sciences, P.O. Box 24162, Al Ain, United Arab Emirates.
  E-mail: samarma@hotmail.com
[3] Department of Biomedical and Molecular Sciences, Queen's University, Kingston, Ontario K7L3N6, Canada.
  E-mail: szewczuk@queensu.ca
* Corresponding author

Glycosylation: An Overview

The glycosylation of membrane proteins is a critical post-translational modification that primarily enables the anchorage of these entities at the cell surface. Glycosylation profiles can render structurally different variations, or glycoforms, of identical proteins based on the arrangement of individual sugars as they are added to the protein backbone during its biosynthesis and transport from the endoplasmic reticulum (ER), through the Golgi apparatus, and finally, to the plasma membrane. In mammalian cells, proteins can have few to several putative N- or O-linked glycosylation sites. N-linked glycosylation involves the addition of monosaccharides to an amino group of an asparagine residue and occurs in the ER. In O-linked glycosylation, glycans can be added to the hydroxyl group of an underlying serine or threonine, which can occur in the ER, Golgi, cytosol or nucleus (van Kooyk and Rabinovich 2008). Glycosylation is enzymatically driven, and can be catalyzed by glycosidases or glycosyltransferases. Glycosidases, all of which are substrate-specific for their target sugars, are important in ridding glycosylated proteins of their sugar molecules by hydrolyzing the glycosidic bonds between them. Glycosyltransferases, on the other hand, are key in synthesizing oligosaccharide chains, and transfer sugars from a nucleotide sugar donor to proteins awaiting post-translational glycosylation. There are nine nucleotide sugar donors: fucose, galactose, N-acetylgalactosamine, glucose, N-acetylglucosamine, glucuronic acid, mannose, xylose, and sialic acid. In addition, there are multiple protein acceptor motifs for glycosyltransferases, all of which can construct glycans in many different stereo-isomeric configurations linked to the donor sugar ring. The first attached monosaccharide can then be linked to other sugars through α or β glycosidic linkages as it forms an oligosaccharide chain (Ohtsubo and Marth 2006).

In this chapter, we focus on sialic acid residues which are the terminal sugars on these oligosaccharide chains, and the sialidase enzymes that catalyze their hydrolysis. Sialidases have several critical roles in the pathophysiology of human diseases, including infection and inflammation. Our interest lies in the glycosylation of cell surface and endogenous toll-like receptors on immune cells, where receptor glycosylation plays a key role in pathogen-molecule ligand recognition and binding. In recent years, we have shown that ligand-induced toll-like receptor activation is elegantly mediated by Neu1 sialidase, the most abundant isoform of this glycosidic enzyme. Here, we review the role of Neu1 sialidase in the activation of toll-like receptors, their downstream signaling events and effector functions.

Sialic Acids and Sialidases

Sialic acids (SAs) are a family of nine-carbon monosaccharides that include neuraminic acid and its derivatives. They form the majority of terminal sugar residues of cell surface N- and O-linked glycans and secreted glycoproteins, and are bound to an underlying galactose residue by either α-2,3-, α-2,6- or α-2,8-glycosidic linkages. Sialic acids were initially thought to function primarily to confer negative charge and hydrophilic properties to vertebrate cell surfaces, and to block underlying galactoses from indiscriminate recognition by receptors. SA-binding proteins are expressed in many organisms that do not themselves have sialic acids; this is thought to be an evolutionary adaptation especially in terms of pathogen infectivity, since sialic acids act as receptors for microbes and toxins. These SA-deficient organisms (particularly those of plant origin) express SA-binding proteins, or lectins, that display exquisite specificity for sialic acids in other species based on their glycosidic linkages (Varki 2007, Varki and Varki 2007). These plant-derived lectins, like *Maackia amurensis* lectin (MAL-2), which specifically binds α-2,3-SA, and *Sambucus nigra* lectin (SNA), which binds α-2,6-SA (Balcan et al. 2008), are very useful tools in studying the role of these sugars on glycoprotein surfaces. In the immune system, sialic acids play well-defined roles, particularly in cell adhesion. Selectins and siglecs (sialic-acid binding immunoglobulin-type lectins) mediate interactions between immune cells. On macrophages, siglec-1 modulates macrophage-driven immune responses and acts as a phagocytic receptor for pathogen-associated sialic acids (Oetke et al. 2006). Sialylation profiles of glycans are important during the thymic development of T cells (Van Dyken and Locksley 2007), and the expression of α-2,6-SAs are upregulated during B cell development (Wuensch et al. 2000), whereas T lymphocyte activation is linked to a downregulation of cell surface sialylation (Nan et al. 2007).

Cellular sialylation is metabolically regulated by sialidase enzymes and sialyltransferases. Endogenous mammalian sialidases (alternatively referred to as neuraminidases), are glycohydrolytic enzymes that catalyze the removal of sialic acid residues from glycoproteins and glycolipids (Miyagi et al. 2004). To date, four types of human sialidases have been characterized, and are classified by their subcellular localization: lysosomal and cell membrane (Neu1), cytosolic (Neu2), plasma membrane-bound (Neu3), and lysosomal or mitochondrial-associated (Neu4). While they share structural similarities, they differ in their functions and substrate specificities (Magesh et al. 2006). Neu1 in lysosomes is associated with lysosomal carboxypeptidase A (protective protein cathepsin A), β-galactosidase, and N-acetyl-galactosamine-6-sulphate sulphatase (Liang et al. 2006). Neu1 functions mainly to regulate lipid storage in lysosomes, but also negatively regulates lysosomal exocytosis in hematopoietic cells where it processes the sialic acids on the lysosomal membrane protein LAMP-1 (Yogalingam et al. 2008). Traditionally, Neu1 has always been classed as a lysosomal enzyme, until its presence was discovered at the surface of cells. Elastin binding protein, involved in elastic fibre deposition, was found to form a complex with Neu1/cathepsin A at the cell surface (Caciotti et al. 2005). In activated lymphocytes, lysosomal sialidase is redistributed to the cell membrane (Lukong et al. 2001). Here, a nine-fold increase in Neu1-specific activity is detected at cell surface, where the Neu1-cathepsin A complex influences signaling that results in the production of interferon gamma (IFNγ) (Nan et al. 2007). Neu1 expression is also upregulated during monocyte differentiation, and is trafficked to the membrane via MHCII-positive vesicles (Liang et al. 2006). More recently, interactions between siglecs and TLRs that were mediated by Neu1 were reported where TLR4 activation by endotoxin triggers Neu1 translocation to the cell surface to disrupt TLR4:Siglec-E interaction (von Minckwitz et al. 2014). Neu1-deficient mice produce markedly less IgE and IgG1 antibodies following immunization with protein antigens, a result of their failure to produce IL-4 cytokines (Chen et al. 1997). Inherited mutations in the *NEU1* gene result in the autosomal recessive disorder, sialidosis, which is categorized by the progressive lysosomal storage of sialylated glycopeptides and oligosaccharides; this presents clinically as either severe neurodegenerative disease, i.e., early-onset (type II sialidosis), or the relatively milder late-onset (type I sialidosis) pathology (Seyrantepe et al. 2003).

Cytosolic Neu2 is usually expressed in low levels in cells, but at higher levels in skeletal muscle (Sato and Miyagi 1996), the liver (Miyagi and Tsuiki 1985), and the thymus (Kotani et al. 2001), as well as potentially playing a significant role in myoblast differentiation (Fanzani et al. 2008). The crystal structure of human Neu2 in its free form as well as in complex with the neuraminidase inhibitor 2-deoxy-2,3-dehydro-N-acetylneuraminic acid (DANA) has been characterized (Chavas et al. 2005).

Neu3 is involved in ganglioside degradation and preferentially targets GM1 gangliosides. In mice, the over-expression of Neu3 has also been implicated in the development of severe insulin-resistant diabetes, and may be an important regulator of insulin sensitivity and glucose tolerance (Yoshizumi et al. 2007).

Neu4 is highly expressed in the mucosal surfaces of the colon, although this expression was markedly reduced in colon cancer, suggesting a role for Neu4 in the maintenance of normal colon mucosa (Yamanami et al. 2007). Additionally, Neu4 can also be localized on the cell surface of macrophages (Finlay et al. 2010).

A Role for Glycosylation in the Innate Immune Response

Given the importance of surface sialylation on immune cells, and the fact that Neu1 sialidase expression can become altered during the development of these cells, a link between glycosylation and cellular activation can be presupposed. In immune cells, toll-like receptors (TLRs) are key in the recognition of highly conserved pathogen-associated molecular patterns (PAMPs) from bacteria, fungi, viruses and parasites. Depending on the specific PAMP-TLR interaction, an intricate TLR-mediated signaling cascade is initiated which translates the rapidly generated innate immune counter attack into delayed adaptive immune responses that result in immunologic memory (Atkinson et al. 2008). The identified human TLRs have specific and well-characterized affinities for their PAMP ligand(s) (Medzhitov and Janeway 1997). Briefly, TLR2, which forms a heterodimer with either TLR1 or TLR6, is key in the immune response to mycobacterial lipoarabinomannan, Gram-positive bacterial peptidoglycans, and zymosan from yeast cell walls (Janssens and Beyaert 2003). TLR3 is activated by double-stranded RNA. TLR4 is a critical component of the Gram-negative bacterial lipopolysaccharide (LPS) receptor complex, along with CD14 and MD2; TLR4 also binds Gram-positive bacterial lipoteichoic acids. TLR5 is the signaling mediator of bacterial flagellin; TLR7 and TLR8 recognize single-stranded RNA; and TLR9 is activated by microbial DNA (Zhang et al. 2009). While ligand specificity and biological function for TLR10 is not known, it is thought to be an anti-inflammatory pattern-recognition receptor (Oosting et al. 2014). Genomic studies have shown that this orphan member of the TLR family can be mapped to a locus that also contains TLR1 and TLR6, both of which are co-receptors for TLR2, suggesting a similar role for TLR10 (Hasan et al. 2005).

TLRs are type I transmembrane glycoproteins found on the plasma membrane or in endosomal compartments of various immune cells including macrophages, dendritic cells, B and T lymphocytes and natural killer cells. They are structurally characterized by: a highly glycosylated extracellular ectodomain, a single transmembrane domain and a cytoplasmic Toll-Interleukin-1 receptor (TIR) homology domain (Choe et al. 2005). PAMP recognition and ligand binding occurs on the ectodomain, while the TIR domain is responsible for activating the TLR signal cascade that ultimately results in the nuclear translocation of NFκB (Leulier and Lemaitre 2008). Ligand binding results in either homo- or hetero-dimerization of TLRs, but it is the resulting juxtaposition of the two TIR domains that initiates the intracellular signaling pathway. This involves the recruitment of various adaptor proteins: MyD88, Mal or TIRAP (MyD88 adaptor-like protein; TIR-associated protein), TRIF (TIR 3 domain-containing adaptor protein-inducing IFN-β) and TRAM (TRIF-related adaptor molecule). Signaling via MyD88 and Mal/TIRAP (MyD88-dependent) induce genes for pro-inflammatory cytokines and chemokines, while TRIF and TRAM (MyD88 independent) signaling induce the interferons (Albiger et al. 2007a,b). All TLRs, with the exception of TLR3, signal through MyD88. Upon ligand-induced TLR dimerization, MyD88 is recruited to and associates with the TIR domain. In the case of TLR2 and TLR4, however, this association is likely mediated by the co-adaptor TIRAP, since cells from TIRAP-knockout mice show defective TLR2 and delayed TLR4 signaling (Yamamoto et al. 2002). MyD88 recruits interleukin-1 receptor-associated kinase 4 (IRAK-4), which is activated by phosphorylation, and further activates IRAK-1. Phosphorylated IRAK-1 associates with TNF receptor-associated factor 6 (TRAF6), which then activates TGF-β-activating kinase 1 (TAK1). TAK1 induces the phosphorylation of IKK-β, which leads to the degradation of IκB and the subsequent activation and nuclear translocation of transcription factor NFκB. MyD88-dependent TLR signaling also activates the MAP kinase signaling pathway which results in the activation of additional transcription factors like AP-1 and IFN regulatory factor (IRF)-5. TLR4, in addition to TLR3, can signal independently of MyD88. Whereas TLR3 signaling requires interaction only with adaptor molecule TRIF, TLR4-mediated signaling requires both TRIF and TRAM. TRIF interacts with TRAF6 or receptor-interacting protein 1 (RIP1), both of which lead to the activation of NFκB. TRIF can also activate TRAF family members-associated NFκB activator (TANK) binding kinase 1 (TBK1) which directly phosphorylates transcription factors IRF-3 and IRF-7, thus allowing for their translocation to the nucleus to induce the expression of the genes for type I interferons (Albiger et al. 2007a,b). This complex TLR signaling is tightly controlled so as not to pose a threat to resident microflora and to avoid an excessive inflammatory response. This is chiefly accomplished by the regulation of protein phosphorylation and degradation, interaction with inhibitory adaptor molecules, or sequesteration (Miggin and O'Neill 2006).

In 2005, the crystal structure of the human TLR3 ectodomain at 2.1 angstroms was characterized (Choe et al. 2005). It revealed a large horseshoe-shaped solenoid assembled from 23 leucine-rich repeats (LRRs), with one surface of this structure being highly glycosylated with 15 potential N-glycosylation sites, whereas glycosylation is completely absent on the other surface, suggesting a possible location for ligand binding and oligomerization. Later that year, the molecular structure of the TLR3 ligand-binding domain was defined (Bell et al. 2005). Early on, because of the inefficiency of the production and crystallization of some LRR proteins like the TLRs, innovative structural analysis strategies had to be employed in addition to sequence analyses. These led to the molecular characterization of TLR1, TLR2, TLR4, TLR6 and TLR10 (Jin et al. 2007). Sharp structural transitions in the LRR domain of these TLRs further divides this region into three subdomains: N-terminal, central, and C-terminal. These structural alterations appear to be important for binding hydrophobic ligands like lipoproteins. TLR3, however, has a structurally flat LRR domain with uniform conformational angles, defined by a single ectodomain that is not divided into subdomains. Although the structures of TLR5, TLR7, TLR8 and TLR9 have not been similarly analyzed, initial comparisons of their LRR domains suggest that they too belong to the single-domain subfamily of

LRR motifs, suggesting that this conformation is important in the recognition of hydrophilic proteins or nucleic acids (Jin and Lee 2008). More recently, crystal structures have been determined for the: ectodomains of human TLRs 1, 2, 3 and 4; mouse TLRs 2, 3, 4 and 6; and zebrafish TLR5; and TIR domains of TLRs 1, 2 and 10 (Tao et al. 2002, Bell et al. 2005, Choe et al. 2005, Jin et al. 2007, Kim et al. 2007, Nyman et al. 2008, Ohto et al. 2012). Evidently, the precise structural complexities of TLRs have important implications for their ligand interactions. It is therefore conceivable that the abundant glycosylation of these receptors may play a key role in their bioactivity.

Glycosylation is thought to contribute to protein stability, and specific glycoforms are involved in key recognition interactions, such as ligand-specific recognition and ligand binding to its cognate receptor. With TLR3 at least, the post-translational N-glycosylations were shown to contribute significantly to the overall mass (about 35%) of the TLR3 ectodomain. TLR3-induced NFκB activation is inhibited in cells treated with tunicamycin, an inhibitor of glycosylation. Additionally, mutations in two different predicted glycosylation sites impaired TLR3 function without altering receptor expression (Sun et al. 2006). MD-2 and CD14, which form a complex with TLR4 for LPS-mediated signaling, are also glycosylated. MD-2 and the amino terminal ectodomain of human TLR4 potentially contain two and nine N-glycosylation sites respectively, based on their sequence analysis. For CD14, four predicted N-glycosylation sites are required for trafficking and ligand interaction (Meng et al. 2008). Studies with TLR4 and MD-2 mutants lacking N-linked glycosylation sites have shown that these are essential to maintaining the functional integrity of the LPS receptor complex (da Silva and Ulevitch 2002). There is also a definitive role for glycosylation in the trafficking of TLR2 and TLR4 from internal compartments to the cell surface, where putative glycosylation sites were shown to be important determinants for the shedding of TLR2 from monocytes (Weber et al. 2004).

Other receptor families also show similar functions for receptor glycosylation. For example, when tumour cells expressing receptor tyrosine kinases, including the epidermal growth factor receptor (EGFR) and the type I insulin-like growth factor receptor (IGF-IR), are treated with tunicamycin, both receptor function and expression are inhibited (Contessa et al. 2008). Microscale deglycosylation assays have showed that both conserved and variable N-glycosylation sites on the nerve growth factor (NGF) binding TrkA receptor played an important dual role: firstly, to localize the TrkA receptor to the plasma membrane, and secondly, to prevent ligand-independent activation (auto-phosphorylation) of TrkA (Watson et al. 1999). Molecular analysis of N-glycosylation site mutant and wild-type forms of the transmembrane human bradykinin B2 receptor (of the G protein coupled receptor family) showed that glycosylation, and particularly sialylation, was critical for receptor stabilization at the cell surface (Michineau et al. 2006). Additionally, when the glycosylation profile of the immunoglobulin G-containing B-cell receptors of peripheral blood lymphocytes from patients with multiple myelomas was compared to normal cells, the degree of sialylation was increased in myeloma cells while expression of galactose and N-acetylglucosamine were not significantly affected (Ilic et al. 2008). It could be speculated, therefore, that for cells involved in disease pathology, receptor glycoproteins may have altered glycosylation profiles. Since most of the major molecules involved in both innate and adaptive responses are glycoproteins, the potential role that these sugars play in immune cell function is myriad.

Neu1 Sialidase in the Activation of Cell Surface TLRs

Insight for the role of glycosylation in TLR activation came from the well-characterized model of the Trk tyrosine-protein kinase receptor family, which functions as a signaling receptor for the neurotrophin family of molecules of nerve growth factor (NGF) and brain-derived neurotrophic factor (BDNF). For TrkA receptors, glycosylation is required to localize receptors to the cell surface where it prevents ligand-independent (auto-)activation of receptors (Watson et al. 1999). The observation that trypanosome *trans*-sialidase and bacterial neuraminidase could activate Trk receptors independent of their cognate ligands was key in inferring a role for endogenous cellular sialidase in the activation of these receptors *in vivo* (Woronowicz et al. 2004). This led to the discovery that Neu1 sialidase localized at the plasma membrane controls the activation of TrkA and TrkB receptors upon binding of their neurotrophin growth factor ligands, NGF and BDNF respectively (Woronowicz et al. 2004, 2007). Here, Neu1 sialidase specifically targets and hydrolyzes sialylα-2,3-linked β-galactosyl residues of TrkA receptors, allowing for their eventual dimerization and activation. It is thought that this desialylation process removes key terminal sialic acids that spatially prevent Trk receptor monomers from auto-dimerization. Once desialylated, Trk receptor dimerization leads to oligomerization, phosphorylation and internalization of Trk dimers with their ligands still bound, thus initiating downstream signalling (Woronowicz et al. 2007).

In the biosynthesis and activation of toll-like receptors, the potential role of Neu1 sialidase is hypothesized to be three-fold: firstly, since glycosylated receptors have a default sorting route, travelling from the endoplasmic reticulum to lysosomal compartments, Neu1 may be involved in dictating the precise pattern of glycosylation on these receptors; secondly, Neu1 could potentially be a requisite intermediate in regulating receptor activation, as in the case of Trk receptors; and thirdly, Neu1 activity could influence the glycosylation pattern of receptors at the cell surface, thus modulating their activity when their cognate ligands are either present or absent. The precise mechanism of how Neu1 influences toll-like receptor activation and cell function in these three contexts is not apparent. However, in recent years, the role of Neu1 as an intermediary in the activation of TLRs has become clearer.

Central to the idea that TLR glycosylation is controlled by the activity of Neu1 sialidase is the localization of Neu1 at the cell surface. Is Neu1 activity detectable at the surface of live, intact cells? To answer this question, a live-cell sialidase assay was developed to visualize Neu1 activity at the plasma membrane (Amith et al. 2010b) (Fig. 1).

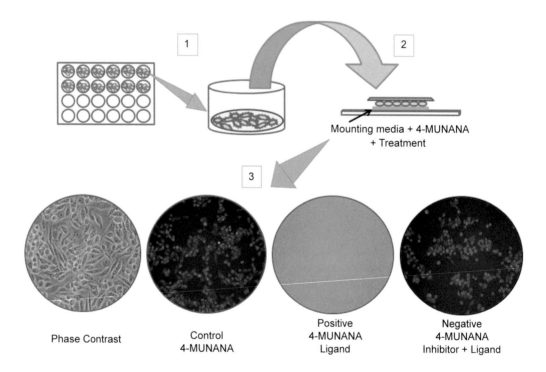

Epi-fluorescent Images at 450 nm – 40X

Figure 1. Live-cell screening assay for sialidase activity: (1) BMC-2 macrophage cells or DC2.4 dendritic cells are allowed to adhere on 12 mm circular glass slides in media containing 10% fetal calf serum for 24 h. Primary bone marrow-derived macrophage cells are grown on 12 mm circular glass slides in RPMI conditioned medium for 7–8 days in a humidified incubator at 37°C and 5% CO_2. (2) After removing media, 0.318 mM 4-MUNANA substrate (2′-(4-methylumbelliferyl)-α-N-acetylneuraminic acid) in Tris buffered saline pH 7.4 is added to cells alone (Control), with receptor ligands (Positive), or with ligand in combination with an inhibitor 200 μM oseltamivir phosphate (Negative). Coverslips are inverted onto glass slides. (3) In the presence of sialidase enzymes, 4-MUNANA is hydrolyzed to give free 4-methylumbelliferone, which has a fluorescence emission at 450 nm (blue color, positive) following excitation at 365 nm. Fluorescent images are taken at 1–2 min after adding substrate using epi-fluorescent microscopy (40x objective).

Briefly, cell surface sialidase activity is detected when 4-MUNANA (2'-(4-methylumbelliferyl)-α-D-N-acetylneuraminic acid), a Neu1-specific fluorogenic substrate, is specifically cleaved and hydrolyzed to 4-methylumbelliferone, which fluoresces with an emission wavelength of 450 nm. This fluorescence is only observed when ligand-receptor interactions occur, wherein Neu1 is induced, for example, when zymosan A binds to TLR2; poly I:C binds to TLR3; or gram-negative bacterial lipopolysaccharide (LPS) binds to TLR4. When these ligands bind to their cognate receptors on the surface of BMC-2 macrophages and DC2.4 dendritic cells, Neu1 sialidase is induced. In the presence of 4-MUNANA, the induced Neu1 sialidase hydrolyzes the fluorogenic substrate, and a visible blue fluorescence is readily observed under the microscope. The fluorescence is rapid but quantifiable, and persists until all the substrate molecules are hydrolyzed. Importantly, Neu1 activity is highly specific for specific ligand-receptor pairs. When HEK293 cells stably expressing either TLR2, TLR3 or TLR4/MD2 on their surface are used in the sialidase assay, the fluorescence of 4-MUNANA as it is cleaved by Neu1 is only detected when cognate ligands are used with their respective TLRs. For example, Neu1 activity of cells expressing TLR4/MD2 is only observed in the presence of LPS; no fluorescence is detected in the presence of zymosan A or poly I:C. Likewise, when parental HEK293 cells which do not normally express these receptors, are used in the assay, no sialidase activity is detected.

Additionally, in primary bone-marrow derived murine macrophages, the same ligand-specific sialidase activity is detected only when ligands are paired with their respective receptors. The only exception is in the case of poly I:C and TLR3. The above mouse and human cell lines display TLR3 (an endogenous TLR) on the cell surface, so when poly I:C binds to TLR3, Neu1 activity is detected. In primary macrophages, TLR3 remains endosomal, and no cell surface Neu1 activity is observed. Confirmation that this cell surface fluorescence is due to sialidase activity came from the use of pharmaceutical sialidase inhibitors, which inhibited any detectable fluorescence upon addition to cells. A variety of known sialidase inhibitors reduced Neu1 activity on the cell surface, including zanamivir, DANA (2-deoxy-2,3-dehydro-N-acetylneuraminic acid), and oseltamivir carboxylate; but only oseltamivir phosphate (Tamiflu®) was able to completely block Neu1 activity. However, none these inhibitors are specifically targeted against Neu1. Further substantiation of the specific involvement of Neu1 in this activation process came from the addition of neutralizing antibodies to these cells in the presence of ligands and their cognate receptors. Here, an inhibition of sialidase-induced fluorescence, akin to that achieved with oseltamivir phosphate, was only seen when an anti-Neu1 antibody was used. This was later confirmed with the immunofluorescent detection of Neu1 at the cell surface of intact cells (Fig. 2).

Interestingly, Neu1 was found to colocalize with TLR4 on the plasma membrane. Neu1 also co-immunoprecipitates with TLR4 in control untreated cells and in cells treated with LPS, but only minimally so when LPS-treated cells are exposed to oseltamivir phosphate. Neu1 was also found to co-immunoprecipitate with TLR2 and TLR3, both in untreated control cells and in cells treated with either zymosan A or poly I:C, respectively. Taken together, these data indicate that Neu1 is in a complex with TLRs at the cell surface, even in the absence of TLR ligands (Amith et al. 2009).

Furthermore, it was demonstrated that LPS-induced MyD88/TLR4 complex formation and subsequent downstream NFκB activation is dependent on the removal of α-2,3-sialyl sugars linked to an underlying β-galactoside residue of TLR4 (Amith et al. 2009). This desialylation process is mediated by the induction of Neu1 sialidase when LPS binds to TLR4 in live primary macrophage cells, and macrophage and dendritic cell lines, but not in primary macrophages isolated from Neu1-deficient mice. In the absence of LPS, exogenous α-2,3 sialyl specific neuraminidase (from *Streptoccocus pneumoniae*) and wild-type *Trypanasoma cruzi* trans-sialidase (TS), but not the catalytically inactive mutant TSΔAsp98-Glu, mediate TLR4 dimerization to facilitate MyD88/TLR4 complex formation and NFκB activation. These same TLR ligand-induced NFκB responses are not observed in parental HEK293 cells deficient in the expression of TLR4, but are re-established in HEK293 cells stably transfected with TLR4/MD2. NFκB activity is also significantly inhibited by α-2,3-sialyl specific *Maackia amurensis* (MAL-2) lectin, α-2,3-sialyl specific galectin-1, and oseltamivir phosphate, but not by α-2,6-sialyl specific *Sambucus nigra* lectin (SNA) (Amith et al. 2010a). Similar to Trk receptors, the above observations also suggest that α-2,3-sialyl residues of TLR receptors are important in creating steric hindrance, preventing TLR monomers on the cell surface from auto-dimerization. In contrast, it was recently reported that α-2,6-sialyl residues of TLR4 may be equally

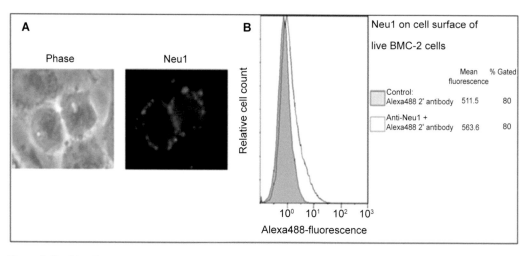

Figure 2. Neu1 localizes on the plasma membrane of intact cells. A. Neu1 on the cell membrane of BMC-2 macrophage cells. Untreated BMC-2 cells were fixed with 4% paraformaldehyde, non-permeabilized and immunostained with anti-Neu1 antibodies followed with Alexa594 conjugated secondary antibody. Stained cells were visualized using epi-fluorescence microscopy at objective 40x. B. Flow cytometry analysis of Neu1 expressed on the cell surface of live BMC-2 cells. Histogram shows staining with rabbit anti-Neu1 antibodies after incubation onice for 15 min and followed with Alexa488 conjugated secondary antibody for additional 15 min onice. Control cells were stained with Alexa488 conjugated secondary antibody for 15 min onice. Cells were analyzed by Beckman Coulter Epics XL-MCL flow cytometry and Expo32 ADC software (Beckman Coulter). Control Alexa488 secondary antibody treated cells are represented by the black-filled histogram. Live cells stained with anti-Neu1 antibody are depicted by the unfilled histogram with the black line. The mean fluorescence for each histogram is indicated for 40000 acquired cells (80% gated). Taken from (Amith et al. 2009) with permission from Glycoconjugate Journal.

important in its activation (Feng et al. 2012a). Using HEK293T cells transfected with plasmids encoding TLR4, CD14, and MD2, as well as a NFκB luciferase reporting system, it was demonstrated that both TLR4 and MD2 are α-2,6 linked sialylated. Here, it is thought that removal of negatively charged sialyl residues from glycans on the TLR4 complex hasten the dimerization of TLR4 monomers required for signaling. It was concluded that sialyl residues on TLR4 modulate LPS responsiveness, likely by facilitating clustering of the homodimers. Additionally, sialic acid, and perhaps other glycosyl species, regulate MD2 activity required for LPS-mediated signaling (Feng et al. 2012b). These findings lend credence to the role endogenous sialidase plays in the activation and regulation of TLR4. Moreover, Neu1 desialylation of these receptor monomers upon LPS binding thus enables TLR4 dimerization and recruitment of MyD88, the signaling event that leads to the nuclear translocation of NFκB, which starts the TLR-mediated immune response, ultimately resulting in cytokine or nitric acid production in response to LPS (Amith et al. 2009). When Neu1-deficient mice are exposed to LPS, their cytokine profiles 5 h post-LPS administration are markedly different from wild-type mice. Neu1-deficient mice produced significantly lower levels of C5a, G-CFS, IL1ra, IL-6, KC (cytokine-induced neutrophil chemoattractant), and MIP2 (macrophage inflammatory protein-2) cytokines in response to LPS compared to the WT mice. Interestingly, THP-1 human monocyte cells show an inhibition of IL-6 and TNFα production in response to LPS when treated with oseltamivir phosphate, suggesting that sialidase activity significantly contributes to the production of pro-inflammatory cytokine in response to LPS (Fig. 3).

Oseltamivir phosphate also significantly inhibits the production of nitric oxide (NO) in DC2.4 dendritic cells in response to LPS or killed *Mycobacterium butyricum*, which activates TLR4 and TLR2, respectively. In primary mouse bone marrow-derived macrophages treated with endotoxin LPS, a significant reduction in NO production was observed in comparison to WT. In comparison, however, primary bone marrow-derived macrophages from cathepsin A-knockin mice (which express a normal Neu1 but inactive cathepsin A), or Neu4 knockout mice, exhibited LPS-induced NO production comparable to that of the WT (Amith et al. 2009) (Fig. 3). These data indicate that the production of both nitric oxide and pro-inflammatory cytokines in immune cells in response to LPS stimulation are at least partially dependent on the induction of Neu1 sialidase.

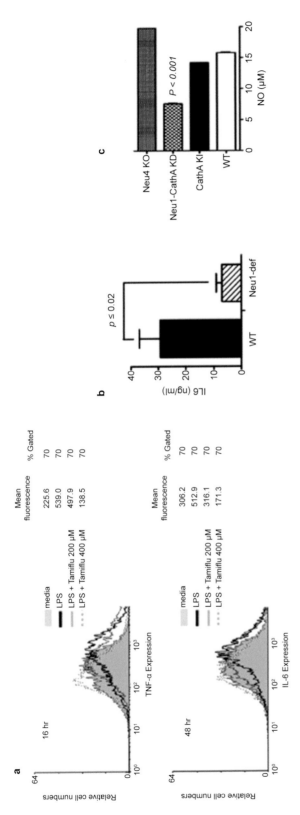

Figure 3. Oseltamivir phosphate, a sialidase inhibitor, reduces cytokine and nitric oxide production in immune cells. (a) Flow cytometric analysis of oseltamivir phosphate inhibition of LPS-induced expression of TNFα (16 h) and IL-6 (48 h) in THP-1 human monocytes. Cells were pretreated with oseltamivir phosphate at indicated doses followed by 3 μg/mL of LPS for 16 h (optimal time for TNFα expression) and for 48 h (optimal time for IL-6 expression) in the presence of Brefeldin A. Untreated control cells are represented by the gray-filled histogram. Cells pretreated with 200 μM or 400 μM of Tamiflu and stimulated with LPS are depicted by the gray-solid line or gray-dashed line, respectively. The mean fluorescence for each histogram is indicated for 10,000 acquired cells (70% gated). (b) *In vivo* LPS-induced serum IL-6 cytokine production in normal, wild-type (WT) and Neu1-deficient mice. Four mice in each group were bled before (no LPS) and 5 h after i.p. injection with 2.5 mg of LPS per mouse. Serum was extracted from blood and immediately analyzed for cytokine array profiling with R&D System Cytokine Array Profiling kit. (c) Nitrite (NO) production by primary BM macrophage cells derived from WT, Neu1-CathA KD (Neu1-deficient), CathA KI (normal Neu1, inactive cathepsin A) and Neu4 KO mice stimulated with LPS. Primary cells (50,000 cells/well) were treated with 1 μg/ml LPS or left untreated in medium for 18 h. Supernatants were used to measure nitric oxide (NO) concentration after subtraction of control cells using the Griess reagent and standard concentration curve. Taken from (Amith et al. 2009) with permission from Glycoconjugate Journal.

While there is evidence to support a role for Neu1 in cell effector functions downstream of TLR activation in addition to its role at the cell surface, the exact mechanism by which ligand binding to TLR induces Neu1 activity was not clear. A clue came from the identification of a membrane signaling paradigm initiated by endotoxin LPS binding to TLR4 to potentiate G protein-coupled receptor (GPCR) signaling via membrane Gαi subunit proteins and matrix metalloproteinase 9 (MMP9) activation to induce Neu1 (Abdulkhalek et al. 2011). Critical to this process is that a Neu1-MMP9 complex is bound to TLR4 on the cell surface of naïve macrophages. Specific inhibition of MMP9 and GPCR Gαi-signaling proteins blocks LPS-induced Neu1 activity and NFκB activation. When MMP9 in primary macrophages is silenced using lentiviral MMP9-targeted shRNA transduction, or siRNA targeted knockdown of MMP9, Neu1 activity and NFκB activation in response to LPS is significantly reduced (Abdulkhalek et al. 2011). Further mechanistic insight into the underlying signaling events that mediate Neu1 induction in response to ligand binding to its cognate TLR, came from studies on GPCR agonists bombesin, bradykinin, lysophosphatidic acid (LPA), cholesterol, angiotensin-1 and -2 inducing Neu1 activity in live macrophage cell lines and primary bone marrow macrophage cells from wild-type mice (Abdulkhalek et al. 2012). This does not occur in cells isolated from Neu1-deficient mice. In addition, the transactivation of TLRs and GPCRs has been suggested previously (Shi et al. 2004, Lattin et al. 2007), but the mechanisms leading up to this was unknown. Using immunocytochemistry and NFκB-dependent secretory alkaline phosphatase (SEAP) analyses, bombesin was found to induce NFκB activation in BMC-2 and RAW-blue macrophage cells, which was inhibited by oseltamivir phosphate, and MMP inhibitors galardin and piperazine, in addition to an anti-MMP9 antibody (Abdulkhalek et al. 2012). The bombesin receptor, neuromedin B (NMBR), was found to form a complex with TLR4 and MMP9. Silencing MMP9 mRNA using siRNA transfection of RAW-blue macrophage cells markedly reduced Neu1 activity associated with bombesin-, bradykinin- and LPA-treated cells compared to the untreated controls (Abdulkhalek et al. 2012). Taken together, these findings uncover a molecular organizational GPCR signaling platform to potentiate Neu1 and MMP9 cross-talk on the cell surface that is essential for the transactivation of TLR4 receptors and subsequent cellular signaling in response to LPS.

Neu1 Sialidase and Endosomal TLRs

Dimerization of the extracellular domain of most mammalian TLRs is essential for their ligand-induced activation. For the majority of TLRs, dimerization is a prerequisite to facilitate MyD88/TLR complex formation and subsequent cellular signaling to activate NF-κB. However, the parameters controlling interactions between the receptors and their ligands have remained poorly defined until now. For the cell-surface TLRs, a novel molecular organizational GPCR signaling platform that potentiates Neu1 sialidase and matrix metalloproteinase 9 (MMP9) cross-talk in the regulation of endotoxin LPS-induced TLR4 receptors and cellular function was recently identified (Abdulkhalek et al. 2011, 2012, Abdulkhalek et al. 2013) (Fig. 4).

In addition, the activity of these TLRs is also regulated by other ligand-related cofactors which are involved in improving ligand recognition by the receptors, such as diacylglyceride sensing by CD36 (Hoebe et al. 2005, Stewart et al. 2010), CD14 (Miyake 2003), and MD-2 (Shimazu et al. 1999, Visintin et al. 2003). However, there is another subset of TLRs, namely TLR3, TLR7, TLR8, and TLR9, which are localized within the endosomal compartments of the cell, that recognize nucleic acids (Blasius and Beutler 2010). It is well known that the distribution of endosomal TLRs in their subcellular compartments are controlled by endoplasmic reticulum (ER) chaperone gp96 (Randow and Seed 2001), protein associated with TLR4 (PRATA/B) (Konno et al. 2006, Wakabayashi et al. 2006, Takahashi et al. 2007), the ER membrane protein, UNC93B (Tabeta et al. 2006, Brinkmann et al. 2007), and the high-mobility group protein B1 (HMGB1) (Ivanov et al. 2007). Nevertheless, the mechanistic process involved in nucleic acid-induced intracellular TLR dimerization and subsequent receptor function is not clear.

Visintin and colleagues studied the molecular mechanism of intracellular TLR7 triggering by using N-nitrose-N9-ethyl urea (ENU)-induced mutations in mice, which identified a crucial role for N-glycosylation target sequence in position 66–68 (N66) within the leucine-rich repeat LRR1 ectodomain (Iavarone et al. 2011). This LRR1 ectodomain contains a putative glycan acceptor site that results in the conversion of threonine 68 to isoleucine (T68I) in TLR7 (Iavarone et al. 2011). This targeted mutation of

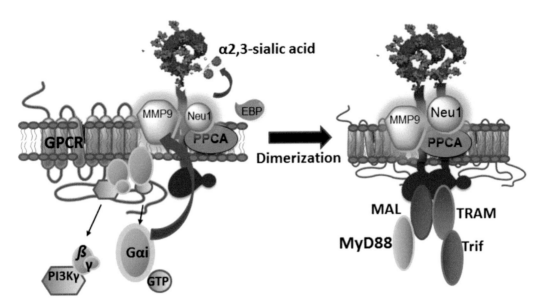

Figure 4. A novel molecular organizational G-protein-coupled receptor (GPCR)-signaling platform potentiates neuraminidase-1 (Neu1) and matrix metalloproteinase 9 (MMP9) cross talk on the cell surface that is essential for the activation of TOLL-like receptors (TLRs). Notes: The ligand-binding TLR potentiates the GPCR-signaling and MMP9 activation in inducing Neu1 sialidase. Activated MMP9 is proposed to remove the elastin-binding protein (EBP) as part of the molecular multienzymatic complex that contains β-galactosidase/Neu1 and protective protein cathepsin A (PPCA). Activated Neu1 hydrolyzes α-2,3sialyl residues of TLR at the ectodomain to facilitate receptor association and recruitment of MAL, TRAM, Trif and MyD88.

Abbreviations: Pi3K, phosphatidylinositol 3-kinase; GTP, guanine triphosphate; MyD88, myeloid differentiation primary response gene-88; MAL, MyD88-adapter-like; Trif, Toll-IL-1 receptordomain-containing adaptor-inducing interferon-β; TRAM, Trif-related adaptor molecule. **Citation:** Taken in part from Research and Reports in Biochemistry 2013: 3 17–30. © 2013 Abdulkhalek et al., publisher and licensee Dove Medical Press Ltd. This is an Open Access article which permits unrestricted non-commercial use, provided the original work is properly cited.

TLR7[rsq1] was found to reside in the N-terminal portion of TLR7, which was found to be in close proximity to the first two insertions relevant for ligand binding. The data from the report showed an impaired ability of TLR7 to signal in response to ssRNA and low molecular weight TLR7 agonist resiquimod (R848), but not its ability to bind to ssRNA. Unexpectedly, this ssRNA binding by the mutant TLR7[rsq1] and lack of signaling implied that the N-glycosylation status of TLR7 is essential for receptor activation and function (Iavarone et al. 2011).

For dimerization, TLR receptors need to undergo conformational changes following ligand binding, which orientate the ectodomains of TLRs for receptor association (Bell et al. 2005, 2006). Indeed, ligand-induced conformational changes have been shown to activate TLR9 receptors in an allosteric manner (Latz et al. 2007). Mutagenesis studies on murine TLR7 and TLR9, showed that these receptors are sensitive to subtle changes in conformation (Peter et al. 2009). The importance of α-2,3-sialyl residues linked to β-galactosides in establishing steric hindrance to receptor dimerization has been established (Woronowicz et al. 2004, Amith et al. 2010a). This entirely new premise was emphasized by using exogenous α2,3-sialyl specific neuraminidases (Amith et al. 2010a) to bring about TLR activation in the absence of their cognate ligands. Primary bone marrow macrophages derived from Neu1-deficient mice treated with a purified recombinant neuraminidase (*C. perfringens*) or recombinant *T. cruzi* trans-sialidase (TS), but not the mutant TSΔAsp98-Glu, induced phosphorylation of NF-κB (Amith et al. 2010a). These results are consistent with other reports (Woronowicz et al. 2007, Jayanth et al. 2010, Amith et al. 2010a) supporting the glycosylation model in corroborating the importance of sialyl α-2,3-linked β-galactosyl residues of TLRs in the initial stages of ligand-induced receptor activation, where Neu1-mediated desialylation of α-2,3-sialyl residues of cell-surface TLR receptors enables receptor dimerization and subsequent cell function (Amith et al. 2010a). Central to this process is that Neu1, and not the other three mammalian sialidases, forms a complex with either TLR2, TLR3 or TLR4 cell-surface receptors in naïve TLR-expressing cells or primary macrophage cells (Amith et al. 2009). The prerequisite desialyation of cell-surface TLR receptors caused by activated Neu1 enables MyD88/TLR4 complex recruitment, NFkB activation and pro-inflammatory responses (Amith et al. 2009, 2010a).

The key players that are involved in the activation of nucleic acid-sensing intracellular TLR7 and TLR9 receptors, against imiquimod and CpG oligodeoxynucleotide (ODN), respectively, was unknown until now. It is noteworthy that TLR7 and TLR9 receptors have the same signaling paradigm depicted in Fig. 4, as described for the cell-surface TLRs (Abdulkhalek et al. 2011, 2012, Abdulkhalek et al. 2013). These reports indicated that Neu1 and MMP9 cross-talk in alliance with GPCR neuromedin-B receptors, forms a complex tethered to the ectodomains of TLR7 and TLR9 receptors. Together, these molecules form a novel organizational GPCR signaling platform that is essential for ligand-induced activation of the intracellular TLRs and their subsequent cellular signaling. Since TLR9 receptors are prone to ligand-induced conformational changes in the ectodomains (Latz et al. 2007), it is proposed that ligand binding to TLR7 and TLR9 receptors initiates a conformational change to potentiate G-protein coupled receptor (GPCR)-signaling via membrane Gα subunit proteins and matrix metalloproteinase 9 (MMP9) activation to induce Neu1 (Abdulkhalek and Szewczuk 2013). Activated Neu1 specifically hydrolyzes α-2,3-sialyl residues linked to β-galactosides on the TLR, the structural perturbation of which triggers the dimeric receptor complex formation to facilitate MyD88/TLR recruitment and subsequent pro-inflammatory cell responses. This concept radically redefines the current dogma(s) governing the essential activating molecules tethered to nucleic acid sensing TLRs. It may also provide novel molecular targets in disease intervention strategies.

For the majority of cell-surface TLR receptors, dimerization is a prerequisite to facilitate MyD88/TLR complex formation and subsequent cellular signaling to activate NF-κB. For intracellular TLR3 receptors, they also form dimers upon interaction of dsRNA. In contrast, the intracellular TLR8 (Zhu et al. 2009) and TLR9 (Latz et al. 2007, Peter et al. 2009) appear to exist as preformed naïve signaling dimers. For TLR9, it is proposed that nucleic acids binding to two distinct binding sites (Rutz et al. 2004, Peter et al. 2009) in the ectodomain of the receptors induce conformational changes which enable subsequent signaling. For TLR7, a receptor signaling platform whereby nucleic acid ligands binding to TLR7 and TLR9 is orchestrated by Neu1 and MMP9 cross-talk in alliance with neuromedin B (NMBR) GPCR has been identified (Abdulkhalek and Szewczuk 2013). This signaling paradigm is essential for nucleic acid activation of intracellular TLR7 and TLR9 receptors. The specific inhibition of Neu1, MMP9, and the heterotrimeric G-protein complex tethered to both TLR7 and TLR9 receptors in live RAW-blue macrophage cells significantly abrogates pro-inflammatory cytokines MCP-1 and TNFα (Fig. 5). Indeed, other studies have shown that ODN induces TNFα and TNFR-II at the transcriptional level. Here, ODN induces MMP9 expression in supernatants obtained from cultured murine RAW264.7 macrophage cells via a TLR9 receptor and a serine/threonine-specific protein kinase B (Akt)-mediated mechanism (Lim et al. 2006, 2007). This ODN-induced MMP9 expression fits well within our novel Neu-1 and MMP9 cross-talk regulating TLR9 receptors (see Fig. 4).

Other reports have shown that ODN stimulation of lung cancer cells induced the secretion of high-mobility group protein B1 (HMGB1) in a dose-dependent manner (Wang et al. 2012). The cancer cell response to HMGB1 stimulation, either alone or acting synergistically with ODN, mediated a MyD88-dependent up-regulation of MMP2, MMP9 and cyclin-dependent kinase-2 (CDK2), which was critically dependent on a 35 kDa transmembrane receptor for advanced glycation end products (RAGE) and TLR4 receptors (Wang et al. 2012). If ODN-induces HMGB1 secretion in these cancer cells, it is possible that HMGB1 may affect ODN-induced NFκB activation via a TLR4 intermediary in macrophage cells. However, other reports provided evidence that this may not be the case. Secreted HMGB1 can be a trigger of inflammation dependent on the complexes it forms with other molecules (Bianchi 2009). Pure recombinant HMGB1 has no proinflammatory activity, but it can form highly inflammatory complexes with ssDNA, LPS, IL-1, and nucleosomes, which interact with TLR9, TLR4, IL-1R, and TLR2 receptors, respectively (Bianchi 2009). Ivanov et al. have identified HMGB1 as an ODN-binding protein, which interacts and pre-associates with TLR9 in the endoplasmic reticulum-Golgi intermediate compartment where it hastens TLR9's redistribution to early endosomes in response to ODN (Ivanov et al. 2007). The extracellular

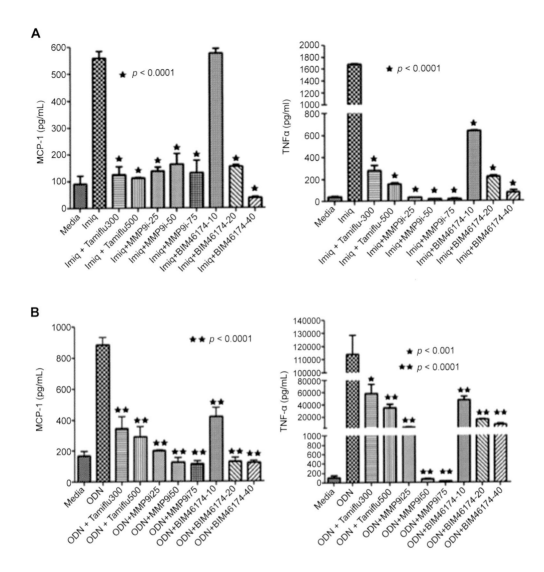

Figure 5. Bio-Plex cytokine microarray profiles in the cell culture supernatants using multiplex color-coded beads. RAW-blue cells were cultured in 96-well microplate at 30,000 cells per well for 24 h followed by pretreatment with Tamiflu, MMP9i and BIM-46174 at the indicated doses in μg/mL for 1 h. The pretreated cells were stimulated for 24 h with either 20 μg/mL imiquimod (A) or 20 μg/mL ODN (B). The Bio-Plex suspension array system was optimized using the xMAP detection technology. The quantitation of the level of TNFα and MCP-1 cytokines in a single well of tissue culture sample was assessed from a standard curve. Each bar in the graphs represents the mean ± S.E. (error bars) of three separate experiments. p values represent significant differences at 99% confidence intervals using the Dunnett's multiple comparison test compared with ligand-treated positive controls. Taken from (Abdulkhalek and Szewczuk 2013) with permission from Elsevier Publishers.

HMGB1 was found to accelerate the delivery of ODNs to its receptor, leading to a TLR9-dependent augmentation of IL-6, IL-12, and TNFα secretion (Ivanov et al. 2007). Using the murine macrophage-like cell lines RAW 264.7 and J774A.1, Pisetsky and colleagues have shown that, under conditions in which ODN1826 activated these cells, as assessed by stimulation of TNF-α and IL-12, it failed to cause HMGB1 release into the media (Jiang et al. 2005). Although unable to induce HMGB1 release by itself, ODN1826 nevertheless potentiated the action of LPS in these macrophage cells (Jiang et al. 2005). These data are consistent with the finding that TLR9 activation associated with ODN1826-treated macrophages,

HEK-293 and HEK-TLR7-HA cells, do not involve HMGB1-induced TLR4 as an intermediary (Abdulkhalek and Szewczuk 2013).

It is evident that TLRs require additional proteins to be activated by their respective ligands. For an example, not only is CD14 associated with MyD88-dependent TLR4 receptors on the cell surface, but it also constitutively interacts with the MyD88-dependent activation of endosomal TLR7 and TLR9 (Baumann et al. 2010). Here, CD14 was necessary for TLR7- and TLR9-dependent induction of pro-inflammatory cytokines *in vitro,* and for TLR9-dependent innate immune responses in mice. In addition, the absence of CD14 led to reduced nucleic acid uptake in macrophages. Using vesicular stomatitis viruses, the report showed that CD14 is dispensable for viral uptake but is required for the triggering of TLR-dependent cytokine responses (Baumann et al. 2010). These findings suggest that CD14 has a dual role in nucleic acid-mediated TLR activation whereby it can promote the selective uptake of nucleic acids and, at the same time, it acts as a co-receptor for endosomal TLR activation. Others have demonstrated another important role for CD14 (Solomon et al. 1998). It can associate with Gi (inhibitory class) and Go (olfactory class) α subunits of G-proteins. The heterotrimeric G proteins were shown to have a specific regulatory function in CD14-associated LPS-induced mitogen-activated protein kinase (MAPK) activation and cytokine production in normal human monocytes (Solomon et al. 1998). A significant decrease in LPS-induced activation of c-Jun-N-terminal kinase (JNK) and p38 kinase was reported with a subsequent loss in the production of TNF-α when THP-1 human monocyte cells were pretreated with Gαi-sensitive pertussis toxin (Ferlito et al. 2002). Using the knockout mouse models of G$\alpha_{12}^{-/-}$ and G$\alpha_{i1/3}^{-/-}$ proteins, Fan et al. showed a significant decrease in TLR ligand-mediated TNF-α and IL-10 production in peritoneal macrophages of the knockout mice compared to wild-type cohort (Fan et al. 2005b). These findings suggest a regulatory role for Gαi proteins in TLR signaling, which is potentially dependent on cellular phenotype (Fan et al. 2005a). In the murine RAW 264.7 macrophage cell line and primary murine macrophages, G protein dysregulation induced by wasp venom-derived peptide mastoparan caused a significant inhibition in LPS-induced TLR4-, but not in TLR2-mediated gene expression (Li et al. 2007). The involvement of heterotrimeric G-protein complex in TLR ligand-mediated receptor function has also been shown for endosomal TLRs (Abdulkhalek and Szewczuk 2013). Using siRNA NMBR knockdown cells and neuromedin B receptor antagonist BIM-23127 and the heterotrimeric G-protein complex antagonist BIM-46174, the results provided evidence for a significant diminution of NF-κB activation and reduced MyD88 recruitment associated with imiquimod- and ODN-stimulated RAW-blue cells. Collectively, the data validated the predicted alliance between nucleic acid sensing TLR7 and TLR9 receptors and NMBR GPCR localized in the late endocytic lysosomal pathway of naïve macrophage cells. This TLR signaling paradigm also predicted that endosomal TLR receptors are in alliance with a functional GPCR signaling complex.

The cross-talk between GPCR and TLR signaling pathways and the GPCR signaling molecules may have uncharacterized functions in macrophage cells (Lattin et al. 2007, Abdulkhalek et al. 2011, 2012, Abdulkhalek et al. 2013). GPCR agonists bombesin, bradykinin, lysophosphatidic acid (LPA), cholesterol, angiotensin-1 and -2, but not thrombin, induce Neu1 activity in live macrophage cell lines and primary bone marrow macrophage cells from wild-type (WT) mice but not from Neu1-deficient mice (Abdulkhalek et al. 2012). Using immunocytochemistry and NFκB-dependent secretory alkaline phosphatase (SEAP) analyses, bombesin induced NFκB activation in BMC-2 and RAW-blue macrophage cells, which was inhibited by MyD88 homodimerization inhibitor, Tamiflu, galardin, piperazine and anti-MMP9 antibody (Abdulkhalek et al. 2012). The bombesin-related receptor, neuromedin B (NMBR), formed a complex with TLR4 and MMP9. Silencing MMP9 mRNA using siRNA transfection of RAW-blue macrophage cells markedly reduced Neu1 activity associated with bombesin-, bradykinin- and LPA-treated cells compared to the untreated controls (Abdulkhalek et al. 2012). The data in the report also indicated that the three different isoforms of NMBR are tethered to TLR4 receptors, but it is the 80 kD isoform of NMBR which formed a complex with MMP9, making it readily available to activate MMP9 on the cell surface of naïve macrophage cells (see Fig. 4). Unexpectedly, the 63 and 80 kDa isoforms of NMBR are eventually lost over time with LPS treatment. The 63 kDa isoform of NMBR is also tethered to the cleaved 65 kDa TLR7 and the cleaved 80 kDa TLR9 receptors with no lost with ligand-stimulation of the cells over 60 min. The reason(s) for this differential activity of the NMBR isoforms is unknown. More importantly, the similarity of the mechanism where NMBR, in alliance with Neu1 and MMP9, regulates TLR4 on the cell surface and the intracellular TLR7 and TLR9 in the endosomal compartments is striking. It is noteworthy that the MMP9/Neu1 complex is separately tethered to TLR4, TLR7 or TLR9 receptors, and it does not shuttle from the cell surface to the endosomal compartments and vice-versa. Firstly, the NMBR/MMP9/Neu1 tripartite complex is already present on TLR4 (Abdulkhalek et al. 2011) and TLR7 and TLR9 receptors in naïve, unstimulated cells. Secondly, imiquimod and ODN stimulation of HEK-293 and HEK-TLR7-HA induce NFκB activation in the absence of the TLR4 intermediary. It is not yet clear how and when this novel regulatory signaling complex is formed on these receptors.

There is an intriguing connection between NMBR GPCR and Neu1/MMP9. The diverse multiple actions of GPCRs regulating TLRs and their translations to human disease requires further investigations to uncover their functional roles in cellular signaling (Abdulkhalek et al. 2013). The regulation and sorting of GPCRs by endocytic membrane trafficking and the potential implications was eloquently reviewed by Hanyaloglu and colleagues (Hanyaloglu and von Zastrow 2008, Jean-Alphonse and Hanyaloglu 2011) and Marchese et al. (Marchese et al. 2008). Achieving a coordinated regulation of multiple receptor-mediated signaling is one of the mandates for GPCRs, which represents the largest family of signaling receptors expressed in animals. GPCRs respond to a wide range of stimuli and exhibit an unprecedented degree of specificity and plasticity in the cellular regulation of mammalian GPCRs by endocytic membrane trafficking (Hanyaloglu and von Zastrow 2008). The diverse physiological roles GPCRs play necessitates further study. For example, there is evidence for disordered GPCR signaling in various pathological conditions, such as (a) dysregulation of GPCR function (Arvanitakis et al. 1998); (b) the 'loss of function' mutation or the 'gain of function' mutation (Spiegel and Weinstein 2004); (c) constitutively active GPCRs, especially those that are tumorigenic *in vitro* and in animal models of human disease, that cause syndromes of hyperfunction and/or tumors in humans, including diseases involving infectious viral agents (Arvanitakis et al. 1998, Tao 2008); and (d) the mutant GPCRs as a cause of human diseases (Schoneberg et al. 2004). To date, over 600 inactivating and almost 100 activating mutations in GPCR have been identified, which have implications in the pathophysiology of more than 30 different human diseases. The number of human disorders is expected to increase given the fact that over 160 GPCRs have been targeted in mice (Schoneberg et al. 2004).

Perhaps, one mechanism by which ligand-induced TLR activation could modify GPCR signaling is by altering the expression of regulator of G protein signaling (RGS) proteins (Shi et al. 2004). Other reports have shown that GPCR sphingosine 1-phosphate S1P1 and S1P3 expressions are induced by LPS in human gingival epithelial cells (HGEC), and these elevated expressions enhanced the influence of S1P in its cooperation with TLR4 to increase cytokine production (Eskan et al. 2008). The relationship between GPCR-signaling and TLRs has been shown for: (a) CC chemokine ligand-2 synergizing with the non-chemokine GPCR ligand fMLP in monocyte chemotaxis (Gouwy et al. 2009); (b) beta-arrestin 2 involvement in complement C1q expression in macrophages (Lattin et al. 2009); (c) leukotriene B4 (LTB4) receptor BTL1 reduction of SOCS1 inhibition of MyD88 expression in mouse macrophages (Serezani et al. 2011); and (d) GPCR-derived cAMP signaling influencing TLR responses in primary macrophages through peptide disruptors of A-kinase anchoring protein (AKAP10) involving prostaglandin E2 (PGE2) (Kim et al. 2011).

Conclusions

The parameters controlling interactions between the TLRs and their ligands still remain poorly defined. We propose that Neu1 is an important intermediary in the initial process of surface and endosomal TLR ligand-induced receptor activations on and adjacent to membranes, and subsequent TLR-mediated cellular function. Central to this process is that Neu1 and MMP9 in alliance with the 80 kDa isoform of GPCR NMBR receptor are separately tethered to TLR4, TLR7 and TLR9 receptors in naïve TLR-expressing cells. This receptor signaling paradigm signifies an unprecedented shift in our understanding of cellular responses in sensing pathogens. The multiplex molecular signaling platform of Neu1, MMP9, and GPCR cross-talk with both cell surface and endosomal TLRs is essential for ligand activation of TLRs and subsequent cellular signaling and pro-inflammatory immune responses.

Acknowledgements

These studies are supported by a grant to M.R.S. from the Natural Sciences and Engineering Research Council of Canada (NSERC). S.R.A. was funded by the Ontario Graduate Scholarship, Robert J. Wilson Fellowship, Queen's University Graduate and Research Awards, and currently, by a Canadian Breast Cancer Foundation Postdoctoral Fellowship Grant. S.A. was the recipient of the R.S. McLaughlin Scholarship, the Ontario Graduate Scholarship, and the Canadian Institutes of Health Research (CIHR) Doctoral Award: Frederick Banting and Charles Best Canada Graduate Scholarship.

Keywords: TOLL-like receptors, Cell surface TLR4, Intracellular TLR7, Intracellular TLR9, Neu1 sialidase, Receptor glycosylation, TLR signaling, GPCR, Matrix metalloproteinase 9, PAMPS, Pro-inflammatory cytokines, Oseltamivir phosphate

References

Abdulkhalek, S., S. R. Amith, S. L. Franchuk, P. Jayanth, M. Guo, T. Finlay et al. 2011. Neu1 sialidase and matrix metalloproteinase-9 cross-talk is essential for Toll-like receptor activation and cellular signaling. J Biol Chem 286: 36532–36549. doi: 10.1074/jbc.M111.237578.

Abdulkhalek, S., M. Guo, S. R. Amith, P. Jayanth and M. R. Szewczuk. 2012. G-protein coupled receptor agonists mediate Neu1 sialidase and matrix metalloproteinase-9 cross-talk to induce transactivation of TOLL-like receptors and cellular signaling. Cell Signal 24: 2035–2042. doi: 10.1016/j.cellsig.2012.06.016.

Abdulkhalek, S., M. Hrynyk and M. R. Szewczuk. 2013. A novel G-protein-coupled receptor-signaling platform and its targeted translation in human disease. Res Rep Biochem 3: 17–30.

Abdulkhalek, S. and M.R. Szewczuk. 2013. Neu1 sialidase and matrix metalloproteinase-9 cross-talk regulates nucleic acid-induced endosomal TOLL-like receptor-7 and -9 activation, cellular signaling and pro-inflammatory responses. Cell Signal 25: 2093–2105. doi: http://dx.doi.org/10.1016/j.cellsig.2013.06.010.

Albiger, B., S. Dahlberg, B. Henriques-Normark and S. Normark. 2007a. Role of the innate immune system in host defence against bacterial infections: focus on the Toll-like receptors. J Intern Med 261: 511–528. doi: 10.1111/j.1365-2796.2007.01821.x.

Albiger, B., S. Dahlberg, A. Sandgren, F. Wartha, K. Beiter, H. Katsuragi et al. 2007b. Toll-like receptor 9 acts at an early stage in host defence against pneumococcal infection. Cell Microbiol 9: 633–644. doi: 10.1111/j.1462-5822.2006.00814.x.

Amith, S. R., P. Jayanth, S. Franchuk, S. Siddiqui, V. Seyrantepe, K. Gee et al. 2009. Dependence of pathogen molecule-induced Toll-like receptor activation and cell function on Neu1 sialidase. Glycoconj J 26: 1197–1212.

Amith, S. R., P. Jayanth, S. Franchuk, T. Finlay, V. Seyrantepe, R. Beyaert et al. 2010a. Neu1 desialylation of sialyl alpha-2,3-linked beta-galactosyl residues of TOLL-like receptor 4 is essential for receptor activation and cellular signaling. Cell Signal 22: 314–324. doi: 10.1016/j.cellsig.2009.09.038.

Amith, S. R, P. Jayanth, T. Finlay, S. Franchuk, A. Gilmour, S. Abdulkhalek et al. 2010b. Detection of Neu1 sialidase activity in regulating Toll-like receptor activation. J Vis Exp 43 http://www.jove.com/index/details.stp?id=2142, doi: 10.3791/2142.

Arvanitakis, L., E. Geras-Raaka and M. C. Gershengorn. 1998. Constitutively signaling G-protein-coupled receptors and human disease. Trends Endocrinol Metab 9: 27–31.

Atkinson, T. M., T. R. Konold and J. J. Glutting. 2008. Patterns of memory: A normative taxonomy of the Wide Range Assessment of Memory and Learning-Second Edition (WRAML-2). J Int Neuropsychol Soc 14: 869–877. doi: 10.1017/S1355617708081137.

Balcan, E., I. Tuglu, M. Sahin and P. Toparlak. 2008. Cell surface glycosylation diversity of embryonic thymic tissues. Acta Histochem 110: 14–25. doi: 10.1016/j.acthis.2007.07.003.

Baumann, C. L., I. M. Aspalter, O. Sharif, A. Pichlmair, S. Bluml, F. Grebien et al. 2010. CD14 is a coreceptor of Toll-like receptors 7 and 9. J Exp Med 207: 2689–2701. doi: 10.1084/jem.20101111.

Bell, J. K., I. Botos, P. R. Hall, J. Askins, J. Shiloach, D. M. Segal et al. 2005. The molecular structure of the Toll-like receptor 3 ligand-binding domain. Proc Natl Acad Sci USA 102: 10976–10980.

Bell, J. K., J. Askins, P. R. Hall, D. R. Davies and D. M. Segal. 2006. The dsRNA binding site of human Toll-like receptor 3. Proc Natl Acad Sci USA 103: 8792–8797.

Bianchi, M. E. 2009. HMGB1 loves company. J Leukoc Biol 86: 573–576. doi: 10.1189/jlb.1008585.

Blasius, A. L. and B. Beutler. 2010. Intracellular toll-like receptors. Immunity 32: 305–315. doi: 10.1016/j.immuni.2010.03.012.

Brinkmann, M. M., E. Spooner, K. Hoebe, B. Beutler, H. L. Ploegh and Y. M. Kim. 2007. The interaction between the ER membrane protein UNC93B and TLR3, TLR7, and TLR9 is crucial for TLR signaling. J Cell Biol 177: 265–275. doi: 10.1083/jcb.200612056.

Caciotti, A., M. A. Donati, A. Boneh, A. d'Azzo, A. Federico, R. Parini et al. 2005. Role of beta-galactosidase and elastin binding protein in lysosomal and nonlysosomal complexes of patients with GM1-gangliosidosis. Human Mutation 25: 285–292.

Chavas, L. M., C. Tringali, P. Fusi, B. Venerando, G. Tettamanti, R. Kato et al. 2005. Crystal structure of the human cytosolic sialidase Neu2. Evidence for the dynamic nature of substrate recognition. J Biol Chem 280: 469–475.

Chen, X. P., E. Y. Enioutina and R. A. Daynes. 1997. The control of IL-4 gene expression in activated murine T lymphocytes: a novel role for neu-1 sialidase. J Immunol 158: 3070–3080.

Choe, J., M. S. Kelker and I. A. Wilson. 2005. Crystal structure of human toll-like receptor 3 (TLR3) ectodomain. Science 309: 581–585. doi: 1115253 [pii] 10.1126/science.1115253.

Contessa, J. N., M. S. Bhojani, H. H. Freeze, A. Rehemtulla and T. S. Lawrence. 2008. Inhibition of N-linked glycosylation disrupts receptor tyrosine kinase signaling in tumor cells. Cancer Res 68: 3803–3809. doi: 10.1158/0008-5472.CAN-07-6389.

da Silva, J. Correia and R. J. Ulevitch. 2002. MD-2 and TLR4 N-linked glycosylations are important for a functional lipopolysaccharide receptor. J Biol Chem 277: 1845–1854.

Eskan, M. A., B. G. Rose, M. R. Benakanakere, Q. Zeng, D. Fujioka, M. H. Martin et al. 2008. TLR4 and S1P receptors cooperate to enhance inflammatory cytokine production in human gingival epithelial cells. Eur J Immunol 38: 1138–1147. doi: 10.1002/eji.200737898.

Fan, H., B. Zingarelli, O. M. Peck, G. Teti, G. E. Tempel, P. V. Halushka et al. 2005a. Lipopolysaccharide- and gram-positive bacteria-induced cellular inflammatory responses: role of heterotrimeric G alpha(i) proteins. Am J Physiol Cell Physiol 289: C293–C301.

Fan, H., B. Zingarelli, O. M. Peck, G. Teti, G. E. Tempel, P. V. Halushka et al. 2005b. Lipopolysaccharide- and gram-positive bacteria-induced cellular inflammatory responses: Role of heterotrimeric G alpha(i) proteins. Am J Physiol Cell Physiol 289: C293–C301.

Fanzani, A., R. Giuliani, F. Colombo, S. Rossi, E. Stoppani, W. Martinet et al. 2008. The enzymatic activity of sialidase Neu2 is inversely regulated during *in vitro* myoblast hypertrophy and atrophy. Biochem Biophys Res Commun 370: 376–381. doi: 10.1016/j.bbrc.2008.03.111.

Feng, C., N. M. Stamatos, A. I. Dragan, A. Medvedev, M. Whitford, L. Zhang et al. 2012a. Sialyl residues modulate LPS-mediated signaling through the Toll-like receptor 4 complex. PLoS One 7: e32359. doi: 10.1371/journal.pone.0032359.

Feng, X. T., J. Leng, Z. Xie, S. L. Li, W. Zhao and Q. L. Tang. 2012b. GPR40: A therapeutic target for mediating insulin secretion (review). Int J Mol Med 30: 1261–1266. doi: 10.3892/ijmm.2012.1142.

Ferlito, M., O. G. Romanenko, K. Guyton, S. Ashton, F. Squadrito, P. V. Halushka et al. 2002. Implication of G alpha i proteins and Src tyrosine kinases in endotoxin-induced signal transduction events and mediator production. J Endotoxin Res 8: 427–435.

Finlay, M. T., S. Abdulkhalek, A. Gilmour, C. Guzzo, P. Jayanth, S. R. Amith et al. 2010. Thymoquinone-induced Neu4 sialidase activates NFκB in macrophage cells and pro-inflammatory cytokines *in vivo*. Glycoconj J 27: 583–600.

Gouwy, M., S. Struyf, H. Verbeke, W. Put, P. Proost, G. Opdenakker et al. 2009. CC chemokine ligand-2 synergizes with the nonchemokine G protein-coupled receptor ligand fMLP in monocyte chemotaxis, and it cooperates with the TLR ligand LPS via induction of CXCL8. J Leukoc Biol 86: 671–680. doi: 10.1189/jlb.1008638.

Hanyaloglu, A. C. and M. von Zastrow. 2008. Regulation of GPCRs by endocytic membrane trafficking and its potential implications. Annu Rev Pharmacol Toxicol 48: 537–568. doi: 10.1146/annurev.pharmtox.48.113006.094830.

Hasan, U., C. Chaffois, C. Gaillard, V. Saulnier, E. Merck, S. Tancredi et al. 2005. Human TLR10 is a functional receptor, expressed by B cells and plasmacytoid dendritic cells, which activates gene transcription through MyD88. J Immunol 174: 2942–2950. doi: 174/5/2942 [pii].

Hoebe, K., P. Georgel, S. Rutschmann, X. Du, S. Mudd, K. Crozat et al. 2005. CD36 is a sensor of diacylglycerides. Nature 433: 523–527. doi: 10.1038/nature03253.

Iavarone, C., K. Ramsauer, A. V. Kubarenko, J. C. Debasitis, I. Leykin, A. N. Weber et al. 2011. A point mutation in the amino terminus of TLR7 abolishes signaling without affecting ligand binding. J Immunol 186: 4213–4222. doi: 10.4049/jimmunol.1003585.

Ilic, V., N. Milosevic-Jovcic, S. Petrovic, D. Markovic, G. Stefanovic and T. Ristic. 2008. Glycosylation of IgG B cell receptor (IgG BCR) in multiple myeloma: Relationship between sialylation and the signal activity of IgG BCR. Glycoconj J 25: 383–392. doi: 10.1007/s10719-007-9101-9.

Ivanov, S., A. M. Dragoi, X. Wang, C. Dallacosta, J. Louten, G. Musco et al. 2007. A novel role for HMGB1 in TLR9-mediated inflammatory responses to CpG-DNA. Blood 110: 1970–1981. doi: 10.1182/blood-2006-09-044776.

Janssens, S. and R. Beyaert. 2003. Role of toll-like receptors in pathogen recognition. Clin Micro Rev 16: 637–646.

Jayanth, Preethi, Schammim Ray Amith, Katrina Gee and Myron R. Szewczuk. 2010. Neu1 sialidase and matrix metalloproteinase-9 cross-talk is essential for neurotrophin activation of Trk receptors and cellular signaling. Cell Signal 22: 1193–1205.

Jean-Alphonse, F. and A. C. Hanyaloglu. 2011. Regulation of GPCR signal networks via membrane trafficking. Mol Cell Endocrinol 331: 205–214. doi: 10.1016/j.mce.2010.07.010.

Jiang, W., J. Li, M. Gallowitsch-Puerta, K. J. Tracey and D. S. Pisetsky. 2005. The effects of CpG DNA on HMGB1 release by murine macrophage cell lines. J Leukoc Biol 78: 930–936. doi: 10.1189/jlb.0405208.

Jin, M. S., S. E. Kim, J. Y. Heo, M. E. Lee, H. M. Kim, S. G. Paik et al. 2007. Crystal structure of the TLR1-TLR2 heterodimer induced by binding of a tri-acylated lipopeptide. Cell 130: 1071–1082. doi: 10.1016/j.cell.2007.09.008.

Jin, M. S. and J. O. Lee. 2008. Structures of TLR-ligand complexes. Curr Opin Immunol 20: 414–419. doi: 10.1016/j.coi.2008.06.002.

Kim, K. W., M. L. Cho, S. H. Lee, H. J. Oh, C. M. Kang, J. H. Ju et al. 2007. Human rheumatoid synovial fibroblasts promote osteoclastogenic activity by activating RANKL via TLR2 and TLR4 activation. Immunol Lett 110: 54–64. doi: 10.1016/j.imlet.2007.03.004.

Kim, S. H., C. H. Serezani, K. Okunishi, Z. Zaslona, D. M. Aronoff and M. Peters-Golden. 2011. Distinct protein kinase a anchoring proteins direct prostaglandin E2 modulation of toll-like receptor signaling in alveolar macrophages. J Biol Chem doi: 10.1074/jbc.M110.187815.

Konno, K., Y. Wakabayashi, S. Akashi-Takamura, T. Ishii, M. Kobayashi, K. Takahashi et al. 2006. A molecule that is associated with toll-like receptor 4 and regulates its cell surface expression. Biochem Biophys Res Commun 339: 1076–1082. doi: 10.1016/j.bbrc.2005.11.123.

Kotani, K., A. Kuroiwa, T. Saito, Y. Matsuda, T. Koda and S. Kijimoto-Ochiai. 2001. Cloning, chromosomal mapping, and characteristic 5'-UTR sequence of murine cytosolic sialidase. Biochem Biophys Res Commun 286: 250–258.

Lattin, J., D. A. Zidar, K. Schroder, S. Kellie, D. A. Hume and M. J. Sweet. 2007. G-protein-coupled receptor expression, function, and signaling in macrophages. J Leukoc Biol 82: 16–32. doi: 10.1189/jlb.0107051.

Lattin, J. E., K. P. Greenwood, N. L. Daly, G. Kelly, D. A. Zidar, R. J. Clark et al. 2009. Beta-arrestin 2 is required for complement C1q expression in macrophages and constrains factor-independent survival. Mol Immunol 47: 340–347. doi: 10.1016/j.molimm.2009.09.012.

Latz, E., A. Verma, A. Visintin, M. Gong, C. M. Sirois, D. C. Klein et al. 2007. Ligand-induced conformational changes allosterically activate Toll-like receptor 9. Nat Immunol 8: 772–779. doi:10.1038/ni1479.

Leulier, F. and B. Lemaitre. 2008. Toll-like receptors—taking an evolutionary approach. Nat Rev Genet 9: 165–178. doi: 10.1038/nrg2303.

Li, D., H. Ji, S. Zaghlul, K. McNamara, M. C. Liang, T. Shimamura et al. 2007. Therapeutic anti-EGFR antibody 806 generates responses in murine *de novo* EGFR mutant-dependent lung carcinomas. J Clin Invest 117: 346–352. doi: 10.1172/jci30446.

Liang, F., V. Seyrantepe, K. Landry, R. Ahmad, A. Ahmad, N. M. Stamatos et al. 2006. Monocyte differentiation up-regulates the expression of the lysosomal sialidase, Neu1, and triggers its targeting to the plasma membrane via major histocompatibility complex class II-positive compartments. JBC 281: 27526–27538.

Lim, E. J., S. H. Lee, J. G. Lee, B. R. Chin, Y. S. Bae, J. R. Kim et al. 2006. Activation of toll-like receptor-9 induces matrix metalloproteinase-9 expression through Akt and tumor necrosis factor-alpha signaling. FEBS Lett 580: 4533–4538.

Lim, E. J., S. H. Lee, J. G. Lee, J. R. Kim, S. S. Yun, S. H. Baek et al. 2007. Toll-like receptor 9 dependent activation of MAPK and NF-kB is required for the CpG ODN-induced matrix metalloproteinase-9 expression. Exp Mol Med 39: 239–245.

Lukong, K. E., V. Seyrantepe, K. Landry, S. Trudel, A. Ahmad, W. A. Gahl et al. 2001. Intracellular distribution of lysosomal sialidase is controlled by the internalization signal in its cytoplasmic tail. JBC 276: 46172–46181.

Magesh, S., T. Suzuki, T. Miyagi, H. Ishida and M. Kiso. 2006. Homology modeling of human sialidase enzymes NEU1, NEU3 and NEU4 based on the crystal structure of NEU2: hints for the design of selective NEU3 inhibitors. J Mol Graph Mod 25: 196–207.

Marchese, A., M. M. Paing, B. R. Temple and J. Trejo. 2008. G protein-coupled receptor sorting to endosomes and lysosomes. Annu Rev Pharmacol Toxicol 48: 601–629. doi: 10.1146/annurev.pharmtox.48.113006.094646.

Medzhitov, R. and C. A. Janeway, Jr. 1997. Innate immunity: Impact on the adaptive immune response. Curr Opin Immunol 9: 4–9.

Meng, J., P. Parroche, D. T. Golenbock and C. J. McKnight. 2008. The differential impact of disulfide bonds and N-linked glycosylation on the stability and function of CD14. J Biol Chem 283: 3376–3384. doi: 10.1074/jbc.M707640200.

Michineau, S., F. Alhenc-Gelas and R. M. Rajerison. 2006. Human bradykinin B2 receptor sialylation and N-glycosylation participate with disulfide bonding in surface receptor dimerization. Biochemistry 45: 2699–2707. doi: 10.1021/bi051674v.

Miggin, S. M. and L. A. O'Neill. 2006. New insights into the regulation of TLR signaling. J Leukoc Biol 80: 220–226.

Miyagi, T. and S. Tsuiki. 1985. Purification and characterization of cytosolic sialidase from rat liver. J Biol Chem 260: 6710–6716.

Miyagi, T., T. Wada, K. Yamaguchi and K. Hata. 2004. Sialidase and malignancy: A minireview. Glycoconj J 20: 189–198.

Miyake, K. 2003. Innate recognition of lipopolysaccharide by CD14 and toll-like receptor 4-MD-2: Unique roles for MD-2. Int Immunopharmacol 3: 119–128.

Nan, X., I. Carubelli and N. M. Stamatos. 2007. Sialidase expression in activated human T lymphocytes influences production of IFN-gamma. J Leukoc Biol 81: 284–296. doi: 10.1189/jlb.1105692.

Nyman, T., P. Stenmark, S. Flodin, I. Johansson, M. Hammarstrom and P. Nordlund. 2008. The crystal structure of the human toll-like receptor 10 cytoplasmic domain reveals a putative signaling dimer. J Biol Chem 283: 11861–11865. doi: 10.1074/jbc.C800001200.

Oetke, C., M. C. Vinson, C. Jones and P. R. Crocker. 2006. Sialoadhesin-deficient mice exhibit subtle changes in B- and T-cell populations and reduced immunoglobulin M levels. Mol Cell Biol 26: 1549–1557. doi: 10.1128/MCB.26.4.1549-1557.2006.

Ohto, U., N. Yamakawa, S. Akashi-Takamura, K. Miyake and T. Shimizu. 2012. Structural analyses of human Toll-like receptor 4 polymorphisms D299G and T399I. J Biol Chem 287: 40611–40617. doi: 10.1074/jbc.M112.404608.

Ohtsubo, K. and J. D. Marth. 2006. Glycosylation in cellular mechanisms of health and disease. Cell 126: 855–867. doi: 10.1016/j.cell.2006.08.019.

Oosting, M., S. C. Cheng, J. M. Bolscher, R. Vestering-Stenger, T. S. Plantinga, I. C. Verschueren et al. 2014. Human TLR10 is an anti-inflammatory pattern-recognition receptor. Proc Natl Acad Sci USA 111: E4478–4484. doi: 10.1073/pnas.1410293111.

Peter, M. E., A. V. Kubarenko, A. N. Weber and A. H. Dalpke. 2009. Identification of an N-terminal recognition site in TLR9 that contributes to CpG-DNA-mediated receptor activation. J Immunol 182: 7690–7697. doi: 10.4049/jimmunol.0900819.

Randow, F. and B. Seed. 2001. Endoplasmic reticulum chaperone gp96 is required for innate immunity but not cell viability. Nat Cell Biol 3: 891–896. doi: 10.1038/ncb1001-891.

Rutz, M., J. Metzger, T. Gellert, P. Luppa, G. B. Lipford, H. Wagner et al. 2004. Toll-like receptor 9 binds single-stranded CpG-DNA in a sequence- and pH-dependent manner. Eur J Immunol 34: 2541–2550. doi: 10.1002/eji.200425218.

Sato, K. and T. Miyagi. 1996. Involvement of an endogenous sialidase in skeletal muscle cell differentiation. Biochem Biophys Res Commun 221: 826–830.

Schoneberg, T., A. Schulz, H. Biebermann, T. Hermsdorf, H. Rompler and K. Sangkuhl. 2004. Mutant G-protein-coupled receptors as a cause of human diseases. Pharmacol Ther 104: 173–206. doi: 10.1016/j.pharmthera.2004.08.008.

Serezani, C. H., C. Lewis, S. Jancar and M. Peters-Golden. 2011. Leukotriene B4 amplifies NF-kappaB activation in mouse macrophages by reducing SOCS1 inhibition of MyD88 expression. J Clin Invest 121: 671–682. doi: 10.1172/jci43302.

Seyrantepe, V., H. Poupetova, R. Froissart, M. T. Zabot, I. Maire and A. V. Pshezhetsky. 2003. Molecular pathology of NEU1 gene in sialidosis. Hum Mutat 22: 343–352. doi: 10.1002/humu.10268.

Shi, G. X., K. Harrison, S. B. Han, C. Moratz and J. H. Kehrl. 2004. Toll-like receptor signaling alters the expression of regulator of G protein signaling proteins in dendritic cells: implications for G protein-coupled receptor signaling. J Immunol 172: 5175–5184.

Shimazu, R., S. Akashi, H. Ogata, Y. Nagai, K. Fukudome, K. Miyake et al. 1999. MD-2, a molecule that confers lipopolysaccharide responsiveness on Toll-like receptor 4. J Exp Med 189: 1777–1782.

Solomon, K. R., E. A. Kurt-Jones, R. A. Saladino, A. M. Stack, I. F. Dunn, M. Ferretti et al. 1998. Heterotrimeric G proteins physically associated with the lipopolysaccharide receptor CD14 modulate both *in vivo* and *in vitro* responses to lipopolysaccharide. J Clin Invest 102: 2019–2027. doi: 10.1172/JCI4317.

Spiegel, A. M. and L. S. Weinstein. 2004. Inherited diseases involving g proteins and g protein-coupled receptors. Annu Rev Med 55: 27–39. doi: 10.1146/annurev.med.55.091902.103843.

Stewart, C. R., L. M. Stuart, K. Wilkinson, J. M. van Gils, J. Deng, A. Halle et al. 2010. CD36 ligands promote sterile inflammation through assembly of a Toll-like receptor 4 and 6 heterodimer. Nat Immunol 11: 155–161. doi: 10.1038/ni.1836.

Sun, J., K. E. Duffy, C. T. Ranjith-Kumar, J. Xiong, R. J. Lamb, J. Santos et al. 2006. Structural and functional analyses of the human Toll-like receptor 3. Role of glycosylation. J Biol Chem 281: 11144–11151.

Tabeta, K., K. Hoebe, E. M. Janssen, X. Du, P. Georgel, K. Crozat et al. 2007. A protein associated with Toll-like receptor (TLR) 4 (PRAT4A) is required for TLR-dependent immune responses. J Exp Med 204: 2963–2976. doi: jem.20071132 [pii] 10.1084/jem.20071132.

Tao, X., Y. Xu, Y. Zheng, A. A. Beg and L. Tong. 2002. An extensively associated dimer in the structure of the C713S mutant of the TIR domain of human TLR2. Biochem Biophys Res Commun 299: 216–221.

Tao, Y. X. 2008. Constitutive activation of G protein-coupled receptors and diseases: insights into mechanisms of activation and therapeutics. Pharmacol Ther 120: 129–148. doi: 10.1016/j.pharmthera.2008.07.005.

Van Dyken, S. J. and R. M. Locksley. 2007. Autoimmunity: altered self-N-glycans trigger innate-mediated autoimmunity. Immunol Cell Biol 85: 572–574. doi: 10.1038/sj.icb.7100122.

van Kooyk, Y. and G. A. Rabinovich. 2008. Protein-glycan interactions in the control of innate and adaptive immune responses. Nat Immunol 9: 593–601. doi: 10.1038/ni.f.203.

Varki, A. 2007. Glycan-based interactions involving vertebrate sialic-acid-recognizing proteins. Nature 446: 1023–1029. doi: 10.1038/nature05816.

Varki, N. M. and A. Varki. 2007. Diversity in cell surface sialic acid presentations: Implications for biology and disease. Lab Invest 87: 851–857. doi: 10.1038/labinvest.3700656.

Visintin, A., E. Latz, B. G. Monks, T. Espevik and D. T. Golenbock. 2003. Lysines 128 and 132 enable lipopolysaccharide binding to MD-2, leading to Toll-like receptor-4 aggregation and signal transduction. J Biol Chem 278: 48313–48320. doi: 10.1074/jbc.M306802200.

von Minckwitz, G., A. Schneeweiss, S. Loibl, C. Salat, C. Denkert, M. Rezai et al. 2014. Neoadjuvant carboplatin in patients with triple-negative and HER2-positive early breast cancer (GeparSixto; GBG 66): A randomised phase 2 trial. Lancet Oncol 15: 747–756. doi: 10.1016/S1470-2045(14)70160-3.

Wakabayashi, Y., M. Kobayashi, S. Akashi-Takamura, N. Tanimura, K. Konno, K. Takahashi et al. 2006. A protein associated with toll-like receptor 4 (PRAT4A) regulates cell surface expression of TLR4. J Immunol 177: 1772–1779. doi: 177/3/1772 [pii].

Wang, C., G. Fei, Z. Liu, Q. Li, Z. Xu and T. Ren. 2012. HMGB1 was a pivotal synergistic effector for CpG oligonucleotide to enhance the progression of human lung cancer cells. Cancer Biol Ther 13: 727–736. doi: 10.4161/cbt.20555.

Watson, F. L., M. A. Porcionatto, A. Bhattacharyya, C. D. Stiles and R. A. Segal. 1999. TrkA glycosylation regulates receptor localization and activity. J Neurobiol 39: 323–336.

Weber, A. N., M. A. Morse and N. J. Gay. 2004. Four N-linked glycosylation sites in human toll-like receptor 2 cooperate to direct efficient biosynthesis and secretion. J Biol Chem 279: 34589–34594. doi: 10.1074/jbc.M403830200.

Wiltshire, B., E. Steinberg, S. Grinstein and B. Beutler. 2006. The Unc93b1 mutation 3d disrupts exogenous antigen presentation and signaling via Toll-like receptors 3, 7 and 9. Nat Immunol 7: 156–164. doi: 10.1038/ni1297.

Woronowicz, A., K. De Vusser, W. Laroy, R. Contreras, S. O. Meakin, G. M. Ross et al. 2004. Trypanosome trans-sialidase targets TrkA tyrosine kinase receptor and induces receptor internalization and activation. Glycobiology 14: 987–998.

Woronowicz, A., S. R. Amith, K. De Vusser, W. Laroy, R. Contreras, S. Basta et al. 2007. Dependence of neurotrophic factor activation of Trk tyrosine kinase receptors on cellular sialidase. Glycobiology 17: 10–24.

Wuensch, S. A., R. Y. Huang, J. Ewing, X. Liang and J. T. Lau. 2000. Murine B cell differentiation is accompanied by programmed expression of multiple novel beta-galactoside alpha2, 6-sialyltransferase mRNA forms. Glycobiology 10: 67–75.

Yamamoto, M., S. Sato, H. Hemmi, H. Sanjo, S. Uematsu, T. Kaisho et al. 2002. Essential role for TIRAP in activation of the signalling cascade shared by TLR2 and TLR4. Nature 420: 324–329.

Yamanami, H., K. Shiozaki, T. Wada, K. Yamaguchi, T. Uemura, Y. Kakugawa et al. 2007. Down-regulation of sialidase NEU4 may contribute to invasive properties of human colon cancers. Cancer Sci 98: 299–307. doi: 10.1111/j.1349-7006.2007.00403.x.

Yogalingam, G., E. J. Bonten, D. van de Vlekkert, H. Hu, S. Moshiach, S. A. Connell et al. 2008. Neuraminidase 1 is a negative regulator of lysosomal exocytosis. Dev Cell 15: 74–86. doi: 10.1016/j.devcel.2008.05.005.

Yoshizumi, S., S. Suzuki, M. Hirai, Y. Hinokio, T. Yamada, T. Yamada et al. 2007. Increased hepatic expression of ganglioside-specific sialidase, NEU3, improves insulin sensitivity and glucose tolerance in mice. Metabolism 56: 420–429. doi: 10.1016/j.metabol.2006.10.027.

Zhang, R., Y. Wu, M. Zhao, C. Liu, L. Zhou, S. Shen et al. 2009. Role of HIF-1alpha in the regulation ACE and ACE2 expression in hypoxic human pulmonary artery smooth muscle cells. Am J Physiol Lung Cell Mol Physiol 297: L631–640. doi: 10.1152/ajplung.90415.2008.

Zhu, J., R. Brownlie, Q. Liu, L. A. Babiuk, A. Potter and G. K. Mutwiri. 2009. Characterization of bovine Toll-like receptor 8: ligand specificity, signaling essential sites and dimerization. Mol Immunol 46: 978–990. doi: 10.1016/j.molimm.2008.09.024.

CHAPTER 10

Novel Insights on Sialyltransferase Regulators of Cancer-associated O-glycans

Charles J. Dimitroff

Introduction

One of the hallmark features of cancer is the abnormal level of glycosylations found on the cell surface. Whether abundantly-expressed, reduced or aberrantly-branched compared with those found on their normal counterparts, cancer cell surface glycans often correlate with type or stage of malignant progression. A cancer cell glycophenotype is dictated by its glycomic gene expression profile consisting of glycosyltransferases, glycosidases, nucleotide-sugar transporters, sulfotransferases and glycan-bearing proteins or lipid. These glycomic factors collaborate in forming cancer-associated glycans and are widely-viewed as causal factors in a cancer cell's virulent behavior. In this chapter, the novel roles of serine/threonine (O)-glycan-modifying α2,6 sialyltransferases controlling lectin-binding interactions and related malignant and metastatic behaviors are reviewed. Recent studies showing that O-glycan modifications by N-acetylgalactosamine:α2,6 sialyltransferases (ST6GalNAc) impact intrinsic malignant potential in a host galectin (Gal)-1- and Gal-3-dependent manner will be highlighted. Related context on the history of cancer-associated glycan discovery and the prospect of glycomic factors as anti-cancer therapeutic targets will also be discussed to provide perspective for these novel findings. In all, the importance and more recognizable roles of Gal-binding cancer cell O-glycans continue to provide new paradigms for cancer research and development of novel cancer therapies.

A Historical Perspective in Cancer Glycan Correlates

The impact of glycobiology on malignant transformation and pathways relating to cancer growth and metastasis is often considered a defining hallmark of cancer (Dube and Bertozzi 2005). Hence, studies on glycobiology and its influence on cancer development are now fixtures in cancer research programs across the world. In these post-genomic and -proteomic eras, there has been a momentous shift towards

Brigham and Women's Hospital, Harvard Medical School, Department of Dermatology, HIM, Rm. 662, 77 Avenue Louis Pasteur, Boston, MA 02115.
E-mail: cdimitroff@rics.bwh.harvard.edu

understanding cancer glycomics—the impact of glycans, glycoconjugates and glycan-forming/-degrading machinery on cancer progression. The influence of glycomics on cancer embodies consequences not only through intrinsic cancer glyco-phenotypes but also through host microenvironmental glycomic factors (Stowell et al. 2015).

Cancer cells selectively harness glycolytic pathways for energy that potentially boost glyco-metabolic activity. The glyco-metabolic activity in cancer cells has been postulated to result in differential glycan levels or in aberrant glycan branching and monosaccharide composition (Dimitroff et al. 1998, Kannagi 2004, Ma and Vosseller 2014). Cancer-associated glycans, thus, may not necessarily be novel, but rather differentially-expressed and frequently confer a particular lectin-binding activity and related malignant behavior. For example, embryonic antigens are one group of cancer-associated glycans with altered expression or uniqueness compared with the normal fully-differentiated cell counterpart.

Aberrancy of Glycosylation as a Hallmark of Cancer Cells

The evolution of our knowledge on the role of glycosylation and cancer development has coincided with the vast improvement in exploratory glycomic tools/methods compared with basic methods first practiced by glycobiologists in the 1950s. Nonetheless, early studies on urine samples from cancer patients revolutionized our understanding of the potential importance of glycobiology on cancer. Changes in the monosaccharide content and length/branching of glycan chains on cancer-associated glycoproteins were first reported in bioassays of as cites and urinary fluids from cancer-bearing rats and humans (Masamune et al. 1957, 1958a,b, 1960, Hakomori et al. 1961, Hakomori and Jeanloz 1961). The pioneering efforts by Drs. H. Masamune and S. Hakomori indicated peculiar aberrancies in the glycosylation and glycoprotein size/levels associated with cancer progression (Masamune et al. 1957, 1958, 1958, 1960, Hakomori et al. 1961, Hakomori and Jeanloz 1961). Observations of larger molecular size, reduced hexose/hexosamine ratios, increased branching and higher overall glycan content on cancer-associated glycoprotein(s) were noted and first modeled as depicted in Fig. 1 (Hakomori and Jeanloz 1961).

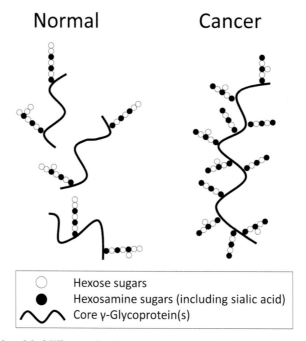

Figure 1. Compositional model of differences in the γ-glycoprotein fraction of urine from normal and cancer patients. Data published in 1961 from Hakomori et al. show that the glycoprotein(s) in fraction 4 of urine from normal or cancer patients is qualitatively and quantitatively different. Notable changes in the cancer-associated glycoprotein(s) compared with normal glycoproteins are: (1) a reduction in the hexose/hexosamine ratio, (2) greater molecular weight of core proteins and (3) greater degree in branching. [This figure was adapted from Hakomori et al. 1961.]

These findings are confirmed and expanded in later works showing that cancer cells intrinsically possess asparagine (N)-linked glycans with increased ß1,6 N-acetylglucosamine (GlcNAc) branching (Reading and Hutchins 1985, Laidler and Litynska 1997, Dennis et al. 1999, Ihara et al. 2004, Dube and Bertozzi 2005, Brooks et al. 2008, Schultz et al. 2012). The critical role of ß1,6 branched antennae on N-glycans in metastasis formation supports their classification as cancer-associated glycans (Dennis et al. 1987, Dennis 1988, Dennis et al. 1989, Dennis 1991).

As more studies on glycomics of cancer emerged through the late 20th century up to the present, data have clearly established that cancer cells also display or secrete elevated levels of sialylated glycosylations (Kannagi et al. 1986, Hoff et al. 1990, Walz et al. 1990, Sugiyama et al. 1992, Chandrasekaran et al. 1995, Kitsuki et al. 1995, Shimodaira et al. 1997, Dimitroff et al. 1998, 1999, Dall'Olio and Chiricolo 2001, Dimitroff et al. 2001, Alpaugh et al. 2002, Dimitroff et al. 2004, Kawaguchi 2005, Descheny et al. 2006, Barthel et al. 2007, Zen et al. 2008, Fujita et al. 2011, Barthel et al. 2013). As examples, expression of sialyl Lewis antigens or $\alpha 2,6$ sialylated GalNAc-serine/threonine (O)-linked glycans in numerous cancer models directly correlate with metastatic potential and poor prognosis (Hakomori 2001, Berriel et al. 2005, Ju et al. 2011, Julien et al. 2012, Ju et al. 2013, Remmers et al. 2013, Ju et al. 2014, Radhakrishnan et al. 2014). The most well-accepted role of the sialyl Lewis antigens on cancer cells is their role in intravascular trafficking and metastatic seeding, as they and their glycoprotein scaffolds, in particular, serve as binding determinants for vascular endothelial (E)-selectin (Dimitroff et al. 1998, Barthel et al. 2007, Jacobs and Sackstein 2011, St. Hill 2011, Schultz et al. 2012). However, whether these sialylated glycans and their protein carriers bind other lectins to impact cancer progression is still poorly understood (Cazet et al. 2010a,b, Bull et al. 2014, Christiansen et al. 2014, Compagno et al. 2014, Dall'Olio et al. 2014).

Contemporary translational glycobiologists are now more than ever poised to leverage new and innovative glycobiological tools and shared institutional resources. Conditional/inducible mouse models of cancer, use of lectin-specific glyco-mimetics and streamlined institutional cores for obtaining human cancer tissues (including metastatic disease) are readily-available for investigating functional aspects of cancer-associated glycomics. National glyco-analytical consortiums, namely the NIH Consortium for Functional Glycomics (www.functionalglycomics.org) and the Emory National Center for Functional Glycomics (www.biochem.emory.edu/emory-ncfg), provide glycome gene expression profiling, MALDI-TOF MS/MS glycan structural analysis and lectin-binding analysis on printed glycan arrays to more rigorously test hypotheses on the role of glycomics in cancer (Damerell et al. 2012, Robinson et al. 2012, Bern et al. 2013, Ruhaak et al. 2013a,b, Campbell et al. 2014, Frost and Li 2014, Hagan et al. 2014, Muthana and Gildersleeve 2014). In all, the future of cancer glycomic studies is well-positioned to evaluate glycomic factors as anti-cancer drug targets.

Glycans and Their Scaffolds Impacting Malignant Behavior

The role of cancer-associated glycans in cancer progression has frequently been linked to the mechanism of intravascular cancer cell trafficking and seeding in distant tissues. An accumulating body of data shows that sialylated Lewis[X] and [A] antigens on distinct membrane protein scaffoldstermed E-, platelet (P)- or leukocyte (L)-selectin ligands are critically involved in metastases formation (Masamune et al. 1960, Dimitroff et al. 1998, Barthel et al. 2007, Jacobs and Sackstein 2011, St. Hill 2011, Schultz et al. 2012). Binding interactions between selectin ligands on cancer cells and E-selectin on vascular endothelial (ECs), P-selectin on platelets or L-selectin on circulating leukocytes elicit dynamic adhesive interactions that encourage cell-cell contact, diapedesis and entry into tissue. Our firm understanding of glyco-molecular mechanisms underlying tissue-specific leukocyte homing has provided testable hypotheses for studies on the role of $\alpha 2,3$ sialyltransferases, $\alpha 1,3$ fucosyltransferases and core 2-mannosyl-ß1,6 N-acetylglucosaminyltransferases along with related membrane protein scaffolds as regulators of metastasis. The standard and variant forms of CD44 (otherwise known as Hematopoietic Cell E- and L-selectin Ligand (HCELL)s and HCELLv, respectively), lysosomal-associated membrane proteins (LAMP)-1 and -2, carcinoembryonic antigen (CEA), E-selectin ligand-1 (ESL-1), P-selectin glycoprotein ligand-1 (PSGL-1), podocalyxin-like protein (PCLP), podocalyxin, MUC-1, MUC-16, CD24 and melanoma cell adhesion molecule (MCAM) have all been shown to display sialyl Lewis[X] or [A] moieties and function as cancer cell selectin ligands

(Aigner et al. 1997, Tomlinson et al. 2000, Dimitroff et al. 2005, Hanley et al. 2005, 2006, Burdick et al. 2006, Alves et al. 2008, Nonomura et al. 2008, Barthel et al. 2009, Thomas et al. 2009a,b, Jacobs and Sackstein 2011, Konstantopoulos and Thomas 2011, Myung et al. 2011, Dallas et al. 2012, Shirure et al. 2012, Barthel et al. 2013, Shirure et al. 2015). Studying the functional role and therapeutic inhibition of cancer-associated selectin ligands remains an active area of cancer glycomic research.

Other well-studied cancer-associated glycans and glycoproteins are those capable of binding galectins—a family of 15 evolutionarily-conserved ß-galactoside-binding S-type lectins. Relative to expression on non-transformed cell counterparts, galectins are typically over expressed or downregulated, depending on the cancer cell model. They also show distinctive expression patterns in immune cell subsets and in endothelial cells (EC) that is further governed by resting or activation status. Upon secretion through non-classical pathways, they are deposited on natural ligands present on cell surfaces or on extracellular matrices (ECM). Galectins characteristically bind ß-galactoside-containing moieties in N- and O-glycans on cell membrane proteins, in ECM glycoconjugates and in membrane glycolipids. The binding specificity of each galectin is governed by the presence or absence of sulfate, sialic acid, fucose, repeating N-acetyllactosamine units or ß1,6 GlcNAc branches on the glycan core juxtaposed to a preferred protein/lipid scaffold (Stowell et al. 2008, Song et al. 2009, Smith et al. 2010, Stowell et al. 2010, Poland et al. 2011, Arthur et al. 2015). In nature, an authentic galectin ligand is conferred when the galectin-binding carbohydrate moiety is presented by a discrete membrane protein/lipid or ECM component (Skrincosky et al. 1993, Zhu et al. 2005, Cedeno-Laurent et al. 2010, Barthel et al. 2011, Cedeno-Laurent et al. 2012a,b, Jouve et al. 2013, Croci et al. 2014, Yazawa et al. 2015). That is, only when a galectin-binding glycan is uniquely displayed by a preferred scaffold can a physiologic galectin 'ligand' activity occur and, in effect, help dictate the ligand specificity for each galectin. Some well-described ligands include CD4, CD7, CD43, CD29, CD45, 90k/MAC-2BP, CD146 (MCAM), CEA, LAMP-1/2, MUC-1, laminin, α3ß1,T-cell immunoglobulin mucin-3 (TIM-3) and T-cell receptor (TCR) complex (Ohannesian et al. 1994, Baum et al. 1995, Ohannesian et al. 1995, Hadari et al. 2000, Tinari et al. 2001, Rabinovich et al. 2002, Kopitz et al. 2003, Bresalier et al. 2004, Krishnan et al. 2005, Hernandez et al. 2006, Liu et al. 2008, Grigorian et al. 2009, Earl et al. 2010, Iacovazzi et al. 2010, Cedeno-Laurent et al. 2012a,b, Clark et al. 2012, Agarwal et al. 2014, Dange et al. 2014, Escoda-Ferran et al. 2014, Yazawa et al. 2015).

Several galectins and their ligands have been found to play a critical role in cancer progression. Data support the concept that galectin–galectin ligand interactions elicit pro-tumorigenic activity by triggering tumor angiogenesis, tumor immunoregulation, homotypic cancer cell aggregation and/or heterotypic adhesion to ECs or ECM (Allen et al. 1990, Woynarowska et al. 1992, Skrincosky et al. 1993, Woynarowska et al. 1994, Takenaka et al. 2004, Yang et al. 2008, Horst and Wagener 2009, Rabinovich and Ilarregui 2009, Salatino and Rabinovich 2011, Cedeno-Laurent and Dimitroff 2012, Dall'Olio et al. 2012, Ito et al. 2012, Rabinovich et al. 2012, Thijssen et al. 2013, Compagno et al. 2014, Griffioen and Thijssen 2014, Hauselmann and Borsig 2014, Murugaesu et al. 2014, Pena et al. 2014, Reticker-Flynn and Bhatia 2014, Yazawa et al. 2015). Considering the repertoire of galectins in humans, galectin (Gal)-1 and Gal-3 have shown the greatest impact on cancer cell behavior. By extension, there is evidence indicating that the major cancer-associated Gal-1 and -3 ligands are membrane proteins LAMP-1/2, MCAM, 90k/MAC-2BP and/or CEA. The poly-N-acetyllactosamines displayed on the ligands' N-glycans and O-glycans have been found to be critical for binding activity (Rosenberg et al. 1991, Skrincosky et al. 1993, Jeng et al. 1994, Ohannesian et al. 1994, Sato and Hughes 1994, Ohannesian et al. 1995, Inohara et al. 1996, Woynarowska et al. 1996, Laidler and Litynska 1997, Andre et al. 1999, Ochieng et al. 1999, Cvejic et al. 2000, Tinari et al. 2001, Krishnan et al. 2005, Song et al. 2009, Srinivasan et al. 2009, Agarwal et al. 2014, Dange et al. 2014). Additionally, Gal-3 exhibits strong binding avidity for Thomsen-Friedenreichantigen (T antigen; Galactoseß1,3N-acetylgalactosamine (Galß1,3GalNAc)) found at high levels on MUC-1 expressed by cancer cells (Bresalier et al. 1996, Byrd and Bresalier 2004, Yu et al. 2007, Zhao et al. 2009, Saeland et al. 2012, Michel et al. 2014).

Studies on the regulatory mechanisms controlling synthesis/degradation of cancer-associated glycans/scaffolds that confer a galectin ligand activity have lagged relative to ligand identification. Nonetheless, one of the most widely-studied glycosyltransferases linked to a galectin-binding phenotype on N-glycans is mannose:ß1,6 N-acetylglucosaminyltransferase V (Mgat5). Mgat5 is a key regulator of poly-N-acetyllactosaminesynthesis on the tetra-antennary arm of N-glycans and related Gal-3-binding activity to the TCR on T cells (Demetriou et al. 2001, Dennis et al. 2002, Morgan et al. 2004, Dennis et al. 2009). Likewise, Mgat5 expression and corresponding poly-N-acetyllactosamine formation on N-glycans plays a key role in Gal-3-binding to cancer cells (Partridge et al. 2004, Takenaka et al. 2004, Lau and Dennis 2008). However, data on how N-glycan poly-N-acetyllactosamines and related Gal-1-binding activities are regulated on cancer cells is incomplete (Dennis et al. 1987, 1989, Lau and Dennis 2008). Regarding regulation of galectin-binding cancer-associated O-glycans, $\alpha2,3$ sialyltransferase-1 (ST3Gal-1) and core 2 ß1,6N-acetylglucosaminyltransferase-1 (GCNT1) have been shown to control the synthesis of Gal-1- and Gal-3-binding poly-N-acetyllactosamine on Core 2 O-glycans (Cabrera et al. 2006, Valenzuela et al. 2007, Tsuboi et al. 2011, Clark et al. 2012, Solatycka et al. 2012, Petrosyan et al. 2014). Transfer of $\alpha2,3$ sialic acid to T antigen by ST3Gal-1 prevents core 2 ß1,6 N-acetylglucosamine (GlcNAc) branching and subsequent poly-N-acetyllactosamine extension, thereby inhibiting Gal-1- and Gal-3-binding. Counter-intuitively, data also suggest that, where Gal-3 selectively binds cancer-associated T antigen, core 2 ß1,6 N-acetylglucosaminyltransferase-2 (GCNT3) actually inhibits Gal-3-binding to TF antigen through core 2 ß1,6 branching activity (Stone et al. 2009, Reticker-Flynn and Bhatia 2014). In all, Mgat5, ST3Gal-1 and GCNT1/3 represent a limited subset of glycosyltransferases shown to regulate cancer-associated N- and O-glycans that bind galectins.

As reviewed here, the pro-tumorigenic roles of Gal-1 and -3 ligands expressed by cancer cells and how they are regulated by $\alpha2,6$ sialyltransferases that transfer sialic acid in an $\alpha2,6$ linkage to N-acetylgalactosamine (GalNAc) on O-glycans are described. Recent studies highlight a key regulatory role of GalNAc: $\alpha2,6$ sialyltransferases (ST6GalNAc) in conferring Gal-1 and Gal-3 binding activity to O-glycans on cancer cells (Murugaesu et al. 2014, Reticker-Flynn and Bhatia 2014, Yazawa et al. 2015). These findings unveil the collaborative importance of galectin ligands and ST6GalNAcs as regulators of cancer cell malignancy and why such glycomic factors represent potential targets for anti-cancer therapy.

N-Acetylgalactosamine α2,6 Sialyltransferases and Cancer

ST6GalNAc Family Members and Acceptor Specificity

There has been a rise of published reports showing that GalNAc:$\alpha2,6$ sialyltransferases (ST6GalNAc) help regulate the formation of Gal-1 and Gal-3 ligand activity on cancer cells and influence malignant behavior. Of the six identified ST6GalNAcs, ST6GalNAc1-4 can transfer N-acetylneuraminic acid (Neu5Ac) in an $\alpha2,6$ linkage to GalNAc on O-glycans (Kurosawa et al. 1994a,b, Ikehara et al. 1999, Lee et al. 1999, Harduin-Lepers et al. 2000, Marcos et al. 2004, Tsuchida et al. 2005), whereas ST6GalNAc5 and ST6GalNAc6 show a preference for transfer of Neu5Ac in an $\alpha2,6$ linkage to GalNAc on glycolipids, namely Neu5Ac2,3Galß1,3GalNAcß1,4Galß1,4Glu-Cer (sialyl-lactotetraosyl-ceramide-G_{M1b}) (Okajima et al. 1999, 2000, Tsuchida et al. 2003). ST6GalNAc3 and ST6GalNAc4 also display $\alpha2,6$ sialyltransferase activity towards G_{M1b} (Lee et al. 1999, Tsuchida et al. 2005).

With regards to acceptor specificity, ST6GalNAc1 and ST6GalNAc2 are capable of generating Neu5Ac$\alpha2,6$GalNAc-Ser/Thr (sialyl-Tn antigen), Galß1,3 (Neu5Ac$\alpha2,6$) GalNAc-Ser/Thr (sialyl-6T antigen) and Neu5Ac$\alpha2,3$Galß1,3 (Neu5Ac$\alpha2,6$) GalNAc-Ser/Thr (disialyl-T antigen) from GalNAc-Ser/Thr (Tn antigen), T antigen (Galß1,3GalNAc-Ser/Thr) and Neu5Ac$\alpha2,3$Galß1,3GalNAc-Ser/Thr (sialyl-T antigen), respectively (Table 1) (Kurosawa et al. 1994a,b, Ikehara et al. 1999, Marcos et al. 2004). However, ST6GalNAc1 shows an acceptor preference for Tn antigen, whereas ST6GalNAc2 favors T antigen and sialyl-T antigen (Table 1). ST6GalNAc3 and ST6GalNAc4 can equally generate disialyl T antigen from sialyl T antigen as well as Neu5Ac2,3Galß1,3(Neu5Ac$\alpha2,6$)GalNAcß1,4Galß1,4Glu-Cer (disialyl-lactotetraosyl-ceramide-$G_{D1\alpha}$) from G_{M1b} (Table 1) (Kurosawa et al. 1994a,b, Lee et al. 1999, Harduin-Lepers et al. 2000, Marcos et al. 2004, Tsuchida et al. 2005). Both ST6GalNAc5 and ST6GalNAc6 show restricted specificity towards G_{M1b} for synthesis of $G_{D1\alpha}$ (Table 1) (Okajima et al. 1999, 2000, Tsuchida et al. 2003). Though the presence or absence of these $\alpha2,6$ sialylated O-glycans (and $G_{D1\alpha}$) have been structurally correlated with certain malignancies (Kudelka et al. 2015), their function in transformation, malignant behavior or metastatic progression is still poorly understood.

Table 1. ST6GalNAc family members and acceptor specificity.

Members	Glycan Acceptor(s)	Sialo-glycan Product(s)	References
ST6GalNAc1	Tn Sialyl-T antigen >>T antigen antigen	SialylDisialyl-Sialyl-Tn antigen >>T antigen 6T antigen	Ikehara et al. 1999, Kurosawa et al. 1994a,b
ST6GalNAc2	T Sialyl-Tn antigen >>T antigen antigen	Sialyl Disialyl-Sialyl-6 T antigen >>T antigen Tn antigen	Kurosawa et al. 1994a,b, Marcos et al. 2004
ST6GalNAc3	Sialyl T antigen Sialyl-Lactotetraosyl-Ceramide (G_{M1b})	Disialyl T antigen Disialyl-Lactotetraosyl-Ceramide (G_{D1a})	Tsuchida et al. 2005, Lee et al. 1999
ST6GalNAc4	Sialyl T antigen Sialyl-Lactotetraosyl-Ceramide (G_{M1b})	Disialyl T antigen Disialyl-Lactotetraosyl-Ceramide (G_{D1a})	Harduin-Lepers et al. 2000, Lee et al. 1999
ST6GalNAc5	Sialyl-Lactotetraosyl-Ceramide (G_{M1b})	Disialyl-Lactotetraosyl-Ceramide (G_{D1a})	Tsuchida et al. 2003, Okajima et al. 1999
ST6GalNAc6	Sialyl-Lactotetraosyl-Ceramide (G_{M1b})	Disialyl-Lactotetraosyl-Ceramide (G_{D1a})	Tsuchida et al. 2003, Okajima et al. 2000

Abbreviations: ST6GalNAc—N-acetylgalactosamine: α2,6 sialyltransferase.

Functional Role in Cancer Progression

Because α2,6 sialyltransferases ST6GalNAc1-4 enzymatically compete with core 2 ß1,6 N-acetylglucosaminyltransferases GCNT1 and GCNT3 for the C-6 position of GalNAc, they can theoretically function as regulators of core 2 poly-N-acetyllactosamine formation and T antigen expression— putative carbohydrate-recognition determinants for Gal-1 and Gal-3, respectively. Furthermore, ST6GalNAc activities could also prevent other galectins from binding, as O-glycans potentially bear ß-galactoside type 1 (Galß1,3GlcNAc), type 2 (Galß1,4GlcNAc) or type 3 (Galß1,3GalNAc) moieties. To this end, recent reports provide strong evidence supporting the regulatory role of ST6GalNAc enzymes in the formation of cancer-associated Gal-1- and Gal-3-binding moieties and related pro-tumorigenic/metastatic activities conferred by interactions with host Gal-1 and Gal-3.

ST6GalNAc2 and Breast Cancer Metastasis

A recent report by Isacke and colleagues reveals the critical role of ST6GalNAc2 as a negative regulator of breast cancer metastasis (Ferrer and Reginato 2014, Murugaesu et al. 2014). Using a functional RNA interference screening method, they identify a short hairpin RNA against ST6GalNAc2 that significantly enhances lung colonization in an experimental murine breast cancer metastasis assay. These data are further strengthened in both experimental and spontaneous metastasis assays using murine mammary cancer cells silenced for ST6GalNAc2 expression, showing that ST6GalNAc2 downregulation augments the frequency and burden of metastases. Furthermore, in experimental metastatic xenograft assays of human breast cancer cells expressing low or high levels of ST6GalNAc2, metastases formation in ST6GalNAc2 high cells is greatly reduced. To establish clinical relevance, data on ST6GalNAc2 expression in estrogen receptor (ER)⁻ vs. ER⁺ breast cancer specimens (and cell lines) demonstrate that ST6GalNAc2 expression is significantly associated with improved survival of patients with ER⁻ breast cancer.

   Importantly, this report examines the role of ST6GalNAc2 and its ability to α2,6 sialylate GalNAc in breast cancer O-glycans and indeed demonstrates that ST6GalNAc2 lowers unmodified (Core 1) T antigen levels, while increasing disialyl T antigen (Murugaesu et al. 2014). Given that T antigen is a well-described Gal-3-binding moiety (Yu et al. 2007, Bian et al. 2011), they provide complementary data that Gal-3-binding activity is heightened in ST6GalNAc2-silenced breast cancer cells. Gal-3's critical role in the context of ST6GalNAc2-silencing is further supported in experimental metastasis assays, in which the high metastatic activity of ST6GalNAc2-silenced breast cancer cells is reversed when similarly silenced for

Gal-3 expression or by treatment with Gal-3 inhibitor, GCS-100 (Chauhan et al. 2005, Streetly et al. 2010). Moreover, data show that Gal-3's pro-metastatic capacity corresponds with low ST6GalNAc2 expression, as evidenced by the improved ability to adhere to endothelial cells or form homotypic cell aggregates.

These data collectively provide a novel glyco-pathogenesis mechanism by which breast cancer-associated O-glycans regulated by ST6GalNAc2 help dictate interactions with Gal-3 to induce a pro-metastatic phenotype. Of clinical importance, using ST6GalNAc2 as a biomarker to rationalize Gal-3 antagonism treatment could be implemented, particularly in ER$^-$ breast cancer patients, who generally have a poorer prognosis than patients with ER$^+$ cancer.

ST6GalNAc4 and Lung Cancer Metastasis

The role of cancer-associated O-glycans related to Gal-3-binding activity and their regulation by another GalNAc: α2,6sialyltransferase, ST6GalNAc4, has recently been described (Reticker-Flynn and Bhatia 2014, Arnal-Estape and Nguyen 2015). Bhatia and colleagues expand on prior work establishing the high capacity of metastatic lung cancer cells to bind ECM component, Gal-3 (Reticker-Flynn et al. 2012), and investigate the role of lung cancer cell Gal-3 ligands (and regulation thereof) on lung cancer metastasis (Reticker-Flynn and Bhatia 2014). In this study, they first identify a relationship between Gal-3 expression in the host liver ('soil') as a pre-requisite for metastatic lung cancer ('seed') activity. The data suggest that a high level of Gal-3 in the pre-metastatic liver niche is largely presented by F4/80$^+$ macrophages. Further analysis of the Gal-3$^+$ leukocytes in lung cancer-bearing mice show that dual Gal-3/CD11b$^+$ cells are indeed elevated in the circulation through induced mobilization by lung cancer-derived IL-6.

To study the functional role between host Gal-3 and lung cancer cell Gal-3 ligands, subsequent experiments explore the relationship between Gal-3 ligand expression/regulation and lung cancer metastasis (Reticker-Flynn and Bhatia 2014). Data show that high Gal-3-binding activity is concomitant with high levels of T antigen expression, the hallmark Gal-3-binding glycan, and that this activity directly corresponds with metastatic potential. In that Gal-3 is unable to bind modified T antigen through Neu5Acα2,3Gal-R, Neu5Acα2,6GalNAc-and/or GlcNAcß1,6GalNAc-R branches, these glyco-modifications have been hypothesized to interfere with maintenance of the T antigen moiety. Indeed, expression array analysis reveals that core 2 ß1,6 GlcNAc-branching enzyme GCNT3 is downregulated in metastatic lung cancer cells. Moreover, expression data show that ST6GalNAc4 is overexpressed in metastatic cells, indicating that ST6GalNAc4's ability to α2,6 sialylate GalNAc on sialyl-T antigen (referred to as capping) may be associated with increased Gal-3 ligand/T antigen levels. These expression data are corroborated with binding results showing that Gal-3 ligand activity is lowered in either GCNT3-overexpressing or ST6GalNAc4-silenced metastatic lung cancer cells. *In vivo* data on ST6GalNAc4-silenced cells further reveal that reduction of Gal-3 ligand corresponds with significantly attenuated metastatic activity. These observations advance the notion that maintenance of cancer-associated Gal-3-binding O-glycans could be controlled by preventing core 2 branching or by capping sialyl-T antigen through GCNT3 or ST6GalNAc4, respectively.

GCNT3's putative role in preventing T antigen is logical through its ability to form core 2 structures. However, ST6GalNAc4's ability to generate disialyl-T antigen from sialyl-T antigen to '*promote*' Gal-3-binding activity is not intuitive. Indeed, the level of T antigen in ST6GalNAc4-silenced cells does not parallel the increase Gal-3 ligand activity. The enhanced Gal-3-binding activity by ST6GalNAc4, therefore, may be due to the presence of fewer core 2 O-glycans and enhanced exposure of T antigen on a select protein scaffold, a defining structural prerequisite for optimal Gal-3 ligand activity. So, while disialyl-T antigen moieties may not directly bind Gal-3, their presence in the context of GCNT3 downregulation (fewer core 2 O-glycans) may indirectly increase Gal-3 ligand activity. O-glycan truncation may, in fact, create a cell surface glycocalyx devoid of steric hindrances caused by core 2 O-glycans, thereby increasing availability to Gal-3-binding T antigen moieties.

ST6GalNAc2 and Melanoma Malignancy

In recent work published by Yazawa et al., results demonstrate a role for α2,6 sialyltransferase ST6GalNAc2 as a negative regulator in forming melanoma-associated O-glycans capable of binding Gal-1 and mediating malignant activity (Yazawa et al. 2015). After establishing that Gal-1 ligands are up-regulated on primary and metastatic melanoma cells compared with epidermal melanocytes in normal skin or benign nevi, biochemical assessments reveal that Gal-1-binding moieties and protein scaffold identities ('Gal-1 ligand') are principally represented by poly-N-acetyllactosamines on N-glycans and by protein scaffold MCAM and to a lesser degree on 90k/MAC-2B, CEA and LAMP-1/2.

While the majority of Gal-1 ligand activity on melanoma cells is found on poly-N-acetyllactosaminyl N-glycans, poly-N-acetyllactosamine-containing O-glycans, also provide a significant level of Gal-1 ligand activity. Considering the newly-established role of ST6GalNAc2 in preventing core 2 O-glycans and lowering Gal-3-binding T antigen moieties on breast cancer cells (Murugaesu et al. 2014), this study explores ST6GalNAc2's role as a putative regulator of Gal-1-binding activity (Yazawa et al. 2015). Since ST6GalNAc2 activity could compete with core 2 ß1,6 GlcNAc branching activity, fewer poly-N-acetyllactosamines on O-glycans may potentially result in attenuated Gal-1 ligand activity. Expression analyses show that ST6GalNAc2, in fact, is markedly downregulated in Gal-1 ligand[+] malignant melanoma cells compared with Gal-1 ligand[-] normal epidermal melanocytes, implicating ST6GalNAc2 as a negative regulator of Gal-1 ligand expression. Binding data show that Gal-1- and *Lycopersicon esculentum* agglutinin (poly-N-acetyllactosamine-specific)-binding to O-glycans are inhibited in melanoma cells overexpressing ST6GalNAc2. Functional data indicate that ST6GalNAc2 suppresses melanoma cell migration on Gal-1 natively expressed in Matrigel and growth of ST6GalNAc2-overexpressing melanomas is severely blunted in mice lacking Gal-1. So, even though Gal-1 ligand activity is predominantly conferred by N-glycans on melanoma cells, these findings indicate that only partial impairment in melanoma cell Gal-1 ligand expression can significantly impact melanoma virulence.

These observations support the notion that ST6GalNAc2 can interfere, in part, with Gal-1 ligand-mediated melanoma malignancy, potentially by preventing poly-N-acetyllactosaminyl O-glycans on melanoma cell Gal-1 ligands. Studies are underway to identify other glycosyltransferase regulators of melanoma-associated Gal-1 ligand activity, such as Mgat5, that may impact the expression of poly-N-acetyllactosamines on N-glycans (Demetriou et al. 2001, Dennis et al. 2002, Partridge et al. 2004).

Conclusions

Model of Novel O-Glycan Structure-Function Relationships in Cancer

The novel roles of ST6GalNAcs in regulating the expression of cancer-associated O-glycans that convey binding interactions with galectins and provoke cancer virulence highlight recent excitement in the cancer glycomics field (Ferrer and Reginato 2014, Murugaesu et al. 2014, Reticker-Flynn and Bhatia 2014, Arnal-Estape and Nguyen 2015, Yazawa et al. 2015). These investigations reinforce the key role of cancer cell O-glycans and how subtle modifications (or lack thereof) by O-glycan-modifying enzymes, namely ST6GalNAcs and GCNT1/3, dictate Gal-1 and Gal-3-binding capacity and downstream consequences on cancer behavior. These data further support the notion that, whether Gal-3 is preferentially binding poly-N-acetyllactosamines on N-glycans or T antigen on O-glycans, the relative abundance of each respective glycan species likely dictates the preferred Gal-3 ligand(s) on a given cancer cell type. Mucinous adenocarcinomas, such as lung, breast and colon cancers, which contain a preponderance of O-glycans relative to N-glycans, provide a distinct Gal-3-binding glycan repertoire that is probably different than that on non-mucinous malignancies. Melanoma cells, for example, display N-glycan poly-N-acetyllactosamines on a select subset of protein scaffolds, namely LAMP-1, that are the preferred Gal-3 ligands (Krishnan et al. 2005, Srinivasan et al. 2009, Agarwal et al. 2014, Dange et al. 2014). A model illustrating ST6GalNAc enzymatic glycan products conferring Gal-1- and Gal-3-binding activity is presented in Fig. 2.

Future Prospects of Cancer Glycomic Research and Therapy

Studies on the discovery and functional role of cancer-associated glycomic factors remain a vital area of cancer research (Gorelik et al. 2001, Barthel et al. 2007, Nakahara and Raz 2008). The role of ST6GalNAc enzymes in regulating O-glycan forms, as reviewed here, reveals the importance in regulating the length

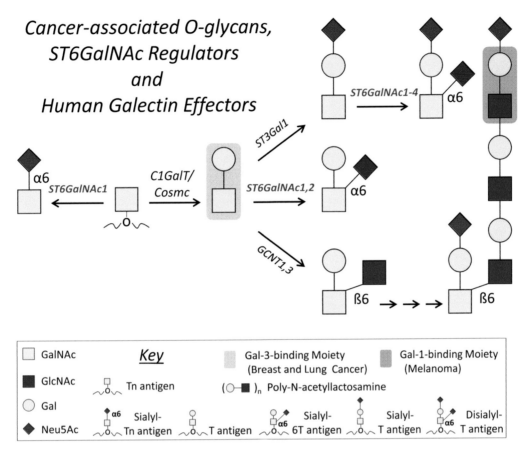

Figure 2. Regulation of O-glycan modifications through ST6GalNAc enzyme activities is associated with Gal-1- and Gal-3-binding and related malignant potential. Recent data indicate that the malignant behavior of breast and lung cancer is regulated, in part, by ST6GalNAc2 and ST6GalNAc4 and related synthesis of Gal-3-binding moieties (Murugaesu et al. 2014, Reticker-Flynn and Bhatia 2014). Similarly, data show that O-glycans-bearing poly-N-acetyllactosamines are regulated by ST6GalNAc2 and help mediate Gal-1 ligand activity and related tumorigenic potential and migratory activity of melanoma cells (Yazawa et al. 2015).

and branching of O-glycans that impact pro-tumorigenic activity dependent on host Gal-1- and/or Gal-3-binding. The advent of sophisticated mouse models of cancer, new and innovative glycomic tools, precise structural mimetics and enhanced human tissue procurement measures are now widely-available to more rigorously dissect how glycomic factors impact cancer progression. Discovering identity, function and enzymatic regulation of glycosylations on cancer cells continues to invigorate efforts to target these factors as anti-cancer therapies. Importantly, glycan-synthetic inhibitors (Woynarowska et al. 1992, 1994, 1996, Dimitroff et al. 1998, 1999, Descheny et al. 2006, Barthel et al. 2007, 2011, Cedeno-Laurent et al. 2012a,b, Dimitroff 2013), glyco-mimetic antagonists (Glinsky et al. 2000, 2003, Thijssen et al. 2006, Giguere et al. 2008, Glinsky and Raz 2009, Stannard et al. 2010, Thijssen et al. 2010, Ito et al. 2011, Salomonsson et al. 2011, Collins et al. 2012, Ito and Ralph 2012, Ito et al. 2012, Bum-Erdene et al. 2013) or neutralizing antibodies (Ouyang et al. 2011, Croci et al. 2012, Laderach et al. 2013, Ouyang et al. 2013, Croci et al. 2014) designed to therapeutically block the function of cancer-associated glycans linked to malignant behaviors are now mainstream and imminent for evaluation in humans.

Clinical development of anti-metastatic agents designed to interfere with cancer cell selectin ligand–selectin interactions has been challenging. Evaluation of such agents is difficult to effectively assess in early Phase I/II clinical trials designed more to examine safety and some biologic effect in cancer patients with late stage disease—when occult micrometastases are likely already established. These therapies need to be safe and well-tolerated, as they will likely be implemented in a maintenance setting on individuals with early stage cancer that have a high probability of progressing to late stage disease. The emerging emphasis on *precision medicine* through genomic screening to help predict progression of disease and/or guide treatment decisions will undoubtedly heighten efforts to develop such agents. Cancer patients presenting with a gene signature suggestive of a virulent phenotype during which cancer cells actively seed distant tissues would be ideal candidates to effectively examine anti-metastatic efficacy. Whether cancer-associated selectin ligands help regulate other pathways, such as pro-survival/migration in primary and metastatic sites, epithelial to mesenchymal transition and pro-angiogenesis, is still poorly understood (Rabinovich and Croci 2012, Croci et al. 2014, Lange et al. 2014), though could potentially reinforce efforts to identify effective therapeutic antagonists.

There are other challenges relating to development of anti-cancer glyco-therapeutics, particularly those biologics that target cancer-associated glycans and glycoproteins that bind galectins. Due to overlapping glycan-binding specificities, identifying antagonists to either Gal-1–Gal-1 ligand or Gal-3–Gal-3 ligand interactions, as examples, should be carefully considered (Gordon-Alonso et al. 2014). Whether using glyco-mimetics to competitively inhibit Gal-1 or -3's carbohydrate-recognition domain or metabolic inhibitors to block Gal-1- or -3-binding glycan synthesis, specificity is critical to develop clinically-useful agents. Blocking other galectin-binding activities with similar binding specificities, such Gal-8 and Gal-9, could have alternative roles in cancer development and immunoprotection (Smetana et al. 2013, Thijssen and Griffioen 2014).

The glyco-mimetic, GCS-100, has been shown to selectively target Gal-3, compete for natural Gal-3 ligand and antagonize Gal-3 ligand-mediated adhesion and downstream intracellular signaling (Chauhan et al. 2005, Streetly et al. 2010, Murugaesu et al. 2014). GCS-100 is a modified citrus pectin pioneered by the Raz laboratory (Inohara and Raz 1994) that is now in clinical development for treating fibrosis in chronic kidney disease and for treating cancer by boosting anti-cancer T cell immunity (http://lajollapharmaceutical.com). The therapeutic potential of GCS-100 is further heightened, as early clinical studies indicate that GCS-100 is well-tolerated and could be used in combination with chemotherapeutic agents (Chauhan et al. 2005, Streetly et al. 2010).

Other recent efforts using neutralizing monoclonal antibodies to carbohydrate-recognition domains of individual galectins, notably Gal-1, have shown promise (Ouyang et al. 2011, Croci et al. 2012, Laderach et al. 2013, Ouyang et al. 2013, Croci et al. 2014). Even though the implied therapeutic targets are interactions between Gal-1 and Gal-1 ligands on T cells or ECs, interference of the pro-tumorigenic role of cancer-associated Gal-1 ligands (Yazawa et al. 2015) further raises the possibility of using humanized antibody forms for clinical utility in cancer patients. Considering the promise of humanized antibodies against immune checkpoint molecules to stimulate anti-cancer immunity (Hodi et al. 2008, Topalian et al. 2012, Hamid et al. 2013, Ott et al. 2013, Ascierto et al. 2014), efforts to develop humanized versions of mono-specific anti-Gal-1 antibodies are warranted. There is an expectation within the glycomics community that neutralizing antibodies against pro-tumorigenic glycomic factors could elicit the same level of clinical effectiveness.

To expedite investigations on glyco-therapeutics, there needs to be an active coordination between cancer glycobiologists, specialists of applied high-throughput molecular discovery and cancer pharmacologists. The future model of glycobiological development for the treatment of cancer is the formation of scientific partnerships between industrial and academic scientists. Each entity can effectively leverage their scientific expertise, research tools and laboratory infrastructure to develop potent and specific glyco-therapeutics in a cost-efficient manner. This type of collaborative relationship provides an opportune circumstance to rapidly test lead candidates in biologically-relevant screening assays and translate their use in *in vivo* settings—namely humans.

Acknowledgements

This work was supported from the National Institutes of Health/National Cancer Institute RO1 grant, CA173610 (C. Dimitroff).

Keywords: sialyltransferase, galectin, cancer-associated glycosylations, glyco-therapeutics

References

Agarwal, A. K., R. P. Gude and R. D. Kalraiya. 2014. Regulation of melanoma metastasis to lungs by cell surface Lysosome Associated Membrane Protein-1 (LAMP1) via galectin-3. Biochem Biophys Res Commun 449(3): 332–7.

Aigner, S., Z. M. Sthoeger, M. Fogel, E. Weber, J. Zarn, M. Ruppert et al. 1997. CD24, a mucin-type glycoprotein, is a ligand for P-selectin on human tumor cells. Blood 89(9): 3385–95.

Allen, H. J., D. Sucato, B. Woynarowska, S. Gottstine, A. Sharma and R. J. Bernacki. 1990. Role of galaptin in ovarian carcinoma adhesion to extracellular matrix *in vitro*. J Cell Biochem 43(1): 43–57.

Alpaugh, M. L., J. S. Tomlinson, Y. Ye and S. H. Barsky. 2002. Relationship of sialyl-Lewis(x/a) underexpression and E-cadherin overexpression in the lymphovascular embolus of inflammatory breast carcinoma. Am J Pathol 161(2): 619–28.

Alves, C. S., M. M. Burdick, S. N. Thomas, P. Pawar and K. Konstantopoulos. 2008. The dual role of CD44 as a functional P-selectin ligand and fibrin receptor in colon carcinoma cell adhesion. Am J Physiol Cell Physiol 294(4): C907–16.

Andre, S., S. Kojima, N. Yamazaki, C. Fink, H. Kaltner, K. Kayser et al. 1999. Galectins-1 and -3 and their ligands in tumor biology. Non-uniform properties in cell-surface presentation and modulation of adhesion to matrix glycoproteins for various tumor cell lines, in biodistribution of free and liposome-bound galectins and in their expression by breast and colorectal carcinomas with/without metastatic propensity. J Cancer Res Clin Oncol 125(8-9): 461–74.

Arnal-Estape, A. and D. X. Nguyen. 2015. Sweets for a bitter end: lung cancer cell-surface protein glycosylation mediates metastatic colonization. Cancer Discov 5(2): 109–11.

Arthur, C. M., L. C. Rodrigues, M. D. Baruffi, H. C. Sullivan, J. Heimburg-Molinaro, D. F. Smith et al. 2015. Examining galectin binding specificity using glycan microarrays. Methods Mol Biol 1207: 115–31.

Ascierto, P. A., A. M. Grimaldi, A. Anderson, C. Bifulco, A. Cochran, C. Garbe et al. 2014. Future perspectives in melanoma research: meeting report from "Melanoma Bridge", Napoli, December 5th–8th 2013. J Transl Med 12(1): 277.

Barthel, S. R., J. D. Gavino, L. Descheny and C. J. Dimitroff. 2007. Targeting selectins and selectin ligands in inflammation and cancer. Expert Opin Ther Targets 11(11): 1473–91.

Barthel, S. R., G. K. Wiese, J. Cho, M. J. Opperman, D. L. Hays, J. Siddiqui et al. 2009. Alpha 1,3 fucosyltransferases are master regulators of prostate cancer cell trafficking. Proc Natl Acad Sci USA 106(46): 19491–6.

Barthel, S. R., A. Antonopoulos, F. Cedeno-Laurent, L. Schaffer, G. Hernandez, S. A. Patil et al. 2011. Peracetylated 4-fluoro-glucosamine reduces the content and repertoire of N- and O-glycans without direct incorporation. J Biol Chem 286(24): 21717–31.

Barthel, S. R., D. L. Hays, E. M. Yazawa, M. Opperman, K. C. Walley, L. Nimrichter et al. 2013. Definition of molecular determinants of prostate cancer cell bone extravasation. Cancer Res 73(2): 942–52.

Baum, L. G., M. Pang, N. L. Perillo, T. Wu, A. Delegeane, C. H. Uittenbogaart et al. 1995. Human thymic epithelial cells express an endogenous lectin, galectin-1, which binds to core 2 O-glycans on thymocytes and T lymphoblastoid cells. J Exp Med 181(3): 877–87.

Bern, M., A. E. Brito, P. C. Pang, A. Rekhi, A. Dell and S. M. Haslam. 2013. Polylactosaminoglycan glycomics: enhancing the detection of high-molecular-weight N-glycans in matrix-assisted laser desorption ionization time-of-flight profiles by matched filtering. Mol Cell Proteomics 12(4): 996–1004.

Berriel, E., M. Hill, J. J. Barcia, L. Ubillos, M. Gonzalez, G. Detjen et al. 2005. Simple mucin-type cancer associated antigens are pre-cancerous biomarkers during 1,2-dimethylhydrazine-induced rat colon carcinogenesis. Oncol Rep 14(1): 219–27.

Bian, C. F., Y. Zhang, H. Sun, D. F. Li and D. C. Wang. 2011. Structural basis for distinct binding properties of the human galectins to Thomsen-Friedenreich antigen. PLoS One 6(9): e25007.

Bresalier, R. S., J. C. Byrd, L. Wang and A. Raz. 1996. Colon cancer mucin: a new ligand for the beta-galactoside-binding protein galectin-3. Cancer Res 56(19): 4354–7.

Bresalier, R. S., J. C. Byrd, D. Tessler, J. Lebel, J. Koomen, D. Hawke et al. 2004. A circulating ligand for galectin-3 is a haptoglobin-related glycoprotein elevated in individuals with colon cancer. Gastroenterology 127(3): 741–8.

Brooks, S. A., T. M. Carter, L. Royle, D. J. Harvey, S. A. Fry, C. Kinch et al. 2008. Altered glycosylation of proteins in cancer: what is the potential for new anti-tumour strategies. Anticancer Agents Med Chem 8(1): 2–21.

Bull, C., M. A. Stoel, M. H. den Brok and G. J. Adema. 2014. Sialic acids sweeten a tumor's life. Cancer Res 74(12): 3199–204.

Bum-Erdene, K., I. A. Gagarinov, P. M. Collins, M. Winger, A. G. Pearson, J. C. Wilson et al. 2013. Investigation into the feasibility of thiodigalactoside as a novel scaffold for galectin-3-specific inhibitors. Chembiochem 14(11): 1331–42.

Burdick, M. M., J. T. Chu, S. Godar and R. Sackstein. 2006. HCELL is the major E- and L-selectin ligand expressed on LS174T colon carcinoma cells. J Biol Chem 281(20): 13899–905.

Byrd, J. C. and R. S. Bresalier. 2004. Mucins and mucin binding proteins in colorectal cancer. Cancer Metastasis Rev 23(1-2): 77–99.

Cabrera, P. V., M. Amano, J. Mitoma, J. Chan, J. Said, M. Fukuda et al. 2006. Haploinsufficiency of C2GnT-I glycosyltransferase renders T lymphoma cells resistant to cell death. Blood 108(7): 2399–406.

Campbell, M. P., R. Ranzinger, T. Lutteke, J. Mariethoz, C. A. Hayes, J. Zhang et al. 2014. Toolboxes for a standardised and systematic study of glycans. BMC Bioinformatics 15 Suppl 1: S9.

Cazet, A., S. Julien, M. Bobowski, J. Burchell and P. Delannoy. 2010a. Tumour-associated carbohydrate antigens in breast cancer. Breast Cancer Res 12(3): 204.

Cazet, A., S. Julien, M. Bobowski, M. A. Krzewinski-Recchi, A. Harduin-Lepers, S. Groux-Degroote et al. 2010b. Consequences of the expression of sialylated antigens in breast cancer. Carbohydr Res 345(10): 1377–83.

Cedeno-Laurent, F., S. R. Barthel, M. J. Opperman, D. M. Lee, R. A. Clark and C. J. Dimitroff. 2010. Development of a nascent galectin-1 chimeric molecule for studying the role of leukocyte galectin-1 ligands and immune disease modulation. J Immunol 185(8): 4659–72.

Cedeno-Laurent, F. and C. J. Dimitroff. 2012. Galectins and their ligands: Negative regulators of anti-tumor immunity. Glycoconj J 29(8-9): 619–25.

Cedeno-Laurent, F., M. Opperman, S. R. Barthel, V. K. Kuchroo and C. J. Dimitroff. 2012a. Galectin-1 triggers an immunoregulatory signature in Th cells functionally defined by IL-10 expression. J Immunol 188(7): 3127–37.

Cedeno-Laurent, F., M. J. Opperman, S. R. Barthel, D. Hays, T. Schatton, Q. Zhan et al. 2012b. Metabolic inhibition of galectin-1-binding carbohydrates accentuates antitumor immunity. J Invest Dermatol 132(2): 410–20.

Chandrasekaran, E. V., R. K. Jain, R. D. Larsen, K. Wlasichuk and K. L. Matta. 1995. Selectin ligands and tumor-associated carbohydrate structures: specificities of alpha 2,3-sialyltransferases in the assembly of 3'-sialyl-6-sialyl/sulfo Lewis a and x, 3'-sialyl-6'-sulfo Lewis x, and 3'-sialyl-6-sialyl/sulfo blood group T-hapten. Biochemistry 34(9): 2925–36.

Chauhan, D., G. Li, K. Podar, T. Hideshima, P. Neri, D. He et al. 2005. A novel carbohydrate-based therapeutic GCS-100 overcomes bortezomib resistance and enhances dexamethasone-induced apoptosis in multiple myeloma cells. Cancer Res 65(18): 8350–8.

Christiansen, M. N., J. Chik, L. Lee, M. Anugraham, J. L. Abrahams and N. H. Packer. 2014. Cell surface protein glycosylation in cancer. Proteomics 14(4-5): 525–46.

Clark, M. C., M. Pang, D. K. Hsu, F. T. Liu, S. de Vos, R. D. Gascoyne et al. 2012. Galectin-3 binds to CD45 on diffuse large B-cell lymphoma cells to regulate susceptibility to cell death. Blood 120(23): 4635–44.

Collins, P. M., C. T. Oberg, H. Leffler, U. J. Nilsson and H. Blanchard. 2012. Taloside inhibitors of galectin-1 and galectin-3. Chem Biol Drug Des 79(3): 339–46.

Compagno, D., L. D. Gentilini, F. M. Jaworski, I. G. Perez, G. Contrufo and D. J. Laderach. 2014. Glycans and galectins in prostate cancer biology, angiogenesis and metastasis. Glycobiology 24(10): 899–906.

Croci, D. O., M. Salatino, N. Rubinstein, J. P. Cerliani, L. E. Cavallin, H. J. Leung et al. 2012. Disrupting galectin-1 interactions with N-glycans suppresses hypoxia-driven angiogenesis and tumorigenesis in Kaposi's sarcoma. J Exp Med 209(11): 1985–2000.

Croci, D. O., J. P. Cerliani, T. Dalotto-Moreno, S. P. Mendez-Huergo, I. D. Mascanfroni, S. Dergan-Dylon et al. 2014. Glycosylation-dependent lectin-receptor interactions preserve angiogenesis in anti-VEGF refractory tumors. Cell 156(4): 744–58.

Cvejic, D., S. Savin, S. Golubovic, I. Paunovic, S. Tatic and M. Havelka. 2000. Galectin-3 and carcinoembryonic antigen expression in medullary thyroid carcinoma: possible relation to tumour progression. Histopathology 37(6): 530–5.

Dall'Olio, F. and M. Chiricolo. 2001. Sialyltransferases in cancer. Glycoconj J 18(11-12): 841–50.

Dall'Olio, F., N. Malagolini, M. Trinchera and M. Chiricolo. 2012. Mechanisms of cancer-associated glycosylation changes. Front Biosci (Landmark Ed) 17: 670–99.

Dall'Olio, F., N. Malagolini, M. Trinchera and M. Chiricolo. 2014. Sialosignaling: Sialyltransferases as engines of self-fueling loops in cancer progression. Biochim Biophys Acta 1840(9): 2752–64.

Dallas, M. R., S. H. Chen, M. M. Streppel, S. Sharma, A. Maitra and K. Konstantopoulos. 2012. Sialofucosylated podocalyxin is a functional E- and L-selectin ligand expressed by metastatic pancreatic cancer cells. Am J Physiol Cell Physiol 303(6): C616–24.

Damerell, D., A. Ceroni, K. Maass, R. Ranzinger, A. Dell and S. M. Haslam. 2012. The GlycanBuilder and GlycoWorkbench glycoinformatics tools: updates and new developments. Biol Chem 393(11): 1357–62.

Dange, M. C., N. Srinivasan, S. K. More, S. M. Bane, A. Upadhya, A. D. Ingle et al. 2014. Galectin-3 expressed on different lung compartments promotes organ specific metastasis by facilitating arrest, extravasation and organ colonization via high affinity ligands on melanoma cells. Clin Exp Metastasis 31(6): 661–73.

Demetriou, M., M. Granovsky, S. Quaggin and J. W. Dennis. 2001. Negative regulation of T-cell activation and autoimmunity by Mgat5 N-glycosylation. Nature 409(6821): 733–9.

Dennis, J. W., S. Laferte, C. Waghorne, M. L. Breitman and R. S. Kerbel. 1987. Beta 1-6 branching of Asn-linked oligosaccharides is directly associated with metastasis. Science 236(4801): 582–5.

Dennis, J. W. 1988. Asn-linked oligosaccharide processing and malignant potential. Cancer Surv 7(4): 573–95.

Dennis, J. W., S. Laferte, S. Yagel and M. L. Breitman. 1989. Asparagine-linked oligosaccharides associated with metastatic cancer. Cancer Cells 1(3): 87–92.

Dennis, J. W. 1991. N-linked oligosaccharide processing and tumor cell biology. Semin Cancer Biol 2(6): 411–20.

Dennis, J. W., M. Granovsky and C. E. Warren. 1999. Glycoprotein glycosylation and cancer progression. Biochim Biophys Acta 1473(1): 21–34.

Dennis, J. W., J. Pawling, P. Cheung, E. Partridge and M. Demetriou. 2002. UDP-N-acetylglucosamine: alpha-6-D-mannoside beta1,6 N-acetylglucosaminyltransferase V (Mgat5) deficient mice. Biochim Biophys Acta 1573(3): 414–22.

Dennis, J. W., K. S. Lau, M. Demetriou and I. R. Nabi. 2009. Adaptive regulation at the cell surface by N-glycosylation. Traffic 10(11): 1569–78.

Descheny, L., M. E. Gainers, B. Walcheck and C. J. Dimitroff. 2006. Ameliorating skin-homing receptors on malignant T cells with a fluorosugar analog of N-acetylglucosamine: P-selectin ligand is a more sensitive target than E-selectin ligand. J Invest Dermatol 126(9): 2065–73.

Dimitroff, C. J., A. Sharma and R. J. Bernacki. 1998. Cancer metastasis: A search for therapeutic inhibition. Cancer Invest 16(4): 279–90.

Dimitroff, C. J., P. Pera, F. Dall'Olio, K. L. Matta, E. V. Chandrasekaran, J. T. Lau et al. 1999. Cell surface n-acetylneuraminic acid alpha2,3-galactoside-dependent intercellular adhesion of human colon cancer cells. Biochem Biophys Res Commun 256(3): 631–6.

Dimitroff, C. J., J. Y. Lee, S. Rafii, R. C. Fuhlbrigge and R. Sackstein. 2001. CD44 is a major E-selectin ligand on human hematopoietic progenitor cells. J Cell Biol 153(6): 1277–86.

Dimitroff, C. J., M. Lechpammer, D. Long-Woodward and J. L. Kutok. 2004. Rolling of human bone-metastatic prostate tumor cells on human bone marrow endothelium under shear flow is mediated by E-selectin. Cancer Res 64(15): 5261–9.

Dimitroff, C. J., L. Descheny, N. Trujillo, R. Kim, V. Nguyen, W. Huang et al. 2005. Identification of leukocyte E-selectin ligands, P-selectin glycoprotein ligand-1 and E-selectin ligand-1, on human metastatic prostate tumor cells. Cancer Res 65(13): 5750–60.

Dimitroff, C. J. 2013. Leveraging fluorinated glucosamine action to boost antitumor immunity. Curr Opin Immunol 25(2): 206–13.

Dube, D. H. and C. R. Bertozzi. 2005. Glycans in cancer and inflammation—potential for therapeutics and diagnostics. Nat Rev Drug Discov 4(6): 477–88.

Earl, L. A., S. Bi and L. G. Baum. 2010. N- and O-glycans modulate galectin-1 binding, CD45 signaling, and T cell death. J Biol Chem 285(4): 2232–44.

Escoda-Ferran, C., E. Carrasco, M. Caballero-Banos, C. Miro-Julia, M. Martinez-Florensa, M. Consuegra-Fernandez et al. 2014. Modulation of CD6 function through interaction with Galectin-1 and -3. FEBS Lett 588(17): 2805–13.

Ferrer, C. M. and M. J. Reginato. 2014. Sticking to sugars at the metastatic site: Sialyltransferase ST6GalNAc2 acts as a breast cancer metastasis suppressor. Cancer Discov 4(3): 275–7.

Frost, D. C. and L. Li. 2014. Recent advances in mass spectrometry-based glycoproteomics. Adv Protein Chem Struct Biol 95: 71–123.

Fujita, T., K. Murayama, T. Hanamura, T. Okada, T. Ito, M. Harada et al. 2011. CSLEX (Sialyl Lewis X) is a useful tumor marker for monitoring of breast cancer patients. Jpn J Clin Oncol 41(3): 394–9.

Giguere, D., M. A. Bonin, P. Cloutier, R. Patnam, C. St-Pierre, S. Sato et al. 2008. Synthesis of stable and selective inhibitors of human galectins-1 and -3. Bioorg Med Chem 16(16): 7811–23.

Glinsky, V. V., M. E. Huflejt, G. V. Glinsky, S. L. Deutscher and T. P. Quinn. 2000. Effects of Thomsen-Friedenreich antigen-specific peptide P-30 on beta-galactoside-mediated homotypic aggregation and adhesion to the endothelium of MDA-MB-435 human breast carcinoma cells. Cancer Res 60(10): 2584–8.

Glinsky, V. V., G. V. Glinsky, O. V. Glinskii, V. H. Huxley, J. R. Turk, V. V. Mossine et al. 2003. Intravascular metastatic cancer cell homotypic aggregation at the sites of primary attachment to the endothelium. Cancer Res 63(13): 3805–11.

Glinsky, V. V. and A. Raz. 2009. Modified citrus pectin anti-metastatic properties: One bullet, multiple targets. Carbohydr Res 344(14): 1788–91.

Gordon-Alonso, M., N. Demotte and P. van der Bruggen. 2014. Sugars boost exhausted tumor-infiltrating lymphocytes by counteracting immunosuppressive activities of galectins. Oncoimmunology 3: e28783.

Gorelik, E., U. Galili and A. Raz. 2001. On the role of cell surface carbohydrates and their binding proteins (lectins) in tumor metastasis. Cancer Metastasis Rev 20(3-4): 245–77.

Griffioen, A. W. and V. L. Thijssen. 2014. Galectins in tumor angiogenesis. Ann Transl Med 2(9): 90.

Grigorian, A., S. Torossian and M. Demetriou. 2009. T-cell growth, cell surface organization, and the galectin-glycoprotein lattice. Immunol Rev 230(1): 232–46.

Hadari, Y. R., R. Arbel-Goren, Y. Levy, A. Amsterdam, R. Alon, R. Zakut et al. 2000. Galectin-8 binding to integrins inhibits cell adhesion and induces apoptosis. J Cell Sci 113(Pt 13): 2385–97.

Hagan, A. K., M. Wang and L. Liu. 2014. Current approaches to glycoprotein analysis. Protein Pept Lett 21(10): 986–99.

Hakomori, S. I. and R. W. Jeanloz. 1961. Isolation and characterization of glycolipids from erythrocytes of human blood A (plus) and B (plus). J Biol Chem 236: 2827–34.

Hakomori, S., T. Ishimoda, H. Kawauti and F. Eidoh. 1961. Isolation, characterization of an abnormal gamma-glycoprotein from urine of patients with cancer. J Biochem 49: 307–16.

Hakomori, S. 2001. Tumor-associated carbohydrate antigens defining tumor malignancy: Basis for development of anti-cancer vaccines. Adv Exp Med Biol 491: 369–402.

Hamid, O., C. Robert, A. Daud, F. S. Hodi, W. J. Hwu, R. Kefford et al. 2013. Safety and tumor responses with lambrolizumab (anti-PD-1) in melanoma. N Engl J Med 369(2): 134–44.

Hanley, W. D., M. M. Burdick, K. Konstantopoulos and R. Sackstein. 2005. CD44 on LS174T colon carcinoma cells possesses E-selectin ligand activity. Cancer Res 65(13): 5812–7.

Hanley, W. D., S. L. Napier, M. M. Burdick, R. L. Schnaar, R. Sackstein and K. Konstantopoulos. 2006. Variant isoforms of CD44 are P- and L-selectin ligands on colon carcinoma cells. FASEB J 20(2): 337–9.

Harduin-Lepers, A., D. C. Stokes, W. F. Steelant, B. Samyn-Petit, M. A. Krzewinski-Recchi, V. Vallejo-Ruiz et al. 2000. Cloning, expression and gene organization of a human Neu5Ac alpha 2-3Gal beta 1-3GalNAc alpha 2,6-sialyltransferase: hST6GalNAcIV. Biochem J 352 Pt 1: 37–48.

Hauselmann, I. and L. Borsig. 2014. Altered tumor-cell glycosylation promotes metastasis. Front Oncol 4: 28.

Hernandez, J. D., J. T. Nguyen, J. He, W. Wang, B. Ardman, J. M. Green et al. 2006. Galectin-1 binds different CD43 glycoforms to cluster CD43 and regulate T cell death. J Immunol 177(8): 5328–36.

Hodi, F. S., M. Butler, D. A. Oble, M. V. Seiden, F. G. Haluska, A. Kruse et al. 2008. Immunologic and clinical effects of antibody blockade of cytotoxic T lymphocyte-associated antigen 4 in previously vaccinated cancer patients. Proc Natl Acad Sci USA 105(8): 3005–10.

Hoff, S. D., T. Irimura, Y. Matsushita, D. M. Ota, K. R. Cleary and S. Hakomori. 1990. Metastatic potential of colon carcinoma. Expression of ABO/Lewis-related antigens. Arch Surg 125(2): 206–9.

Horst, A. K. and C. Wagener. 2009. Bitter sweetness of complexity. Top Curr Chem 288: 1–15.

Iacovazzi, P. A., M. Notarnicola, M. G. Caruso, V. Guerra, S. Frisullo and D. F. Altomare. 2010. Serum levels of galectin-3 and its ligand 90k/mac-2bp in colorectal cancer patients. Immunopharmacol Immunotoxicol 32(1): 160–4.

Ihara, S., E. Miyoshi, S. Nakahara, H. Sakiyama, H. Ihara, A. Akinaga et al. 2004. Addition of beta1-6 GlcNAc branching to the oligosaccharide attached to Asn 772 in the serine protease domain of matriptase plays a pivotal role in its stability and resistance against trypsin. Glycobiology 14(2): 139–46.

Ikehara, Y., N. Kojima, N. Kurosawa, T. Kudo, M. Kono, S. Nishihara et al. 1999. Cloning and expression of a human gene encoding an N-acetylgalactosamine-alpha2,6-sialyltransferase (ST6GalNAc I): a candidate for synthesis of cancer-associated sialyl-Tn antigens. Glycobiology 9(11): 1213–24.

Inohara, H. and A. Raz. 1994. Effects of natural complex carbohydrate (citrus pectin) on murine melanoma cell properties related to galectin-3 functions. Glycoconj J 11(6): 527–32.

Inohara, H., S. Akahani, K. Koths and A. Raz. 1996. Interactions between galectin-3 and Mac-2-binding protein mediate cell-cell adhesion. Cancer Res 56(19): 4530–4.

Ito, K., S. A. Scott, S. Cutler, L. F. Dong, J. Neuzil, H. Blanchard et al. 2011. Thiodigalactoside inhibits murine cancers by concurrently blocking effects of galectin-1 on immune dysregulation, angiogenesis and protection against oxidative stress. Angiogenesis 14(3): 293–307.

Ito, K. and S. J. Ralph. 2012. Inhibiting galectin-1 reduces murine lung metastasis with increased CD4(+) and CD8(+) T cells and reduced cancer cell adherence. Clin Exp Metastasis 29(6): 561–72.

Ito, K., K. Stannard, E. Gabutero, A. M. Clark, S. Y. Neo, S. Onturk et al. 2012. Galectin-1 as a potent target for cancer therapy: role in the tumor microenvironment. Cancer Metastasis Rev 31(3-4): 763–78.

Jacobs, P. P. and R. Sackstein. 2011. CD44 and HCELL: preventing hematogenous metastasis at step 1. FEBS Lett 585(20): 3148–58.

Jeng, K. C., L. G. Frigeri and F. T. Liu. 1994. An endogenous lectin, galectin-3 (epsilon BP/Mac-2), potentiates IL-1 production by human monocytes. Immunol Lett 42(3): 113–6.

Jouve, N., N. Despoix, M. Espeli, L. Gauthier, S. Cypowyj, K. Fallague et al. 2013. The involvement of CD146 and its novel ligand Galectin-1 in apoptotic regulation of endothelial cells. J Biol Chem 288(4): 2571–9.

Ju, T., V. I. Otto and R. D. Cummings. 2011. The Tn antigen-structural simplicity and biological complexity. Angew Chem Int Ed Engl 50(8): 1770–91.

Ju, T., Y. Wang, R. P. Aryal, S. D. Lehoux, X. Ding, M. R. Kudelka et al. 2013. Tn and sialyl-Tn antigens, aberrant O-glycomics as human disease markers. Proteomics Clin Appl. 7(9-10): 618–31.

Ju, T., R. P. Aryal, M. R. Kudelka, Y. Wang and R. D. Cummings. 2014. The Cosmc connection to the Tn antigen in cancer. Cancer Biomark 14(1): 63–81.

Julien, S., P. A. Videira and P. Delannoy. 2012. Sialyl-tn in cancer: (how) did we miss the target? Biomolecules 2(4): 435–66.

Kannagi, R., Y. Fukushi, T. Tachikawa, A. Noda, S. Shin, K. Shigeta et al. 1986. Quantitative and qualitative characterization of human cancer-associated serum glycoprotein antigens expressing fucosyl or sialyl-fucosyl type 2 chain polylactosamine. Cancer Res 46(5): 2619–26.

Kannagi, R. 2004. Molecular mechanism for cancer-associated induction of sialyl Lewis X and sialyl Lewis A expression-The Warburg effect revisited. Glycoconj J 20(5): 353–64.

Kawaguchi, T. 2005. Cancer metastasis: characterization and identification of the behavior of metastatic tumor cells and the cell adhesion molecules, including carbohydrates. Curr Drug Targets Cardiovasc Haematol Disord 5(1): 39–64.

Kitsuki, H., M. Katano, T. Morisaki and M. Torisu. 1995. CEA-mediated homotypic aggregation of human colorectal carcinoma cells in a malignant effusion. Cancer Lett 88(1): 7–13.

Konstantopoulos, K. and S. N. Thomas. 2011. Hematogenous metastasis: Roles of CD44v and alternative sialofucosylated selectin ligands. Adv Exp Med Biol 705: 601–19.

Kopitz, J., S. Andre, C. von Reitzenstein, K. Versluis, H. Kaltner, R. J. Pieters et al. 2003. Homodimeric galectin-7 (p53-induced gene 1) is a negative growth regulator for human neuroblastoma cells. Oncogene 22(40): 6277–88.

Krishnan, V., S. M. Bane, P. D. Kawle, K. N. Naresh and R. D. Kalraiya. 2005. Altered melanoma cell surface glycosylation mediates organ specific adhesion and metastasis via lectin receptors on the lung vascular endothelium. Clin Exp Metastasis 22(1): 11–24.

Kudelka, M. R., T. Ju, J. Heimburg-Molinaro and R. D. Cummings. 2015. Simple sugars to complex disease-mucin-type o-glycans in cancer. Adv Cancer Res 126: 53–135.

Kurosawa, N., T. Hamamoto, Y. C. Lee, T. Nakaoka, N. Kojima and S. Tsuji. 1994a. Molecular cloning and expression of GalNAc alpha 2,6-sialyltransferase. J Biol Chem 269(2): 1402–9.

Kurosawa, N., N. Kojima, M. Inoue, T. Hamamoto and S. Tsuji. 1994b. Cloning and expression of Gal beta 1,3GalNAc-specific GalNAc alpha 2,6-sialyltransferase. J Biol Chem 269(29): 19048–53.

Laderach, D. J., L. D. Gentilini, L. Giribaldi, V. C. Delgado, L. Nugnes, D. O. Croci et al. 2013. A unique galectin signature in human prostate cancer progression suggests galectin-1 as a key target for treatment of advanced disease. Cancer Res 73(1): 86–96.

Laidler, P. and A. Litynska. 1997. Tumor cell N-glycans in metastasis. Acta Biochim Pol 44(2): 343–57.

Lange, T., T. R. Samatov, A. G. Tonevitsky and U. Schumacher. 2014. Importance of altered glycoprotein-bound N- and O-glycans for epithelial-to-mesenchymal transition and adhesion of cancer cells. Carbohydr Res 389: 39–45.

Lau, K. S. and J. W. Dennis. 2008. N-Glycans in cancer progression. Glycobiology 18(10): 750–60.

Lee, Y. C., M. Kaufmann, S. Kitazume-Kawaguchi, M. Kono, S. Takashima, N. Kurosawa et al. 1999. Molecular cloning and functional expression of two members of mouse NeuAcalpha2,3Galbeta1,3GalNAc GalNAcalpha2,6-sialyltransferase family, ST6GalNAc III and IV. J Biol Chem 274(17): 11958–67.

Liu, S. D., C. C. Whiting, T. Tomassian, M. Pang, S. J. Bissel, L. G. Baum et al. 2008. Endogenous galectin-1 enforces class I-restricted TCR functional fate decisions in thymocytes. Blood 112(1): 120–30.

Ma, Z. and K. Vosseller. 2014. Cancer metabolism and elevated O-GlcNAc in oncogenic signaling. J Biol Chem 289(50): 34457–65.

Marcos, N. T., S. Pinho, C. Grandela, A. Cruz, B. Samyn-Petit, A. Harduin-Lepers et al. 2004. Role of the human ST6GalNAc-I and ST6GalNAc-II in the synthesis of the cancer-associated sialyl-Tn antigen. Cancer Res 64(19): 7050–7.

Masamune, H., S. Tsuiki, S. Kamiyama, Sin-Iti Abe, M. Haga, H. Kawasaki et al. 1957. A toxohormone from cancerous ascitic fluid; preliminary note. Tohoku J Exp Med 67(1): 10.

Masamune, H., S. Hakomori, H. Kaketa and S. Abe. 1958a. Toxohormones without KIK-potency from urines, cancerous and normal; preliminary note. Tohoku J Exp Med 67(4): 334.

Masamune, H., S. Hakomori, H. Kaketa, H. Sinohara and S. Abe. 1958b. Chemical nature of toxohormone (Nakahara). 3. KIK-in-active toxohormones from urines, cancerous and normal. Tohoku J Exp Med 68(1): 63–73.

Masamune, H., H. Kawasaki and H. Sinohara. 1960. Anemia-inducing substances from stomach cancer tissue. I. On a dialyzable active substance. Tohoku J Exp Med 72: 348–55.

Michel, A. K., P. Nangia-Makker, A. Raz and M. J. Cloninger. 2014. Lactose-functionalized dendrimers arbitrate the interaction of galectin-3/MUC1 mediated cancer cellular aggregation. Chembiochem 15(14): 2106–12.

Morgan, R., G. Gao, J. Pawling, J. W. Dennis, M. Demetriou and B. Li. 2004. N-acetylglucosaminyltransferase V (Mgat5)-mediated N-glycosylation negatively regulates Th1 cytokine production by T cells. J Immunol 173(12): 7200–8.

Murugaesu, N., M. Iravani, A. van Weverwijk, A. Ivetic, D. A. Johnson, A. Antonopoulos et al. 2014. An *in vivo* functional screen identifies ST6GalNAc2 sialyltransferase as a breast cancer metastasis suppressor. Cancer Discov 4(3): 304–17.

Muthana, S. M. and J. C. Gildersleeve. 2014. Glycan microarrays: powerful tools for biomarker discovery. Cancer Biomark 14(1): 29–41.

Myung, J. H., K. A. Gajjar, R. M. Pearson, C. A. Launiere, D. T. Eddington and S. Hong. 2011. Direct measurements on CD24-mediated rolling of human breast cancer MCF-7 cells on E-selectin. Anal Chem 83(3): 1078–83.

Nakahara, S. and A. Raz. 2008. Biological modulation by lectins and their ligands in tumor progression and metastasis. Anticancer Agents Med Chem 8(1): 22–36.

Nonomura, C., J. Kikuchi, N. Kiyokawa, H. Ozaki, K. Mitsunaga, H. Ando et al. 2008. CD43, but not P-selectin glycoprotein ligand-1, functions as an E-selectin counter-receptor in human pre-B-cell leukemia NALL-1. Cancer Res 68(3): 790–9.

Ochieng, J., P. Warfield, B. Green-Jarvis and I. Fentie. 1999. Galectin-3 regulates the adhesive interaction between breast carcinoma cells and elastin. J Cell Biochem 75(3): 505–14.

Ohannesian, D. W., D. Lotan and R. Lotan. 1994. Concomitant increases in galectin-1 and its glycoconjugate ligands (carcinoembryonic antigen, lamp-1, and lamp-2) in cultured human colon carcinoma cells by sodium butyrate. Cancer Res 54(22): 5992–6000.

Ohannesian, D. W., D. Lotan, P. Thomas, J. M. Jessup, M. Fukuda, H. J. Gabius et al. 1995. Carcinoembryonic antigen and other glycoconjugates act as ligands for galectin-3 in human colon carcinoma cells. Cancer Res 55(10): 2191–9.

Okajima, T., S. Fukumoto, H. Ito, M. Kiso, Y. Hirabayashi, T. Urano et al. 1999. Molecular cloning of brain-specific GD1alpha synthase (ST6GalNAc V) containing CAG/Glutamine repeats. J Biol Chem 274(43): 30557–62.

Okajima, T., H. H. Chen, H. Ito, M. Kiso, T. Tai, K. Furukawa et al. 2000. Molecular cloning and expression of mouse GD1alpha/GT1aalpha/GQ1balpha synthase (ST6GalNAc VI) gene. J Biol Chem 275(10): 6717–23.

Ott, P. A., F. S. Hodi and C. Robert. 2013. CTLA-4 and PD-1/PD-L1 blockade: New immunotherapeutic modalities with durable clinical benefit in melanoma patients. Clin Cancer Res 19(19): 5300–9.

Ouyang, J., P. Juszczynski, S. J. Rodig, M. R. Green, E. O'Donnell, T. Currie et al. 2011. Viral induction and targeted inhibition of galectin-1 in EBV+ posttransplant lymphoproliferative disorders. Blood 117(16): 4315–22.

Ouyang, J., A. Plutschow, E. Pogge von Strandmann, K. S. Reiners, S. Ponader, G. A. Rabinovich et al. 2013. Galectin-1 serum levels reflect tumor burden and adverse clinical features in classical Hodgkin lymphoma. Blood 121(17): 3431–3.

Partridge, E. A., C. Le Roy, G. M. Di Guglielmo, J. Pawling, P. Cheung, M. Granovsky et al. 2004. Regulation of cytokine receptors by Golgi N-glycan processing and endocytosis. Science 306(5693): 120–4.

Pena, C., L. Mirandola, J. A. Figueroa, N. Hosiriluck, N. Suvorava, K. Trotter et al. 2014. Galectins as therapeutic targets for hematological malignancies: A hopeful sweetness. Ann Transl Med 2(9): 87.

Petrosyan, A., M. S. Holzapfel, D. E. Muirhead and P. W. Cheng. 2014. Restoration of compact Golgi morphology in advanced prostate cancer enhances susceptibility to galectin-1-induced apoptosis by modifying mucin o-glycan synthesis. Mol Cancer Res 12(12): 1704–16.

Poland, P. A., C. Rondanino, C. L. Kinlough, J. Heimburg-Molinaro, C. M. Arthur, S. R. Stowell et al. 2011. Identification and characterization of endogenous galectins expressed in Madin Darby canine kidney cells. J Biol Chem 286(8): 6780–90.

Rabinovich, G. A., L. G. Baum, N. Tinari, R. Paganelli, C. Natoli, F. T. Liu et al. 2002. Galectins and their ligands: amplifiers, silencers or tuners of the inflammatory response? Trends Immunol 23(6): 313–20.

Rabinovich, G. A. and J. M. Ilarregui. 2009. Conveying glycan information into T-cell homeostatic programs: A challenging role for galectin-1 in inflammatory and tumor microenvironments. Immunol Rev 230(1): 144–59.

Rabinovich, G. A. and D. O. Croci. 2012. Regulatory circuits mediated by lectin-glycan interactions in autoimmunity and cancer. Immunity 36(3): 322–35.

Rabinovich, G. A., Y. van Kooyk and B. A. Cobb. 2012. Glycobiology of immune responses. Ann N Y Acad Sci 1253: 1–15.

Radhakrishnan, P., S. Dabelsteen, F. B. Madsen, C. Francavilla, K. L. Kopp, C. Steentoft et al. 2014. Immature truncated O-glycophenotype of cancer directly induces oncogenic features. Proc Natl Acad Sci USA 111(39): E4066–75.

Reading, C. L. and J. T. Hutchins. 1985. Carbohydrate structure in tumor immunity. Cancer Metastasis Rev 4(3): 221–60.

Remmers, N., J. M. Anderson, E. M. Linde, D. J. DiMaio, A. J. Lazenby, H. H. Wandall et al. 2013. Aberrant expression of mucin core proteins and o-linked glycans associated with progression of pancreatic cancer. Clin Cancer Res 19(8): 1981–93.

Reticker-Flynn, N. E., D. F. Malta, M. M. Winslow, J. M. Lamar, M. J. Xu, G. H. Underhill et al. 2012. A combinatorial extracellular matrix platform identifies cell-extracellular matrix interactions that correlate with metastasis. Nat Commun 3: 1122.

Reticker-Flynn, N. E. and S. N. Bhatia. 2014. Aberrant glycosylation promotes lung cancer metastasis through adhesion to galectins in the metastatic niche. Cancer Discov 5(2): 168–181.

Robinson, L. N., C. Artpradit, R. Raman, Z. H. Shriver, M. Ruchirawat and R. Sasisekharan. 2012. Harnessing glycomics technologies: integrating structure with function for glycan characterization. Electrophoresis 33(5): 797–814.

Rosenberg, I., B. J. Cherayil, K. J. Isselbacher and S. Pillai. 1991. Mac-2-binding glycoproteins. Putative ligands for a cytosolic beta-galactoside lectin. J Biol Chem 266(28): 18731–6.

Ruhaak, L. R., S. Miyamoto and C. B. Lebrilla. 2013a. Developments in the identification of glycan biomarkers for the detection of cancer. Mol Cell Proteomics 12(4): 846–55.

Ruhaak, L. R., U. T. Nguyen, C. Stroble, S. L. Taylor, A. Taguchi, S. M. Hanash et al. 2013b. Enrichment strategies in glycomics-based lung cancer biomarker development. Proteomics Clin Appl. 7(9-10): 664–76.

Saeland, E., A. I. Belo, S. Mongera, I. van Die, G. A. Meijer and Y. van Kooyk. 2012. Differential glycosylation of MUC1 and CEACAM5 between normal mucosa and tumour tissue of colon cancer patients. Int J Cancer 131(1): 117–28.

Salatino, M. and G. A. Rabinovich. 2011. Fine-tuning antitumor responses through the control of galectin-glycan interactions: An overview. Methods Mol Biol 677: 355–74.

Salomonsson, E., V. L. Thijssen, A. W. Griffioen, U. J. Nilsson and H. Leffler. 2011. The anti-angiogenic peptide anginex greatly enhances galectin-1 binding affinity for glycoproteins. J Biol Chem 286(16): 13801–4.

Sato, S. and R. C. Hughes. 1994. Regulation of secretion and surface expression of Mac-2, a galactoside-binding protein of macrophages. J Biol Chem 269(6): 4424–30.

Schultz, M. J., A. F. Swindall and S. L. Bellis. 2012. Regulation of the metastatic cell phenotype by sialylated glycans. Cancer Metastasis Rev 31(3-4): 501–18.

Shimodaira, K., J. Nakayama, N. Nakamura, O. Hasebe, T. Katsuyama and M. Fukuda. 1997. Carcinoma-associated expression of core 2 beta-1,6-N-acetylglucosaminyltransferase gene in human colorectal cancer: Role of O-glycans in tumor progression. Cancer Res 57(23): 5201–6.

Shirure, V. S., N. M. Reynolds and M. M. Burdick. 2012. Mac-2 binding protein is a novel E-selectin ligand expressed by breast cancer cells. PLoS One 7(9): e44529.

Shirure, V. S., T. Liu, L. F. Delgadillo, C. M. Cuckler, D. F. Tees, F. Benencia et al. 2015. CD44 variant isoforms expressed by breast cancer cells are functional E-selectin ligands under flow conditions. Am J Physiol Cell Physiol 308(1): C68–78.

Skrincosky, D. M., H. J. Allen and R. J. Bernacki. 1993. Galaptin-mediated adhesion of human ovarian carcinoma A121 cells and detection of cellular galaptin-binding glycoproteins. Cancer Res 53(11): 2667–75.

Smetana, K., Jr., S. Andre, H. Kaltner, J. Kopitz and H. J. Gabius. 2013. Context-dependent multifunctionality of galectin-1: A challenge for defining the lectin as therapeutic target. Expert Opin Ther Targets 17(4): 379–92.

Smith, D. F., X. Song and R. D. Cummings. 2010. Use of glycan microarrays to explore specificity of glycan-binding proteins. Methods Enzymol 480: 417–44.

Solatycka, A., T. Owczarek, F. Piller, V. Piller, B. Pula, L. Wojciech et al. 2012. MUC1 in human and murine mammary carcinoma cells decreases the expression of core 2 beta1,6-N-acetylglucosaminyltransferase and beta-galactoside alpha2,3-sialyltransferase. Glycobiology 22(8): 1042–54.

Song, X., B. Xia, S. R. Stowell, Y. Lasanajak, D. F. Smith and R. D. Cummings. 2009. Novel fluorescent glycan microarray strategy reveals ligands for galectins. Chem Biol 16(1): 36–47.

Srinivasan, N., S. M. Bane, S. D. Ahire, A. D. Ingle and R. D. Kalraiya. 2009. Poly N-acetyllactosamine substitutions on N- and not O-oligosaccharides or Thomsen-Friedenreich antigen facilitate lung specific metastasis of melanoma cells via galectin-3. Glycoconj J 26(4): 445–56.

St Hill, C. A. 2011. Interactions between endothelial selectins and cancer cells regulate metastasis. Front Biosci (Landmark Ed) 16: 3233–51.

Stannard, K. A., P. M. Collins, K. Ito, E. M. Sullivan, S. A. Scott, E. Gabutero et al. 2010. Galectin inhibitory disaccharides promote tumour immunity in a breast cancer model. Cancer Lett 299(2): 95–110.

Stone, E. L., M. N. Ismail, S. H. Lee, Y. Luu, K. Ramirez, S. M. Haslam et al. 2009. Glycosyltransferase function in core 2-type protein O glycosylation. Mol Cell Biol 29(13): 3770–82.

Stowell, S. R., C. M. Arthur, P. Mehta, K. A. Slanina, O. Blixt, H. Leffler et al. 2008. Galectin-1, -2, and -3 exhibit differential recognition of sialylated glycans and blood group antigens. J Biol Chem 283(15): 10109–23.

Stowell, S. R., C. M. Arthur, M. Dias-Baruffi, L. C. Rodrigues, J. P. Gourdine, J. Heimburg-Molinaro et al. 2010. Innate immune lectins kill bacteria expressing blood group antigen. Nat Med 16(3): 295–301.

Stowell, S. R., T. Ju and R. D. Cummings. 2015. Protein glycosylation in cancer. Annu Rev Pathol 10: 473–510.

Streetly, M. J., L. Maharaj, S. Joel, S. A. Schey, J. G. Gribben and F. E. Cotter. 2010. GCS-100, a novel galectin-3 antagonist, modulates MCL-1, NOXA, and cell cycle to induce myeloma cell death. Blood 115(19): 3939–48.

Sugiyama, K., T. Kawai, N. Nagata and M. Suzuki. 1992. Tumor-associated carbohydrate antigens in primary pulmonary adenocarcinomas and their metastases. Hum Pathol 23(8): 900–4.

Takenaka, Y., T. Fukumori and A. Raz. 2004. Galectin-3 and metastasis. Glycoconj J 19(7-9): 543–9.

Thijssen, V. L., R. Postel, R. J. Brandwijk, R. P. Dings, I. Nesmelova, S. Satijn et al. 2006. Galectin-1 is essential in tumor angiogenesis and is a target for antiangiogenesis therapy. Proc Natl Acad Sci USA 103(43): 15975–80.

Thijssen, V. L., B. Barkan, H. Shoji, I. M. Aries, V. Mathieu, L. Deltour et al. 2010. Tumor cells secrete galectin-1 to enhance endothelial cell activity. Cancer Res 70(15): 6216–24.

Thijssen, V. L., G. A. Rabinovich and A. W. Griffioen. 2013. Vascular galectins: Regulators of tumor progression and targets for cancer therapy. Cytokine Growth Factor Rev 24(6): 547–58.

Thijssen, V. L. and A. W. Griffioen. 2014. Galectin-1 and -9 in angiogenesis: A sweet couple. Glycobiology 24(10): 915–20.

Thomas, S. N., R. L. Schnaar and K. Konstantopoulos. 2009a. Podocalyxin-like protein is an E-/L-selectin ligand on colon carcinoma cells: comparative biochemical properties of selectin ligands in host and tumor cells. Am J Physiol Cell Physiol 296(3): C505–13.

Thomas, S. N., Z. Tong, K. J. Stebe and K. Konstantopoulos. 2009b. Identification, characterization and utilization of tumor cell selectin ligands in the design of colon cancer diagnostics. Biorheology 46(3): 207–25.

Tinari, N., I. Kuwabara, M. E. Huflejt, P. F. Shen, S. Iacobelli and F. T. Liu. 2001. Glycoprotein 90K/MAC-2BP interacts with galectin-1 and mediates galectin-1-induced cell aggregation. Int J Cancer 91(2): 167–72.

Tomlinson, J., J. L. Wang, S. H. Barsky, M. C. Lee, J. Bischoff and M. Nguyen. 2000. Human colon cancer cells express multiple glycoprotein ligands for E-selectin. Int J Oncol 16(2): 347–53.

Topalian, S. L., F. S. Hodi, J. R. Brahmer, S. N. Gettinger, D. C. Smith, D. F. McDermott et al. 2012. Safety, activity, and immune correlates of anti-PD-1 antibody in cancer. N Engl J Med 366(26): 2443–54.

Tsuboi, S., M. Sutoh, S. Hatakeyama, N. Hiraoka, T. Habuchi, Y. Horikawa et al. 2011. A novel strategy for evasion of NK cell immunity by tumours expressing core2 O-glycans. EMBO J 30(15): 3173–85.

Tsuchida, A., T. Okajima, K. Furukawa, T. Ando, H. Ishida, A. Yoshida et al. 2003. Synthesis of disialyl Lewis a (Le(a)) structure in colon cancer cell lines by a sialyltransferase, ST6GalNAc VI, responsible for the synthesis of alpha-series gangliosides. J Biol Chem 278(25): 22787–94.

Tsuchida, A., M. Ogiso, Y. Nakamura, M. Kiso, K. Furukawa and K. Furukawa. 2005. Molecular cloning and expression of human ST6GalNAc III: Restricted tissue distribution and substrate specificity. J Biochem 138(3): 237–43.

Valenzuela, H. F., K. E. Pace, P. V. Cabrera, R. White, K. Porvari, H. Kaija et al. 2007. O-glycosylation regulates LNCaP prostate cancer cell susceptibility to apoptosis induced by galectin-1. Cancer Res 67(13): 6155–62.

Walz, G., A. Aruffo, W. Kolanus, M. Bevilacqua and B. Seed. 1990. Recognition by ELAM-1 of the sialyl-Lex determinant on myeloid and tumor cells. Science 250(4984): 1132–5.

Woynarowska, B., H. Wikiel, M. Sharma, N. Carpenter, G. W. Fleet and R. J. Bernacki. 1992. Inhibition of human ovarian carcinoma cell- and hexosaminidase-mediated degradation of extracellular matrix by sugar analogs. Anticancer Res 12(1): 161–6.

Woynarowska, B., D. M. Skrincosky, A. Haag, M. Sharma, K. Matta and R. J. Bernacki. 1994. Inhibition of lectin-mediated ovarian tumor cell adhesion by sugar analogs. J Biol Chem 269(36): 22797–803.

Woynarowska, B., C. J. Dimitroff, M. Sharma, K. L. Matta and R. J. Bernacki. 1996. Inhibition of human HT-29 colon carcinoma cell adhesion by a 4-fluoro-glucosamine analogue. Glycoconj J 13(4): 663–74.

Yang, R. Y., G. A. Rabinovich and F. T. Liu. 2008. Galectins: Structure, function and therapeutic potential. Expert Rev Mol Med 10: e17.

Yazawa, E. M., J. E. Geddes-Sweeney, F. Cedeno-Laurent, K. C. Walley, S. R. Barthel, M. J. Opperman et al. 2015. Melanoma cell galectin-1 ligands functionally correlate with malignant potential. J Invest Dermatol 135(7): 1849–62.

Yu, L. G., N. Andrews, Q. Zhao, D. McKean, J. F. Williams, L. J. Connor et al. 2007. Galectin-3 interaction with Thomsen-Friedenreich disaccharide on cancer-associated MUC1 causes increased cancer cell endothelial adhesion. J Biol Chem 282(1): 773–81.

Zen, K., D. Q. Liu, Y. L. Guo, C. Wang, J. Shan, M. Fang et al. 2008. CD44v4 is a major E-selectin ligand that mediates breast cancer cell transendothelial migration. PLoS One 3(3): e1826.

Zhao, Q., X. Guo, G. B. Nash, P. C. Stone, J. Hilkens, J. M. Rhodes et al. 2009. Circulating galectin-3 promotes metastasis by modifying MUC1 localization on cancer cell surface. Cancer Res 69(17): 6799–806.

Zhu, C., A. C. Anderson, A. Schubart, H. Xiong, J. Imitola, S. J. Khoury et al. 2005. The Tim-3 ligand galectin-9 negatively regulates T helper type 1 immunity. Nat Immunol 6(12): 1245–52.

CHAPTER 11

Pectins as Biological Modulators of Human Physiological Reactions[#]

Sergey V. Popov

Introduction. General Information about Pectins

Pectins are complicated heteropolysaccharides belonging to the group of acidic plant polysaccharides, glycanogalacturonans (Ovodov 2009). Pectin is well known to be an important component of the primary cell wall and intercellular substance (middle lamella) of higher terrestrial plants, sea grasses and some freshwater algae (Popper 2008). The primary plant cell wall is composed of a mixture of cellulose, hemicellulose, and pectin, while the middle lamella can be considered as an extension of this matrix material from which the cellulose are lacking. Pectic substances make up about 30 percentage of the dry matter of the primary cell wall and are the primary macromolecules of the middle lamella. In the plant cell wall several dozen chains of cellulose interconnected by hydrogen and van der Waals forces form linear microfibril. Molecules of hemicelluloses, which include xyloglucan, xylans, glucuronoarabonoxilans, gluco-, galacto-, and galactoglucomannans are situated between these microfibrils forming network with the molecules of cellulose (Burton et al. 2010). The entire network of cellulose microfibrils and linking them hemicelluloses is immersed in a matrix of pectic substances. It acts as the cementing agent for the fibrils, provides them with effective tensile and keeps the cell walls of adjacent cells glued together. Pectins contribute to the mechanical strength, porosity, adhesion and stiffness of the cell wall and have been implicated in many processes, including wall slippage, extension and intercellular signaling. In total, pectin functions in plants have been thoroughly investigated (Palin and Geitmann 2012, Wolf and Greiner 2012, Komarova et al. 2014, Yokawa and Baluska 2015).

The plant cell wall represents a dynamic system whose state depends on many external and internal parameters. Therefore, the structure of pectic substances depends on numerous parameters and may substantially change during the growth and vegetation of the plant, whereas the dynamic character of pectin structures is ensured by the non-regular structural pattern of the sugar chain containing various macromolecular fragments in the linear and branched regions. The linear region consists of units of 1,4-α-D-galacturonan, which represent the backbone of all pectins. These units are bound to each other with one or two α-L-rhamnopyranose residues by 1,2-linkages. The ramified region is represented by different heteropolysaccharides (Fig.).

Institute of Physiology, Komi Science Centre, The Urals Branch of the Russian Academy of Sciences, 50, Pervomaiskaya str., Syktyvkar, 167982, Russia.
E-mail: popov@physiol.komisc.ru
[#] This chapter is dedicated to the memory of Professor Yury S. Ovodov (1937–2014).

Linear region   **Ramified region**

Homogalacturonan   *Rhamnogalacturonan*   *Rhamnogalacturonan-I*   *Xylogalacturonan*

$$\left.\!\!\!\!\!\left[\!\!\rightarrow\!4\text{-}\alpha\text{-D-Gal}p\text{A}(1\!\!\right]\!\!\!\!\!\!\rightarrow\!4)\text{-}\alpha\text{-D-Gal}p\text{A}(1\!\rightarrow\!2)\text{-}\alpha\text{-L-Rha}p(1\!\longrightarrow\!4)\text{-}\alpha\text{-D-Gal}p\text{A}(1\!\rightarrow\!4)\text{-}\alpha\text{-L-Rha}p(1\!\rightarrow\!4)\text{-}\alpha\text{-D-Gal}p\text{A}(1\!\rightarrow\right.$$

Side chains: β-D-Xyl*p*(1

α-L-Ara*f*(1→5)-α-L-Ara*f*(1→...

β-D-Gal*p*(1→3)-β-D-Gal*p*(1→4)-β-D-Gal*p*(1→...

→6)-β-D-Gal*p*(1→6)-β-D-Gal*p*(1→...

α-L-Ara*f*(1→5)-α-L-Ara*f*(1

Figure. Schematic representation of the main structural elements of pectin.

The fragments of linear and ramified regions are assumed to be covalently connected (Coenen et al. 2007, Caffall and Mohnen 2009). Pectins isolated from plant tissue have been shown to represent a heterogeneous mixture of pectic polysaccharides that appeared to be the structural constituents of the native macromolecule. Homogalacturonan (HG), rhamnogalacturonan-I (RG-I), xylogalacturonan, and apiogalacturonan are the primary pectic polysaccharides (Voragen et al. 2009, Round et al. 2010). Moreover, the pectin polysaccharides are different for various plants. Galacturonan differs in the degree of methyl esterification (DE) and molecular weight (Mw), rhamnogalacturonan differs in the fine structure of the branched chains that consist of galactose, arabinose and other sugars, and xylo- and apiogalacturonans differ in the degree of branching.

As a ubiquitous component of fruits and vegetables, pectin is a natural component of the human diet. The content of pectin has been determined in the most fruits and vegetables. Pectin content ranged from 0.1 to 4 g per 100 g fresh weight (Table 1).

The daily mean intake of pectin by an individual estimated in German cohorts (n = 4,021) equal to 6.3–7.4 g per day (Linseisen et al. 2003). The mean dietary intake of pectin in US population (n = 29,104) was measured to be in a range from 0.7 (children of age 2–11 mon) to 2.0 (adults of age 60–69 yr) g per day (Bialostosky et al. 2002). Urban residents of Siberia (Russia) have been found to consume from 1.2–1.6 (1,905 women) to 2.0–2.1 (2,190 men) g of pectin per day (Simonova et al. 2006). The joint Food and Agriculture Organization/World Health Organization committee consider pectin to be a safe additive with no limits on daily intake. The pectin backbone consisting of 1,4-linked α-D-galacturonic acid (GalA) residues is well known to be resistant in the human stomach and small intestine and to be fermented in the large bowel by colonic bacteria. So, pectin is considered as a constituent of dietary fiber (Lattimer and Haub 2010, Dhingra et al. 2012).

Overall, the relative ease of isolation and valuable physical properties of pectins make their practical application attractive (Table 2).

In the food industry, pectin is used in a range of processed food products as a gelling, stabilizing, or thickening agent in products such as jam, yogurt drinks, fruity milk drinks, confectionaries, desserts and ice cream. Some of the more important modern uses include pectins as fillers in low calorie food products and dietary fat replacements. Due to its biodegradability, biocompatibility and edibility, pectin is a suitable polymeric matrix for the elaboration of edible films that are intended to be active food packaging (Espitia et al. 2014).

Pectin has promising pharmaceutical uses due to its low toxicity and water solubility. Pectin hydrogels have been used in tablet formulations as a binding agent and have been used in controlled-release matrix tablet formulations (Sriamornsak 2003). The modern lead pectin-based drug delivery product appears to be a fentanyl nasal spray formulation, which has successfully met the primary objective in a pivotal Phase III clinical study as treatment for breakthrough pain that is induced by chemoradiotherapy in head and neck cancer (Watts and Smith 2009).

Table 1. Pectin content[#] of some fruits and vegetables.

Plant foods	Rani and Kawatra 1994*	Baker 1997**	Mahattanatawee et al. 2006**	Prasana et al. 2007**
Apple	3.85	0.14 ÷ 1.15	0.25 ÷ 0.63	0.5 ÷ 1.6
Apricot	-	0.42 ÷ 1.32	-	-
Avocado	-	-	-	0.73
Banana	-	0.44 ÷ 1.02	0.44 ÷ 1.02	0.7 ÷ 1.2
Cabbage	1.14	-	-	-
Carrot	1.46	0.63 ÷ 1.01	-	-
Cherries	-	0.01 ÷ 1.15	0.44 ÷ 1.02	0.24 ÷ 0.54
Guava	10.4	-	0.77	0.26 ÷ 1.2
Grape	-	0.12 ÷ 0.80	0.7 ÷ 0.8	-
Grapefruit	-	0.24 ÷ 0.65	0.65	-
Lemon	-	0.63	-	2.5 ÷ 4.0
Litchi	-	-	0.48	0.42
Mango	-	-	0.48	0.66 ÷ 1.5
Orange	-	0.25 ÷ 0.76	0.57	1.35
Papaya	-	-	0.6	-
Passion fruit	-	-	-	0.5
Pea	0.72	-	-	-
Peach	-	-	-	0.1 ÷ 0.9
Pineapple	-	-	-	0.04 ÷ 0.13
Plum	5.78	-	-	-
Strawberry	-	-	-	0.14 ÷ 0.44
Tomato	-	-	-	0.2 ÷ 0.6

[#] - g per 100 g dry (*) and fresh (**) weight basis.

Table 2. Uses of pectin.

Food Industry	*Agriculture*
- gelling agent;	- microbial culture media;
- thickening agent;	- animal foods;
- stabilizer;	- insecticides;
- decolorization agent;	- plant growth factors.
- fat replacement;	
- edible films.	
Biomedicine	*Technical Applications*
- drug carriers;	- soil conservation;
- biomaterials;	- cigarette manufacture;
- prophylactic substances.	- paper substitutes;
	- plasticizers.

Pectin, due to its simple and cytocompatible gelling mechanism, has been exploited for different biomaterial applications, including wound healing, tissue engineering, dentistry, and skin-care products (Endress 1991). Pectin hydrogels were found to have a large potential for bone tissue engineering applications because they promote the nucleation of a mineral phase if they are immersed in adequate physiological solutions, with the formation of biomimetic constructs that better mimic the natural architecture of the bone. A wide variety of hydrocolloid pectin-based wound dressings has been patented and is currently commercially available. These are mainly composed of adhesive, absorbent polymers, pectin gelling agents and sodium carboxy-methylcellulose. The hydrophilic pectin particles react within the dressing with the wound fluid to form a soft gel over the wound bed, thus removing or controlling exudates in the wounds. The acid environment that is obtained with pectin solubilization can further act as a bacterial or viral barrier. In addition, pectin hydrogels provide improved systems of loading and releasing drugs, i.e., antibiotics, pain relievers and/or tissue repair factors at the site of action (Munarin et al. 2012). Nanocomposite biomaterial that is based on pectin was recently proposed as implantable electrodes (Amarnath et al. 2014).

In various other ways, pectic substances have been involved in cigarette manufacturing, agricultural industries, soil conservation, textile production and other uses (Endress 1991).

Finally, pectin has been found to be useful in the prevention and therapy of a variety of diseases. Pectins have been shown to possess hypolipidemic, hypoglycemic, anti-cancer, anti-infective, anti-ulcer, immunostimulating, anti-inflammatory, antioxidant and other effects. The enormous literature on the physiological activity of pectin includes clinical and epidemiological observations as well as experimental studies with different animal models and cell test systems.

A long history of use in the food industry and physiological activity leads to the development of functional foods that contain pectin. Functional foods (specific nutrients and/or food components) should beneficially affect one or more target functions in the body. The development of functional foods based on pectin requires understanding the effects of pectin on the physiological processes. However, the existent reviews on pectin seldom provide satisfying information. First, conclusions on the health benefits of pectin have often been postulated from experimental animal studies. Second, the therapeutic function pectins has been mechanistically suspected to be due to its role as dietary fiber. Indeed, a large amount of experimental and epidemiological data has attributed many disorders and diseases to the lack of dietary fiber in the diet. These conditions include type-2 diabetes, overweight and obesity, cardiovascular disease, colon cancer and various gastrointestinal disorders (Anderson et al. 2009, Kendall et al. 2010, Papathanasopoulos and Camilleri 2010). However, dietary fiber is a term that reflects a heterogeneous group of non-digestible compounds that differ in their chemical structure and physicochemical properties. Dietary fiber studies appear to have not distinguished the specific physiological effects of pectin.

This chapter summarizes the data on the physiological effects of individual pectins in human studies only. The pectin investigations with animals or isolated cells *in vitro* as well as the studies that use pectin mixed with other substances or crude pectin-rich extracts are not presented here. A short overview of the history of studies on the chemistry and medicinal uses of pectin is initially provided followed by a review of the health beneficial effects of pectin consumption. Finally, the physiological processes that underlie the action of pectin are described.

Historical Overview

Pectins were first identified by the French scientists Braconnot and Payen in 1825 (Braconnot 1825a,b). The word "Pectin" originated from the Greek word "Pectos", which means "gelled". Initially, the study of the chemical nature of these substances and their role in plants progressed very slowly. Intensive study on pectin began after the organization of pectin manufacturing. The first pectin plant (Douglas Pectin Co., Fairport, New York) that extracted pectin from apple peelings was built in 1919. For the first four yr, pectin was sold to commercial processors; it was placed on the retail market in 1923.

Early studies on the structure of pectins are summarized in a magnificent review (Hirst 1942). In 1917, it was first found that pectin is very labile toward alkali and produces mainly D-GalA in acidic and enzymatic hydrolysis. Pectins were long considered to be structurally close to the related polysaccharides of low molecular weight. Only in 1936 was it clearly shown that pectin is a mixture of high molecular weight polysaccharides, which are constructed similar to cellulose, i.e., composed of long linear carbohydrate chains but of α-1,4-linked residues of D-GalA. In 1935, Henglein offered one of the first nomenclatures of the pectic polysaccharides, dividing them into two groups: pectic acid and pectin (Henglein 1958). The first group, in his view, consisted of polymer homologues of polygalacturonic acid (PGA) that were devoid of methoxyl groups. Pectin was a partially or fully methylesterified PGA. Highly (H-pectin) and low (L-pectin) esterified pectins possess a DE of more and less than 50 percentage, respectively. Under the pectins, he proposed to imply a mixture of pectins with concomitant polysaccharides. The first attempt to develop a formal nomenclature for pectin was made in 1944 by a special committee on the nomenclature of polysaccharides, when it was still believed that pectins are polygalacturonic acid partially esterified with methanol. Based on this approach, it was suggested to distinguish pectin and pectic acid. Pectic acid is a galacturonan that contains carboxyl groups esterified with methanol, whereas pectic acid is a galacturonan with free carboxyl groups.

For a long time, the study of pectin was restricted to galacturonan obtained from a variety of sources (Kertesz 1951) isolated using sufficiently severe methods of extraction. Therefore, the pectin substances were considered to be a mixture of galacturonan and the related neutral polysaccharides composed of D-galactose and L-arabinose residues. Harsh methods of pectin isolation, in particular using the extraction solutions of organic and inorganic acids, led to the production of so-called "commercial pectin", the main sources of which were wastes from processing apples, sugar beets, citrus and other produce (Henglein 1958).

Already in the late 1940s, it was found that the composition of the galacturonic backbone of pectins includes residues of L-rhamnose. Rhamnose (Rha) has been suggested to play an essential role in the establishment of the architectonics of the macromolecule of pectin. Many studies on partial acid and enzymatic hydrolysis of pectin led to the isolation of aldobiuronic acid, α-D-GalpA1→2L-Rha, and the three saccharide α-D-GalpA1→2-α-L-Rhap1→2-L-Rha. These studies led to the conclusion that L-rhamnopyranose residues incorporate into a galacturonan chain with α-1,2-bonds and separated blocks of linear galacturonan. Thus, all of the pectin polysaccharides belong to the class rhamnogalacturonans. Only in the late 1950s to early 1960s, when the isolation of pectin used milder methods, was it suggested that the pectin polysaccharides contain not only the backbone of linear galacturonan but also numerous side chains, which form branched regions of the macromolecule (Aspinall 1980).

The last 50 years were dedicated mainly to the definition of the structural characteristics of pectins of various plants. The overall structure of the pectin macromolecule was proposed. The reader is referred to some excellent recent reviews on the chemical structure and functional features of pectins (Coenen et al. 2007, Caffall and Mohnen 2009, Voragen et al. 2009, Round et al. 2010).

Therapeutic uses of pectic substances have a long history as well. Braconnot, who discovered and named pectic acid in 1825, observed its reactions with heavy metals and suggested its use as an antidote for heavy metal poisoning. The detoxification potential of pectin appeared to be based on the knowledge that glucuronic acid of mucin, chondroitin, heparin and other compounds plays a very prominent role in detoxification of the body. The uronic acid of pectin was suggested to act similarly to glucuronic acid of endogenous polysaccharides (Manville et al. 1936).

Pectin therapy for diarrheal disorders had been a natural outgrowth of the well-known apple therapy. In traditional medicine in Europe, the treatment of diarrhea used the "apple diet", which consisted of eating only apples for a few days (Rowley 1934). A number of studies reported merit of the raw apple diet in diarrhea of infancy and childhood. Malyoth in 1934 referred to a series of approximately twenty-five papers published in various journals dating back to 1928, all pertaining to the use of apples for the treatment of gastro-intestinal disturbances. He suggested that the efficacy of raw apple was due to its pectin content. In 1936, he made a comparative study of the effect of pure pectin derived from apple and raw apple, recommending the former only when the latter fails. Hunt (1936) concurred with this opinion, employing a raw apple diet and pectin-agar mixture. In the same year, Winters and Tompkins (1936) in controlled experiments observed that pectin-agar in a mixture of dextrimaltose is far more effective than scraped raw apple in the treatment of infant diarrhea. The experiment showed a reduction in the number of liquid stools, the disappearance of blood in the stools, a general gain in weight, effectiveness in maintaining water balance, an improvement in the general condition of the patient, and facilitation of the transition from the special to a general diet. They also noted that Flexner and Sonne dysenteries responded more slowly and were more apt to recur than did other types of diarrheas. Manville et al. (1937) also concluded following an intensive study of the properties of pectin that it is the most likely component of apple to provide the anti-diarrheal capacity. Pectin was widely used as an effective anti-diarrheal agent before the discovery and introduction of antibiotics in medical practice.

The use of pectin in connection with gastric ulcers appeared to be a logical extension of its use with diarrhea and dysentery (Olsen 1940). The study of pectin as a prophylactic and curative agent for peptic ulcers was also initiated because pectin has a chemical similarity to mucin in that both contain uronic acid and are similar in their physical properties. It was theorized that pectin might have an effect that corresponds to that of mucin (Winters et al. 1939). A soothing and healing effect of pectin was shown on the inflamed and ulcerated gastro-intestinal tract (Manville et al. 1937). The main theory of pectin therapy claimed that "pectin removes the exotoxic products of bacterial growth, thereby relieving the system from the absorption of these products and allowing the bloodstream defenses to concentrate on the bacterial invasion" (Olsen 1940). Principal emphasis had also been placed on the bactericidal action of pectin (Manville and Sullivan 1940).

The observation that pectin solution had a bactericidal effect appeared to stimulate the use of pectin therapy for surgical dressing, especially in cases of infected wounds and burns. Haynes and co-authors (Haynes et al. 1937) reported results of successful treatment of wounds by pectin, including osteomyelitis and other deep wounds that had not responded well to the accepted methods of treatment.

The origin of the use of pectin to accelerate blood clotting is rather obscure. Apparently, first, Hirsch (Hirsch 1924) noted the similar role of H ion changes in both the clotting of blood and the gelling of pectin. Pectins were intensively studied and used as a component in hemostatic formulations during the 1940s and 1950s (Hartman et al. 1941, McClure et al. 1944). However, the further introduction of pectin in medicine as a basis for blood substitutes did not occur due to the instability of the chemical composition and the difficulty of the standardization of pectin preparations.

On reviewing the historical background, it can be stated that almost all of the current ideas about pectin originated from the first decades of pectin investigation. Two types of ideas appeared to initiate investigations of pectin for medicinal usage. First, pectin was examined as a constituent of known physiologically active plant material. Second, pectin was studied as an analog of other structure-related molecules. Interestingly, the originally formed duality appeared to continue throughout the modern history of pectin. One group of studies considers pectin to be a physiologically active component of plant food. Studies of the other group are devoted to the elucidation of the physiological activity of isolated pectins, especially commercial ones.

Effects of the Oral Intake of Pectin in Humans

Pectin Lowers Cholesterol

Cholesterol lowering appeared to be the most prominent and investigated effect of pectin. The suggestion that dietary pectin might influence the intestinal absorption or excretion of cholesterol arose from two early ideas. The first idea was that pectin could form a colloidal mass in which cholesterol and fat could be adsorbed or dispersed. The second idea was that pectin lowering the pH of the intestinal contents might affect the growth of certain bacteria that are known to participate in the conversion of cholesterol to other sterols (Lin et al. 1957). In 1961, Keys et al. published the first human study that suggested that pectin supplementation lowered serum total cholesterol concentrations. A significant reduction in the blood cholesterol by pectin intake was then reported in studies that used a wide variety of subjects and experimental conditions. The most important studies with healthy and hypercholesterolemic individuals are summarized in Table 3.

The results of most of these studies were positive. Generally, it could be demonstrated that six to 15 g of pectin per day taken for three to six wk can reduce the cholesterol level significantly, by 10 to approximately 18 percentages. When all of the available studies were summarized, it was reported from a meta-analysis that pectin decreased the total and low-density lipoprotein (LDL) cholesterol (LDL-C) concentrations by, respectively, –0.070 mmol/L and –0.055 mmol/L (Brown et al. 1999). The diets were either controlled or self-selected, without influencing the result. Better results were obtained if pectin was completely hydrated in a food product compared to powdered pectin mixed with food. The cholesterol-lowering effect was proportional to the amount of dietary cholesterol in the blood. Pectin did not significantly alter the serum high-density lipoprotein (HDL) cholesterol and triacylglycerol levels.

Table 3. Pectin and serum total cholesterol.

Reference	Subjects	Time	Pectin, g per d	Effect, %
Keys et al. 1961	24 healthy	3 wk	15	−5
Palmer and Dixon 1966	16 healthy	4 wk	2 ÷ 10	−6
Durrington et al. 1976	12 healthy	3 wk	12	−8
Kay and Truswell 1977	9 healthy	3 wk	15	−13
Miettinen and Tarpila 1977	2 healthy	2 wk	40 ÷ 50	0
	6 hyper-cholesterolaemic	2 wk	40 ÷ 50	−13
Jenkins et al. 1979	22 healthy	3 wk	31	−13
Stasse-Wolthuis et al. 1979	62 healthy	5 wk	9	−7
Stasse-Wolthuis et al. 1980	62 healthy	5 wk	15	−10
Judd and Truswell 1982	10 healthy	3 wk	15	−16 ÷ −18
Challen et al. 1983	6 healthy	3 wk	36	−10
Vargo et al. 1985	10 healthy	2 wk	15	−7
Hillman et al. 1985	10 healthy	8 wk	12	0
Cerda 1988	27 healthy	4 wk	15	−8
Remer et al. 1996	6 healthy	4 d	15 ÷ 30	0
Veldman et al. 1997	10 hyper-cholesterolaemic	4 wk	15	−9
Sheehan et al. 1997	15 non-insulin diabetics	4 wk	15	−7
Wu et al. 2003	9 healthy	3 wk	15	−13
Schwab et al. 2006	22 abnormal glucose metabolism	12 wk	16	0
Brouns et al. 2012	10 mild-cholesterolaemic	4 wk	15	−7 ÷ −10
Sirtori et al. 2012	25 hyper-cholesterolaemic	4 wk	10	−5 ÷ −6

It should be noted that pectin was not well-characterized in most of the mentioned studies. As a result, recent Scientific Opinion on the substantiation of health claims related to pectin, including cholesterol lowering, does not consider pectin characterization to be a likely factor that contributes to the observed physiological effect (Brouns et al. 2012). However, in a study (Brouns et al. 2012), it was clearly demonstrated that pectin characteristics such as DE and Mw affect cholesterol lowering. Cross-over studies were completed in mildly hyper-cholesterolemic persons who received 15 g per day of well-characterized pectins of different sources and types. High DE and high Mw were found to be important for the cholesterol lowering effect. The relative LDL-C lowering was as follows: citrus pectin DE-70 = apple pectin DE-70 (7–10 percentage reduction versus control) > apple pectin DE-35 = citrus pectin DE-35 > low-MW pectin DE-70 > citrus pectin DE-0. The sources could also be important; for example, citrus and apple DE-70 pectins were more effective than orange pulp fiber DE-70.

The major biological mechanisms that were proposed to explain the cholesterol-reducing effects of pectin include the prevention of bile acid and/or cholesterol re-absorption and the inhibition of hepatic cholesterol synthesis by fermentation products (Gunnes and Gidley 2010). Pectin could also lower the cholesterol levels through its effects on postprandial glycemia. Reducing the rate of intestinal absorption of glucose is expected to decrease the insulin production by the pancreas. Because insulin is an activator of 3-hydroxy 3-methylglutaryl co-enzyme A reductase (HMG-Co AR), it is possible that reduced insulin levels could lead to a decrease in the cholesterol synthesis. However, that insulin changes result in lowered cholesterol concentrations has never been demonstrated in humans.

Pectin Enhances Glucose Tolerance

Early studies on the fate of ingested pectin demonstrated clearly that pectin was decomposed in the colon but not in the small intestine (Werch and Ivy 1941). This feature of the "digestibility" of pectin allowed pectin to belong to the group of unabsorbable carbohydrates and stimulated interest in its study as an anti-diabetic agent. Studies with healthy volunteers and diabetics have shown that pectic substances lower the postprandial blood glucose level (Table 4).

Table 4. Pectin and postprandial glycaemia and insulinaemia.

Reference	Subjects	Test meal	Pectin, g	Glucose level, %	Insulin level, %
Jenkins et al. 1977	8 healthy	marmalade	10	−9	Sign. lower
Jenkins et al. 1978	6 healthy	carbohydrate solution	14.5	−15	0
Holt et al. 1979	7 healthy	glucose solution	14.5	−24	not determined
Wahlqvist et al. 1979	7 healthy	jelly	10	0	0
Jenkins et al. 1980	11 gastric surgery patients	glucose solution	14.5	−41	−61
Vaaler et al. 1980	8 insulin-dependent diabetics	complex breakfast	15	−56	not determined
Williams et al. 1980	7 non insulin-dependent diabetics	complex breakfast	10	−22	0
Leeds et al. 1981	12 dumping syndrom	glucose solution	10.5	−38	−50
Speth et al. 1983	9 gastric surgery patients	complex breakfast	4.2	0	0
Siddhu et al. 1989	5 healthy	glucose, casein, corn oil	20	−45 ÷ −73	−25
Siddhu et al. 1990	6 healthy	glucose, casein, corn oil	20	−42 ÷ −43	−20
Siddhu et al. 1991	6 healthy	glucose, casein, corn oil	20	−20 ÷ −25	−48
Ranganathan et al. 1994	6 healthy	glucose solution	30	0	−63
Brenelli et al. 1997	10 healthy	glucose solution	40	−8	−40
Sanaka et al. 2007	10 healthy	protein-carbohydrate solution	5.2	0	not determined
Shimoyama et al. 2007	11 healthy	enteral nutrition solution	1.4	+12	+30

Supplementation of more than 10 g pectin to the test meal was found to decrease the glucose response by 8–73 percentages. However, there are not any additional recent studies that confirm this effect. Data on the effect on blood glucose of sustained pectin ingestion are also contradictory. A diet supplemented with 20 g pectin per day for four wk was found to decrease the incremental area under the glucose tolerance curve in 12 non-insulin-dependent diabetic patients (Schwartz et al. 1988). A significant inverse association was found between the incremental area under the curve and the intake of pectin in the Zutphen Study, where the oral glucose tolerance test was conducted in 394 non-diabetic men (Feskens and Kromhout 1990). However, Gardner et al. (1984) did not find an effect of five g of pectin received for 3 mon on the glycemic stability of 17 diabetic subjects. Pectin failed to have an effect on the postprandial plasma glucose concentrations when administered at 16 g per day to subjects with an abnormal glucose metabolism for 12 wk (Schwab et al. 2006). Pectin (10 g) given with meals for 18 d did not have an effect on either the serum glucose or insulin (Gold et al. 1980). In a study (Wanders et al. 2014b), fasting glucose concentrations were even higher after repeated exposure to 10 g daily pectin for 15 d. These results can be accounted for by sugar impurities in the commercial pectins, which are often added to the product to improve and stabilize the gelling capacities.

The exact mechanism by which pectin attenuates the glycemic and insulinemic responses is not known. Pectin could affect the glucose level by various mechanisms that include delayed gastric emptying, increased satiety, modified neural and hormonal signals in the gut, slowed down or diminished the absorption of glucose, or an altered fermentation pattern in the large intestine.

Pectin Increases Satiety

Satiety is defined as the condition of being satisfied after consuming a meal, which prevents the onset of a subsequent meal. Interest in the modulation of satiety by pectin appears to have originated from thinking about the mechanism of pectin's effect on cholesterol and glucose levels. Additionally, epidemiological studies have suggested that there is an inverse relationship between dietary fiber intake and body weight, which exists through the overall mechanism of improving satiety (Slavin 2005, Anderson et al. 2009, Wanders et al. 2011).

Di Lorenzo et al. (1988) compared a treatment of 15 g of pectin vs. 15 g of methylcellulose on the gastric emptying time and satiety in nine obese participants. Pectin was found to increase the subject's sensation of satiety. Pectin was shown to increase satiety and decreased subsequent energy intake in doses as low as five g in healthy US Army adults. This effect lasted up to four hr after ingesting pectin mixed with orange juice (Tiwary et al. 1997). However, adding five g of apple pectin to apple juice failed to enhance satiety in another study (Flood-Obbagy and Rolls 2009). These contrasting results could be interpreted by the fact that measures of satiety can be influenced by the time interval between the beverage consumption and the next test meal. In the study of Perrigue et al. (2010), the participants consumed beverages that contained eight g of pectin, either 90 min before or 15 min before lunch. Beverages with added pectin reduced the energy intakes at lunch relative to beverages without pectin. A short delay (15 min) between beverage consumption and a subsequent meal was associated with higher satiety ratings.

Pectin has been found to increase satiety after both single and repeated exposure (Wanders et al. 2014b). The participants consumed test foods that contained 10 g of gel-forming pectin once daily for 15 consecutive days. Satiety ratings that were measured on days one and 15 were higher as a result of the pectin intake.

The different types of pectin have been found to possess different effects on human satiety. Orange juice solutions were formulated to be either low or high viscosity using low- (LM), high- (HM) and LM amidated (LMA) pectins (Logan et al. 2014). The LM low and high viscosity pectin beverages were associated with the greatest effects on the subjective ratings of satiety. The HM pectin treatments had an effect on only some of the satiety parameters, despite being present at a higher concentration and at the same initial viscosity as the LM pectin. The LMA pectin treatments had no significant effect compared to the control beverage.

Another study reported different physicochemical properties of the same pectin, including different methods of supplementation, impacted appetite and energy intake (Wanders et al. 2014a). Subjects consumed dairy-based liquid test products that contained (10 g) no pectin, bulking pectin, viscous pectin, or gelled pectin. The gelled pectin was also supplemented as capsules and as liquid. Physicochemical properties such as the viscosity and water holding capacity of the test products were measured as being very different. The preload viscosity was larger for gelled > viscous > bulking > no pectin and was larger for gelled > liquid > capsules. Appetite was reduced after the ingestion of gelled pectin compared to bulking, viscous and no pectin. Regarding the methods of supplementation, appetite was reduced after ingestion of the gelled test product compared to after capsules and liquid.

Viscous or gel-forming pectins are suggested to affect satiety by various mechanisms, which could include increased oral exposure (i.e., the presence of food in the oral cavity), delayed gastric emptying as well as modified neural and hormonal signals in the gut.

Pectin Promotes Gastrointestinal Health

The potential value of pectin as an antidiarrheal agent was touted by both Europeans and Americans in the early 20th century. An antidiarrheal effect of pectin was considered to result from its bactericidal action. The development of a pectin preparation for the treatment of infectious diarrhea was strongly inhibited by the discovery of antibiotics. However, later, pectin was recommended in combination with kaolin (kaopectate) in a liquid suspension that was given in a dose of one to two ounces after every bowel movement. The kaolin-pectin was said to act by adsorbing "irritans" and was included in the Compendium of Pharmaceuticals and Specialties (Kinnear 1964, Cimolai and Carter 1991). According to Kasi et al. (1995), 46 percent of the doctors in Pakistan prescribed commercially prepared mixtures of kaolin and pectin or neomycin and pectin for diarrhea treatment. However, more recently, most clinicians have discouraged the use of kaopectate in the treatment of diarrhea primarily because of a lack of supportive evidence. Moreover, the safety information about kaolin and pectin is limited, especially in relation to possible electrolyte disturbances or the decreased bioavailability of other drugs. At least 13 developing countries have, thus, banned, deregistered, or restricted the use of products that contain kaolin and pectin as a result of the WHO report of 1992 (Lexchin 1994).

Nevertheless, several modern studies provide evidence for the benefit of pectin treatment in diarrhea and other gastrointestinal disorders. Pectin was found to reduce the rate of diarrhea in critically ill tube-fed patients who were receiving antibiotics (Schultz et al. 2000). Diarrhea is known to be one of the most common complications in patients who receive tube-feeding formulas. Supplementing the isotonic tube-feeding formula has earlier been shown to reduce the incidence of liquid stools and promote a normalization of colonic fluid composition (Zimmaro et al. 1989). A multicenter, randomized, double-blind, placebo-controlled parallel study that enrolled 255 patients demonstrated clearly the beneficial influence of a pectin-chamomile preparation for the treatment of diarrhea in children (Becker et al. 2006). However, the study did not demonstrate the effectiveness of pectin alone because the effectiveness of only the combination and not the single ingredients was compared to a placebo.

In a double-blind trial (Rabbani et al. 2001), boys five–12 mon of age were given a rice-based diet that contained pectin at a dose of four g/kg body weight or the rice-diet alone. By day three posttreatment, significantly more children who were receiving pectin recovered from diarrhea than controls (55 and 15 percentage, respectively). By day four, these proportions correspondingly increased to 78 and 23 percentage, respectively. Pectin significantly reduced the amounts of stool, oral rehydration solution, intravenous fluid, and number of vomiting episodes, as well as the diarrheal duration.

Rapid gastric emptying has been described in some duodenal ulcer subjects. Pectin was proposed to possess an anti-ulcer effect because pectin was known to slow down gastric emptying. However, pectin that was administered at a dose of 10 g for six mon did not reduce the incidence of duodenal ulcer relapse in a controlled study with 109 patients (Kang et al. 1988).

Pectin solution is reported to increase the viscosity of a liquid nutrient even when it is infused separately into the stomach when the liquid nutrient is being supplied. The combined usage of a pectin solution with a liquid nutrient has been reported to prevent gastro-esophageal reflux of liquid nutrient and diarrhea that are induced by the rapid infusion of nutrients in patients who were undergoing percutaneous endoscopic gastrostomy feeding. The efficacy of pectin solution for the prevention of gastro-esophageal reflux has also been shown in comparison with the usage of a half-solid nutrient with high viscosity, although there was no significant difference in the total number of reflux events between the two nutrient delivery methods. In contrast to the delivery of half-solid nutrients with a high viscosity, pectin solution can be easily infused into the stomach via a percutaneous endoscopic gastrostomy tube, and it can increase the viscosity of the intragastric liquid nutrient (Adachi et al. 2012). Increasing the viscosity of an enteral solution with pectin has been observed to decrease gastro-esophageal reflux and improve vomiting and respiratory symptoms in children with cerebral palsy (Miyazawa et al. 2008). The effectiveness of a pectin-based formula has been found to be significantly inferior to that of a pharmaceutical product (esomeprazole) as an agent for the treatment of gastro-esophageal reflux disease (Farup et al. 2009).

Anti-tumor and Anti-inflammation Effects of Pectin

There is extensive experimental data with animal models regarding the anti-tumor, anti-inflammatory and immunomodulatory properties of pectins. However, human studies on the role of pectin in cancerogenesis, inflammation and immunity are rare.

The idea of the anti-tumor effect of pectin is based on the observation that dietary fiber decreases the risk of cancer (Kendall et al. 2010). The possible role of dietary fiber in the development of colon cancer in humans became of particular interest following epidemiologic descriptions of its occurrence in different populations. For example, the frequency of cancer in 7th Day Adventists is two times lower than in Californians. Members of this religion are vegetarians and consume two to three times more pectin (Kurup et al. 1984, Ross et al. 1990). The American Cancer Society suggests that adults eat five servings of fruits and vegetables each day to prevent cancer risk, which indicates a potential and essential fruit pectin role in cancer prevention (Kushi et al. 2006). Binding bile acids, the production of short chain fatty acids (SFCA) and the inhibition of inflammation have been suggested to represent the mechanism for the anti-cancer potential of pectin. The relative importance of pectin as a component of dietary fiber in the development of human cancer, however, remains to be determined.

A large body of literature suggests the anti-tumor potential of modified citrus pectin (MCP). MCP is commonly produced from commercial citrus pectin using temperature and pH modification, which yields a pectin that contains preferentially the branched regions of galactan chains and reduced arabinogalactan chains. An anti-tumor effect of MCP was examined in different cell lines and in different animal models but was demonstrated in only two human studies. Guess et al. (2003) investigated the tolerability and effect of MCP on the prostate specific antigen (PSA) doubling time in prostate cancer patients. MCP was administered orally at a dosage of 14.4 g per day in three divided doses. It was found that the PSA doubling time increased in seven of 10 men (70 percentages) after taking MCP for 12 mon. MCP was well tolerated by all 10 of the evaluable patients. In a prospective pilot trial by Azemar et al. (2007), the tolerability, clinical benefit and antitumoral efficacy of MCP were assessed in 49 patients with various solid tumors that were in an advanced state progression. The treatment consisted of the oral intake of five g MCP per day for eight wk. All of the patients tolerated the therapy well without any severe therapy-related adverse events. Twenty per cent of the patients had an overall clinical benefit response that was associated with stabilization or improvement in life quality. One patient who suffered from metastasized prostate carcinoma showed a 50 percentage decrease in serum PSA level after 16 wk of treatment, which was associated with a significant increase in clinical benefit and quality of life and a decrease in pain. The mechanism of anti-tumor effect of MCP was announced to involve interaction of galactose residues of MCP with galectin-3 receptors on the cancer cells. However this mechanism has not been demonstrated in humans yet.

The assumption that pectin possesses an anti-inflammatory effect results also from the anti-inflammatory effect of dietary fiber (Kaczmarczyk et al. 2012). Indeed, the concentration of C-reactive protein has been measured to be equal to 1.5 and 2.4 mg/L in individuals who consume daily 20 and eight g of dietary fiber, respectively (Ridker et al. 2000). In addition, pectins have been found to exert anti-inflammatory action in various experimental animal models. Human studies of pectin's effects on inflammation are scarce relative to the animal literature. Relieving systemic inflammation has been found to be associated with the anti-diarrheal action of pectin in patients with irritable bowel syndrome (Xu et al. 2015). At baseline, patients with irritable bowel syndrome demonstrated an abnormal interleukin (IL)-10/IL-12 ratio, which was normalized by pectin feeding. However, citrus pectin did not affect the inflammatory markers of high-sensitivity C-reactive protein or plasma homocysteine (Brouns et al. 2012). Pectin was found to decrease the migration activity of leukocytes stimulated with physical exercise stress (Paderin and Nikitina 2012). However, the rise in plasma tumor necrosis factor-α (TNF-α) concentration induced by exercise was higher after the consumption of 3.6 g pectin. The pectic polysaccharide *Angelica sinensis* has been shown to decrease serum IL-1β, IL-6 and TNF-α levels in middle-aged women. The pectin-treatment group received oral pectin at a dose of 150 mg/kg body weight three times a day before a meal for three mon (Juan et al. 2009). The pectic polysaccharide in soy sauce has been found to improve the quality of life in patients with seasonal allergic rhinitis (Kobayashi et al. 2005).

There are no human studies that clarify the mechanisms of the anti-cancer and anti-inflammatory effects of pectin.

Physiological Processes that are Affected by Pectin

Entero-Hepatic Circulation

Evidence suggests that pectin could interfere with lipid and/or bile acid metabolism, influencing the 'Entero-hepatic Pathway', which consists of liver, small intestine and colon. Pectin has been suggested to reduce the (re)absorption of bile acids/cholesterol by binding them during the formation of micelles in the intestinal lumen. Alternatively, it has been suggested that pectin could form a thick unstirred water layer in the intestinal lumen that acts as a physical barrier, thereby also decreasing the (re)absorption of fats, including cholesterol and bile acids. This circumstance would lead to an increased fecal output of these two components followed by a decrease in its back-resorption into the liver. As a result, the hepatic conversion of cholesterol into bile acids increases, and the hepatic pools of free cholesterol decrease. This arrangement leads to increased endogenous cholesterol synthesis and the upregulation of hepatic LDL-C receptors, thereby reducing circulating blood cholesterol. Knowing that the human body produces more cholesterol than the intake from daily food, it is obvious that breaking down the entero-hepatic circle is a very effective way of reducing serum cholesterol. Several human studies have explored this mechanism. Citrus pectin (15 g per day) added for three wk to metabolically controlled diets reduced the plasma cholesterol concentrations by a mean of 13 percentage and increased the fecal fat excretion by 44 percentage, neutral steroids by 17 percentage and fecal bile acids by 33 percentage (Kay and Truswell 1977). A significant decrease in the serum cholesterol by pectin administered to normolipidemic and hyperlipidemic patients was associated with an increased excretion of fecal bile acids and total steroids (Miettinen and Tarpila 1977). Acid steroid concentration and excretion and the mean β-glucuronidase activity were increased by six and 35 percentage, respectively, when the subjects were fed 15 g of citrus pectin (Ross and Leklem 1981). An addition of 15 g of citrus pectin to the diet of ileostomy patients increased bile acid excretion by 35 percentage and net cholesterol excretion by 14 percentage (Bosaeus et al. 1986). After pectin supplementation (12 g per day) for four wk, the mean percentage of deoxycholate acid increased significantly by 39 percentage (Hillman et al. 1986).

Gastric Emptying

Delayed gastric emptying has been shown to result from an increase in the meal viscosity. In a number of studies, it has been shown that high amounts of viscous pectin delayed gastric emptying in both normal subjects and patients (Table 5).

Depending on the type of test meal times, gastric emptying varies from 60 to 160 min. Pectin increases these times by 14–64 min. However, a delay in gastric emptying was not observed in all of the studies. The glucose meal emptied from the stomach was reduced by pectin supplementation in patients with dumping syndrome, but pectin had no effect on the gastric emptying of the healthy volunteers (Lawaetz et al. 1983).

Table 5. Pectin and gastric emptying.

Reference	Subjects	Method	Pectin, g	Effect
Holt et al. 1979	7 healthy	scintigraphy	14.5	delay twofold
Schwartz et al. 1982	7 healthy	scintigraphy	20 g/d 4 wk	delay twofold
Nguyen et al. 1982	6 healthy	scintigraphy	15	no effect
Flourie et al. 1985	12 healthy	scintigraphy	15 5	delay 26% no effect
Kasper et al. 1985	healthy	scintigraphy	4	no effect
Shafer et al. 1985	10 healthy	scintigraphy	10	no effect
Sandhu et al. 1987	6 healthy	scintigraphy	15	delay
Di Lorenzo et al. 1988	9 obese	scintigraphy	15	delay 63%
Schwartz et al. 1988	12 diabetics	scintigraphy	20 g/d 4 wk	delay 43%
Iftikhar et al. 1994	10 healthy	scintigraphy		no effect
Sanaka et al. 2007	10 healthy	breath test	5.2	delay 8%
Shimoyama et al. 2007	11 healthy	breath test	1.4	increasing
Sakamoto et al. 2011	6 healthy	breath test	16	delay 39%
Atia et al. 2011	6 jeiunocolonic anastomosis	scintigraphy	4	no effect
Wanders et al. 2014a	29 healthy	breath test	10	delay

In one study (Iftikhar et al. 1994), the times for the stomach to empty half of a radiolabeled meal were similar after both the pectin and a placebo. However, pectin delayed the emptying of the last 20 percentage of the meal. The individual sensitivity of volunteers to pectin supplementation has been demonstrated (Shafer et al. 1985). In another study (Shimoyama et al. 2007), the gastric emptying coefficient was even increased by adding pectin to the enteral nutrition. Pectin failed to have an effect on gastric emptying when administered at doses of four–five g (Flourie et al. 1985). The consumption of at least 14 g per day of pectin is necessary to have a significant effect on the gastric emptying delay. Amounts of less than 10 g per day of pectin are suggested to not be effective, with one exception, which is when pectin delayed gastric emptying at a dose of 5.2 g (Sanaka et al. 2007). The time at which half the ultimate pulmonary recovery of $[^{13}CO_2]$ is exhaled was 2.60 and 2.84 h for the control and the pectin meal, respectively. The effects of pectin on gastric emptying appeared to differ as a function of the pectin properties. The effects of gelled pectin that delayed gastric emptying were significant compared to viscous pectin, bulking pectin and a nonpectin control. Additionally, the same gelled pectin delayed gastric emptying more when it was consumed as a gel, compared to when it was consumed in the form of capsules or in a liquid form (Wanders et al. 2014).

The ability of pectin to form a gel or thicken a solution followed by a delay in gastric emptying is thought to be the likely mechanism behind pectin's effects on satiety and glucose intake.

Absorption of Nutrients and Intestinal Permeability

There is ample evidence that the physical state of the food matrix plays a key role in the accessibility and biochemical stability of many food components. Viscous pectin solution has been, thus, assumed to influence the bioavailability of the molecules in the intestinal content. Moreover, pectin has been suspected of impairing nutrients and drug absorption because charged polysaccharides such as pectin, through their carboxyl groups, have been well known to bind to various organic and inorganic molecules *in vitro*.

The effect of citrus pectin (15 g) on the absorption of nutrients in the small intestine was shown in ileostomy patients (Sandberg et al. 1983). During the pectin period, there was a significant increase in the amount of nitrogen, fat, ash, Na and K found in the ileostomy content. The apparent absorption of Fe decreased significantly, while that of P, Ca, Mg and Zn remained unchanged. There are some results on the capacity of pectin to reduce the absorption of vitamins (Keltz et al. 1978, Spiricheva et al. 2011). The increase in plasma β-carotene concentration after the intake of a controlled meal with β-carotene was significantly reduced by 12 g citrus pectin in female subjects (Rock and Swendseid 1992). Citrus pectin has been shown to reduce the bioavailability of β-carotene, lycopene and lutein (Riedl et al. 1999). Apple pectin has been shown to significantly lower the duration of niacin-induced flushing, and it produced nonsignificant but positive improvement in all of the other major flushing parameters compared with a placebo (Moriarty et al. 2013). Niacin, or vitamin B3, when used at high doses, can safely and significantly modify all of the major lipid parameters. However, the use of niacin to reduce cardiovascular events is greatly limited due to adverse events, in particular cutaneous flushing that primarily involves the face, torso, and upper extremities. Apple pectin appears to limit the flushing parameters differently when compared with aspirin therapy. The mechanism by which pectin mitigates niacin-induced flushing is the result of apple pectin slowing the absorption of niacin and further extending its release.

In addition to gastric emptying, pectin in the intestine might inhibit the processes that are associated with digestion and the absorption of available carbohydrates and, thereby, decrease the rate of glucose absorption into the hepatic portal vein. This effect appears to constitute physical dietary carbohydrates becoming caught up in the highly viscous network of pectin gel, making them less accessible to digestive enzymes and slowing down their diffusion toward the small intestine. High methoxy apple pectin has been found to impair intestinal glucose absorption by means of an increased unstirred layer resistance (Flourie et al. 1984).

In this study, the effect of intraluminal pectin solution at concentrations of 6–15 g/L was evaluated in healthy volunteers by the intestinal perfusion technique under an occlusive balloon. In totally pancreatectomized patients, the supplementation of pectin reduced the effect of the pancreatic enzyme preparation. In the same patients, pectin reduced the amylase activity of jejunal aspirates after a test meal (Isaksson et al. 1984).

The modulation of intestinal permeability could mediate the anti-diarrheal effect of pectin. Rabbani et al. (2004) found that the antidiarrheal effects of pectin are associated with an improvement in the small intestine's permeability. The lactulose–mannitol test was used to assess whether the antidiarrheal effects of pectin are associated with a change in the intestinal permeability and integrity. This test is based on the differential permeability of two nonmetabolizing sugar molecules that have low (mannitol; Mw, 180) and high (lactulose; Mw, 340) Mw; their renal excretions are determined in urine after an oral dose. Because persistent diarrhea is associated with villous atrophy and a reduction in both the mucosal surface area and number of cells, paracellular transport of large molecules through tight junctions is increased, and that of small molecules is decreased. Thus, a dual sugar test gives an indirect but reliable indication of the mucosal integrity in this disease. Treatment with pectin significantly reduced lactulose recovery, increased mannitol recovery, and decreased the lactulose–mannitol ratio, which indicates an improvement in the permeability. Permeability changes were associated with a 50 percentage reduction in the stool weights, which correlated strongly with the lactulose–mannitol ratio.

Indirect Mechanisms

Pectin has been suggested to exert a considerable effect on the microbiota composition and fecal SCFA production, the concentration of which in the colon is important for maintaining gut and overall health.

In a randomized controlled trial (Xu et al. 2014), the efficacy of the supplementation of 24 g per day pectin for four wk was evaluated in 80 adults who had slow-transit constipation. The colonic transit time and constipation score decreased after pectin treatment. In a related study (Xu et al. 2015), the efficacy of pectin was found in the treatment of diarrhea predominant irritable bowel syndrome. The stool frequency and disease-specific scores were reduced after treatment with 24 g pectin for six wk. Pectin was found to stimulate *Bifidobacterium* sp. and decrease *Clostridium* sp. fecal bacterial populations in both groups of patients. Similar results were earlier obtained in healthy males (Drasar and Jenkins 1976). Pectin has been found to decrease the clinical symptoms and improve the microbiocenosis structure in patients with a syndrome of irritated intestines (Fluer et al. 2006).

Human fecal and breath gas measurements indicate that pectin consumption increases the SCFA concentration in feces and blood (Spiller et al. 1980, Fleming and Rodriguez 1983, Pomare et al. 1985). It has been proposed that SCFA, especially propionate, depletes plasma cholesterol by inhibiting the hepatic cholesterol metabolism via a reduction in the activity of HMG-CoAR a rate-limiting enzyme in cholesterol biosynthesis. However, this hypothesis mainly originates from animal studies, while properly controlled intervention studies in humans are scarce. Moreover, data on the effects of SCFA production in the colon on serum lipids in humans are still conflicting.

The mechanism by which pectin brings about an antidiarrheal effect has also been suggested to be mediated by the production of colonic SCFA (butyrate, acetate, propionate), which is assumed to possess colonotrophic effects. Specifically, butyrate is an energy source for colonocytes, and it regulates colonocyte proliferation. Furthermore, butyrate upregulates one of the sodium-hydrogen exchangers (NH3), thus enhancing the water and sodium absorption (Kocoshis 2010). Other mechanism for the trophic action of pectin could result from the stimulation of gastrointestinal smooth muscle cells, which provide peristalsis due to the high viscosity of the bolus-containing pectin. The activity of smooth muscle cells increases the blood circulation in the intestinal wall and then causes hypertrophy of the intestinal tissue.

It should be noted that the methodology to measure SCFA appears to be established. However, fecal measures of SCFA do not allow for continuous sampling and have yet to be applied at the population level. Indirect measures of SCFA production (breath gas evolution, peripheral blood SCFA) can be obtained in real time but are not very informative overall changes in the fermentation of pectin.

Methanol (MeOH) that is derived from dietary pectin has been recently shown to regulate human gene activity (Shindyapina et al. 2014). Two hr after citrus pectin intake (six g), the MeOH content increased by almost two times in volunteers' plasma. A full-genome analysis of white blood cells in the volunteers revealed 106 up-regulated and 17 down-regulated genes after pectin intake. Among them, 32 were selected for analysis, which found that MeOH concentration changes affect the expression of genes for intercellular communication in leukocytes. Interestingly, most of the identified genes were somehow involved in Alzheimer's disease. The regulation of gene transcriptional activity with MeOH derived from dietary pectin undoubtedly represents a new possible mechanism of the physiological activity of pectin, which requires further investigation.

Carbohydrate antigen-specific antibodies appeared to be one more possible mediator of the effect of pectin on the body. The idea that pectin is capable of inducing the production of human natural antibodies arose from the investigation of complement-activating activity of pectic polysaccharides from herbal medicines. Normal human serum is usually used to assess the activation of the complement system *in vitro* through the classical pathway. The polysaccharide activity was significantly reduced when immunoglobulin (Ig)G-depleted normal human serum was used. Therefore, Kiohara et al. (2006) analyzed the presence of antibodies in human sera that react with pharmacologically active pectic polysaccharides that were isolated from plants that are used in traditional Japanese herbal (Kampo) medicine. The sera from healthy volunteers were shown to contain IgM, IgG, IgA and secretory IgA class antibodies, which react with the active pectic polysaccharides to different degrees. The reacting IgG antibody in normal human serum recognized the ramified regions (RG core with carbohydrate side-chains) of the pectic polysaccharides. Importantly, the reacting IgG antibody showed cross-reactivity with autoantigens, such as single-strand DNA, myosin and tubulin. It was recently found that the serum levels of antibodies that are capable of recognizing PGA strongly correlate with rheumatoid arthritis in humans. The measurements of PGA-specific antibodies in sera are comparable to rheumatoid factors and anti-cyclic citrullinated peptide antibodies as serological diagnostic markers for rheumatoid arthritis in terms of the sensitivity and specificity. Immunohistochemical staining results indicate that the PGA-antibodies selectively bound synovial membrane cells and chondrocytes in the joints of humans (Dai et al. 2014). The data indicate that the PGA–cross-reactive moiety represents a major autoantigen in the joints and can be targeted by autoantibodies that are capable of triggering arthritogenic responses. Clearly, pectin ingestion studies are required to show that dietary pectin induces a production of PGA antibodies that are circulated in the blood.

Conclusions and Future Directions

The health effects of pectin have been postulated for two centuries. A large body of literature exists on this subject, including clinical observations and experimental studies with different animal models and cell systems. This chapter summarizes the data on the beneficial effects of pectin obtained in human studies only. The next aim is to identify the physiological processes that underlie the action of pectin.

The effects based on the ability of the pectin to induce a viscous or gelled gastro-intestinal content appear to represent the most studied effects of pectin on humans. Many studies demonstrate that pectin affects lipid metabolism, enhances glucose tolerance, increases satiety and promotes gastrointestinal health. Importantly, most of the data mentioned in the review were obtained using commercial pectins. Although the majority of plant tissues contain pectins, their industrial production is almost entirely based on only a few sources, such as citrus peel and apple pomace. The structure of common commercial pectins appears to be rather simple. The conditions of the industrial production of pectin are optimized to improve the content of the linear PG fragments, which are necessary for the gelation of pectins. Commercial apple and citrus pectins are considered to be devoid of the side-branched sugar chains. In view of the present knowledge on the complexity of the structure of the entire pectin macromolecule, it is timely and important to study the role of pectins that contain both linear and branch areas in human health. Therefore, the first problem to be solved is to investigate the physiological effects of native pectins of different plants.

The second item that requires investigation is the physiological effects of pectin at lower doses. Indeed, most of the data summarized here were obtained using an intake of at least 10 g of pectin. It is not clear whether low pectin doses that failed to increase the viscosity of the gastrointestinal content could affect any other physiological processes.

Paradoxically, clinical and epidemiological data for a protective role for pectin in human cancer and inflammation are weak. Only a few human trials reported on the anti-cancer, anti-inflammatory, and anti-allergic effects of ingested pectin. The mechanism of these effects is not clear. The proposed interaction of galactose residues of MCP with galectin-3 has not been demonstrated in humans yet. Therefore, the third actual direction of pectin research should be to conduct extensive human studies on the anti-cancer and anti-inflammatory effects of pectin.

The mechanism of the physiological effects of pectin is thought to be realized inside the gastrointestinal tract because pectin is not digested and is not absorbed into the blood stream. The main physiological processes that are affected by pectin appear to be entero-hepatic recirculation, gastric emptying and the absorption of nutrients. Indirectly, pectin is considered to influence the body's metabolism through having an effect on the gut microbiota by increasing the population of healthy microflora and stimulating the production of SCFA.

The MeOH-mediated regulation of gene transcriptional activity after pectin ingestion appears to represent a new possible mechanism for the physiological activity of pectin. In addition to digestive and gastrointestinal processes, other physiological functions, such as cognitive functions, could be proposed to be influenced by pectin.

Another indirect possible mechanism that should be studied is the production by the human immune system of autoantibodies against pectic polysaccharide chains. These antibodies could be involved in both physiological and pathological processes. Studies of the effects of pectin on immunity are of special interest because of the importance of the immune system in human health. The suggestion that pectin could increase weakened immunity or decrease undesirable immune reactions requires investigation, although it is not supported well by epidemiological or human intervention data.

It is suggested that future research on the effect of pectin on physiological functions will provide valuable insight into undefined mechanisms and could lead to new strategies to derive the greatest benefit from the rational use of dietary pectin.

Keywords: Pectin, Physiological effects, Cholesterol level, Glucose tolerance, Satiety, Gastric emptying, Anti-tumor effect, Anti-inflammatory effect, Entero-hepatic circulation, Nutrient absorption

References

Adachi, K., K. Furuta, M. Aimi, K. Fukazawa, S. Shimura, S. Ohara et al. 2012. Efficacy of pectin solution for preventing gastro-esophageal reflux events in patients with percutaneous endoscopic gastrostomy. J Clin Biochem Nutr 50: 190–194.

Amarnath, C. A., N. Venkatesan, M. Doble and S. N. Sawant. 2014. Water dispersible Ag@polyaniline-pectin as supercapacitor electrode for physiological environment. J Mater Chem B 2: 5012–5019.

Anderson, J. W., P. Baird, R. H. Davis, S. Ferreri, M. Knudsen, A. Koraym et al. 2009. Health benefits of dietary fiber. Nutr Rev 67: 188–205.

Aspinall, G. O. 1980. Chemistry of cell wall polysaccharides. pp. 473–500. *In*: Preiss, J. (ed.). The Biochemistry of Plants. Academic Press, New York, USA.

Atia, A., F. Girard-Pipau, X. Hebuterne, W. G. Spies, A. Guardiola, C. W. Ahn et al. 2011. Macronutrient absorption characteristics in humans with short bowel syndrome and jejunocolonic anastomosis: Starch is the most important carbohydrate substrate, although pectin supplementation may modestly enhance short chain fatty acid production and fluid absorption. J Parenter Enteral Nutr 35: 229–240.

Azemar, M., B. Hildenbrand, B. Haering, M. E. Heim and C. Unger. 2007. Clinical benefit in patients with advanced solid tumors treated with modified citrus pectin: a prospective pilot study. Clin Med Oncol 1: 73–80.

Baker, R. A. 1997. Reassessment of some fruit and vegetable pectin levels. J Food Sci 62: 225–229.

Becker, B., U. Kuhn and B. Hardewig-Budny. 2006. Double-blind, randomized evaluation of clinical efficacy and tolerability of an apple pectin-chamomile extract in children with unspecific diarrhea. Arzneimittelforschung 56: 387–393.

Bialostosky, K., J. D. Wright, J. Kennedy-Stephenson, M. McDowell and C. L. Johnson. 2002. Dietary intake of macronutrients micronutrients and other dietary constituents: United States 1988–94. National Center for Health Statistics. Vital Health Stat 11: 1–168.

Bosaeus, I., N. G. Carlsson, A. S. Sandberg and H. Andersson. 1986. Effect of wheat bran and pectin on bile acid and cholesterol excretion in ileostomy patients. Hum Nutr Clin Nutr 40: 429–440.

Braconnot, M. N. 1825a. Nouvelles observations sur l'acide pectique. Ann Chim Phys 28: 96–102.

Braconnot, M. N. 1825b. Recherches sur un nouvel acide universellement répardu dans tous les végétaux. Ann Chim Phys 28: 173–178.

Brenelli, S. L., S. D. Campos and M. J. Saad. 1997. Viscosity of gums *in vitro* and their ability to reduce postprandial hyperglycemia in normal subjects. Braz J Med Biol Res 30: 1437–1440.

Brouns, F., E. Theuwissen, A. Adam, M. Bell, A. Berger and R. P. Mensink. 2012. Cholesterol-lowering properties of different pectin types in mildly hyper-cholesterolemic men and women. Eur J Clin Nutr 66: 591–599.

Brown, L., B. Rosner, W. W. Willett and F. M. Sacks. 1999. Cholesterol-lowering effects of dietary fiber: A meta-analysis. Am J Clin Nutr 69: 30–42.

Burton, R. A., M. J. Gidley and G. B. Fincher. 2010. Heterogeneity in the chemistry, structure and function of plant cell walls. Nat Chem Bio 6: 724–732.

Caffall, K. H. and D. Mohnen. 2009. The structure, function, and biosynthesis of plant cell wall pectic polysaccharides. Carbohydr Res 344: 1879–1900.

Cerda, J. J. 1988. The role of grapefruit pectin in health and disease. Trans Am Climatol Assoc 99: 203–213.

Challen, A. D., W. J. Branch and J. H. Cummings. 1983. The effect of pectin and wheat bran on platelet function and haemostatis in man. 37: 209–217.

Cimolai, N. and J. E. Carter. 1991. Antidiarrheal agents: More to the apple sauce than you might think. Can Fam Physician 37: 185–187.

Coenen, G. J., E. J. Bakx, R. P. Verhoef, H. A. Schols and A. G. J. Voragen. 2007. Identification of the connecting linkage between homo- or xylogalacturonan and rhamnogalacturonan type I. Carbohydr Polym 70: 224–235.

Dai, H., H. L. Dong, F. Y. Gong, S. L. Sun, X. Y. Liu, Z. G. Li et al. 2014. Disease association and arthritogenic potential of circulating antibodies against the alpha 1,4-polygalacturonic acid moiety. J Immunol 192: 4533–4540.

Dhingra, D., M. Michael, H. Rajput and R. T. Patil. 2012. Dietary fibre in foods: A review. J Food Sci Technol 49: 255–266.

Di Lorenzo, C., C. M. Williams, F. Hajnal and J. E. Valenzuela. 1988. Pectin delays gastric emptying and increases satiety in obese subjects. Gastroenterology 95: 1211–1215.

Drasar, B. S. and D. J. A. Jenkins. 1976. Bacteria, diet, and large bowel cancer. Am J Clin Nutr 29: 1410–1416.

Durrington, P. N., A. P. Manning, C. H. Bolton and M. Hartog. 1976. Effect of pectin on serum lipids and lipoproteins, whole-gut transit-time, and stool weight. Lancet 2: 394–396.

Endress, H. -U. 1991. Nonfood uses of pectin. pp. 251–268. *In*: Walter, R. H. (ed.). The Chemistry and Technology of Pectin. Academic Press, San Diego, USA.

Espitia, P. J. P., W. -X. Du, R. J. Avena-Bustillos, N. F. F. Soares and T. H. McHugh. 2014. Edible folms from pectin: Physical-mechanical and antimicrobial properties—A review. Food Hydrocoll 35: 287–296.

Farup, P. G., M. Heibert and V. Hoeg. 2009. Alternative vs. conventional treatment given on-demand for gastroesophageal reflux disease: A randomized controlled trial. BMC Compl Altern Med 9: 3.

Feskens, E. J. and D. Kromhout. 1990. Habitual dietary intake and glucose tolerance in euglycaemic men: the Zutphen study. Int J Epidem 19: 953–959.

Fleming, S. E. and M. A. Rodriguez. 1983. Influence of dietary fiber on fecal excretion of volatile fatty acids by human adults. J Nutr 113: 1613–1625.

Flood-Obbagy, J. E. and B. J. Rolls. 2009. The effect of fruit in different forms on energy intake and satiety at a meal. Appetite 52: 416–422.

Flourie, B., N. Vidon, C. H. Florent and J. -J. Bernier. 1984. Effect of pectin on jejunal glucose absorption and unstirred layer thickness in normal man. 25: 936–941.

Flourie, B., N. Vidon, J. -A. Chayvialle, R. Palma, C. Franchisseur and J. -J. Bernier. 1985. Effect of increased amounts of pectin on a solid-liquid meal digestion in healthy man. Am J Clin Nutr 42: 495–503.

Fluer, F. S., G. G. Kuznetsova, S. Batishcheva, V. N. Matushevsaia and G. A. Donskaia. 2006. Influence of the food products, enriched with pectin, on properties of potentially pathogenic representatives of the microflora of the large intestine. Vopr Pitan 75: 46–49 [In Russian].

Gardner, D. F., L. Schwartz, M. Krista and T. J. Merimee. 1984. Dietary pectin and glycemic control in diabetes. Diabetes Care 7: 143–146.

Gold, L. A., J. P. McCourt and T. J. Merimee. 1980. Pectin: An examination in normal subjects. Diab Care 3: 50–52.

Guess, B. W., M. C. Scholz, S. B. Strum, R. Y. Lam, H. J. Johnson and R. I. Jennrich. 2003. Modified citrus pectin MCP increases the prostate-specific antigen doubling time in men with prostate cancer: a phase II pilot study. Prost Canc Prost Dis 6: 301–304.

Gunnes, P. and M. J. Gidley. 2010. Mechanisms underlying the cholesterol-lowering properties of soluble dietary fibre polysaccharides. Food Funct 1: 149–155.

Hartman, F. W., V. Schelling, H. N. Harking and B. Brush. 1941. Pectin solution as a blood substitute. Ann Surg 114: 212–225.

Haynes, E., C. A. Tompkins, G. Washburn and M. Winters. 1937. Bactericidal action of pectin. Exp Biol Med 36: 839–840.

Henglein, F. A. 1958. Die Uron and Polyuronsäuren. Handbuch der Pflanzenphysiologie. Bd VI: 405–464.

Hillman, L. C., S. G. Peters, C. A. Fisher and E. W. Pomare. 1985. The effects of the fiber components pectin, cellulose and lignin on serum cholesterol levels. Am J Clin Nutr 42: 495–213.

Hillman, L. C., S. G. Peters, C. A. Fisher and E. W. Pomare. 1986. Effects of the fibre components pectin, cellulose, and lignin on bile salt metabolism and biliary lipid composition in man. Gut 27: 29–36.

Hirsch, E. F. 1924. Change in the hydrogen ion concentration of the blood with coagulation. J Biol Chem 61: 795–805.

Hirst, E. L. 1942. Recent progress in the chemistry of pectic materials and plant gums. J Chem Soc 2: 70–78.

Holt, S., R. C. Heading, D. C. Carter, L. F. Prescott and P. Tothill. 1979. Effect of gel fibre on gastric emptying and absorption of glucose and paracetamol. Lancet 1: 636–639.

Hunt, J. S. 1936. Observation on the use of raw apple diet and pectin-agar mixtures in pediatric diarrheas. Arch Pediat 53: 736–738.

Iftikhar, S. Y., N. Washington, C. G. Wilson, I. A. Macdonald and M. D. Homer-Ward. 1994. The effect of pectin on the gastric emptying rates and blood glucose levels after a test meal. J Pharm Pharmacol 46: 851–853.

Isaksson, G., I. Lundquist, B. Akesson and I. Ihse. 1984. Effects of pectin and wheat bran on intraluminal pancreatic enzyme activities and on fat absorption as examined with the triolein breath test in patients with pancreatic insufficiency. Scand J Gastroenterol 19: 467–472.

Jenkins, D. J., A. R. Leeds, M. A. Gassull, B. Cochet and G. M. Alberti. 1977. Decrease in postprandial insulin and glucose concentrations by agar and pectin. Ann Intern Med 86: 20–23.

Jenkins, D. J., T. M. S. Wolever, A. R. Leeds, M. A. Gassull, P. Haisman and J. Dilawari. 1978. Dietary fibres, fibre analogues, and glucose tolerance: importance of viscosity. British Med J 1: 1392–1394.

Jenkins, D. J., D. Reynolds, A. R. Leeds, A. L. Waller and J. H. Cummings. 1979. Hypocholesterolemic action of dietary fiber unrelated to fecal bulking effect. Am J Clin Nutr 32: 2430–2435.

Jenkins, D. J., S. R. Bloom, R. H. Albuquerque, A. R. Leeds, D. L. Sarson and G. L. Metz. 1980. Pectin and complications after gastric surgery: normalization of postprandial glucose and endocrine responses. Gut 21: 574–579.

Juan, J., G. Yingjie and N. Aijun. 2009. Extraction, characterization of *Angelica sinensis* polysaccharides and modulatory effect of the polysaccharides and Tai Chi exercise on oxidative injury in middle-aged women subjects. Carbohydr Polym 77: 384–388.

Judd, P. A. and A. S. Truswell. 1982. Comparison of the effects of high- and low-methoxyl pectins on blood and faecal lipids in man. Br J Nutr 48: 451–458.

Kaczmarczyk, M., M. J. Miller and G. G. Freund. 2012. The health benefits of dietary fiber: beyond the usual suspects of type 2 diabetes, cardiovascular disease and colon cancer. Metabolism 61: 1058–1066.

Kang, J. Y., H. H. Tay, R. Guan, M. V. Math, I. Yap and S. J. Labrooy. 1988. Dietary supplementation with pectin in the maintenance treatment of duodenal ulcer. A controlled study. Scand J Gastroenterol 23: 95–99.

Kasi, M., P. Kausar, R. Naz and L. C. Miller. 1995. Treatment of diarrhoea in infants by medical doctors in Balochistan, Pakistan. J Diarrheal Dis Res 13: 238–241.

Kasper, H., C. Eilles, C. Reiners and J. Schrezenmeir. 1985. The influence of dietary fiber on gastric transit time. Hepatogastroenterology 32: 69–71.

Kay, R. M. and A. S. Truswell. 1977. Effect of citrus pectin on blood lipids and fecal steroid excretion in man. Am J Clin Nutr 30: 171–175.

Keltz, F. R., C. Kies and H. M. Fox. 1978. Urinary ascorbic acid excretion in the human as affected by dietary fiber and zinc. Am J Clin Nutr 31: 1167–1171.

Kendall, C. W. C., A. Esfahani and D. J. A. Jenkins. 2010. The link between dietary fibre and human health. Fd Hydrocoll 24: 42–48.

Kertesz, Z. Y. 1951. The Pectic Substances. Interscience Publishers, New York.

Keys, A., F. Grande and J. T. Anderson. 1961. Fiber and pectin in the diet and serum cholesterol concentration in man. Exp Biol Med 106: 555–558.

Kinnear, D. G. 1964. Drugs used in the symptomatic treatment of diarrhea. Canad Med Ass J 91: 971–972.

Kiohara, H., T. Matsumoto, T. Nagai, S. -J. Kim and H. Yamada. 2006. The presence of natural human antibodies reactive against pharmacologically active pectic polysaccharides from herbal medicines. Phytomedicine 13: 494–500.

Kobayashi, M., H. Matsushita, R. -I. Tsukiyama, M. Saito and T. Sugita. 2005. Shoyu polysaccharides from soy sauce improve quality of life for patients with seasonal allergic rhinitis: a double-blind placebo-controlled clinical study. Intern J Mol Med 15: 463–467.

Kocoshis, S. A. 2010. Medical management of pediatric intestinal failure. Sem Ped Surg 19: 20–26.

Komarova, T. V., E. V. Sheshukova and Y. L. Dorokhov. 2014. Cell wall methanol as a signal in plant immunity. Front Plant Sci 5: 101.

Kurup, P. A., N. Jayakumari, M. Indira, G. M. Kurup, T. Vargheese, A. Mathew et al. 1984. Diet, nutrition intake, and metabolism in populations at high and low risk for colon cancer. Composition, intake, and excretion of fiber constituents. 40: 942–946.

Kushi, L. H., T. Byers, C. Doyle, E. V. Bandera, M. McCullough, T. Cansler et al. 2006. American cancer society guidelines on nutrition and physical activity for cancer prevention: reducing the risk of cancer with healthy food choices and physical activity. CA Cancer J Clin 56: 254–281.

Lattimer, J. M. and M. D. Haub. 2010. Effects of dietary fiber and its components on metabolic health. Nutrients 2: 1266–1289.

Lawaetz, O., A. M. Blackburn, S. R. Bloom, Y. Aritas and D. N. Ralphs. 1983. Effect of pectin on gastric emptying and gut hormone release in the dumping syndrome. Scand J Gastroenterol 18: 327–336.

Leeds, A. R., D. N. Ralphs, F. Ebied, G. Metz and J. B. Dilawari. 1981. Pectin in the dumping syndrome: Reduction of symptoms and plasma volume changes. Lancet 1: 1075–1078.

Lexchin, J. 1994. Agents against pediatric diarrhea. Can Fam Physician 40: 2082–2087.

Lin, T. M., K. S. Kim, E. Karvinen and A. C. Ivy. 1957. Effect of dietary pectin, "protopectin" and gum Arabic on cholesterol excretion in rats. Am J Physiol 188: 66–70.

Linseisen, J., M. B. Schulze, M. Saadatian-Elahi, A. Kroke, A. B. Miller and H. Boeing. 2003. Quantity and quality of dietary fat, carbohydrate, and fiber intake in the German EPIC cohorts. Ann Nutr Metab 47: 37–46.

Logan, K., A. J. Wright and H. D. Goff. 2014. Correlating the structure and *in vitro* digestion viscosities of different pectin fibers to *in vivo* human satiety. Food Funct 6: 63–71.

Mahattanatawee, K., J. A. Manthey, G. Luzio, S. T. Talcott, K. Goodner and E. A. Baldwin. 2006. Total antioxidant activity and fiber content of select Florida-grown tropical fruits. J Agric Food Chem 54: 7355–7363.

Manville, I. A., E. M. Bradway and A. S. McMinis. 1936. Pectin as a detoxication mechanism. Am J Dig Dis 3: 570–572.

Manville, I. A., E. M. Bradway and A. S. McMinis. 1937. The use of apple powder in the treatment of diarrheal conditions and its rationale. Can Med Assoc J 36: 252–257.

Manville, I. A. and N. P. Sullivan. 1940. Relationship of the diet to the self-regulatory defense mechanism. Am J Dig Dis 7: 111–114.

McClure, R. D., K. W. Warren and L. S. Fallis. 1944. Intravenous pectin solution in the prophylaxis and treatment of shock. Can Med Assoc J 51: 206–210.

Miettinen, T. A. and S. Tarpila. 1977. Effect of pectin on serum cholesterol, fecal bile acids and biliary lipids in normolipidemic and hyperlipidemic individuals. Clin Chim Acta 79: 471–477.

Miyazawa, R., T. Tomomasa, H. Kaneko, H. Arakawa, N. Shimizu and A. Morikawa. 2008. Effects of pectin liquid on gastroesophageal reflux disease in children with cerebral palsy. BMC Gastroenterol 8: 11.

Moriarty, P. M., J. Backes, J. -A. Dutton, J. He, J. F. Ruisinger and K. Schmelzle. 2013. Apple pectin for the reduction of niacin-induced flushing. J Clin Lipidol 7: 140–146.

Munarin, F., M. C. Tanzi and P. Petrini. 2012. Advances in biomedical applications of pectin gels. Intern J Biol Macromol 51: 681–689.

Nguyen, K. N., J. D. Welsh, C. V. Manion and V. J. Ficken. 1982. Effect of fiber on breath hydrogen response and symptoms after oral lactose malabsorbers. Am J Clin Nutr 35: 1347–1351.

Olsen, A. G. 1940. Pectin therapy and pectin types. Am J Dig Dis 7: 515–519.

Ovodov, Yu. S. 2009. Current information about pectin substances. Rus J Bioorgan Chem 35: 269–284.

Paderin, N. M. and I. R. Nikitina. 2012. Effects of pectin polysaccharides on leukocytes migration into the oral cavity during exercise. Bull Exp Biol Med 152: 603–605.

Palin, R. and A. Geitmann. 2012. The role of pectin in plant morphogenesis. Biosystems 109: 397–402.

Palmer, G. H. and D. G. Dixon. 1966. Effect of pectin dose on serum cholesterol levels. Am J Clin Nutr 18: 437–442.

Papathanasopoulos, A. and M. Camilleri. 2010. Dietary fiber supplements: Effects in obesity and metabolic syndrome and relationship to gastrointestinal functions. Gastroenterology 138: 65–72.

Perrigue, M., B. Carter, S. A. Roberts and A. Drewnowski. 2010. A low-calorie beverage supplemented with low-viscosity pectin reduces energy intake at a subsequent meal. J Food Sci 75: H300–H305.

Pomare, E. W., W. J. Branch and J. H. Cummings. 1985. Carbohydrate fermentation in the human colon and its relation to acetate concentrations in venous blood. J Clin Ivest 75: 1448–1454.

Popper, Z. A. 2008. Evolution and diversity of green plant cell walls. Curr Op Plant Biol 11: 286–292.

Prasana, V., T. N. Prabha and R. N. Tharanathan. 2007. Fruit ripening phenomena—An overview. Crit Rev Food Sci Nutr 47: 1–19.

Rabbani, G. H., T. Teka, B. Zaman, N. Majid, M. Khatun and G. J. Fuchs. 2001. Clinical studies in persistent diarrhea: dietary management with green banana or pectin in Bangladeshi children. 121: 554–560.

Rabbani, G. H., T. Teka, S. K. Saha, B. Zaman, N. Majid, M. Khatun et al. 2004. Green banana and pectin improve small intestinal permeability and reduce fluid loss in Bangladeshi children with persistent diarrhea. Dig Dis Sci 49: 475–484.

Ranganathan, S., M. Champ, C. Pechard, P. Blanchard, M. Nguyen et al. 1994. Comparative study of the acute effects of resistant starch and dietary fibers on metabolic indexes in men. Am J Clin Nutr 59: 879–883.

Rani, B. and A. Kawatra. 1994. Fibre constituents of some foods. Plant Foods Hum Nutr 45: 343–347.

Remer, T., K. Pietrzik and F. Manz. 1996. The short-term effect of dietary pectin on plasma levels and renal excretion of dehydroepiandrosterone sulfate. Z Ernahrungswiss 35: 32–38.

Ridker, P. M., N. Rifai, M. J. Stampfer and C. H. Hennekens. 2000. Plasma concentration of interleukin-6 and the risk of future myocardial infarction among apparently healthy men. Circulation 101: 1767–1772.

Riedl, J., J. Linseisen, J. Hoffmann and G. Wolfram. 1999. Some dietary fibers reduce the absorption of carotenoids in women. J Nutr 129: 2170–2176.

Rock, C. L. and M. E. Swendseid. 1992. Plasma β-carotene response in humans after meals supplemented with dietary pectin. Am J Clin Nutr 55: 96–99.

Ross, J. K. and J. E. Leklem. 1981. The effect of dietary citrus pectin on the excretion of human fecal neutral and acid steroids and the activity of 7α-dehydroxylase and β-glucouronidase. Am J Clin Nutr 34: 2068–2077.

Ross, J. K., D. J. Pusateri and T. D. Shultz. 1990. Dietary and hormonal evaluation of men at different risks for prostate cancer: Fiber intake, excretion, and composition, with *in vitro* evidence for an association between steroid hormones and specific fiber components. Am J Clin Nutr 51: 365–370.

Round, A. N., N. M. Rigby, A. J. MacDougall and V. J. Morris. 2010. A new view of pectin structure revealed by acid hydrolysis and atomic force microscopy. Carbohydr Res 345: 487–497.

Rowley, J. L. 1934. Raw apple diet. Am J Nurs 34: 682–684.

Sakamoto, Y., Y. Sekino, E. Yamada, H. Ohkubo, T. Higurashi, E. Sakai et al. 2011. Mosapride accelerates the delayed gastric emptying of high-viscosity liquids: A crossover study using continuous real-time 13C breath test (BreathID system). J Neurogastroenterol Motil 17: 395–401.

Sanaka, M., T. Yamamoto, H. Anjiki, K. Nagasawa and Y. Kuyama. 2007. Effects of agar and pectin on gastric emptying and post-prandial glycaemic profiles in healthy human volunteers. Clin Exp Pharmacol Physiol 34: 1151–1155.

Sandberg, A. S., R. Ahderinne, H. Andersson, B. Hallgren and L. Hulten. 1983. The effect of citrus pectin on the absorption of nutrients in the small intestine. Hum Nutr Clin Nutr 37: 171–183.

Sandhu, K. S., M. M. el Samahi, J. Mena, C. P. Dooley and J. E. Valenzuela. 1987. Effect of pectin on gastric emptying and gastroduodenal motility in normal subjects. Gastroenterology 92: 486–492.

Schultz, A. A., B. Ashby-Hughes, R. Taylor, D. E. Gillis and M. Wilkins. 2000. Effects of pectin on diarrhea in critically ill tube-fed patients receiving antibiotics. Am J Crit Care 9: 403–411.

Schwab, U., A. Louheranta, A. Torronen and M. Uusitupa. 2006. Impact of sugar beet pectin and polydextrose on fasting and postprandial glycemia and fasting concentrations of serum total and lipoprotein lipids in meddle-aged subjects with abnormal glucose metabolism. Eur J Clin Nutr 60: 1073–1080.

Schwartz, S. E., R. A. Levine, A. Singh, J. R. Scheidecker and N. S. Track. 1982. Sustained pectin ingestion delays gastric emptying. Gastroenterology 83: 812–817.

Schwartz, S. E., R. A. Levine, R. S. Weinstock, S. Petokas, C. A. Mills and F. D. Thomas. 1988. Sustained pectin ingestion: effect on gastric emptying and glucose tolerance in non-insulin-dependent diabetic patients. Am J Clin Nutr 48: 1413–1417.

Shafer, R. B., A. S. Levine, J. M. Marlette and J. E. Morley. 1985. Do calories, osmolality, or calcium determine gastric emptying? Am J Physiol 248: R479–483.

Sheehan, J. P., I. W. Wei, M. Ulchaker and K. Y. Tserng. 1997. Effect of high fiber intake in fish oil-treated patients with non-insulin-dependent diabetes mellitus. Am J Clin Nutr 660: 1183–1187.

Shindyapina, A. V., I. V. Petrunia, T. V. Komarova, E. V. Sheshukova, V. S. Kosorukov, G. I. Kiryanov et al. 2014. Dietary methanol regulates human gene activity. 9: e102837.

Shimoyama, Y., M. Kusano, O. Kawamura, H. Zai, S. Kuribayashi, T. Higuchi et al. 2007. High-viscosity liquid meal accelerates gastric emptying. Neurogastroenterol Motil 19: 879–886.

Siddhu, A., S. Sad, R. L. Bijlani, M. G. Karmarkar and U. Nayar. 1989. Modulation of postprandial glycaemia and insulinaemia by pectin in mixed nutrient combinations. Indian J Physiol Pharmacol 33: 77–83.

Siddhu, A., S. Sad, R. L. Bijlani, M. G. Karmarkar and U. Nayar. 1990. Nutrient interaction in relation to glycaemic response in isocarbohydrate and isocaloric meals. Indian J Physiol Pharmacol 34: 171–178.

Siddhu, A., S. Sad, R. L. Bijlani, M. G. Karmarkar and U. Nayar. 1991. Modulation of postprandial glycaemia and insulinaemia by dietary fat. Indian J Physiol Pharmacol 35: 99–105.

Simonova, G. I., Yu. P. Nikitin, O. M. Bragina, L. V. Sherbakova and S. K. Malutina. 2006. Actual nutrition and health of the population of Siberia: Results of two decades of epidemiological studies. Bull SB RAMS 4: 22–30.

Sirtori, C. R., M. Triolo, R. Bosiso, A. Bondioli, L. Calabresi, V. De Vergori et al. 2012. Hypocholesterolaemic effects of lupin protein and pea protein/fibre combinations in moderately hypercholesterolaemic individuals. Br J Nutr 107: 1176–1183.

Slavin, J. L. 2005. Dietary fiber and body weight. Nutrition 21: 411–418.

Speth, P. A., J. B. Jansen and C. B. Lamers. 1983. Effect of acarbose, pectin, a combination of acarbose with pectin, and placebo on postprandial reactive hypoglycaemia after gastric surgery. Gut 24: 798–802.

Spiller, G. A., M. C. Chernoff, R. A. Hill, J. E. Gates, J. J. Nassar and E. A. Shipley. 1980. Effect of purified cellulose, pectin, and a low-residue diet on fecal volatile fatty acids, transit time, and fecal weight in humans. Am J Clin Nutr 33: 754–759.

Spiricheva, T. V., V. B. Spirichev, V. M. Kodentsova, N. A. Beketova, O. G. Pereverzeva, O. V. Kosheleva et al. 2011. Effectiveness of use in preventive nutrition the food products with contents of pectin and vitamins. Vopr Pitan 80: 47–55 [In Russian].

Sriamornsak, P. 2003. Chemistry of pectin and its pharmaceutical uses: A review. Silpakorn Univer Intern J 3: 206–228.

Stasse-Wolthuis, M., M. B. Katan, R. J. J. Hermus and J. G. Hautvast. 1979. Increase of serum cholesterol in man fed bran diet. Atherosclerosis 34: 87–91.

Stasse-Wolthuis, M., F. F. A. Albers, J. G. C. van Jeveren, J. W. de Jong, J. Hautvast and R. J. J. Hermus. 1980. Influence of dietary fiber from vegetables and fruits, bran or citrus pectin on serum lipids, fecal lipids, and colonic function. Am J Clin Nutr 33: 1745–1756.

Tiwary, C. M., J. A. Ward and B. A. Jackson. 1997. Effect of pectin on satiety in healthy US Army adults. J Am Coll Nutr 16: 423–428.

Vaaler, S., K. F. Hanssen and O. Aagenaes. 1980. Effects of different kinds of fibre on postprandial blood glucose in insulin-dependent diabetics. Acta Med Scand 208: 389–391.

Vargo, D., R. Doyle and M. H. Floch. 1985. Colonic bacterial flora and serum cholesterol: alterations induced by dietary citrus pectin. Am J Gastroenterol 80: 361–364.

Veldman, F. J., C. H. Nair, H. H. Vorster, W. J. Vermaak, J. C. Jerling, W. Oosthuizen et al. 1997. Dietary pectin influences fibrin network structure in hypercholesterolaemic subjects. Thromb Res 86: 183–196.

Voragen, A. G. J., G. J. Coenen, R. P. Verhoef and H. A. Schols. 2009. Pectin, a versatile polysaccharide present in plant cell walls. Struct Chem 20: 263–275.

Wahlqvist, M. L., M. J. Morris, G. O. Littlejohn, A. Bond and R. V. Jackson. 1979. The effects of dietary fibre on glucose tolerance in healthy males. Aust N Z J Med 9: 154–158.

Wanders, A. J., J. J. G. C. van den Borne, C. de Graaf, T. Hulshof, M. C. Jonathan, M. Kristensen et al. 2011. Effects of dietary fibre on subjective appetite, energy intake and body weight: a systematic review of randomized controlled trials. Obes Rev 12: 724–739.

Wanders, A. J., E. J. M. Feskens, M. C. Jonathan, H. A. Schols, C. de Graaf and M. Mars. 2014a. Pectin is not pectin: A randomized trial on the effect of different physicochemical properties of dietary fiber on appetite and energy intake. Physiol Behav 128: 212–219.

Wanders, A. J., M. Mars, K. J. Borgonjen-van den Berg, C. de Graaf and E. J. Feskens. 2014b. Satiety and energy intake after single and repeated exposure to gel-forming dietary fiber: Post-ingestive effects. Int J Obes (Lond) 38: 794–800.

Watts, P. and A. Smith. 2009. PecSys: *in situ* gelling system for optimized nasal drug delivery. Expert Opin Drug Deliv 6: 543–552.

Werch, S. C. and A. C. Ivy. 1941. On the fate of ingested pectin. Am J Dig Dis 8: 101–105.

Williams, D. R., W. P. James and I. E. Evans. 1980. Dietary fibre supplementation of a 'normal' breakfast administered to diabetics. Diabetologia 18: 379–383.

Winters, M. and C. A. Tompkins. 1936. A pectin-agar preparation for treatment of diarrhea of infants. Am J Dis Child 52: 259–265.

Winters, M., G. A. Peters and G. W. Crook. 1939. Pectin as a prophylactic and curative agent for peptic ulcers produced experimentally with cinchophen. Am J Dig Dis 6: 13–15.

Wolf, S. and S. Greiner. 2012. Growth control by cell wall pectins. Protoplasma 249: S169–175.

Wu, H., K. M. Dwyer, Z. Fan, A. Shircore, J. Fan and J. H. Dwyer. 2003. Dietary fiber and progression of atherosclerosis: the Los Angeles Atherosclerosis Study. Am J Clin Nutr 78: 1085–1091.

Xu, L., W. Yu, J. Jiang and N. Li. 2014. Clinical benefits after soluble fiber supplementation: a randomized clinical trial in adults with slow-transit constipation. Zhonghua Wei Chang Ke Za Zhi 94: 3813–3816 [In Chinese].

Xu, L., W. Yu, J. Jiang, X. Feng and N. Li. 2015. Efficacy of pectin in the treatment of diarrhea predominant irritable bowel syndrome. Zhonghua Wei Chang Ke Za Zhi 18: 267–271 [In Chinese].

Yokawa, K. and F. Baluska. 2015. Pectins, ROS homeostasis and UV-B responses in plant roots. Phytochemistry 112: 80–83.

Zimmaro, D. M., R. H. Rolandelli, M. J. Koruda, R. G. Settle, T. P. Stein and J. L. Rombeau. 1989. Isotonic tube feeding formula induces liquid stool in normal subjects: reversal by pectin. J Parenter Enteral Nutr 13: 117–123.

CHAPTER 12

Glycobiology of Human Milk in Health and Disease

YingYing He[a] and David S. Newburg[b],*

Introduction

A major evolutionary advantage of mammals is the investment by females toward the survival of their offspring by providing milk to their infants via the mammary gland (Newburg 2013). Mammary glands are epidermal prominences evolved from ancient apocrine glands of the skin that are specialized to provide fluid for the infant. The maturation and activation of the gland is under hormonal control. Mammary glands experience three developmental stages: embryonic, pubertal, and mature adult. In the embryonic stage, milk ducts form from overlying ectoderm; ectodermal cells migrate along the ducts to coalesce into epithelial placodes, which differentiate into the mammary bud, mammary sprout, and the rudimentary gland. The next qualitative maturation of the mammary gland occurs in puberty, when branching morphogenesis and lumen formation are the major events. This matures into a complex secretory organ of epithelial cells, adipocytes, vascular endothelial cells, and a variety of immune cells. Upon pregnancy, mammary glands undergo further morphological change and differentiation as they prepare for lactation (Watson and Khaled 2008). Lactation, the production of milk, is strictly controlled by hormones, such as progesterone, estrogen, prolactin, growth hormone, adrenocorticotropic hormone (ACTH), thyroid stimulating hormone (TSH), and many others (Capuco and Akers 2009). The stages of modification of the adult breast for lactation are initiated during pregnancy, culminate with lactation, and end at weaning with involution of the breast, reversing many of the stages of lactogenesis until the next pregnancy.

Milk is an ideal mixture of nutrients for the species of offspring for which it is intended. As the first food, it provides the proteins and fats needed for the structural expansion of growth, the energy supply to support such growth. Moreover, it also contains hundreds of thousands of distinct bioactive molecules that protect against infection and inflammation, contribute to immune maturation, organ development, and healthy microbial colonization of the neonatal gut (Ballard and Morrow 2013). The needs of the infant change during development, and the components of milk change qualitatively and quantitatively across lactation (Chaturvedi et al. 2001). That notwithstanding, human milk always includes: (1) live cells, including macrophages (over 80% of the cells in colostrum), neutrophils, T cells (CD8[+] and CD4[+]CCR5[+]), stem cells, and milk bacteria (Speer et al. 1985, Sabbaj et al. 2002, Ichikawa et al. 2003, Kourtis et al. 2007, Hunt

Program in Glycobiology, Department of Biology, Boston College, 140 Commonwealth Ave, Chestnut Hill, MA, USA-02467.
[a] E-mail: yingying.he@bc.edu
[b] E-mail: david.newburg@bc.edu

et al. 2011, Hassiotou et al. 2012, Bode et al. 2014, Hassiotou et al. 2014, Khodayar-Pardo et al. 2014). (2) Bioactive molecules, including antibodies (secretory IgA, IgM, IgG, IgE and IgD), hormones, cytokines, chemokines, glycans (Kverka et al. 2007, Garofalo 2010, Cerini and Aldrovandi 2013, Lonnerdal 2014, He et al. 2015), and enzymes including glycosidases and glycosyltransferases (Wiederschain and Newburg 1996, 2001). Each species has unique patterns of specific carbohydrates, and human milk is notable in its high content of glycans. Indeed, human milk seems to be the most heavily glycosylated fluid of the human body. Furthermore, each individual mother has a somewhat unique complement of glycans in her milk.

Lactose and oligosaccharides represent approximately 6.8 and 1% of the milk, respectively; other sources of human milk glycans include glycoproteins, glycopeptides, glycolipids, and monosaccharides. The glycan composition of human milk is summarized in Table 1.

Lactose is the predominant carbohydrate in human milk, with a concentration consistently around 67–68 g/liter in mature milk. Lactose is digested into glucose and galactose by lactase (β-galactosidase), and glucose can be used as a source of energy in all cell types to support cell functions (Lonnerdal et al. 1976, Jenness 1979, Mitoulas et al. 2002, Newburg et al. 2012, Newburg 2013).

Human milk oligosaccharides (HMOS) are a heterogeneous mixture of complex carbohydrate structures appended to a lactose or a polylactosamine backbone (Kunz et al. 2000). After fat and lactose, HMOSs are the third most abundant solid component of human milk with a concentration of 5–15 g/liter (Newburg et al. 2005). To date, over 200 individual oligosaccharides have been defined in HMOSs. The indigestible oligosaccharides exhibit biological activities that include pathogen inhibition, promotion of beneficial bacterial growth, stimulation of immune system development, and quenching inflammation. Bacterial and viral binding to their glycosylated host receptors can be competitively inhibited by HMOS whose moieties are structural homologs to the receptors. Likewise, binding of bacterial toxins whose targets are glycans can be inhibited. Conversely, HMOS can promote growth of beneficial bacterial, that is, the prebiotic activities of HMOS promote growth of mutualists in the gut, which in turn limit growth of pathobionts.

HMOS can also directly modulate signaling processes, which can stimulate immune system development and quench potentially devastating inflammation at the mucosal surface during early colonization.

Almost all of the proteins in human milk are glycoproteins. Well-defined glycan structures were described in β-casein, α-lactalbumin, mucins, secretory immunoglobulin A (sIgA), bile salt-stimulated lipase (BSSL), lactoferrin, and lactoperoxidase (Table 1). Milk glycoproteins vary in size, structure and abundance. Glycoproteins concentrations vary over a wide range: the level of β-casein is approximately 5000 mg/liter; levels of lactoferrin vary from 1000–7000 mg/liter; the level of lactadherin is close to 100 mg/liter. Some glycoproteins occur in human milk at trace levels. For example, lactoperoxidase concentrations are approximately 0.77 mg/liter (Shin et al. 2001).

The total monosaccharide content in human milk is 500–900 mg/liter, which contains glucose, galactose, L-fucose and N-acetyl neuraminic acid (sialic acid) (Coppa et al. 1993). The concentration of each monosaccharide can change dynamically and vary widely among individuals. For example, glucose is the most abundant monosaccharide in human milk. Its concentration increases from 30 mg/liter on the first day of lactation (colostrum) to 260 mg/liter after the 15th day of lactation (mature milk); but after weaning, the milk glucose level declines (Newburg and Neubauer 1995).

Human milk glycolipids include sphingomyelin, gangliosides, and neutral glycolipids (glucosylceramide, galactosylceramide, lactosylceramide, globotriosyl-ceramide, globoside). Sphingolipids, lipids based on a long-chain nitrogenous base complexed with a long-chain fatty acid through an amide linkage, are the most prevalent components for membranous structures of the human milk fat globule membrane. Human milk sphingomyelin level is around 110 μM (Bouhours and Bouhours 1981). Gangliosides, containing negatively charged sialic acid on their carbohydrate moiety, are components in the outer leaflet of the plasma membrane. The total ganglioside content of human milk is 15–20 mg/liter. GD3 is the predominant ganglioside in early human milk with a concentration of approximately 2.7 mg/liter, while GM3 is predominant late in lactation with a concentration up to 8.1 mg/liter. The level of neutral glycolipids is around 20–25 mg/liter. The concentration of globotriosylceramide (Gb3) is around 123 nM, and the concentration of globoside (Gb4) is ~91 nM. Both the sialic acid-containing ganglioside (GM1) and the globo-series neutral glycolipids strongly bind to bacteria toxins, each to its specific toxin, suggesting a central role of human milk glycolipids in the protection of infants against damage by bacterial infections.

Table 1. Human milk glycans (Newburg 2013, Peterson et al. 2013).

Human milk glycans	Concentration
Lactose	68 g/liter
Human milk oligosaccharides (HMOSs)	5–15 g/liter
Glycoproteins	
β-Casein	4670±890 mg/L
Mucins	729±75 mg/L
sIgA	200–6200 mg/L
BSSL	100–200 mg/L
Lactoferrin	1000–7000 mg/L
Lactadherin	93±10 mg/L
Lactoperoxidase	0.77 mg/L
Monosaccharides	500–900 mg/L
Glucose	30–260 mg/L
Galactose	30–260 mg/L
L-fucose	1 mg/L
Sialic acid (N-acetylneuraminic acid, Neu5Ac)	40 mg/L
Glycolipids	11.6 mg/L
Sphingomyelin	110 μM
Total gangliosides (sialic acid glycolipids)	15–20 mg/L
GM1	12 μg/L
GM2	250 μg/L
GM3	8.1 mg/L
GD3	2.7 mg/L
Neutral glycolipids	20–25 mg/L
Glucosylceramide	32 μg/L
Galactosylceramide	235 μg/L
Lactosylceramide	133 μg/L
Gb3 (globotriosylceramide)	123 nM
Gb4 (globoside)	91 nM

The presence and patterns of these glycans in human milk vary depending upon the stage of lactation and the maternal genetic polymorphisms that control glycosyltransferases (Le Pendu 2004, Newburg 2013). The synthesis of milk glycans utilizes significant metabolic energy from the mother when producing her milk, but, other than lactose, these glycans are indigestible, and therefore do not make a biologically meaningful contribution to the nutritional needs of the infant. Human milk glycans, as found in the glycoproteins presented in Table 1, have many other documented functions: (1) Inhibition of pathogen binding to the intestinal mucosa (Fig. 1A). (2) A prebiotic effect of stimulating the growth of mutualist bacteria of the microbiota (Fig. 1B); these mutualists and their fermentation products can, in turn, (a) inhibit pathogens, (b) modulate signaling and inflammation, and (c) the fermentation products can be absorbed and utilized as a source of energy. (3) Human milk glycans modulate immune system development and attenuate disproportionate inflammation (Fig. 1C). These functions support intestinal postnatal growth, stimulate mucosal immune system development, and direct the ontogeny of colonization, which may synergistically protect infants from diseases. Human milk glycans and their homologs are now being synthesized and tested as novel prophylactic or therapeutic agents for a range of infections, chronic dysbiosis, and deleterious inflammatory conditions.

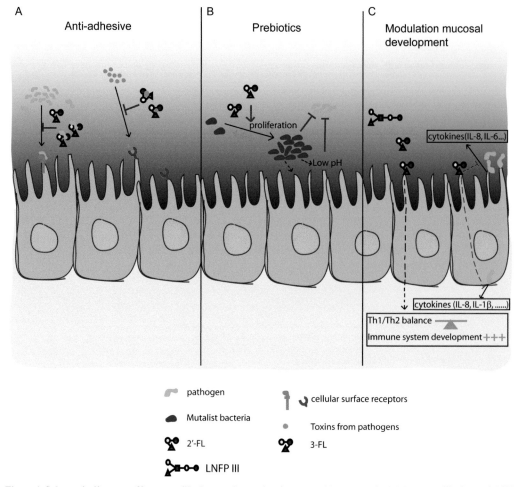

Figure 1. Schematic diagram of human milk glycans that maintain mucosal homeostasis. (A) Human milk glycans inhibit binding by pathogen and pathogenic toxins to the intestinal mucosa. (B) Human milk glycans, especially HMOS, exhibit prebiotic effects. (C) Human milk glycans modulate mucosal development and suppress excess inflammation.

Antimicrobial and Antiviral Activity of Human Milk

HMOS are Anti-adhesive and Inhibit Microbial and Microbial Toxin Binding

Bacterial adhesion is the first essential step for a pathogen to infect a host. Human milk is an innate immune system that contains many components that inhibit many types and stages of pathogenesis. Pathogen binding inhibition is attributed to the structural homology between the human milk glycans and gut glycan receptors that are specifically bound by bacterial adhesins or viral capsids. When human milk glycans competitively bind bacteria, this limits the ability of the pathogen to bind the mucosal surface of neonatal infant (Ruiz-Palacios et al. 2003, Morrow et al. 2004, Newburg et al. 2005). Several anti-adhesive molecules, including fucosylated oligosaccharides, lactadherin, mucin1, glycosaminoglycans, and GM1, have been defined in human milk.

Campylobacter jejuni (C. jejuni), a bacterium carried by many types of birds including domestic fowl, is the most common agent of bacteria-induced diarrhea worldwide. The fucosylated H-2 epitope is widely thought to be the major determinant of susceptibility to *C. jejuni* infection based on these experimental results: (1) *C. jejuni* has high avidity for the fucosylated antigen H-2 (Fucα1,2Galβ1,4GlcNAc); (2)

monoclonal antibodies against the H-2 epitope inhibit *C. jejuni* binding. (3) Overexpression of H-2 fucosylated antigen on Chinese hamster ovary cells transforms these cells from a *C. jejuni* unbound cells to a *C. jejuni* bound cells. (4) Ligands that bind to H-2 epitope, such as *Ulex europaeus* agglutinin and *Lotus tetragonolobus* lectins, inhibit *C. jejuni* adhesion.

Human milk contains the H-2 epitope in many forms, and they compete with H-2 epitopes of the host cell surface receptors for binding to *C. jejuni*, preventing *C. jejuni* adhesion to the host. The clinical relevance of this phenomenon is supported by oral administration of HMOSs inhibiting *C. jejuni* colonization in mice *in vivo*. In *ex vivo* experiments, HMOSs also inhibit invasive, pathogenic *C. jejuni* from binding to human intestinal mucosa. In transgenic female mice, introducing the α1,2-fucosyltransferase gene (FUT1) induces 2-linked fucose antigen (H-2 epitope) expression in their mammary glands and milk, which protects their pups from an inoculum of *C. jejuni* (Ruiz-Palacios et al. 1990). 2'-fucosyllactose (2'-FL), the most prevalent of the milk oligosaccharides, is a major source of H-2 epitope in human milk. A study of the relevance of breastfeeding and diarrhea was performed in a prospective study of a human cohort of 93 breastfeeding mother-infant pairs during the first two years of the newborn's life: *C. jejuni* diarrhea occurred less often in infants whose mother's milk contained high levels of 2'-FL (Ruiz-Palacios et al. 2003, Newburg et al. 2005), strongly supporting the relevance of 2'-FL in protecting infants. However, the final proof will be feeding pure 2'-FL directly to infants in a prospective study to measure its ability to lower the risk of diarrhea.

Mucins are major components of the extracellular matrix. These heavily glycosylated proteins contain ~80% carbohydrate. The carbohydrate moieties contain N-acetylgalactosamine, N-acetylglucosamine, fucose, galactose, sialic acid, and traces of mannose and sulfate. Moderately branched oligosaccharide chains contain 5–15 monomers and attach to the protein core by O-glycosidic bonds. The mucin protein core contains a central glycosylated region with STP (serine, threonine and proline) repeats and terminal cysteine rich domains (Rama and Turner 2006). The 20 recognized members of the mucin family are divided into three subfamilies: Secreted gel-forming mucins, including MUC2, 5AC, 5B, 6, and 19; Secreted non-gel-forming mucins, including MUC7; and cellular surface mucins, including MUC1, 3A/B, 4, 12, 13, 15, 16, 17, and 20 (Linden et al. 2008, Liu and Newburg 2013). These high-molecular-mass glycoproteins are present on the apical membrane of all mucosal epithelial cells. They are a constituent of the glycocalyx epithelial shield, a barrier that limits access of other cells, large molecules, and pathogens to the mucosal cell surface.

The major human milk mucins are MUC1 and MUC4. MUC1 and 4 are able to bind *Salmonella* (Liu et al. 2012); MUC1 can bind HIV, rotavirus, *E. coli* and *Salmonella typhimurium* (Schroten et al. 1992, Yolken et al. 1992, Saeland et al. 2009, Liu et al. 2012). This mucin binding may protect the mucosa, with the sialic acid moiety interacting with pathogens and inhibiting pathogen binding to its infant host cell surface glycan receptor. Other human milk glycans containing a sialic acid moiety also inhibit pathogens. For example, sialyllactose inhibits *E. coli*, *P. aeruginosa*, *Aspergillus fumigatus conidia*, and *Helicobacter pylori* (Schroten et al. 1992, Virkola et al. 1993, Stins et al. 1994, Bouchara et al. 1997, Mysore et al. 1999). Glycolipid GM1 limits the adhesion of *enterotoxigenic E. coli* to Caco-2 cells to less than 20% of the positive control. GM3 depresses adhesion of *enterotoxigenic E. coli* and *enteropathogenic E. coli in vitro* (Idota and Kawakami 1995).

Besides competing with cell surface receptors to bind pathogenic bacteria, human milk glycans are able to bind microbial toxins. Stable toxin is one of two major pathogenic agents whereby *enterotoxigenic E. coli* (ETEC) infection causes diarrhea in children. Human milk α1,2-linked fucosylated glycans inhibit ETEC stable toxin (Newburg et al. 2005). The major component responsible for STa binding inhibition is present at a concentration of 30 ppm in human milk (Newburg et al. 1995a). In prospective clinical studies, infants who developed diarrhea associated with ST of *E. coli* were consuming milk with significantly lower 2-linked oligosaccharides than those of the remaining infants. Glycolipids can also strongly bind to toxins. For example, GM1 is known to bind to cholera toxin, labile toxin of ETEC, and a similar toxin from *C. jejuni* (Newburg 2013). Gb3 binds to Shiga-like toxin produced by some *enterohemorrhagic E. coli*. Gb4 binds to a variant of Shiga-like toxin. This binding by glycans protects the host.

Inhibition of Microbial Growth

Human milk per se suppresses bacterial growth. Levels of pathogens do not increase in human milk stored for 8 hours at room temperature, for 3 days at 4°C, or for a year at –20°C (Lawrence 1999). Human milk not only exhibits antimicrobial activity, but it actually inhibits pathogen growth. The anti-microbial activities of human milk stored for 48 hours were measured as a reduction (~80%) in pathogenic *E. coli* that originally was present as a contaminant in freshly collected and stored milks (Martinez-Costa et al. 2007, Hill and Newburg 2015). In fresh human milk, anti-microbial activities are present as lymphocytes, milk glycans, and antibodies, and their presence in milk may protect the breasts as well as the nursing infant from pathogen infection.

Specific glycans (carbohydrate moieties of a glycoconjugate) found in human milk that exhibit anti-microbial activities include IgG and lactoferrin. Human milk IgG, a 150-kDa-glycosylation protein, is one major type of antibody that is present at low concentrations in colostrum and mature milk. IgG is an important component of opsonization; IgG-coating of pathogen surfaces triggers pathogen recognition and ingestion by phagocytic immune cells, including by the polymorphonuclear leukocytes in human milk, which leads to sequentially phagocytosis and the intracellular killing of pathogen (Murphy et al. 1983).

One of the most studied antimicrobial glycans in human milk is lactoferrin, which inhibits fungi (*Candida albicans*), protozoa, viruses, and a wide range of bacteria, including *Escherichia coli*, *Staphylococcus albus*, *Staphylococcus aureus*, *Pseudomonas aeruginosa*, *Bacillus stearothermophilus*, *Bacillus subtilis*, *Vibrio cholerae* and *Streptococcus mutans* (Brock 1980, Newburg and Walker 2007, Adlerova et al. 2008). Human milk lactoferrin is a glycoprotein consisting of a single polypeptide chain of molecular weight 75–90 kDa with iron binding activity (Brock 1980). Ferric ion can be transferred to bacterial surfaces by bacterial siderophores that bind the iron with high affinity. Bacteria require this iron, and the chelation of iron by lactoferrin limits the iron available to bacteria, resulting in a rapid loss of capacity to form colonies. Lactoferrin antimicrobial activity is also a consequence of its ability to bind to the lipid A moiety of bacterial lipopolysaccharide (LPS), causing release of LPS from bacteria, thereby inducing cytoplasmic membrane permeability (Orsi 2004). Lactoferrin blocks bacterial biofilm development, inhibits bacterial adhesion, colonization, and intracellular invasion, and induces the apoptosis of infected cells (Brock 1980, Orsi 2004).

Inhibition of Viral Replication

Noroviruses, which include Norwalk virus and the various Norwalk-like viruses, is a major genus of the caliciviruses family. Noroviruses are a principal cause of diarrhea in humans, especially in infants (Newburg et al. 2005). Noroviruses utilize human histo-blood group antigens as receptors. The fucosylα-1,2-epitope is essential for binding by many noroviruses strains. (1) Norwalk virus binds to individuals with secretor phenotype but not non-secretor phenotype. (2) Target tissue treated with α-1,2-fucosidase loses the ability to bind Norwalk virus. (3) H-1 and H-3 monoclonal antibodies inhibit norovirus binding. Binding by Norwalk virus *in vitro* is specifically inhibited by the human milk oligosaccharide lacto-N-difucohexaose (LDFH-I). The clinical relevance was tested in a cohort of mother-infant pairs, and the level of LDFH-I in the milk consumed by the infants is inversely related to the risk of norovirus-associated diarrhea in breastfed infants. Thus, high content of LDFH-I in milk protects infants against norovirus diarrhea (Newburg 2013).

Rotavirus causes more than 50% of cases of gastroenteritis in infants and young children worldwide (Yolken et al. 1992). A macromolecular component of human milk, lactadherin, inhibits rotavirus replication *in vitro* and prevents the development of gastroenteritis from rotavirus infection. Lactadherin is a 46 kDa mucin-associated glycoprotein of the human milk fat globule membrane that contains sialic acid. Many human strains of rotavirus bind to sialic acid-containing receptors; their binding and infection is inhibited by sialylated glycans. A crude human milk mucin fraction inhibited rotavirus replication and prevented experimental gastroenteritis, and the activity was attributed to the presence of lactadherin (Newburg et al. 1998). Lactadherin binds specifically to rotavirus, inhibits rotavirus replication, and protects against symptoms of rotavirus infection, but loses its inhibitory activity when the sialic acid is removed (Newburg et al. 1998). In a newborn piglet model, human milk oligosaccharides shorten rotavirus-induced diarrhea (Li et al. 2014). *In vitro*, sialic acid-dependent porcine OSU strain rotavirus binding or infectivity/replication were inhibited by 3'-sialyllactose (3'-SL) and 6'-sialyllactose (6'-SL).

HIV. The binding of envelope glycoprotein gp120 of Human Immunodeficiency Virus (HIV) to its host cell CD4 receptor is the essential first step in HIV infection. The human milk glycosaminoglycan (GAG) fraction inhibits this binding and blocks HIV infection (Newburg et al. 1995b). Some human milk glycans, including human milk bile salt-stimulated lipase (BSSL) (90–316 kDa) and the milk oligosaccharide lacto-N-fucopentaose III (LNFP III), bind to Dendritic Cell-Specific Intracellular adhesion molecule-3-Grabbing Non-integrin (DC-SIGN) and inhibit DC-SIGN mediated HIV type 1 transfer to $CD4^+$ lymphocytes (Blackberg and Hernell 1981, Stromqvist et al. 1997, Naarding et al. 2005).

Like the bacterial enteropathogens, viral pathogens also utilize host cell surface glycosylated molecules as their receptors to bind and invade its host cells; the specificity of binding defines the target tissues and species specificity of the pathogen. Milk soluble glycans containing the epitope to which a pathogen will, through binding the bacterial adhesion or viral capsid, competitively inhibit pathogen binding to the host, thereby protecting against infection.

Prebiotic Activity of HMOS

Feces are one of the more dense populations of microbes in nature, and contain more than 10^{12} bacteria/gram fecal content. The large number of microorganisms at the surface of human intestines consist of over 500 species, with the majority being in phyla *Bacteroidetes*, *Firmicutes* and *Proteobacteria* (Ley et al. 2006). The intestinal microbiota is now increasingly recognized as playing important physiologic functions in the gut, especially in immune system regulation (Round and Mazmanian 2009). Beneficial bacteria of the gut microbiota, such as *Bifidobacteria* and *Lactobacilli*, are known as probiotics when they are deliberately added to the diet. The other approach to increasing their numbers in the gut are to feed indigestible dietary glycans, prebiotics, which when consumed orally, arrive intact in the distal intestine where they selectively support growth of a beneficial microbiota, including common probiotics, that benefit host health by improving fecal quality, reducing risks of gastrointestinal infections, and decreasing incidence of allergic symptoms (Rinne et al. 2005). The mucosal surface contains no enzyme that can digest HMOSs. Therefore HMOSs pass through the small intestine and arrive at the heavily colonized distal intestine, where key predominant species of the microbiota metabolized HMOSs. *Bifidobacterium* is a genus with high concentration in breast-fed infant gut. The ability of *Bifidobacterium* to metabolize HMOS is attributed to clustered genes within conserved loci that allow oligosaccharide processing and transport. These genes typically contain regulatory elements, ABC transporters, carbohydrate binding proteins, and glycoside hydrolases (Ouwehand et al. 2002). The broad strategies for consuming milk glycans can vary among different strains. For example, *Bif. infantis* consumes two short chain oligosaccharides lacto-*N*-tetraose (LNT) (Gal*β*1-3GlcNAc*β*1-3Gal*β*1-4Glc) and lacto-*N*-neotetraose (LNnT) (Gal*β*1-4GlcNAc*β*1-3Gal*β*1-4Glc). LNT and LNnT are imported into the *Bif. infantis* cell, where intracellular glycoside hydrolases degrade them to monosaccharides that enter the fructose-6-phosphate phosphoketolase central metabolic pathway (Ouwehand et al. 2002). In contrast, *Bif. bifidum* cleave LNT into two disaccharides (LNB and lactose) outside the cells using extracellular lacto-*N*-biosidase. After the cleavage, LNB is imported into cell plasma (Sela and Mills 2010).

The intestinal microbiota also contain pathobionts, such as *C. jejuni* and *E. coli*, whose overgrowth is often associated with human intestinal diseases including diarrhea or/and intestinal inflammation (Chow et al. 2011, Ayres et al. 2012, Chassaing et al. 2014). The intestinal microbiota must be balanced delicately for proper development of the host and maintenance of intestinal homeostasis. Emerging data suggest that disruption of the gut microbial ecosystem, termed dysbiosis, can significantly compromise digestive/absorptive capacity, epithelial barrier function, healthy metabolic function, and a proper immune response to injury and infection. Causes of microbial dysbiosis include enteric or systemic infection, mucosal injury, nutritional deficiency, and antibiotic treatment (Dupaul-Chicoine et al. 2013).

Of course, the major source of prebiotics for the breastfed infant is the glycan fraction of human milk, the major component of which is the HMOS. After weaning, the major source of prebiotics becomes the indigestible soluble glycans from plants. In 25 major isolates of the human intestinal microbiota, HMOSs most strongly stimulate growth of *Bifidobacteria* spp. and *Bacteroides* spp. (Yu et al. 2013b). The principle human milk oligosaccharide 2'-fucosyllactose (2'-FL) exhibit prebiotic properties on cultured infant microbiota (Yu et al. 2013a). Feeding 2'-FL and 3-fucosyllactose (3-FL) to mice increased the levels of bacteria of the *Porphyromonadaceae* family, more precisely members of the genus *Barnesiella*, in the lumen of the gut (Weiss et al. 2014). Galactosyloligosaccharides (GOS) are prepared artificially from trangalactosylation of lactose to produce a mixture that is used as a prebiotic, but GOS can also refer to the galactosyllactoses found primarily in human colostrum. Perhaps the latter should be designated hGOS. The synthetic GOS exhibits prebiotic activities, as exemplified by the stimulation of growth of beneficial microorganisms in the gastrointestinal tract (Peacock et al. 2013, Miyazaki et al. 2014). GOS supplements have also been demonstrated to be effective prebiotics for adults and for infants (Sierra et al. 2015). Human milk lactoferrin exhibits prebiotic properties by promoting growth of *Bifidobacterium* spp. *in vitro* (Arnold et al. 1980, Petschow et al. 1999).

When metabolizing prebiotics, mutualist bacteria ferment the glycans into small organic acids, including short chain fatty acids and lactate (Ward et al. 2006, Schwab and Ganzle 2011, Yu et al. 2013a). These organic acids acidify the gut and thereby inhibit colonization by pathogens, making a major contribution to health benefits for the host.

Human Milk Inhibits Inflammation

Breastfeeding is associated with a lower incidence of inflammatory diseases. Breastfed neonates have a lower risk of necrotizing enterocolitis (NEC) than those fed artificial formula, and the decrease in NEC risk is proportional to the amount of human milk that comprises the infant diet. Consistent with these associations, human milk components reduce the degree of NEC-like symptoms in the NEC neonatal rat model (Jantscher-Krenn et al. 2012). In a murine model of Inflammatory Bowel Disease (IBD), in which colitis is induced chemically, the incidence and severity of inflammation is reduced in mice receiving components of human milk (Grazioso et al. 1997). Overall, few components have been found in human milk that initiate or prolong inflammation, but many have now been identified that attenuate overwhelming inflammation (Grazioso et al. 1997). The ability of milk components to quench inflammatory signaling balances the tendency of immature gut of neonatal infants to overreact to inflammatory stimuli. The immature gut of premature infants is prone to overexpress innate inflammatory genes, such as NF-κB, MyD88, TLR2, TLR4, and TRAF, with scant expression of negative feedback regulator genes (Nanthakumar et al. 2011). The high concentrations of compounds in colostrum that lower inflammatory signaling in the gut suggest that the differences in milk composition over the course of lactation may be temporally coordinated with early maturation of function in the maturing intestinal mucosa. Moreover, breastfed infants have a lower risk of IBD in later life (Acheson and True Love 1961, Whorwell et al. 1979, Bergstrand and Hellers 1983, Ekbom et al. 1990, McGuire and Anthony 2003, Klement et al. 2004, Barclay et al. 2009).

The lower risk of IBD in individuals who had been breastfed during infancy may relate to the ability of human milk components to guide early colonization of the gut; breastfed infants are thought to have an early predominance of bifidobacteria that is greater than seen in formula-fed infant microbiota; an initial predominance of bifidobacteria and bacteroidetes may help in developing a robust microbiota whose benefits can persist into later life. For example, gut colonization by mutualists induces expression of the *fut2* gene in the intestinal mucosa, resulting in greater fucosylation of the mucosal surface, supporting stronger colonization by fucose-utilizing denizens of the microbiota. Such interkingdom communication may underlie long-term benefits of consuming breastmilk at an early age, thereby lowering risk later in life of intestinal inflammatory disorders, including IBD (Nanthakumar et al. 2000, Meng et al. 2007). Human milk glycans also affect the development and differentiation of the immune system, and play the anti-inflammatory roles directly by affecting the inflammatory signaling pathways (Grazioso et al. 1997). These can also contribute to acute and chronic resilience to various forms of intestinal insult.

Three types of bioactivity of HMOS can contribute to a reduction in inflammation in the intestinal mucosa. HMOS anti-adhesive properties inhibit the ability of pathogens to bind to their receptors of the surface of the intestinal epithelial cell, thereby reducing infection, and this, of course, reduces the need for an inflammatory response. HMOS are also strongly prebiotic, promoting colonization by mutualists, which occupy the surface of the mucosa, reducing the availability of the surface receptors to pathogen binding. The dominance of mutualists also promotes homeostasis of the microbiota and of the intestinal mucosa, adding to the resilience of the gut to inflammatory stimuli. More recently, data has emerged that HMOSs directly attenuate specific inflammatory pathways while also stimulating development and maturation of the intestinal innate immune system. In immature human intestine *ex vivo*, colostrum HMOS (cHMOS) modulated expression of several intracellular signaling networks responsible for production of cytokines associated with cell trafficking and maturation of lymphoid tissue (He et al. 2014b). The ability of cHMOS to improve the balance between Th1 and Th2 enhances defense against pathogen infection and attenuates susceptibility to food allergy and autoimmune diseases (Chen et al. 2014, He et al. 2014b). The human milk oligosaccharide lacto-N-fucopentaose III (LNFP III) contains the Lewis X (Le^x) epitope, and strongly promotes a Th2 response *in vivo*. LNFP III induces recruitment of a population of suppressor macrophages and accelerates maturation of dendritic cells; these phenomena are mediated through TLR4 dependent activation of extracellular signal-regulated kinase (ERK) and mitogen-activated protein kinase (MAPK) (Thomas et al. 2003). Another example of direct stimulation of immune signaling by HMOS is the ability of sialyl (α2,3) lactose (3SL) to arouse mesenteric lymph node CD11c$^+$ dendritic cells and cause them to release cytokines that expand Th1 and Th17 T cells (Kurakevich et al. 2013).

Several anti-inflammatory HMOSs have been defined. Disialyllacto-N-tetraose (DSLNT) suppresses NEC-like inflammation in neonatal rats (Jantscher-Krenn et al. 2012). cHMOS modulate TLR3, TLR5 and IL-1β dependent PAMP signaling pathways, depressing acute phase inflammatory cytokine protein expression (Chen et al. 2014). One oligosaccharide found in especially high concentrations in colostrum relative to mature milk, 3'-galactosyllactose (3'-GL), specifically quenches polyinosine-polycytidylic acid (the TLR3 ligand)-induced IL-8 levels (Chen et al. 2014). 2'-FL, the principle oligosaccharide in most human milk, decreases CD14 mRNA transcription and the amount of CD14 bound to membrane; these changes quench the inflammation elicited by type I pili *E. coli* infection (He et al. 2014a).

Bioactive Glycoproteins: Lactoferrin and Lactadherin

Human milk lactoferrin strongly inhibits inflammatory cytokine production at local sites of inflammation of gastrointestinal tract (Haversen et al. 2002). *In vivo*, lactoferrin protects against intestinal infection and inflammation (Venkatesh and Abrams 2010). In VLBW and ELBW preterm infants, oral administration of lactoferrin reduces the risk of late-onset sepsis (Pammi and Abrams 2015). Although treatment with lactoferrin *in vitro* can activate TRAF-6-dependent NF-κB, a TLR4 proinflammatory signaling pathway, lactoferrin simultaneously inhibits the ability of lipopolysaccharide binding protein (LBP) to adhere to TLR4; the net result is that lactoferrin inhibits LPS-stimulated TLR4 signaling and depresses endotoxemia (Legrand et al. 2005, Ando et al. 2010).

The human milk glycoprotein lactadherin can attenuate inflammation *in vivo*. In mice with DSS induced colitis, administration of lactadherin significantly ameliorated colitis and promoted mucosal repair (Chogle et al. 2011); these protective effects were attributed to its acceleration of mucosal healing. Moreover, lactadherin can also directly attenuate inflammatory processes. For example, lactoferrin elicits IL-10 and TGF-β release from regulatory T cells, which are generally anti-inflammatory and promote intestinal dendritic cell development (Zhou et al. 2010, Chogle et al. 2011, Kusunoki et al. 2012, Garcia et al. 2013). Lactadherin enhances the ability of macrophages to phagocytize apoptotic cells, thereby ameliorating inflammatory process induced by NF-κB and MAP kinases (Aziz et al. 2011). The activation of STAT3-SOCS3 pathways is activated by lactadherin, thereby directly quenching LPS-induced TNF-α production (Aziz et al. 2011, Chogle et al. 2011, Kusunoki et al. 2012).

The activities of these two glycoproteins are robust and well studied, but other glycoproteins of human milk may also have activities that are currently not as well recognized.

Glycolipids

Human milk gangliosides have a role in the healthy development of the neonatal intestinal immune system. *In vivo*, administration of milk derived GM3 and GD3 has been shown to differentially influence dendritic cell maturation and downstream effects, suggesting a role in the early postnatal modulation of oral tolerance (Bronnum et al. 2005). Moreover, dietary gangliosides stimulate proliferation of cytokine-secreting lymphocytes and production of IgA-secreting cells of the small intestine, thereby activating the intestinal immune system (Rueda 2007). In an *ex vivo* infant model of necrotizing enterocolitis, LPS exposure and hypoxia elevate pro-inflammatory signals, including nitric oxide, IL-1β, IL-6 and IL-8; gangliosides suppress the induction of these signals, thereby protecting the mucosa (Schnabl et al. 2009).

Other Bioactive Human Milk Glycans

Galactose from human milk lactose was hypothesized to support infant brain development because in humans, nursing coincides with the most rapid period of myelination in the brain. Myelin formation requires large amounts of the galactose-containing molecules galactoceramide and sulfatide; by providing the preformed galactose precursor, human milk could be ensuring that the availability of galactose does not become limiting to brain development (Newburg and Neubauer 1995). Mucosal growth and repair is another rapidly occurring process that coincides with nursing. Human milk is rich in mucins. Mucins associate with small peptides, including the trefoils in human milk, to form active complexes that protect and repair the mucus layer of the intestinal mucosa (Shirazi et al. 2000). Most of the lactadherin in milk is found complexed with mucin, and lactadherin also promotes mucosal wound healing.

Glycans of Bovine Milk

Bovine milk has a much lower concentration of oligosaccharides than human milk, and the majority of the molecules are simpler in structure than those found in human milk, particularly in mature milk relative to early milk (colostrum) (Tao et al. 2009). The human milk oligosaccharides are predominantly fucosylated, while the bovine oligosaccharides are mostly sialylated (Tao et al. 2009, Barile et al. 2010). The macromolecule glycosylation of human milk is also richer in fucose than the glycosylated macromolecules of bovine milk, and those of human milk are more richly glycosylated.

The sialylated bovine milk oligosaccharides can be thought of as analogous to HMOSs, with a similar protective role, but against pathogens that utilize sialylated receptors for infecting the calf (Gopal and Gill 2000, Tao et al. 2008, 2009). The sialylated oligosaccharides of bovine colostrum may also have a prebiotic role, but presumably for a microbiota that is more adapted to the calf gut. However, mature bovine milk contains only trace amounts of these glycans, and had been considered a poor source of oligosaccharides for human or animal use. In addition, the evaluation of bovine milk OS as a substitute for HMOS has been hindered by the lack of precise analytical methods to accurately characterize and quantify these oligosaccharides. Recently, a high-throughput strategy to annotate the human and bovine milk glycomes by using high accuracy MS has been developed (Ninonuevo and Lebrilla 2009). Using these novel techniques, dairy streams including whey permeate from cheese production have been identified as novel sources of oligosaccharides that may have functions analogous to some of the activities of HMOSs (Barile et al. 2009). Although the concentrations of these molecules are low, the volumes available from the dairy industry are enormous, making bovine milk a potentially useful source of commercially viable analogs of some of the glycans of human milk.

Lactose

Lactose is the primary sugar of the milks of most species, but colostrum contains sparse amounts of this sugar (Newburg et al. 2012). Mature term human milk contains ~6.7 g/dL of lactose (Ballard and Morrow 2013). The milk of mothers who produce higher quantities tend to have lower concentrations of fat and protein, but higher concentrations of lactose (Ballard and Morrow 2013). Lactose can be hydrolyzed into galactose and glucose by lactase (β-D-galactosidase) secreted by intestinal villi or, if not, can be fermented by bacteria in the colon. The glucose and galactose released by lactase is transported through the portal vein to the liver, where galactose can be converted to glucose (Pereira 2014). In most mammals, the production of lactase gradually declines with decreased consumption of milk at maturity.

Artificial Formula and Glycans

Substitutes for human milk have been used through the ages, with the most popular being milk of other species, often supplemented with a source of extra calories. For example, a formula based on bovine milk with added wheat flour, malt flour and potassium bicarbonate was available in 1867. Since then, some pediatricians devised improved formulas, with subsequent changes as new understanding of infant nutrition emerged. By the 1950s, application of nutritional science to artificial infant formulas resulted in improvements that, accompanied with improved hygiene, resulted in better weight gain. However, even after the improvements of the late 20th century, such as addition of polyunsaturated fatty acids docosahexaenoic acid and arachidonic acid, artificially fed infants in heavily populated areas of the world were at three- to 10-fold higher risk of disease, especially enteric infections leading to diarrhea (Newburg and Walker 2007). Recent reports associate artificial feeding of neonates with subsequent chronic diseases of later life, especially those with an autoimmune component (Newburg and Walker 2007), are consistent with protective effects and immunomodulatory activities that are unique to constituents of human milk. For example, we have identified three major functions of human milk glycans: pathogen inhibition, prebiotic function, and immune modulation. Bovine milk lacks many of the human milk oligosaccharides.

Some infant formula-producing companies have tested readily available inexpensive alternatives to HMOS, such as mixtures of galactosyloligosaccharides (GOS) and fructosyloligosaccharides (FOS) whose prebiotic effects promote a bacterial microbiota that more closely resembles that bifidobacteria-rich microbiota of breast-fed infants (Moro et al. 2002, Costalos et al. 2008). GOS/FOS supplemented formulae have also been reported to modulate the immune system in mice (Vos et al. 2006), reduce the incidence for infectious episodes (Arslanoglu et al. 2007), and suppress risk of atopic dermatitis in infants (Moro et al. 2006). However, the use of GOS/FOS is still controversial. Formula supplemented with GOS/inulin increases bacterial translocation in artificially reared newborn rats (Barrat et al. 2008). A diet supplemented with FOS increased *Salmonella enteritidis* counts and infection-induced diarrhea, and enhanced *Salmonella* translocation (Ten Bruggencate et al. 2003). In some studies, FOS impaired intestinal epithelial barrier function (Ten Bruggencate et al. 2005), but in others FOS did not affect colonic permeability (Barrat et al. 2008). Further improvement of artificial formulas may follow a more complete understanding of mechanisms of HMOS activity, and of their synthesis in quality and quantity suitable for human consumption.

Synthesis of Human Milk Glycans

Infants needing supplementation with HMOS include those fed artificial infant formula, those whose mothers have genotypes that preclude synthesis of specific HMOS, and potentially those dependent on donor milk whose fortification does not include oligosaccharides. As HMOS occur in appreciable quantities only in human milk, supplementation requires synthesis as an alternate source. Several approaches have been attempted. Naturally existing human milk glycans are synthesized through posttranslational processes, and are difficult to isolate, which limits the ease with which their synthesis can be transferred into the mammary glands of dairy animals. Moreover, the amounts necessary for human use as a supplement for breastfeeding, artificial formulas, or weaning are large. Laboratory synthesis of HMOSs had been based on chemical synthesis, enzymatic synthesis, chemical-enzymatic synthesis, or fermentation technology.

Chemical Synthesis of Glycans

Chemical synthesis of glycans starts with blocking all of the hydroxyl groups on the acceptor sugar except that to be reacted with the next sugar to form the glycoside linkage (Flowers 1978, Sinay 1998). The other sugar of the glycoside must also be blocked on all hydroxyl groups except for the relevant hydroxyl group that is required to react with the first sugar. The new molecule must be purified from the mixture of excess reagents and byproducts before repeating the process to add another sugar to grow the glycan chain. This tedious procedure can be automated, but even so, the size of the sugars is limited by side reactions. Fortunately, for most bioactive glycans from human milk, the minimum active moieties consist of 3 to 9 sugars. With automation, many of the combinations of diverse molecules can be produced and can allow structure-function relationships to be systematically explored. A major advantage of chemical synthesis is the ability to synthesize modified versions of molecules quickly. However, the number of synthesis steps (more than 20) required can be daunting; and the coupling and decoupling reactions and minimizing waste are hard to monitor. At the present time, procedures are fairly promising for making simple human oligosaccharides, but for larger molecules and more difficult linkages, the low yields become limiting. Another promising approach to chemical synthesis of the human milk glycans is the use of fluorocarbon tags for the efficient recovery of product (Roychoudhury and Pohl 2014a). Derivatization with fluorocarbon tags with recovery by solid phase extraction on fluorocarbon-derivatized silica (F-SPE) could provide synthetic sugars for use in microarrays for determining binding characteristics of known structures (Roychoudhury and Pohl 2014b).

Chemo-enzymatic Synthesis of Oligosaccharides

Chemo-enzymatic sequential synthesis involves utilizing glycosyltransferases, usually expressed through genetically engineered cells, to glycosylate a synthetic oligosaccharide precursor by a sequential series of glycosyltransferases to build more complex glycan moieties (Koeller and Wong 2000). This technology allows synthesis of branched oligosaccharides, including N-glycans of biological significance. The technology uses a core pentasaccharide that is modified at critical branching positions by orthogonal protecting groups. This allows selective attachment of unique saccharide structures by chemical glycosylation. Antenna compounds can be extended by glycosyltransferases to give large numbers of highly asymmetrical substituted multiantennary glycans. Libraries of asymmetrically substituted glycans make it possible to fabricate the next generation of glycan microarrays (Wang et al. 2013), which has been applied in the N-glycan synthesis (Wang et al. 2013) and synthetic SLeX (Soriano del Amo et al. 2010). A glycan-related enzyme expression repository was created to express all human glycosyltransferases and glycoside hydrolases as soluble, secreted catalytic domain constructs.

A related oligosaccharide synthesis is a cell-free "superbead" process. Each synthetic enzyme is attached to a bead; each bead adds a unique sugar to the substrate. The beads are assembled into a reactor column. As the substrate passes through the column, specific sugars are transferred from the appropriate nucleotide sugars to the substrate in the proper sequence, allowing synthesis of Galβ1,4GlcNAc and globotriose, among others (Zhang et al. 2003).

Pertinent to this approach, an enzyme that efficiently fucosylted sugar substrates was cloned and characterized (Engels and Elling 2014).

Synthesis by Metabolic Engineering Fermentation Technology

The synthesis strategy utilizing metabolic engineering is to put the needed transferases into *E. coli*, including the synthesis of nucleotide sugars, and culture in the presence of simple nutrients needed by bacteria. Examples of this approach are the 'superbug' of the Wang laboratory, where all needed biosynthetic genes are cloned into a single artificial gene cluster which, when inserted, generates human milk oligosaccharides by fermentation (Chen et al. 2002). Although HMOS produced by superbugs may not be compatible with medical application, this synthesis method produces oligosaccharides in a very clean reaction with a higher yield in a more energy efficient way than by chemo-enzymatic synthesis. This approach has been applied to a variety of synthetic and biochemical procedures.

In another approach, the genes and their level of expression are controlled more closely by transfecting them stepwise into a microorganism. For example, lacZ-strains of *E. coli*, which overexpressed the β1,3 N-acetylglucosaminyltransferase lgtA gene of Neisseria meningitides, produce 6 g/L trisaccharide

(GlcNAcβ1-3Galβ1-4Glc). When β1,4galactosyltransferase lgtB gene of N. meningitides was coexpressed with lgtA, the trisaccharide was further converted to lacto-N-neotetraose (Galβ1-4GlcNAcβ1-3Galβ1-4Glc) and lacto-N-neohexaose with a yield higher than 5 g/ L (Priem et al. 2002).

Similarly, fucosyltransferase is inserted into the microbe and it is fed lactose and fucose to produce a fucosylated trisaccharide (Dumon et al. 2006). In a more recent approach, enzymes for synthesis of GDP-fucose from glucose are inserted, and lactose is included in the medium so that it is fucosylated after entering the cell. Using this type of engineering, *E. coli* produce about 40 g/L of 2'-FL into the medium during fermentation, and the 2'-FL can be purified from the medium with 95% to 98% purity after only a few steps of purification. Using this approach, bacteria have been engineered to individually synthesize each of 15 human milk oligosaccharides, including 2'-FL, 3-FL, LDFT, 6'-SL, LNnT, and LNT (Newburg and Grave 2014).

Conclusions

Human milk is the best food for infants, as the exclusive food for 4–6 months, and continuing as an important part of mixed feeding thereafter. The nutrient content supports optimum (not the largest) body weight gain, and is now recognized as providing many bioactive components that inhibit pathogens, promote growth of a microbiome rich in mutualists, modulate mucosal inflammation, and promote development of many aspects of the enteric immune system. The multiplicity and high content of glycans in human milk includes lactose, HMOS, glycoproteins, glycosaminoproteoglycans, glycolipids and monosaccharides. In addition to helping support brain growth, the aspect of infant development with the greatest need for exogenous nutrients, human milk glycans protect the neonate from gastrointestinal diseases and their sequelae, thereby avoiding the channeling of nutrients from development to defensive processes. Three major biological activities of milk glycans include: Firstly, protection from pathogen infection through competing with mucosal cell surface receptorepitopes that are the targets for pathogens and pathogenic toxins, or, for sIgs directly suppressing pathogenic microbes. Secondly, human milk glycans, especially HMOS, are prebiotic, promoting growth of mutualist microbes of the gut microbiota, which contribute toward maintenance of mucosa homeostasis. In immature gut, human milk glycans also stimulate mucosal development and soothe exaggerated inflammation. Individual components that play important roles in human milk protection have been identified. Synthesis of human milk glycans, especially of individual HMOSs, has been successfully achieved in the laboratory. This recent availability now facilitates studies on mechanisms of action and will allow clinical trials of pure molecules as nutritional supplements. Human milk glycans for prophylaxis and treatment of neonatal diseases and chronic gut inflammation is very promising. Further knowledge concerning the components of human milk, including enzymes, hormones, activators, and inhibitors, that includes their dynamic changes over the course of lactation and mechanisms whereby they exert metabolic control on the nursing infant, are on the horizon. Additional understanding of the unique active components of this exceptional and complex biological fluid, human milk, is highly likely to result in even more promising novel prophylactic and therapeutic candidate molecules.

Acknowledgements

Partially supported by NIH grants R01HD059140, U01AI075563, and P01HD013021. We thank Dr. Charles E. Isaacs, New York Institute for Basic Research, for reviewing and editing this chapter.

Keywords: Human milk, oligosaccharides, glycans, bioactive, prebiotic, antimicrobial, adhesion, inflammation, synthesis, weaning, microbiota

References

Acheson, E. D. and S. C. True Love. 1961. Early weaning in the aetiology of ulcerative colitis. A study of feeding in infancy in cases and controls. Br Med J 2: 929–933.
Adlerova, L., A. Bartoskova and M. Faldyna. 2008. Lactoferrin: A review. Vet Med 9: 457–465.

Ando, K., K. Hasegawa, K. Shindo, T. Furusawa, T. Fujino, K. Kikugawa et al. 2010. Human lactoferrin activates NF-kappaB through the Toll-like receptor 4 pathway while it interferes with the lipopolysaccharide-stimulated TLR4 signaling. FEBS J 277: 2051–2066.

Arnold, R. R., M. Brewer and J. J. Gauthier. 1980. Bactericidal activity of human lactoferrin: Sensitivity of a variety of microorganisms. Infect Immun 28: 893–898.

Arslanoglu, S., G. E. Moro and G. Boehm. 2007. Early supplementation of prebiotic oligosaccharides protects formula-fed infants against infections during the first 6 months of life. J Nutr 137: 2420–2424.

Ayres, J. S., N. J. Trinidad and R. E. Vance. 2012. Lethal inflammasome activation by a multidrug-resistant pathobiont upon antibiotic disruption of the microbiota. Nat Med 18: 799–806.

Aziz, M., A. Jacob, A. Matsuda and P. Wang. 2011. Review: Milk fat globule-EGF factor 8 expression, function and plausible signal transduction in resolving inflammation. Apoptosis 16: 1077–1086.

Ballard, O. and A. L. Morrow. 2013. Human milk composition: Nutrients and bioactive factors. Pediatr Clin North Am 60: 49–74.

Barclay, A. R., R. K. Russell, M. L. Wilson, W. H. Gilmour, J. Satsangi and D. C. Wilson. 2009. Systematic review: The role of breastfeeding in the development of pediatric inflammatory bowel disease. J Pediatr 155: 421–426.

Barrat, E., C. Michel, G. Poupeau, A. David-Sochard, M. Rival, A. Pagniez et al. 2008. Supplementation with galactooligosaccharides and inulin increases bacterial translocation in artificially reared newborn rats. Pediatr Res 64: 34–39.

Barile, D., N. Tao, C. B. Lebrilla, J. D. Coisson, M. Arlorio and J. B. German. 2009. Permeate from cheese whey ultrafiltration is a source of milk oligosaccharides. Int Dairy J 19: 524–530.

Barile, D., M. Marotta, C. Chu, R. Mehra, R. Grimm, C. B. Lebrilla et al. 2010. Neutral and acidic oligosaccharides in Holstein-Friesian colostrum during the first 3 days of lactation measured by high performance liquid chromatography on a microfluidic chip and time-of-flight mass spectrometry. J Dairy Sci 93: 3940–3949.

Bergstrand, O. and G. Hellers. 1983. Breast-feeding during infancy in patients who later develop Crohn's disease. Scand J Gastroenterol 18: 903–906.

Blackberg, L. and O. Hernell. 1981. The bile-salt-stimulated lipase in human milk. Purification and characterization. Eur J Biochem 116: 221–225.

Bode, L., M. McGuire, J. M. Rodriguez, D. T. Geddes, F. Hassiotou, P. E. Hartmann et al. 2014. It's alive: Microbes and cells in human milk and their potential benefits to mother and infant. Adv Nutr 5: 571–573.

Bouchara, J., P. M. Sanchez, A. Chevailler, A. Marot-Leblond, J. C. Lissitzky, G. Tronchin et al. 1997. Sialic acid-dependent recognition of laminin and fibrinogen by Aspergillus fumigatus conidia. Infect Immun 65: 2717–2724.

Bouhours, J. F. and D. Bouhours. 1981. Ceramide structure of sphingomyelin from human milk fat globule membrane. Lipids 16: 726–731.

Brock, J. H. 1980. Lactoferrin in human milk: Its role in iron absorption and protection against enteric infection in the newborn infant. Arch Dis Child 55: 417–421.

Bronnum, H., T. Seested, L. I. Hellgren, S. Brix and H. Frokiaer. 2005. Milk-derived GM(3) and GD(3) differentially inhibit dendritic cell maturation and effector functionalities. Scand J Immunol 61: 551–557.

Capuco, A. V. and R. M. Akers. 2009. The origin and evolution of lactation. J Biol 8: 37.

Cerini, C. and G. M. Aldrovandi. 2013. Breast milk: Proactive immunomodulation and mucosal protection against viruses and other pathogens. Future Virology 8: 1127–1134.

Chassaing, B., O. Koren, F. A. Carvalho, R. E. Ley and A. T. Gewirtz. 2014. AIEC pathobiont instigates chronic colitis in susceptible hosts by altering microbiota composition. Gut 63: 1069–1080.

Chaturvedi, P., C. D. Warren, M. Altaye, A. L. Morrow, G. Ruiz-Palacios, L. K. Pickering et al. 2001. Fucosylated human milk oligosaccharides vary between individuals and over the course of lactation. Glycobiology 11: 365–372.

Chen, X., Z. Liu, J. Zhang, W. Zhang, P. Kowal and P. G. Wang. 2002. Reassembled Biosynthetic pathway for large-scale carbohydrate synthesis: a-Gal epitope producing "Superbug". Chembiochem 3: 47–53.

Chen, A. C., M. Y. Chung, J. H. Chang and H. C. Lin. 2014. Pathogenesis implication for necrotizing enterocolitis prevention in preterm very-low-birth-weight infants. J Pediatr Gastroenterol Nutr 58: 7–11.

Chogle, A., H. F. Bu, X. Wang, J. B. Brown, P. M. Chou and X. D. Tan. 2011. Milk fat globule-EGF factor 8 is a critical protein for healing of dextran sodium sulfate-induced acute colitis in mice. Mol Med 17: 502–507.

Chow, J., H. Tang and S. K. Mazmanian. 2011. Pathobionts of the gastrointestinal microbiota and inflammatory disease. Curr Opin Immunol 23: 473–480.

Coppa, G. V., O. Gabrielli, P. Pierani, C. Catassi, A. Carlucci and P. L. Giorgi. 1993. Changes in carbohydrate composition in human milk over 4 months of lactation. Pediatrics 91: 637–641.

Costalos, C., A. Kapiki, M. Apostolou and E. Papathoma. 2008. The effect of a prebiotic supplemented formula on growth and stool microbiology of term infants. Early Hum Dev 84: 45–49.

Dumon, C., C. Bosso, J. P. Utille, A. Heyraud and E. Samain. 2006. Production of Lewis x tetrasaccharides by metabolically engineered *Escherichia coli*. Chembiochem 7: 359–365.

Dupaul-Chicoine, J., M. Dagenais and M. Saleh. 2013. Crosstalk between the intestinal microbiota and the innate immune system in intestinal homeostasis and inflammatory bowel disease. Inflamm. Bowel Dis 19: 2227–2237.

Ekbom, A., H. O. Adami, C. G. Helmick, A. Jonzon and M. M. Zack. 1990. Perinatal risk factors for inflammatory bowel disease: A case-control study. Am J Epidemiol 132: 1111–1119.

Engels, L. and L. Elling. 2014. WbgL: A novel bacterial alpha 1,2-fucosyltransferase for the synthesis of 2'-fucosyllactose. Glycobiology 24: 170–178.

Flowers, H. M. 1978. Chemical synthesis of oligosaccharides. Methods Enzymol 50: 93–121.

Garcia, C., R. D. Duan, V. Brevaut-Malaty, C. Gire, V. Millet, U. Simeoni et al. 2013. Bioactive compounds in human milk and intestinal health and maturity in preterm newborn: An overview. Cell Mol Biol (Noisy-le-grand) 59: 108–131.

Garofalo, R. 2010. Cytokines in human milk. J Pediatr 156: S36–40.

Gopal, P. K. and H. S. Gill. 2000. Oligosaccharides and glycoconjugates in bovine milk and colostrum. Br J Nutr 84 Suppl 1: S69–74.

Grazioso, C. F., A. L. Werner, D. W. Alling, P. R. Bishop and E. S. Buescher. 1997. Antiinflammatory effects of human milk on chemically induced colitis in rats. Pediatr Res 42: 639–643.

Hassiotou, F., A. Beltran, E. Chetwynd, A. M. Stuebe, A. J. Twigger, P. Metzger et al. 2012. Breast milk is a novel source of stem cells with multilineage differentiation potential. Stem Cells 30: 2164–2174.

Hassiotou, F., B. Heath, O. Ocal, L. Filgueira, D. Geddes, P. Hartmann et al. 2014. Breastmilk stem cell transfer from mother to neonatal organs (216.4). FASEB J 28.

Haversen, L., B. G. Ohlsson, M. Hahn-Zoric, L. A. Hanson and I. Mattsby-Baltzer. 2002. Lactoferrin down-regulates the LPS-induced cytokine production in monocytic cells via NF-kappa B. Cell Immunol 220: 83–95.

He, Y., S. Liu, D. E. Kling, S. Leone, N. T. Lawlor, Y. Huang et al. 2014a. The human milk oligosaccharide 2'-fucosyllactose modulates CD14 expression in human enterocytes, thereby attenuating LPS-induced inflammation. Gut [Epub ahead of print]. PMID: 25431457.

He, Y., S. Liu, S. Leone and D. S. Newburg. 2014b. Human colostrum oligosaccharides modulate major immunologic pathways of immature human intestine. Mucosal Immunol 7: 1326–1339.

He, Y., N. T. Lawlor and D. S. Newburg. 2015. Human milk components that curb Toll-like receptor-mediated gut inflammation (in preparation).

Hill, D. R. and D. S. Newburg. 2015. Clinical applications of bioactive milk components. Nutr Rev [Epub ahead of print]. PMID: 26011900.

Hunt, K. M., J. A. Foster, L. J. Forney, U. M. Schutte, D. L. Beck, Z. Abdo et al. 2011. Characterization of the diversity and temporal stability of bacterial communities in human milk. PLoS One 6: e21313.

Ichikawa, M., M. Sugita, M. Takahashi, M. Satomi, T. Takeshita, T. Araki et al. 2003. Breast milk macrophages spontaneously produce granulocyte-macrophage colony-stimulating factor and differentiate into dendritic cells in the presence of exogenous interleukin-4 alone. Immunology 108: 189–195.

Idota, T. and H. Kawakami. 1995. Inhibitory effects of milk gangliosides on the adhesion of *Escherichia coli* to human intestinal carcinoma cells. Biosci Biotechnol Biochem 59: 69–72.

Jantscher-Krenn, E., M. Zherebtsov, C. Nissan, K. Goth, Y. S. Guner, N. Naidu et al. 2012. The human milk oligosaccharide disialyllacto-N-tetraose prevents necrotising enterocolitis in neonatal rats. Gut 61: 1417–1425.

Jenness, R. 1979. The composition of human milk. Semin Perinatol 3: 225–239.

Khodayar-Pardo, P., L. Mira-Pascual, M. C. Collado and C. Martinez-Costa. 2014. Impact of lactation stage, gestational age and mode of delivery on breast milk microbiota. J Perinatol 34: 599–605.

Klement, E., R. V. Cohen, J. Boxman, A. Joseph and S. Reif. 2004. Breastfeeding and risk of inflammatory bowel disease: A systematic review with meta-analysis. Am J Clin Nutr 80: 1342–1352.

Koeller, K. M. and C. H. Wong. 2000. Synthesis of complex carbohydrates and glycoconjugates: Enzyme-based and programmable one-pot strategies. Chem Rev 100: 4465–4494.

Kourtis, A. P., C. C. Ibegbu, R. Theiler, Y. X. Xu, P. Bansil, D. J. Jamieson et al. 2007. Breast milk CD4+ T cells express high levels of C chemokine receptor 5 and CXC chemokine receptor 4 and are preserved in HIV-infected mothers receiving highly active antiretroviral therapy. J Infect Dis 195: 965–972.

Kunz, C., S. Rudloff, W. Baier, N. Klein and S. Strobel. 2000. Oligosaccharides in human milk: Structural, functional, and metabolic aspects. Annu Rev Nutr 20: 699–722.

Kurakevich, E., T. Hennet, M. Hausmann, G. Rogler and L. Borsig. 2013. Milk oligosaccharide sialyl(alpha2,3)lactose activates intestinal CD11c+ cells through TLR4. Proc Natl Acad Sci U S A 110: 17444–17449.

Kusunoki, R., S. Ishihara, M. Aziz, A. Oka, Y. Tada and Y. Kinoshita. 2012. Roles of milk fat globule-epidermal growth factor 8 in intestinal inflammation. Digestion 85: 103–107.

Kverka, M., J. Burianova, R. Lodinova-ZadnikovaI. Kocourkova, J. Cinova, L. Tuckova et al. 2007. Cytokine profiling in human colostrum and milk by protein array. Clin Chem 53: 955–962.

Lawrence, R. A. 1999. Storage of human milk and the influence of procedures on immunological components of human milk. Acta Paediatr Suppl 88: 14–18.

Le Pendu, J. 2004. Histo-blood group antigen and human milk oligosaccharides: Genetic polymorphism and risk of infectious diseases. Adv Exp Med Biol 554: 135–143.

Legrand, D., E. Elass, M. Carpentier and J. Mazurier. 2005. Lactoferrin: A modulator of immune and inflammatory responses. Cell Mol Life Sci 62: 2549–2559.

Ley, R. E., P. J. Turnbaugh, S. Klein and J. I. Gordon. 2006. Microbial ecology: Human gut microbes associated with obesity. Nature 444: 1022–1023.

Li, M., M. H. Monaco, M. Wang, S. S. Comstock, T. B. Kuhlenschmidt, G. C. Fahey, Jr. et al. 2014. Human milk oligosaccharides shorten rotavirus-induced diarrhea and modulate piglet mucosal immunity and colonic microbiota. ISME J 8: 1609–1620.

Linden, S. K., P. Sutton, N. G. Karlsson, V. Korolik and M. A. McGuckin. 2008. Mucins in the mucosal barrier to infection. Mucosal Immunol 1: 183–197.

Liu, B., Z. Yu, C. Chen, D. E. Kling and D. S. Newburg. 2012. Human milk mucin 1 and mucin 4 inhibit *Salmonella enterica* serovar Typhimurium invasion of human intestinal epithelial cells *in vitro*. J Nutr 142: 1504–1509.

Liu, B. and D. S. Newburg. 2013. Human milk glycoproteins protect infants against human pathogens. Breastfeed Med 8: 354–362.

Lonnerdal, B., E. Forsum and L. Hambraeus. 1976. A longitudinal study of the protein, nitrogen, and lactose contents of human milk from Swedish well-nourished mothers. Am J Clin Nutr 29: 1127–1133.

Lonnerdal, B. 2014. Infant formula and infant nutrition: Bioactive proteins of human milk and implications for composition of infant formulas. Am J Clin Nutr 99: 712S–717S.

Martinez-Costa, C., M. D. Silvestre, M. C. Lopez, A. Plaza, M. Miranda and R. Guijarro. 2007. Effects of refrigeration on the bactericidal activity of human milk: A preliminary study. J Pediatr Gastroenterol Nutr 45: 275–277.

McGuire, W. and M. Y. Anthony. 2003. Donor human milk versus formula for preventing necrotising enterocolitis in preterm infants: Systematic review. Arch Dis Child Fetal Neonatal Ed 88: F11–14.

Meng, D., D. S. Newburg, C. Young, A. Baker, S. L. Tonkonogy, R. B. Sartor et al. 2007. Bacterial symbionts induce a FUT2-dependent fucosylated niche on colonic epithelium via ERK and JNK signaling. Am J Physiol Gastrointest Liver Physiol 293: G780–787.

Mitoulas, L. R., J. C. Kent, D. B. Cox, R. A. Owens, J. L. Sherriff and P. E. Hartmann. 2002. Variation in fat, lactose and protein in human milk over 24 h and throughout the first year of lactation. Br J Nutr 88: 29–37.

Miyazaki, K., N. Masuoka, M. Kano and R. Iizuka. 2014. Bifidobacterium fermented milk and galacto-oligosaccharides lead to improved skin health by decreasing phenols production by gut microbiota. Benef Microbes 5: 121–128.

Moro, G., I. Minoli, M. Mosca, S. Fanaro, J. Jelinek, B. Stahl et al. 2002. Dosage-related bifidogenic effects of galacto- and fructooligosaccharides in formula-fed term infants. J Pediatr Gastroenterol Nutr 34: 291–295.

Moro, G., S. Arslanoglu, B. Stahl, J. Jelinek, U. Wahn and G. Boehm. 2006. A mixture of prebiotic oligosaccharides reduces the incidence of atopic dermatitis during the first six months of age. Arch Dis Child 91: 814–819.

Morrow, A. L., G. M. Ruiz-Palacios, M. Altaye, X. Jiang, M. L. Guerrero, K. Meinzen-Derr et al. 2004. Human milk oligosaccharides are associated with protection against diarrhea in breast-fed infants. J Pediatr 145: 297–303.

Murphy, J. F., M. L. Neale and N. Matthews. 1983. Antimicrobial properties of preterm breast milk cells. Arch Dis Child 58: 198–200.

Mysore, J. V., T. Wigginton, P. M. Simon, D. Zopf, L. M. Heman-Ackah and A. Dubois. 1999. Treatment of Helicobacter pylori infection in rhesus monkeys using a novel antiadhesion compound. Gastroenterology 117: 1316–1325.

Naarding, M. A., I. S. Ludwig, F. Groot, B. Berkhout, T. B. Geijtenbeek, G. Pollakis et al. 2005. Lewis X component in human milk binds DC-SIGN and inhibits HIV-1 transfer to CD4$^+$ T lymphocytes. J Clin Invest 115: 3256–3264.

Nanthakumar, N. N., R. D. Fusunyan, I. Sanderson and W. A. Walker. 2000. Inflammation in the developing human intestine: A possible pathophysiologic contribution to necrotizing enterocolitis. Proc Natl Acad Sci USA 97: 6043–6048.

Nanthakumar, N. N., D. Meng, A. M. Goldstein, W. Zhu, L. Lu, R. Uauy et al. 2011. The mechanism of excessive intestinal inflammation in necrotizing enterocolitis: An immature innate immune response. PLoS One 6: e17776.

Newburg, D. S. and S. H. Neubauer. 1995. Analytical measurement of carbohydrates in milk. pp. 274–349. *In*: Jensen, R. G. (ed.). Handbook of Milk Composition. Academic Press, San Diego, California, USA.

Newburg, D. S., P. Chaturvedi, J. K. Crane, T. G. Cleary and L. K. Pickering. 1995a. Fucosylated oligosaccharides of human milk inhibits stable toxin of *Escherichia coli*. pp. 199–226. *In*: Agrawal, V.P., Sharma C. B., Sah A. and Zingde M.D. (eds.). Complex Carbohydrates and Advances in Biosciences, Muzaffarnagar, India: Society of Biosciences.

Newburg, D. S., R. J. Linhardt, S. A. Ampofo and R. H. Yolken. 1995b. Human milk glycosaminoglycans inhibit HIV glycoprotein gp120 binding to its host cell CD4 receptor. J Nutr 125: 419–424.

Newburg, D. S., J. A. Peterson, G. M. Ruiz-Palacios, D. O. Matson, A. L. Morrow, J. Shults et al. 1998. Role of human-milk lactadherin in protection against symptomatic rotavirus infection. Lancet 351: 1160–1164.

Newburg, D. S., G. M. Ruiz-Palacios and A. L. Morrow. 2005. Human milk glycans protect infants against enteric pathogens. Annu Rev Nutr 25: 37–58.

Newburg, D. S. and W. A. Walker. 2007. Protection of the neonate by the innate immune system of developing gut and of human milk. Pediatr Res 61: 2–8.

Newburg, D. S., C. Chen and G. Wiederschain. 2012. Analysis of human milk lactose. pp. 570–588. *In*: Preedy, V. (ed.). Dietary Sugars: Chemistry, Analysis, Function, and Effects. Series: Food and Nutritional Components in Focus. The Royal Society of Chemistry, Cambridge, UK.

Newburg, D. S. 2013. Glycobiology of human milk. Biochemistry (Mosc) 78: 771–785.

Newburg, D. S. and G. Grave. 2014. Recent advances in human milk glycobiology. Pediatr Res 75: 675–679.

Ninonuevo, M. R. and C. B. Lebrilla. 2009. Mass spectrometric methods for analysis of oligosaccharides in human milk. Nutr Rev 67 Suppl 2: S216–226.

Orsi, N. 2004. The antimicrobial activity of lactoferrin: Current status and perspectives. Biometals 17: 189–196.

Ouwehand, A. C., S. Salminen and E. Isolauri. 2002. Probiotics: An overview of beneficial effects. Antonie Van Leeuwenhoek 82: 279–289.

Pammi, M. and S. A. Abrams. 2015. Oral lactoferrin for the prevention of sepsis and necrotizing enterocolitis in preterm infants. Cochrane Database Syst Rev 2: Cd007137.

Peacock, K. S., L. R. Ruhaak, M. K. Tsui, D. A. Mills and C. B. Lebrilla. 2013. Isomer-specific consumption of galactooligosaccharides by bifidobacterial species. J Agric Food Chem 61: 12612–12619.

Pereira, P. C. 2014. Milk nutritional composition and its role in human health. Nutrition 30: 619–627.

Peterson, R., W. Y. Cheah, J. Grinyer and N. Packer. 2013. Glycoconjugates in human milk: Protecting infants from disease. Glycobiology 23: 1425–1438.

Petschow, B. W., R. D. Talbott and R. P. Batema. 1999. Ability of lactoferrin to promote the growth of *Bifidobacterium* spp. *in vitro* is independent of receptor binding capacity and iron saturation level. J Med Microbiol 48: 541–549.

Priem, B., M. Gilbert, W. W. Wakarchuk, A. Heyraud and E. Samain. 2002. A new fermentation process allows large-scale production of human milk oligosaccharides by metabolically engineered bacteria. Glycobiology 12: 235–240.

Rama, B. and B. S. Turner. 2006. Mucin structure, aggregation, physiological functions and biomedical applications. Curr Opin Colloid Interface Sci 11: 164–170.

Rinne, M., M. Kalliomaki, H. Arvilommi, S. Salminen and E. Isolauri. 2005. Effect of probiotics and breastfeeding on the bifidobacterium and lactobacillus/enterococcus microbiota and humoral immune responses. J Pediatr 147: 186–191.

Round, J. L. and S. K. Mazmanian. 2009. The gut microbiota shapes intestinal immune responses during health and disease. Nat Rev Immunol 9: 313–323.

Roychoudhury, R. and N. L. Pohl. 2014a. Light fluorous-tag-assisted synthesis of oligosaccharides, in modern synthetic methods. pp. 221–239. *In*: Werz, D. B. and S. Vidal (eds.). Carbohydrate Chemistry: From Monosaccharides to Complex Glycoconjugates. Wiley-VCH Verlag GmbH & Co. KGaA, Weinheim, Germany.

Roychoudhury, R. and N. L. Pohl. 2014b. Synthesis of fluorous photolabile aldehyde and carbamate and alkyl carbamate protecting groups for carbohydrate-associated amines. Org Lett 16: 1156–1159.

Rueda, R. 2007. The role of dietary gangliosides on immunity and the prevention of infection. Br J Nutr 98 Suppl 1: S68–73.

Ruiz-Palacios, G. M., J. J. Calva, L. K. Pickering, Y. Lopez-Vidal, P. Volkow, H. Pezzarossi et al. 1990. Protection of breast-fed infants against campylobacter diarrhea by antibodies in human milk. J Pediatr 116: 707–713.

Ruiz-Palacios, G. M., L. E. Cervantes, P. Ramos, B. Chavez-Munguia and D. S. Newburg. 2003. *Campylobacter jejuni* binds intestinal H(O) antigen (Fuc alpha 1, 2Gal beta 1, 4GlcNAc), and fucosyloligosaccharides of human milk inhibit its binding and infection. J Biol Chem 278: 14112–14120.

Sabbaj, S. B., H. Edwards, M. K. Ghosh, K. Semrau, S. Cheelo, D. M. Thea et al. 2002. Human immunodeficiency virus-specific CD8(+) T cells in human breast milk. J Virol 76: 7365–7373.

Saeland, E., M. A. de Jong, A. A. Nabatov, H. Kalay, T. B. Geijtenbeek and Y. van Kooyk. 2009. MUC1 in human milk blocks transmission of human immunodeficiency virus from dendritic cells to T cells. Mol Immunol 46: 2309–2316.

Schnabl, K. L., B. Larsen, J. E. VanAerde, G. Lees, M. Evans, M. Belosevic et al. 2009. Gangliosides protect bowel in an infant model of necrotizing enterocolitis by suppressing proinflammatory signals. J Pediatr Gastroenterol Nutr 49: 382–392.

Schroten, H., F. G. Hanisch, R. Plogmann, J. Hacker, G. Uhlenbruck, R. Nobis-Bosch et al. 1992. Inhibition of adhesion of S-fimbriated *Escherichia coli* to buccal epithelial cells by human milk fat globule membrane components: a novel aspect of the protective function of mucins in the nonimmunoglobulin fraction. Infect Immun 60: 2893–2899.

Schwab, C. and M. Ganzle. 2011. Lactic acid bacteria fermentation of human milk oligosaccharide components, human milk oligosaccharides and galactooligosaccharides. FEMS Microbiol Lett 315: 141–148.

Sela, D. A. and D. A. Mills. 2010. Nursing our microbiota: Molecular linkages between bifidobacteria and milk oligosaccharides. Trends Microbiol 18: 298–307.

Shin, K., H. Hayasawa and B. Lonnerdal. 2001. Purification and quantification of lactoperoxidase in human milk with use of immunoadsorbents with antibodies against recombinant human lactoperoxidase. Am J Clin Nutr 73: 984–989.

Shirazi, T., R. J. Longman, A. P. Corfield and C. S. Probert. 2000. Mucins and inflammatory bowel disease. Postgrad Med J 76: 473–478.

Sierra, C., M. J. Bernal, J. Blasco, R. Martinez, J. D. Ortuno et al. 2015. Prebiotic effect during the first year of life in healthy infants fed formula containing GOS as the only prebiotic: a multicentre, randomised, double-blind and placebo-controlled trial. Eur J Nutr 54: 89–99.

Sinay, P. 1998. Chemical synthesis of oligosaccharide mimetics. Pure & Appl Chem 70: 407–410.

Soriano del Amo, D., W. Wang, C. Besanceney, T. Zheng, Y. He, B. Gerwe et al. 2010. Chemoenzymatic synthesis of the sialyl Lewis X glycan and its derivatives. Carbohydr Res 345: 1107–1113.

Speer, C. P., R. Schatz and M. Gahr. 1985. Function of breast milk macrophages. Monatsschr Kinderheilkd 133: 913–917.

Stins, M. F., N. V. Prasadarao, L. Ibric, C. A. Wass, P. Luckett and K. S. Kim. 1994. Binding characteristics of S fimbriated *Escherichia coli* to isolated brain microvascular endothelial cells. Am J Pathol 145: 1228–1236.

Stromqvist, M., O. Hernell, L. Hansson, K. Lindgren, A. Skytt, L. Lundberg et al. 1997. Naturally occurring variants of human milk bile salt-stimulated lipase. Arch Biochem Biophys 347: 30–36.

Tao, N., E. J. DePeters, S. Freeman, J. B. German, R. Grimm and C. B. Lebrilla. 2008. Bovine milk glycome. J Dairy Sci 91: 3768–3778.

Tao, N., E. J. DePeters, J. B. German, R. Grimm and C. B. Lebrilla. 2009. Variations in bovine milk oligosaccharides during early and middle lactation stages analyzed by high-performance liquid chromatography-chip/mass spectrometry. J Dairy Sci 92: 2991–3001.

Ten Bruggencate, S. J., I. M. Bovee-Oudenhoven, M. L. Lettink-Wissink and R. Van der Meer. 2003. Dietary fructo-oligosaccharides dose-dependently increase translocation of salmonella in rats. J Nutr 133: 2313–2318.

Ten Bruggencate, S. J., I. M. Bovee-Oudenhoven, M. L. Lettink-Wissink and R. Van der Meer. 2005. Dietary fructooligosaccharides increase intestinal permeability in rats. J Nutr 135: 837–842.

Thomas, P. G., M. R. Carter, O. Atochina, A. A. Da'Dara, D. Piskorska, E. McGuire et al. 2003. Maturation of dendritic cell 2 phenotype by a helminth glycan uses a Toll-like receptor 4-dependent mechanism. J Immunol 171: 5837–5841.

Venkatesh, M. P. and S. A. Abrams. 2010. Oral lactoferrin for the prevention of sepsis and necrotizing enterocolitis in preterm infants. Cochrane Database Syst Rev 5: Cd007137.

Virkola, R., J. Parkkinen, J. Hacker and T. K. Korhonen. 1993. Sialyloligosaccharide chains of laminin as an extracellular matrix target for S fimbriae of *Escherichia coli*. Infect Immun 61: 4480–4484.

Vos, A. P., M. Haarman, A. Buco, M. Govers, J. Knol, J. Garssen et al. 2006. A specific prebiotic oligosaccharide mixture stimulates delayed-type hypersensitivity in a murine influenza vaccination model. Int Immunopharmacol 6: 1277–1286.

Wang, Z., Z. S. Chinoy, S. G. Ambre, W. Peng, R. McBride, R. P. de Vries et al. 2013. A general strategy for the chemoenzymatic synthesis of asymmetrically branched N-glycans. Science 341: 379–383.

Ward, R. E., M. Ninonuevo, D. A. Mills, C. B. Lebrilla and J. B. German. 2006. *In vitro* fermentation of breast milk oligosaccharides by Bifidobacterium infantis and Lactobacillus gasseri. Appl Environ Microbiol 72: 4497–4499.

Watson, C. J. and W. T. Khaled. 2008. Mammary development in the embryo and adult: a journey of morphogenesis and commitment. Development 135: 995–1003.

Weiss, G. A., C. Chassard and T. Hennet. 2014. Selective proliferation of intestinal Barnesiella under fucosyllactose supplementation in mice. Br J Nutr 111: 1602–1610.

Whorwell, P. J., G. Holdstock, G. M. Whorwell and R. Wright. 1979. Bottle feeding, early gastroenteritis, and inflammatory bowel disease. Br Med J 1: 382.

Wiederschain, G. Y. and D. S. Newburg. 1996. Compartmentalization of fucosyltransferase and alpha-L-fucosidase in human milk. Biochem Mol Med 58: 211–220.

Wiederschain, G. Y. and D. S. Newburg. 2001. Glycoconjugate stability in human milk: Glycosidase activities and sugar release. J Nutr Biochem 12: 559–564.

Yolken, R. H., J. A. Peterson, S. L. Vonderfecht, E. T. Fouts, K. Midthun and D. S. Newburg. 1992. Human milk mucin inhibits rotavirus replication and prevents experimental gastroenteritis. J Clin Invest 90: 1984–1991.

Yu, Z. T., C. Chen, D. E. Kling, B. Liu, J. M. McCoy, M. Merighi et al. 2013a. The principal fucosylated oligosaccharides of human milk exhibit prebiotic properties on cultured infant microbiota. Glycobiology 23: 169–177.

Yu, Z. T., C. Chen and D. S. Newburg. 2013b. Utilization of major fucosylated and sialylated human milk oligosaccharides by isolated human gut microbes. Glycobiology 23: 1281–1292.

Zhang, J., X. Chen, J. Shao, Z. Liu, P. Kowal, Y. Lu et al. 2003. Synthesis of galactose-containing oligosaccharides through superbeads and superbug approaches: Substrate recognition along different biosynthetic pathways. Methods Enzymol 362: 106–124.

Zhou, Y. J., J. Gao, H. M. Yang, X. L. Yuan, T. X. Chen and Z. J. He. 2010. The role of the lactadherin in promoting intestinal DCs development *in vivo* and *vitro*. Clin Dev Immunol 2010: 357541.

CHAPTER 13

Molecular Mechanisms Underlying the Association between Gaucher Disease and Parkinson's Disease

Gali Maor[a] and *Mia Horowitz**

Introduction and Overview

Gaucher disease (GD), an inherited lysosomal storage disorder characterized by impaired activity of the lysosomal enzyme β-glucocerebrosidase (GCase), results from mutations in the corresponding GBA gene. Due to the impaired activity of mutant GCase, there is accumulation of lysosomal glucosylceramide, which ultimately leads to lysosomal dysfunction (Beutler 1980, Beutler and Dale 1982, Brady 1982, Beutler and Gelbart 1996, Beutler 1999). Due to its heterogeneity, GD was divided into three types: type 1, primarily a non-neurological disease; type 2, the acute neuronopathic disease; and type 3, the sub-acute neuronopathic disease (Hruska et al. 2008). The hallmark of GD is reduced lysosomal GCase activity and elevation in glucosylceramide levels mainly in monocyte derived cells. The reduced lysosomal GCase activity reflects the fact that mutant GCase variants are recognized in the endoplasmic reticulum ER as misfolded, and are retained there by the ER quality control machinery, in an attempt to correctly fold the mutant molecules. This ER retention leads to ER stress and eventually to ER stress response, known as the unfolded protein response (UPR), and ER associated degradation (ERAD) (Kono et al. 2010), which involves retrotranslocation of the mutant molecules through the ER membrane into the cytosol where they undergo ubiquitination and proteasomal degradation. The level of ERAD is directly correlated to disease severity (Ron and Horowitz 2005, Mu et al. 2008, Maor et al. 2013).

In recent years, a large number of independent studies documented the association between GD and Parkinson's disease (PD) (Neudorfer et al. 1996, Machaczka et al. 1999, Tayebi et al. 2001, Bembi et al. 2003, Tayebi et al. 2003, Aharon-Peretz et al. 2004, Lwin et al. 2004, Aharon-Peretz et al. 2005, Clark et al. 2005, Eblan et al. 2005, Sato et al. 2005, Schlossmacher et al. 2005, Sidransky 2005, Zimran et al. 2005, Eblan et al. 2006, Spitz et al. 2006, Clark et al. 2007, Tan et al. 2007, Wu et al. 2007, Ziegler et al. 2007, Goker-Alpan et al. 2008, Mitsui et al. 2009, Nishioka et al. 2009, Sidransky et al. 2009a,b, Bultron et al. 2010, Saunders-Pullman et al. 2010, Velayati et al. 2010, Cullen et al. 2011, Rosenbloom et al. 2011). PD is the second most common neurodegenerative disorder that usually affects individuals

Department of Cell Research and immunology, Life Sciences, Tel Aviv University, Levanon St., Ramat Aviv, 6997801, Israel.
[a] E-mail: galifit@gmail.com
* Corresponding author: horwitzm@post.tau.ac.il

above the age of 60. The disease is characterized by the loss of dopaminergic cells in the substantia nigra pars compacta, which results in movement disorder with resting tremor, stiffness, postural instability and bradykinesia (Shulman et al. 2011).

The first finding of late neurological involvement in type 1 GD was presented by Miller et al. (1973). The authors described two siblings with type 1 GD who developed movement disturbance and abnormal encephalogram. McKeran et al. (1973) described a 45 years old woman with type 1 GD with stiffness in her lower body, who later on presented stooped posture and bradykinesia, all known clinical signs of PD (McKeran et al. 1985). In 1996, six cases of patients with type 1 GD and development of parkinsonian signs were described (Neudorfer et al. 1996) and further reports of patients with type 1 GD who developed parkinsonian signs have been accumulating since.

On the basis of the sporadic published cases of GD patients with PD, two genetic studies were performed among PD patients, screening for GBA mutations (Tayebi et al. 2001, Aharon-Peretz et al. 2004). These studies led to the recognition that there is an association between GD and PD and to a remarkable multicenter analysis of GCase mutations in PD (Sidransky et al. 2009a). Other multicenter publications followed, all pointing to the observation that the GD carrier frequency among PD patients is much higher than that in the general population. It is well established today that mutation in the GBA gene is the most common familial cause for PD (Aharon-Peretz et al. 2004, Lwin et al. 2004, Aharon-Peretz et al. 2005, Clark et al. 2005, Eblan et al. 2005, Sato et al. 2005, Eblan et al. 2006, Clark et al. 2007, Tan et al. 2007, Wu et al. 2007, Hruska et al. 2008, Mitsui et al. 2009, Nishioka et al. 2009, Sidransky et al. 2009a,b, Bultron et al. 2010, Cullen et al. 2011, Rosenbloom et al. 2011, Asselta et al. 2014, Romo-Gutierrez et al. 2015).

Interestingly, GD associated PD involves aggregation of α-synuclein (Yap et al. 2011, Hruska et al. 2006, Goker-Alpan et al. 2010, Cullen et al. 2011, Kinghorn 2011, Mazzulli et al. 2011, Sardi et al. 2011, Xu et al. 2011, Murphy et al. 2014). Alpha-synuclein, one of the hallmarks in autopsies from brains of PD patients, is a 140 amino acids cytoplasmic protein, which is highly expressed in the central nervous system and is concentrated in the presynaptic terminals. It is mainly expressed in neurons and to a lesser extent in glial cells. Its suggested role is in maintaining a supply of synaptic vesicles in mature presynaptic terminals (Kim et al. 2014). Post-translational modifications of α-synuclein, including phosphorylation, ubiquitination and nitration, impact on its functionality and its tendency to aggregate (Giasson et al. 2000, Okochi et al. 2000, Nakamura et al. 2001, Nonaka et al. 2005, Anderson et al. 2006, House et al. 2006). Lewy bodies are cytoplasmic inclusions containing aggregated α-synuclein that appear in brains of patients with synucleinopathies, including PD patients (Kruger et al. 2000). In Dementia with Lewy Bodies (DLBs) 90% of insoluble α-synuclein is phosphorylated on serine129, suggesting that this post-translational modification is directly associated with α-synuclein aggregation. Aggregated Lewy body associated α-synuclein is also nitrated. Lewy bodies are cytoplasmic inclusions containing aggregated α-synuclein (Simmons and Lewy 1948, Gibb and Less 1988, Lees 2012, Kalia et al. 2013). They appear in brains of patients with synucleinopathies including PD patients (Kruger et al. 2000).

Intracellular removal (degradation) of α-synuclein takes place via both lysosomal and proteasomal degradation. Degradation of α-synuclein in the proteasomal pathway depends on its SIAH mediated ubiquitination (Okochi et al. 2000, Nakamura et al. 2001, Nonaka et al. 2005, Anderson et al. 2006, House et al. 2006), whereas its lysosomal degradation depends on its autophagy and fusion of autophagosomes with lysosomes, where α-synuclein is degraded by cathepsin D (Cullen et al. 2009). Transport of cathepsin D requires the retromer, a complex that participates in vesicular shuttling from the Golgi apparatus to the lysosomes and back. Lately, the D620N mutation in VPS35, a retromer specific protein, was identified. It has been suggested that this mutation abrogates normal shuttling of cathepsin D from the Golgi apparatus to the lysosomes, thus leading to lysosomal aggregation of α-synuclein and development of PD (Follett et al. 2014). Brain autopsies that derived from GD patients who developed PD also displayed abnormal oligomerization and fibrillization, as well as higher levels of insoluble α-synuclein oligomers (Tayebi et al. 2003, Wong et al. 2004, Clark et al. 2009, Choi et al. 2011).

Since carriers of GD mutations develop PD at a frequency significantly higher than that of the general population, mutation in the GBA allele is a predisposing factor in the development of PD. This is a dominant trait, like development of breast cancer in women carrying a BRCA1 mutation. Thus, not every woman with a BRCA1 mutation will develop breast cancer, however, the chances of a carrier of a BRCA1 mutation to develop breast cancer are much higher than that of a non-carrier woman (Venkitaraman 2002). Dominance can result from haploinsufficiency or from gain of function (Griffiths et al. 2000). Haploinsufficiency attests a situation where only one normal allele does not produce enough products, leading to development of clinical disease signs. Gain of function refers to a gene product with a deleterious cellular effect. Below we present publications arguing that one or both account for the association between GD and PD.

Work from our laboratory has shown, using a transgenic fly model, that expression of a mutant GBA allele is enough to cause ER stress and ER stress response which leads to degeneration of dopaminergic cells. In a parallel work, another laboratory has shown that expression of a mutant GBA allele in the fly eye leads to neurodegeneration (Suzuki et al. 2013). It also seems that in brain sections of sporadic PD patients there is decreased GCase activity, which may result from misfolding of normal GCase. It is possible that this is an age related phenomenon, which leads to ER stress and UPR, impaired autophagy, mitophagy and eventually leads to death of the very vulnerable dopaminergic cells.

Insufficient GCase Activity

Haploinsufficiency describes the presence of decreased lysosomal GCase activity, leading to lysosomal impairment and dysfunction and the development of PD. In 2011, Mazzulli et al. were the first to suggest the contribution of glucosylceramide metabolism to the development of PD in GD patients or carriers of GD mutations. The authors argued that the accumulation of glucosylceramide caused by impaired lysosomal activity of mutant GCase promotes lysosomal formation of toxic α-synuclein oligomers. The authors first showed that reducing GCase activity by 50% in mouse cortical neurons led to a fourfold increase in the amount of accumulated glucosylceramide as tested by mass spectroscopy. Knock down (KD) of GCase led to a general lysosomal inhibition, increase in the levels of α-synuclein oligomers and to neurotoxicity in neuroglioma cell line (H4), expressing WT α-synuclein under control of tetracycline inducible promotor (Mazzulli et al. 2011). Since in none of the mentioned experiments was mutant GBA allele present, the results strongly implicated accumulation of lysosomal glucosylceramide as the cause for development of PD. This result is surprising as no substrate accumulation has ever been documented in any tissue or cells that derived from carriers of GD mutations. In induced pluripotent stem (iPS) dopaminergic neurons, carrying endogenous N370S/84GG GD mutations, there was a decrease in proteolysis and concomitant α-synuclein accumulation, which could result from the presence of mutant GCase. The authors proposed a feedback mechanism in which elevated levels of toxic α-synuclein lead to depletion of GCase and further stabilization of α-synuclein oligomers through glucosylceramide accumulation (Mazzulli et al. 2011).

Sardi et al. (Sardi et al. 2011) argued that both loss of function and gain of function mechanisms underlie the association between GD and PD. The authors used knock-in mutant mice, homozygous for the D409V mutation, to show α-synuclein aggregation in hippocampal neurons and inflammation. No glucosylceramide accumulation was noted in the cerebral cortex and cerebellum of these mice, but elevated levels of toxic glucosylsphingosine were recorded. The animals developed cognition impairment, pointing to development of parkinsonian signs. These results suggested a loss of function model for development of PD in GD patients. Hyppocampal administration of recombinant AAV viral vector expressing wild type GCase corrected the α-synuclein aggregation and the memory deficit (Sardi et al. 2011). It is worth mentioning that the clinical signs described for the animals resemble neuronopathic GD, which ameliorates with enzymatic treatment, and not necessarily cognition impairment, associated with PD (Lees and Smith 1983, Boyd et al. 1991, Hobson and Meara 1999, Johnson et al. 2004, Lee et al. 2012, Meireles and Massano 2012, Bocanegra et al. 2014).

Bae et al. (Bae et al. 2015) introduced nonsense mutations into the GBA gene of SHSY5Y cells, using ZFN targeted mutagenesis (Lloyd et al. 2005), and created GBA–/– cells. They found lysosomal dysfunction in these cells by examining the accumulation of p62, a marker for autophagy, and of ubiquitinated proteins. They also found a significantly higher staining of lysosomes and slower dextran degradation, pointing to lysosomal dysfunction in the GBA–/– cells. These cells also exhibited aggregation of α-synuclein (Bae et al. 2015).

It is worth mentioning that none of the presented studies showed active development of PD in any animal model due to reduced lysosomal GCase activity, glucosylceramide accumulation or lysosomal dysfunction.

In several very recent publications loss of GCase activity and a concomitant increase in glucosylceramide has been documented in older individuals who developed PD, in comparison to non-PD patients (Chiasserini et al. 2015, Sardi et al. 2015). We hypothesize that under normal conditions non-mutated misfolded GCase molecules are refolded by the ER quality control (ERQC) machinery. At older ages, however, this ability of the ERQC reduces, leading to retention of more misfolded wild type GCase molecules in the ER. This ER retention causes ER stress and evokes the ER stress response, leading to death of dopaminergic cells and development of PD. Such misfolded molecules can be removed from the ER by chemical chaperones, a strategy that has been successfully employed lately in a mouse model of synucleinopathy (Richter et al. 2014).

Contribution of Mutant GCase to Development of PD through Gain of Function Mechanism

Evidence for gain of function, induced by mutant GCase, as the cause for development of PD was first provided in a study by Cullen et al. (2011). The authors showed that transient over-expression of different mutant GBA variants in MES23.5 and PC12 cells, expressing wild-type α-synuclein, promoted accumulation of α-synuclein in a time- and dose-dependent manner that was independent of GCase enzyme activity status. To determine whether the effect of mutant GBA on α-synuclein could be ameliorated pharmacologically, the cells were treated with rapamycin, which induces macroautophagy. Rapamycin significantly reduced α-synuclein accumulation in the mutant GBA expressing cells, strongly suggesting that autophagy is upregulated in the presence of mutant GCase. Isofagomine, a pharmacological chaperone for mutant GCase, had the same effect in the cells expressing the mutant GBA alleles (Cullen et al. 2011).

The effect of a mutant GBA allele on α-synuclein degradation was tested in primary cortical neurons that derived from mice heterozygous for the L444P (Tsuji et al. 1987) mutation, expressing different variants of human α-synuclein (Fishbein et al. 2014). The L444P mutation reduced the A53T mutant α-synuclein degradation and triggered its accumulation in the cells. In mice transgenic for the human A53T mutant α-synuclein and heterozygous for the L444P mutant allele there were deficits in motor and gastrointestinal neurons, compared to mice expressing only the human mutant α-synuclein. These results highlight the importance of mutant GCase in downregulation degradation of α-synuclein.

Another aspect of the involvement of mutant GCase in the development of PD is quality control of the enzyme in the cells and its many effects on different cellular functions. In 2005, it was first shown that mutant GCase variants undergo ER retention and that a certain fraction of the mutant enzymes, depending on the degree of misfolding, undergoes ER associated degradation (Ron and Horowitz 2005, Kono et al. 2010). This ER retention and ERAD of mutant GCase was later supported by the effective use of chemical chaperones as agents to improve GCase activity and reduce cell stress. GD is one of a growing number of diseases in which ER retention is a predominant feature, including several lysosomal diseases, such as Fabry disease, Tay-Sachs and α-Mannosidosis (Mu et al. 2008), as well as non-lysosomal diseases, such as Cystic Fibrosis (Gilbert et al. 1998) and alpha-1 antitrypsin deficiency (Carlson et al. 1988, Hosokawa et al. 2007, Araki and Nagata 2011).

ER retention and ERAD of mutant GCase variants were also studied as a factor that promotes development of PD in GD patients and carriers of GD mutations. In 2010 Ron et al. (Ron et al. 2010) showed that mutant GCase variants undergo parkin mediated ubiquitination and proteasomal degradation. Parkin is an E3 ubiquitin ligase associated with familial autosomal recessive juvenile PD. Interestingly, mutant GCase variants compete with endogenous parkin substrates, whose accumulation is deleterious to cells, like PARkin Interacting Substrate (PARIS) and ARTS. Under normal conditions, PARIS undergoes parkin-mediated ubiquitination and proteasomal degradation in the cytoplasm. However, when non-ubiquitinated PARIS accumulates in the cytoplasm, it shuttles to the nucleus and represses transcription of PGC1a, NRF1 and ATPase5β, major regulators of mitochondria biogenesis (Castillo-Quan 2011, Shin et al. 2011). PARIS is upregulated in brains of PD patients, where levels of NRF1, PGC1a and ATPase5β are downregulated. In GD derived skin fibroblasts, as well as in SHSY5Y neuroblastoma derived cells, expressing the human mutant GCase variants N370S L444P, the levels of the three PARIS-regulated proteins is decreased as well. ARTS, is a pro-apoptotic protein that undergoes parkin mediated proteasomal degradation. Its accumulation leads to apoptosis (Kemeny et al. 2012). Thus, accumulation of parkin substrates due to the presence of mutant GCase that undergoes parkin-mediated degradation may play a role in the development of PD in carriers of GD mutations or in GD patients. Interestingly, parkin was also shown to mediate α-synuclein autophagy (Lonskaya et al. 2013).

Two studies have shown a direct association between the presence of a mutant GBA allele, leading to ER stress and ER stress response (UPR), and development of neurodegeneration, using Drosophila melanogaster as a model system. These studies strongly supported gain of function association between mutant GCase and development of PD (Maor et al. 2013, Suzuki et al. 2013). Thus, Maor et al. (2013) used transgenic Drosophila to express human mutant N370S and L444P GCase variants in the dopaminergic cells of the fly. The authors showed that the presence of mutant GCase variants, but not of the normal counterpart, leads to accumulation of misfolded protein in the ER, ER stress and UPR. Eventually, these processes led to death of dopaminergic cells and motor impairment in the flies. Suzuki et al. showed the same neurodegeneration processes following expression of the R120W and the recNci mutant variants (Eyal et al. 1990, Hong et al. 1990) in Drosophila eyes. This neurodegeneration could be partially rescued by growing the flies on a medium containing ambroxol (Suzuki et al. 2013). Ambroxol is one of many pharmacological chaperones used to remove unfolded mutant GCase from the ER (Maegawa et al. 2009, Shanmuganathan and Britz-McKibbin 2011, Babajani et al. 2012, Bendikov-Bar et al. 2013, Zimran et al. 2013, McNeill et al. 2014). Pharmacological chaperones are low molecular weight compounds, which specifically bind proteins and induce their refolding, thus restoring their function and preventing their degradation and retention in the ER (Cortez and Sim 2014). The partial phenotypic rescue by Ambroxol therefore further supports a gain of function mode of action of the mutant GCase variants.

Conclusions

A large number of publications prove the association between GD and PD. Both GD patients and carriers of GD mutations have a significantly higher propensity than the general population to develop PD. Since carriers of GD mutations develop PD, a dominant effect of the GBA mutation should be considered, either gain of function or haploinsufficiency. We present data arguing that one or both account for the association between GD and PD. Work from our laboratory has shown, using a transgenic fly model, that expression of a mutant GBA allele is enough to cause ER stress and ER stress response which leads to degeneration of dopaminergic cells. In a parallel work, another laboratory has shown that expression of a mutant GBA allele in the fly eye leads to neurodegeneration. It also seems that in brain sections of sporadic PD patients there is decreased GCase activity, which may result from misfolding of normal GCase. It is possible that this is an age related phenomenon, which leads to ER stress and UPR, impaired autophagy, mitophagy and eventually leads to death of the very vulnerable dopaminergic cells.

Acknowledgements

The research in M.H.'s lab on the association between Gaucher disease and Parkinson's disease is supported by funding from the Israel Science Foundation (ISF), by Teva Pharmaceutical Industries Ltd as part of the Israeli National Network of Excellence in Neuroscience (NNE) and by Pfizer IIR. We thank Dr. Sigal Rencus-Lazar for critical reading of the manuscript.

Keywords: Gaucher disease, glucocerebrosidase, ER stress, UPR, Parkinson's disease

References

Aharon-Peretz, J., H. Rosenbaum and R. Gershoni-Baruch. 2004. Mutations in the glucocerebrosidase gene and Parkinson's disease in Ashkenazi Jews. N Engl J Med 351: 1972–1977.

Aharon-Peretz, J., S. Badarny, H. Rosenbaum and R. Gershoni-Baruch. 2005. Mutations in the glucocerebrosidase gene and Parkinson disease: Phenotype-genotype correlation. Neurology 65: 1460–1461.

Anderson, J. P., D. E. Walker, J. M. Goldstein, R. de Laat, K. Banducci, R. J. Caccavello et al. 2006. Phosphorylation of Ser-129 is the dominant pathological modification of alpha-synuclein in familial and sporadic Lewy body disease. J Biol Chem 281: 29739–29752.

Araki, K. and K. Nagata. 2011. Protein folding and quality control in the ER. Cold Spring Harb Perspect Biol 3: a007526.

Asselta, R., V. Rimoldi, C. Siri, R. Cilia, I. Guella, S. Tesei et al. 2014. Glucocerebrosidase mutations in primary parkinsonism. Parkinsonism Relat Disord 20: 1215–1220.

Babajani, G., M. B. Tropak, D. J. Mahuran and A. R. Kermode. 2012. Pharmacological chaperones facilitate the post-ER transport of recombinant N370S mutant beta-glucocerebrosidase in plant cells: evidence that N370S is a folding mutant. Mol Genet Metab 106: 323–329.

Bae, E. J., N. Y. Yang, C. Lee, H. J. Lee, S. Kim, S. P. Sardi et al. 2015. Loss of glucocerebrosidase 1 activity causes lysosomal dysfunction and alpha-synuclein aggregation. Exp Mol Med 47: e153.

Bembi, B., S. Zambito Marsala, E. Sidransky, G. Ciana, M. Carrozzi, M. Zorzon et al. 2003. Gaucher's disease with Parkinson's disease: Clinical and pathological aspects. Neurology 61: 99–101.

Bendikov-Bar, I., G. Maor, M. Filocamo and M. Horowitz. 2013. Ambroxol as a pharmacological chaperone for mutant glucocerebrosidase. Blood Cells Mol Dis 50: 141–145.

Beutler, E. 1980. Gaucher's disease. Compr Ther 6: 65–68.

Beutler, E. and G. L. Dale. 1982. Gaucher disease: A century of delineation and research. Enzyme replacement therapy: model and clinical studies. Prog Clin Biol Res 95: 703–716.

Beutler, E. and T. Gelbart. 1996. Glucocerebrosidase (Gaucher disease). Hum Mutat 8: 207–213.

Beutler, E. 1999. Gaucher disease. Arch Intern Med 159: 881–882.

Bocanegra, Y., N. Trujillo-Orrego and D. Pineda. 2014. Dementia and mild cognitive impairment in Parkinson's disease: A review. Rev Neurol 59: 555–569.

Boyd, J. L., C. A. Cruickshank, C. W. Kenn, P. Madeley, R. H. Mindham, A. G. Oswald et al. 1991. Cognitive impairment and dementia in Parkinson's disease: A controlled study. Psychol Med 21: 911–921.

Brady, R. O. 1982. Lysosomal storage diseases. Pharmacol Ther 19: 327–336.

Bultron, G., K. Kacena, D. Pearson, M. Boxer, R. Yang, S. Sathe et al. 2010. The risk of Parkinson's disease in type 1 Gaucher disease. J Inherit Metab Dis 33: 167–173.

Carlson, J. A., B. B. Rogers, R. N. Sifers, H. K. Hawkins, M. J. Finegold and S. L. Woo. 1988. Multiple tissues express alpha 1-antitrypsin in transgenic mice and man. J Clin Invest 82: 26–36.

Castillo-Quan, J. I. 2011. Parkin' control: Regulation of PGC-1alpha through PARIS in Parkinson's disease. Dis Model Mech 4: 427–429.

Chiasserini, D., S. Paciotti, P. Eusebi, E. Persichetti, A. Tasegian, M. Kurzawa-Akanbi et al. 2015. Selective loss of glucocerebrosidase activity in sporadic Parkinson's disease and dementia with Lewy bodies. Mol Neurodegener 10: 15.

Choi, J. H., B. Stubblefield, M. R. Cookson, E. Goldin, A. Velayati, N. Tayebi et al. 2011. Aggregation of alpha-synuclein in brain samples from subjects with glucocerebrosidase mutations. Mol Genet Metab 104: 185–188.

Clark, L. N., A. Nicolai, S. Afridi, J. Harris, H. Mejia-Santana, L. Strug et al. 2005. Pilot association study of the beta-glucocerebrosidase N370S allele and Parkinson's disease in subjects of Jewish ethnicity. Mov Disord 20: 100–103.

Clark, L. N., B. M. Ross, Y. Wang, H. Mejia-Santana, J. Harris, E. D. Louis et al. 2007. Mutations in the glucocerebrosidase gene are associated with early-onset Parkinson disease. Neurology 69: 1270–1277.

Clark, L. N., L. A. Kartsaklis, R. Wolf Gilbert, B. Dorado, B. M. Ross, S. Kisselev et al. 2009. Association of glucocerebrosidase mutations with dementia with Lewy bodies. Arch Neurol 66: 578–583.

Cortez, L. and V. Sim. 2014. The therapeutic potential of chemical chaperones in protein folding diseases. Prion 8: 197–202.

Cullen, V., M. Lindfors, J. Ng, A. Paetau, E. Swinton, P. Kolodziej et al. 2009. Cathepsin D expression level affects alpha-synuclein processing, aggregation, and toxicity *in vivo*. Mol Brain 2: 5.

Cullen, V., S. P. Sardi, J. Ng, Y. H. Xu, Y. Sun, J. J. Tomlinson et al. 2011. Acid beta-glucosidase mutants linked to Gaucher disease, Parkinson disease, and Lewy body dementia alter alpha-synuclein processing. Ann Neurol 69: 940–953.

Eblan, M. J., J. M. Walker and E. Sidransky. 2005. The glucocerebrosidase gene and Parkinson's disease in Ashkenazi Jews. N Engl J Med 352: 728–731.

Eblan, M. J., S. Scholz, B. Stubblefield, U. Gutti, O. Goker-Alpan, K. S. Hruska et al. 2006. Glucocerebrosidase mutations are not found in association with LRRK2 G2019S in subjects with parkinsonism. Neurosci Lett 404: 163–165.

Eyal, N., S. Wilder and M. Horowitz. 1990. Prevalent and rare mutations among Gaucher patients. Gene 96: 277–283.

Fishbein, I., Y. M. Kuo, B. I. Giasson and R. L. Nussbaum. 2014. Augmentation of phenotype in a transgenic Parkinson mouse heterozygous for a Gaucher mutation. Brain 137: 3235–3247.

Follett, J., S. J. Norwood, N. A. Hamilton, M. Mohan, O. Kovtun, S. Tay et al. 2014. The Vps35 D620N mutation linked to Parkinson's disease disrupts the cargo sorting function of retromer. Traffic 15: 230–244.

Giasson, B. I., J. E. Duda, I. V. Murray, Q. Chen, J. M. Souza, H. I. Hurtig et al. 2000. Oxidative damage linked to neurodegeneration by selective alpha-synuclein nitration in synucleinopathy lesions. Science 290: 985–989.

Gibb, W. R. and A. J. Lees. 1988. The relevance of the Lewy body to the pathogenesis of idiopathic Parkinson's disease. J Neurol Neurosurg Psychiatry 51: 745–752.

Gilbert, A., M. Jadot, E. Leontieva, S. Wattiaux-De Coninck and R. Wattiaux. 1998. Delta F508 CFTR localizes in the endoplasmic reticulum-Golgi intermediate compartment in cystic fibrosis cells. Exp Cell Res 242: 144–152.

Goker-Alpan, O., G. Lopez, J. Vithayathil, J. Davis, M. Hallett and E. Sidransky. 2008. The spectrum of parkinsonian manifestations associated with glucocerebrosidase mutations. Arch Neurol 65: 1353–1357.

Goker-Alpan, O., B. K. Stubblefield, B. I. Giasson and E. Sidransky. 2010. Glucocerebrosidase is present in alpha-synuclein inclusions in Lewy body disorders. Acta Neuropathol 120: 641–649.

Griffiths, A., J. Miller, D. Suzuki, R. Lewontin and W. Gelbart. 2000. An Introduction to Genetic Analysis, 7th Edition. W.H Freeman, New York.

Hobson, P. and J. Meara. 1999. The detection of dementia and cognitive impairment in a community population of elderly people with Parkinson's disease by use of the CAMCOG neuropsychological test. Age Ageing 28: 39–43.

Hong, C. M., T. Ohashi, X. J. Yu, S. Weiler and J. A. Barranger. 1990. Sequence of two alleles responsible for Gaucher disease. DNA Cell Biol 9: 233–241.

Hosokawa, N., Z. You, L. O. Tremblay, K. Nagata and A. Herscovics. 2007. Stimulation of ERAD of misfolded null Hong Kong alpha1-antitrypsin by Golgi alpha1,2-mannosidases. Biochem Biophys Res Commun 362: 626–632.

House, C. M., N. C. Hancock, A. Moller, B. A. Cromer, V. Fedorov, D. D. Bowtell et al. 2006. Elucidation of the substrate binding site of Siah ubiquitin ligase. Structure 14: 695–701.

Hruska, K. S., O. Goker-Alpan and E. Sidransky. 2006. Gaucher disease and the synucleinopathies. J Biomed Biotechnol 2006: 78549.

Hruska, K. S., M. E. LaMarca, C. R. Scott and E. Sidransky. 2008. Gaucher disease: Mutation and polymorphism spectrum in the glucocerebrosidase gene (GBA). Hum Mutat 29: 567–583.

Johnson, A. M., Q. J. Almeida, C. Stough, J. C. Thompson, R. Singarayer and M. S. Jog. 2004. Visual inspection time in Parkinson's disease: deficits in early stages of cognitive processing. Neuropsychologia 42: 577–583.

Kalia, L. V., S. K. Kalia, P. J. McLean, A. M. Lozano and A. E. Lang. 2013. alpha-Synuclein oligomers and clinical implications for Parkinson disease. Ann Neurol 73: 155–169.

Kemeny, S., D. Dery, Y. Loboda, M. Rovner, T. Lev, D. Zuri et al. 2012. Parkin promotes degradation of the mitochondrial pro-apoptotic ARTS protein. PLoS One 7: e38837.

Kim, W. S., K. Kagedal and G. M. Halliday. 2014. Alpha-synuclein biology in Lewy body diseases. Alzheimers Res Ther 6: 73.

Kinghorn, K. J. 2011. Pathological looping in the synucleinopathies: investigating the link between Parkinson's disease and Gaucher disease. Dis Model Mech 4: 713–715.

Kono, S., Y. Ouchi, T. Terada, H. Ida, M. Suzuki and H. Miyajima. 2010. Functional brain imaging in glucocerebrosidase mutation carriers with and without parkinsonism. Mov Disord 25: 1823–1829.

Kruger, R., T. Muller and O. Riess. 2000. Involvement of alpha-synuclein in Parkinson's disease and other neurodegenerative disorders. J Neural Transm 107: 31–40.

Lee, W. J., C. F. Tsai, S. Gauthier, S. J. Wang and J. L. Fuh. 2012. The association between cognitive impairment and neuropsychiatric symptoms in patients with Parkinson's disease dementia. Int Psychogeriatr 24: 1980–1987.

Lees, A. J. and E. Smith. 1983. Cognitive deficits in the early stages of Parkinson's disease. Brain 106(Pt 2): 257–270.

Lees, A. J. 2012. Impact Commentaries. A modern perspective on the top 100 cited JNNP papers of all time: The relevance of the Lewy body to the pathogenesis of idiopathic Parkinson's disease: accuracy of clinical diagnosis of idiopathic Parkinson's disease. J Neurol Neurosurg Psychiatry 83: 954–955.

Lloyd, A., C. L. Plaisier, D. Carroll and G. N. Drews. 2005. Targeted mutagenesis using zinc-finger nucleases in Arabidopsis. Proc Natl Acad Sci USA 102: 2232–2237.

Lonskaya, I., M. L. Hebron, N. K. Algarzae, N. Desforges and C. E. Moussa. 2013. Decreased parkin solubility is associated with impairment of autophagy in the nigrostriatum of sporadic Parkinson's disease. Neuroscience 232: 90–105.

Lwin, A., E. Orvisky, O. Goker-Alpan, M. E. LaMarca and E. Sidransky. 2004. Glucocerebrosidase mutations in subjects with parkinsonism. Mol Genet Metab 81: 70–73.

Machaczka, M., M. Rucinska, A. B. Skotnickiand W. Jurczak. 1999. Parkinson's syndrome preceding clinical manifestation of Gaucher's disease. Am J Hematol 61: 216–217.

Maegawa, G. H., M. B. Tropak, J. D. Buttner, B. A. Rigat, M. Fuller, D. Pandit et al. 2009. Identification and characterization of ambroxol as an enzyme enhancement agent for Gaucher disease. J Biol Chem 284: 23502–23516.

Maor, G., S. Rencus-Lazar, M. Filocamo, H. Steller, D. Segal and M. Horowitz. 2013. Unfolded protein response in Gaucher disease: From human to Drosophila. Orphanet J Rare Dis 8: 140.

Mazzulli, J. R., Y. H. Xu, Y. Sun, A. L. Knight, P. J. McLean, G. A. Caldwell et al. 2011. Gaucher disease glucocerebrosidase and alpha-synuclein form a bidirectional pathogenic loop in synucleinopathies. Cell 146: 37–52.

McKeran, R. O., P. Bradbury, D. Taylor and G. Stern. 1985. Neurological involvement in type 1 (adult) Gaucher's disease. J Neurol Neurosurg Psychiatry 48: 172–175.

McNeill, A., J. Magalhaes, C. Shen, K. Y. Chau, D. Hughes, A. Mehta et al. 2014. Ambroxol improves lysosomal biochemistry in glucocerebrosidase mutation-linked Parkinson disease cells. Brain 137: 1481–1495.

Meireles, J. and J. Massano. 2012. Cognitive impairment and dementia in Parkinson's disease: clinical features, diagnosis, and management. Front Neurol 3: 88.

Miller, J. D., R. McCluer and J. N. Kanfer. 1973. Gaucher's disease: neurologic disorder in adult siblings. Ann Intern Med 78: 883–887.

Mitsui, J., I. Mizuta, A. Toyoda, R. Ashida, Y. Takahashi, J. Goto et al. 2009. Mutations for Gaucher disease confer high susceptibility to Parkinson disease. Arch Neurol 66: 571–576.

Mu, T. W., D. S. Ong, Y. J. Wang, W. E. Balch, J. R. Yates, 3rd, L. Segatori et al. 2008. Chemical and biological approaches synergize to ameliorate protein-folding diseases. Cell 134: 769–781.

Murphy, K. E., A. M. Gysbers, S. K. Abbott, N. Tayebi, W. S. Kim, E. Sidransky et al. 2014. Reduced glucocerebrosidase is associated with increased alpha-synuclein in sporadic Parkinson's disease. Brain 137: 834–848.

Nakamura, T., H. Yamashita, T. Takahashi and S. Nakamura. 2001. Activated Fyn phosphorylates alpha-synuclein at tyrosine residue 125. Biochem Biophys Res Commun 280: 1085–1092.

Neudorfer, O., N. Giladi, D. Elstein, A. Abrahamov, T. Turezkite, E. Aghai et al. 1996. Occurrence of Parkinson's syndrome in type I Gaucher disease. QJM 89: 691–694.

Nishioka, K., C. Vilarino-Guell, S. A. Cobb, J. M. Kachergus, O. A. Ross, C. Wider et al. 2009. Glucocerebrosidase mutations are not a common risk factor for Parkinson disease in North Africa. Neurosci Lett. 477(2): 57–60.

Nonaka, T., T. Iwatsubo and M. Hasegawa. 2005. Ubiquitination of alpha-synuclein. Biochemistry (Mosc) 44: 361–368.

Okochi, M., J. Walter, A. Koyama, S. Nakajo, M. Baba, T. Iwatsubo et al. 2000. Constitutive phosphorylation of the Parkinson's disease associated alpha-synuclein. J Biol Chem 275: 390–397.

Richter, F., S. M. Fleming, M. Watson, V. Lemesre, L. Pellegrino, B. Ranes et al. 2014. A GCase chaperone improves motor function in a mouse model of synucleinopathy. Neurotherapeutics 11: 840–856.

Romo-Gutierrez, D., P. Yescas, M. Lopez-Lopez and M. C. Boll. 2015. [Genetic factors associated with dementia in parkinson's disease (PD)]. Gac Med Mex 151: 110–118.

Ron, I. and M. Horowitz. 2005. ER retention and degradation as the molecular basis underlying Gaucher disease heterogeneity. Hum Mol Genet 14: 2387–2398.

Ron, I., D. Rapaport and M. Horowitz. 2010. Interaction between parkin and mutant glucocerebrosidase variants: A possible link between Parkinson disease and Gaucher disease. Hum Mol Genet 19: 3771–3781.

Rosenbloom, B., M. Balwani, J. M. Bronstein, E. Kolodny, S. Sathe, A. R. Gwosdow et al. 2011. The incidence of Parkinsonism in patients with type 1 Gaucher disease: Data from the ICGG Gaucher Registry. Blood Cells Mol Dis 46: 95–102.

Sardi, S. P., J. Clarke, C. Kinnecom, T. J. Tamsett, L. Li, L. M. Stanek et al. 2011. CNS expression of glucocerebrosidase corrects alpha-synuclein pathology and memory in a mouse model of Gaucher-related synucleinopathy. Proc Natl Acad Sci USA 108: 12101–12106.

Sardi, S. P., S. H. Cheng and L. S. Shihabuddin. 2015. Gaucher-related synucleinopathies: the examination of sporadic neurodegeneration from a rare (disease) angle. Prog Neurobiol 125: 47–62.

Sato, C., A. Morgan, A. E. Lang, S. Salehi-Rad, T. Kawarai, Y. Meng et al. 2005. Analysis of the glucocerebrosidase gene in Parkinson's disease. Mov Disord 20: 367–370.

Saunders-Pullman, R., J. Hagenah, V. Dhawan, K. Stanley, G. Pastores, S. Sathe et al. 2010. Gaucher disease ascertained through a Parkinson's center: Imaging and clinical characterization. Mov Disord 25: 1364–1372.

Schlossmacher, M. G., V. Cullen and J. Muthing. 2005. The glucocerebrosidase gene and Parkinson's disease in Ashkenazi Jews. N Engl J Med 352: 728–731.

Shanmuganathan, M. and P. Britz-McKibbin. 2011. Inhibitor screening of pharmacological chaperones for lysosomal beta-glucocerebrosidase by capillary electrophoresis. Anal Bioanal Chem 399: 2843–2853.

Shin, J. H., H. S. Ko, H. Kang, Y. Lee, Y. I. Lee, O. Pletinkova et al. 2011. PARIS (ZNF746) repression of PGC-1alpha contributes to neurodegeneration in Parkinson's disease. Cell 144: 689–702.

Shulman, J. M., P. L. De Jager and M. B. Feany. 2011. Parkinson's disease: Genetics and pathogenesis. Annu Rev Pathol 6: 193–222.

Sidransky, E. 2005. Gaucher disease and parkinsonism. Mol Genet Metab 84: 302–304.

Sidransky, E., M. A. Nalls, J. O. Aasly, J. Aharon-Peretz, G. Annesi, E. R. Barbosa et al. 2009a. Multicenter analysis of glucocerebrosidase mutations in Parkinson's disease. N Engl J Med 361: 1651–1661.

Sidransky, E., T. Samaddar and N. Tayebi. 2009b. Mutations in GBA are associated with familial Parkinson disease susceptibility and age at onset. Neurology 73: 1425–1426.

Simmons, M. W. and R. B. Lewy. 1948. Foreign body in the postnasal space; report of a case. Laryngoscope 58: 1324–1330.

Spitz, M., R. Rozenberg, P. A. Silveira and E. R. Barbosa. 2006. Parkinsonism in type 1 Gaucher's disease. J Neurol Neurosurg Psychiatry 77: 709–710.

Suzuki, T., M. Shimoda, K. Ito, S. Hanai, H. Aizawa, T. Kato et al. 2013. Expression of human Gaucher disease gene GBA generates neurodevelopmental defects and ER stress in Drosophila eye. PLoS One 8: e69147.

Tan, E. K., J. Tong, S. Fook-Chong, Y. Yih, M. C. Wong, R. Pavanni et al. 2007. Glucocerebrosidase mutations and risk of Parkinson disease in Chinese patients. Arch Neurol 64: 1056–1058.

Tayebi, N., M. Callahan, V. Madike, B. K. Stubblefield, E. Orvisky, D. Krasnewich et al. 2001. Gaucher disease and parkinsonism: A phenotypic and genotypic characterization. Mol Genet Metab 73: 313–321.

Tayebi, N., J. Walker, B. Stubblefield, E. Orvisky, M. E. LaMarca, K. Wong et al. 2003. Gaucher disease with parkinsonian manifestations: Does glucocerebrosidase deficiency contribute to a vulnerability to parkinsonism? Mol Genet Metab 79: 104–109.

Tsuji, S., P. V. Choudary, B. M. Martin, B. K. Stubblefield, J. A. Mayor, J. A. Barranger et al. 1987. A mutation in the human glucocerebrosidase gene in neuronopathic Gaucher's disease. N Engl J Med 316: 570–575.

Velayati, A., W. H. Yu and E. Sidransky. 2010. The role of glucocerebrosidase mutations in Parkinson disease and Lewy body disorders. Curr Neurol Neurosci Rep 10: 190–198.

Venkitaraman, A. R. 2002. Cancer susceptibility and the functions of BRCA1 and BRCA2. Cell 108: 171–182.

Wong, K., E. Sidransky, A. Verma, T. Mixon, G. D. Sandberg, L. K. Wakefield et al. 2004. Neuropathology provides clues to the pathophysiology of Gaucher disease. Mol Genet Metab 82: 192–207.

Wu, Y. R., C. M. Chen, C. Y. Chao, L. S. Ro, R. K. Lyu, K. H. Chang et al. 2007. Glucocerebrosidase gene mutation is a risk factor for early onset of Parkinson disease among Taiwanese. J Neurol Neurosurg Psychiatry 78: 977–979.

Xu, Y. H., Y. Sun, H. Ran, B. Quinn, D. Witte and G. A. Grabowski. 2011. Accumulation and distribution of alpha-synuclein and ubiquitin in the CNS of Gaucher disease mouse models. Mol Genet Metab 102: 436–447.

Yap, T. L., J. M. Gruschus, A. Velayati, W. Westbroek, E. Goldin, N. Moaven et al. 2011. {alpha}-synuclein interacts with Glucocerebrosidase providing a molecular link between Parkinson and Gaucher diseases. J Biol Chem 286(32): 28080–8.

Ziegler, S. G., M. J. Eblan, U. Gutti, K. S. Hruska, B. K. Stubblefield, O. Goker-Alpan et al. 2007. Glucocerebrosidase mutations in Chinese subjects from Taiwan with sporadic Parkinson disease. Mol Genet Metab 91: 195–200.

Zimran, A., O. Neudorfer and D. Elstein. 2005. The glucocerebrosidase gene and Parkinson's disease in Ashkenazi Jews. N Engl J Med 352: 728–731.

Zimran, A., G. Altarescu and D. Elstein. 2013. Pilot study using ambroxol as a pharmacological chaperone in type 1 Gaucher disease. Blood Cells Mol Dis 50: 134–137.

CHAPTER 14

Differential Expression and Function of Linear and Branched Polylactosamine N-linked Glycans in the Nervous System

Gerald A. Schwarting

Introduction

N-acetyl-lactosamine (LN) and N-acetyl-polylactosamine (PLN) are glycans that are components of lipids, O- and N-linked glycoproteins and proteoglycans and are expressed in most if not all cells and tissues in mammals. LN can be expressed as the terminal structure of an oligosaccharide chain, but is often further modified by the addition of fucose, sialic acid and sulfate. Extended LN chains are produced by the repeated alternating addition of β1,4Galactose (β1,4Gal) and β1,3 N-Acetylglucosamine (β1,3GlcNAc) to generate PLN glycans. Although they have been extensively studied for many years, their structures and functions remain unknown for the most part. On red blood cells PLNs serve as scaffolds for many carbohydrate antigens such as ABO, Le^X, Le^Y and sLe^X blood groups. LNs and PLNs are of considerable interest because of their ability to interact with a large family of endogenous lectins, the galectins. A great deal of what we know about lactosamine function comes from studies of galectin-1, which preferentially binds to lactosamine on N- and O-glycans. Thus, LN and PLN can affect biological systems in two ways: by directly modulating the properties of the proteins to which they are attached; and by interacting with galectins and other glycan binding proteins.

There are seven known β1,3GlcNAc transferases in mice with different levels of activity, patterns of expression, and substrate preferences. Although LN is widely expressed, LN containing glycan structures vary considerably depending on the specific GlcNAc transferase expressed in combination with uniqueprotein or lipid backbone structures. Branched N-linked PLN glycans are complex structures that occur only in cells that express the β1,6GlcNAc transferase (GCNT2) blood group-I glycosyltransferase in combination with one of the seven β1,3GlcNAc transferases. Although GCNT2 is expressed at very high levels in sensory neurons in the peripheral nervous system and in the cerebellum of the central nervous system, interest in LN and PLN has been largely focused on their possible roles in the immune system and as regulators of tumor progression and metastasis. From a disease perspective, cancer has been one of the most active topics in glycan research because of the many examples of altered glycosylation patterns

Department of Cell and Developmental Biology, University of Massachusetts Medical School, 55 Lake Avenue North, Worcester, MA 01655.
E-mail: gerald.schwarting@umassmed.edu

observed in animal models and in human tumors. Changing levels of glycosyltransferases can lead to modified N-glycan expression, and one of the most common changes seen is the increase in N-linked branching, which can in turn lead to the increase in terminal epitopes associated with transformed cells. Indeed, inhibiting the synthesis of complex tri- and tetra-antennary N-linked glycan structures has been shown to reduce solid tumor growth (Goss et al. 1997), suggesting that targeting early stages in N-linked glycan synthesis may be a potential anti-cancer treatment.

It is worth noting that many studies of congenital disorders of glycosylation (CDG) reveal that although they are multisystem disorders, the nervous system is most often moderately or severely affected. Recently, studies in knockout mice have shown that the loss of LN and PLN glycans on important glycoproteins in the nervous system causes severe axon guidance defects and aberrant cell-matrix interactions. Here, we review studies on LN and PLN focusing on recent progress in their expression and function in the developing nervous system. Important questions that remain unanswered, particularly in the nervous system, are the identity of proteins that specifically express high levels of PLNs and how these glycans modify the unique properties of the individual proteins. One of the major determinants of N-linked PLN appears to be the restricted co-expression of β3GnT2 and GCNT2, but other factors include the structural features of the unique neuronal proteins being glycosylated, and the number of N-linked sites on those proteins that express PLN. Importantly, expression and function of specific PLN-modified proteins may be conserved, implicating LN and PLN in diseases involving nervous system development.

Synthesis and Expression of N-linked Lactosamine and Polylactosamine

Lactosamine (LN) and Polylactosamine (PLN) Structures

Figure 1 shows the structures of the three types of LN containing glycoproteins that are expressed in mammalian tissues as N-linked glycans. Simple LNs contain one or two disaccharide units, and linear PLNs contain three or more lactosamine disaccharide units. Simple lactosamine and linear polylactosamine are often further modified by the addition of fucose, sialic acid, and sulfate (not shown). N-linked glycans can contain up to 4 antennae and lactosamine units can be added to each of the four branches. Mgat5 (also known as GnT V and GlcNAc-T V), is a β1,6GlcNAc transferase, creating a branch on α-mannose, and is required for the synthesis of tetra-antennary N-linked glycans. In the absence of Mgat5, lactosamine glycans are produced as di- and tri-antennary N-linked glycoproteins rather than as tri- and tetra-antennary glycans

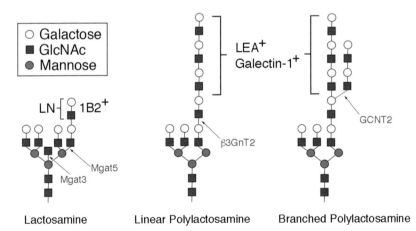

Figure 1. Structures of tri- and tetra-antennary N-linked glycans expressing lactosamine (LN) units. LN can be expressed as one or two units (left) or as a linear chain of 3 or more LN units (center). Prior addition of bisecting GlcNAc by Mgat3 inhibits action of Mgat5, thus tetra-antennary structures with a bisecting GlcNAc (left) are unlikely to occur in significant amounts. Mgat5 is required to produce tetra-antennary glycans but linear and branched PLN glycans can be made as tri-antennary structures. The expression of branched N-linked polylactosamine is dependent on GCNT2. LEA and galectin-1 bind preferentially to long repeating LN units.

(Cummings and Kornfeld 1984). Addition of a bisecting GlcNAc by Mgat3 (see Fig. 1) is considered to be an antagonist of tetra-antennary N-glycan expression because it renders the substrate inaccessible to Mgat5 action (Schachter 1986, Fukuta et al. 2000).

As indicated in Fig. 1, β3GnT2 is the major enzyme responsible for addition of β1,3GlcNAc to N-linked glycans and is the key enzyme in the synthesis of simple lactosamine and linear polylactosamine on N-linked glycans. The 1B2 monoclonal antibody has proven useful for its reactivity with lactosamine on glycolipids and with simple lactosamine on N-linked glycans but not with branched polylactosamine containing glycans (Young et al. 1981).

When initially cloned (Zhou et al. 1999), β3GnT2 was named β3GnT1 to distinguish it from iGnT (Sasaki et al. 1997). Subsequent nomenclature updates occurred, changing the name of iGnT to β3GnT1 and β3GnT1 (Zhou et al. 1999) to β3GnT2. β3GnT1 (iGnT), which since 1997 was thought to be a key regulator of LN and PLN expression in many cells and tissues, has now been shown to be a β4-glucuronyltransferase, and has no activity related to LN or PLN synthesis (Willer et al. 2014, Praissman et al. 2014). Thus the gene previously named iGnT and β3GnT1 is now named B4GAT1. The enzyme activity associated with iGnT gene expression (Magnet and Fukuda 1997, Sasaki et al. 1997, Ujita et al. 1999a,b) is now unclear.

The expression of branched PLN on N-linked glycans is dependent on the β1,6GlcNAc transferase (IGnT), creating a branch on β-galactose. Branched PLN structures thus can be significantly larger and more complex than linear PLN (see Fig. 1). Few large complex N-linked PLNs have been structurally characterized, in part because of the difficulty in distinguishing linear PLN from branched PLN. Identifying reagents that distinguish simple lactosamine from polylactosamine has been difficult.

Lycoperiscon esculentum lectin (LEA or tomato lectin) binds longer chain LN repeats with greater affinity than with simple lactosamine units but it reacts with both linear and branched PLNs (Leppänen et al. 2005). It will agglutinate group O RBCs and all neuraminidase treated RBCs. In humans and in mice LEA is used as marker for microglial cells (Billiards et al. 2006), which are macrophage lineage cells in the brain. Although rarely used, *Datura stramonium* agglutinin (DSA), which has a similar binding specificity to LEA lectin, was used to show that approximately one half of the tri-antennary structures normally contained PLN glycans. In cells that were unable to make tetra-antennary structures, the amount of total PLN was reduced, presumably due to the loss of the 4th antenna. Other useful reagents are some human cold-reactive autoantibodies (reviewed by Cooling 2010) that react with blood group I glycolipids but individual antisera appear to have somewhat differing specificities (Feizi et al. 1979). Other plant lectins, including pokeweed agglutinin, have been used to react specifically with either linear or branched PLN, but their specificities are also difficult to verify (Irimura and Nicolson 1984).

Recent studies in the nervous system have demonstrated that the expression of LN and PLN on N-linked glycoproteins play important roles in cellular signaling (Henion et al. 2005, 2011, 2013, Henion and Schwarting 2014). Histochemical analysis (Fig. 2) shows that 1B2 antibodies react with about 20% of glomeruli (axon terminals) in the olfactory bulb of adult mice. In contrast, LEA reacts strongly with nearly all glomeruli in wild-type mice. In *β3GnT2* knockout mice, LEA reactivity is largely absent, whereas 1B2 reactivity is increased dramatically. These results suggest that β3GnT2 regulates the synthesis of linear N-linked PLN (Henion and Schwarting 2014). Furthermore, although no other β3GnT is upregulated to compensate for the loss of β3GnT2 expression in mutant mice, low levels of other β3GnTs such as β3GnT8 may account for residual expression of simple LN structures in the absence of β3GnT2. In addition, simple LN as defined by 1B2 reactivity is highly expressed by most if not all glomeruli in *β3GnT2*$^{-/-}$ mice. These results also suggest that there is a reciprocal relationship between simple LN and PLN such that β3GnT2 and GCNT2 act together to convert simple LN to linear and branched PLN, respectively.

Simple Lactosamine (LN) and Linear Polylactosamine (PLN) Synthesis and Expression

Simple lactosamine (LN) synthesis requires β1,4-galatosyltransferase (β4GalT) and β3GnT enzyme activities to form the Galβ1-4GlcNAcβ1-3-R disaccharide unit. There are currently seven known β4GalTs expressed in mice, each exhibiting differing specificities towards glycoprotein, glycolipid and proteoglycan acceptors. The best characterized member of the β4GalT family, β4GalT1, has broad activity towards terminal GlcNAc structures on N-glycans and is widely expressed in mammals. In addition, many tissues

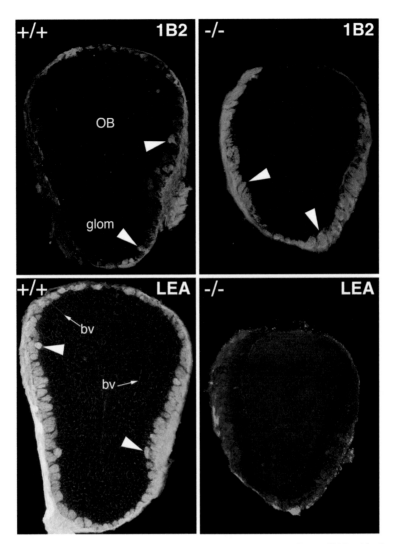

Figure 2. Reciprocal relationship between 1B2 antibody reactive and LEA reactive glomeruli (glom) in the adult olfactory bulb (OB). In *β3GnT2*[+/+] mice, 1B2 reacts weakly with about 20% of all glomeruli, whereas LEA reacts strongly with most glomeruli. In *β3GnT2*[–/–] mice, all glomeruli are strongly 1B2 reactive but are mostly LEA negative. Blood vessels (bv) are also highly LEA reactive in wild-type mice but are LEA negative in null mice (Henion and Schwarting 2014).

express several β4GalT activities, suggesting that one or more of these are present in most cells for synthesizing PLN. In general, the availability of β4GalT activity does appear to be the primary determinant for linear lactosamine expression on N-glycans. However, there are seven β3GnTs that are differentially expressed and have different substrate specificities (Zhou et al. 1999, Shiraishi et al. 2001, Togayachi et al. 2001, Hiruma et al. 2004, Ishida et al. 2005). β3GnT1 was originally named iGnT because it was the first enzyme described that was capable of the synthesis of lactosamine units characteristic of the i blood group antigen (Sasaki et al. 1997). The enzymatic activity of β3GnT1 was questionable however, and it was finally shown that the protein has no N-acetylglucosaminyltransferase activity and is, in fact, a β4-glucuronyltransferase (Willer et al. 2014, Praissman et al. 2014). The implications of β3GnT1 having no role in LN or PLN synthesis are discussed below in more detail. β3GnT2 is believed to be the main enzyme regulating the synthesis of N-linked lactosamine and is expressed most prominently in the peripheral nervous system (Shiraishi et al. 2001, Henion et al. 2005). β3GnT8 also synthesizes N-linked lactosamine and is expressed in many tissues in mice (Ishida et al. 2005) but is believed to have much weaker activity than β3GnT2 (Togayachi et al. 2010). β3GnT3 and β3GnT6 are involved in O-linked lactosamine synthesis. Both enzymes are principally expressed in mouse stomach, intestine, colon, trachea and esophagus (Shiraishi et al. 2001, Iwai et al. 2002). β3GnT5 synthesizes lactosamine on glycolipids (Henion et al. 2001, Togayachi et al. 2001) and β3GnT7 produces lactosamine on keratan sulfate glycosaminoglycans and is mainly expressed in colon and placenta in mice (Kataoka and Huh 2002).

In most cases, the expression of these β3GnT genes has not been examined at the individual tissue level using techniques that detail cell-specific expression. Classical methodologies, such as Northern blotting, as well as RT-qPCR analysis can sometimes be problematic for mRNAs that are broadly expressed in blood vessels that vascularize all tissues. For example, β3GnT2 expression determined by RT-qPCR and Northern analysis initially showed broad expression in most tissues examined (Zhou et al. 1999, Shiraishi et al. 2001). *In situ* hybridization studies, by contrast, show that β3GnT2 mRNA is highly expressed in sensory neurons of the peripheral nervous system of mice including olfactory neurons, trigeminal neurons, dorsal root ganglion neurons and also other cranial ganglia (Henion et al. 2005). Other studies also show that *in situ* hybridization analyses provide invaluable evidence that β3GnTs can be expressed in a highly restricted fashion. For example, in adult mouse cerebellum, β3GnT5 is expressed only in Purkinje cells, not in granule cells or in glia (Henion et al. 2001).

Branched Polylactosamine Synthesis and Expression in Mice

The expression of N-linked branched PLN chains requires the β1-6 N-acetylglucosaminyltransferase branching enzyme named IGnT, in addition to β4GalT and β3GnT activity (see Fig. 1). Since most mammalian tissues are likely to express β4GalT activity together with one or more of the 7β3GnTs, PLN expression is also often said to be ubiquitous. IGnT activity was initially reported in rat tissue (Gu et al. 1992) then cloned and analyzed in several reports from the Fukuda laboratory (Bierhuizen et al. 1993, Ujita et al. 1999a,b, Yeh et al. 1999). The gene that encodes the IGnT enzyme, GCNT2 is expressed in brain, kidney, intestine, lung, spleen and thymus in adult mice (Magnet and Fukuda 1997), and it was concluded from Northern blots that it was expressed by glial cells in the cerebellum of adult mice (Sasaki et al. 1997). *In situ* hybridization studies demonstrate that GCNT2 expression is more restricted than previously thought (Henion and Schwarting 2014). It is principally expressed in sensory neurons in the olfactory system, in cranial ganglia, in the spinal cord, dorsal root ganglia and the cerebellum. These studies also suggest that branched PLN expression is highly restricted in the developing and adult mouse. Interestingly, GCNT2 expression in the embryonic mouse is very similar to the expression of β3GnT2, the enzyme responsible for the expression of the majority of N-linked PLN glycans (Henion and Schwarting 2014).

HEK293 cells were cultured in order to study LEA$^+$ PLN synthesis and expression (Fig. 3). Mock transfected cells are weakly LEA positive suggesting that one or more of the β3GnT genes, including β3GnT2 and β3GnT8 may be expressed endogenously by these cells. In HEK293 cells transfected with β3GnT2, LEA reactivity increased due to the expression of N-linked PLN (Henion and Schwarting 2014). Co-transfection of β3GnT2 and Mgat5 did not increase LEA reactivity compared to transfection with β3GnT2 alone. However, co-transfection of β3GnT2 and GCNT2 greatly increased LEA$^+$ N-linked glycan synthesis and expression.

These results demonstrate that β3GnT2 and GCNT2 together are required for high level expression of LEA$^+$ glycans on the cell surface (Henion and Schwarting 2014). Studies with Mgat5 have demonstrated that PLN modification of cell surface glycoproteins can enhance their retention at the cell surface (Dennis et al. 2009). Our results demonstrate that co-expression of β3GnT2 and GCNT2 is a clear determinant for increasing PLN in transfected cells and *in vivo*, which may potentially enhance their functions in cell signaling or adhesion within the relatively restricted number of tissues in which they are coexpressed (Henion and Schwarting 2014). Studies that have examined Mgat5-dependent glycosylation have not traditionally used LEA as a measure PLN extension. Very likely, significant differences exist between Mgat5 and GCNT2 in terms of both the specific proteins they glycosylate as well as PLN length, branching and terminal modifications. It would be interesting to see how these differences influence galectin interactions and cell retention for specific proteins using cell-based signaling assays. The glycosyltransferase activities of cells expressing optimal levels of LEA-positive and galectin-reactive, N-linked glycans would likely

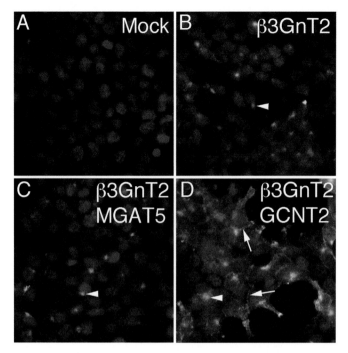

Figure 3. GCNT2 enhances cell surface expression of PLN. HEK293 cells were transfected with glycosyltransferases involved in the synthesis of LEA⁺, N-linked LN and PLN. (A) Mock transfected cells did not react with LEA. (B) β3GnT2 produced weak LEA reactivity (arrowheads) and Mgat5 (C) had little effect on LEA reactivity in cells that expressed β3GnT2. (D) Co-expression of β3GnT2 and GCNT2 induced significantly enhanced LEA reactivity throughout the cell but particularly at the cell surface (arrows) (Henion and Schwarting 2014).

include high levels of β3GnT2, GCNT2 and Mgat5 and low levels of Mgat3 and other LN modifying enzymes like ST6Gal1. Although expression of PLN is said to be ubiquitous, proteins expressing branched, N-linked PLNs that are unmodified by sialic acid, fucose or sulfate may be quite rare.

Human Ii Blood Groups

There is a long-standing interest in the expression and function of LN and PLN. The distinction between the two glycans originated with the discovery of the Ii blood group system. I and i are developmentally regulated red blood cell (RBC) antigens that were first described in 1956 (Wiener et al. 1956). Newborns are typically i positive and I negative but during neonatal development I increases. i_{adult} is a rare phenotype resulting from the loss of the IGnT glycosyltransferase, encoded by the GCNT2 locus. IGnT is a β1,6GlcNAc transferase that is required for the synthesis of branched polylactosamine structures on N-linked glycans. For example Band 3, a protein that is heavily expressed on erythrocytes contains an N-glycan that is composed of more than 20 to 25 lactosamine units (Fukuda et al. 1984). N-linked PLNs from rabbit erythrocytes have also been analyzed in detail. They are composed of bi- and tri-antennary glycans and are usually capped by α-galactose (Sutton-Smith et al. 2007). In both cases, PLN structures are characterized by multiple branches, but nearly all branches consist of single lactosamine units. Furthermore, to emphasize the point that GCNT2 dependent glycans are not ubiquitously expressed, glycophorin A, another major RBC protein, does not contain PLN glycans. GCNT2 dependent glycans can be expressed on N-linked glycoproteins such as Band 3, on O-linked glycoproteins, glycosphingolipids and keratan sulfates.

Mutations in the GCNT2 gene have been reported to be associated with congenital cataracts. The I locus is composed of 5 exons giving rise to 3 isoforms of the enzyme (Yu et al. 2003). The most common transcript uses exons E1A, E2 and E3. A second transcript GCNT2B is expressed in the lens and brain. A third transcript, GCNT2C is expressed only in reticulocytes and is responsible for the expression of

PLN on RBC. Thus, mutations in exon E1C lead to an adult RBC phenotype without cataracts whereas mutations in exons E2 and E3 result in congenital cataracts. RT-PCR analysis of human RNA extracted from various tissue samples indicates that the isoforms are differentially expressed in humans.

Naturally occurring antibodies and monoclonal antibodies have been used to study Ii reactivity (Feizi et al. 1979, Feizi 1981, reviewed by Cooling 2010). By definition anti-i antibodies react with cord blood but not adult RBC, and anti-I antibodies react with adult RBCs but not cord blood. Anti-i antibodies require at least two lactosamine units and are sensitive to endo-β-galactoside treatment that cleaves the individual lactosamine units. Anti-i blood group reactivity is often enhanced by protease treatment. The minimum requirement for anti-I reactivity is a β1,6-branched lactosamine unit that is not sensitive to endo-β-galactosidase treatment. Individual anti-I antibodies are somewhat heterogeneous as shown by their reactivity with a panel of glycolipids (Feizi et al. 1979). Some anti-I antibodies require a Gal-βGlcNAc-β1,3 branch, whereas others require both β1,3 and β1,6 branches.

Function of N-linked Lactosamine and Polylactosamine

Interactions of LN and PLN with Galectins

Lactosamine containing glycans are of considerable potential interest because they have the ability to interact with members of the galectin family of lactosamine binding proteins. Galectins are proteins that share sequence similarities and recognize galactose, LN and PLN containing glycans (Rabinovich et al. 2002). Galectin-1 and galectin-3 are the most studied members of this family and there is considerable evidence that they both play important roles in T cell survival (Clark et al. 2012). Several leukocyte surface glycoproteins, including CD7, CD43 and CD45 have been identified that are recognized by galectin-1 (Galvan et al. 2000, Pace et al. 2000). In addition, even though galectin-1 induced T-cell death is not CD45 dependent, the core 2 GnT2 enzyme greatly enhances CD45 dependent cell death presumably by increasing its expression of O-linked LN (Galvan et al. 2000, Nguyen et al. 2001). In contrast, cells expressing Mgat5 did not induce susceptibility to galectin-1 apoptosis, suggesting that addition of β1,6GlcNAc to mannose does not influence LN expression in these cells. N-linked glycans were also shown to participate in galectin-1 apoptosis, however. When the sialyltransferase, ST6Gal-1 was overexpressed and α2,6-linked sialic acid on the N-linked glycans of CD45 was increased, galectin-1 binding was reduced (Earl et al. 2010). Increased α2,6 sialic acid may decrease galectin-1 binding to other receptors as well, such as CD7, a receptor that is required for galectin-1 apoptosis in human T cells (Amano et al. 2003).

In spite of these elegant studies, complete O- and N-linked structures on thymocytes and T cells remain to be determined. Comprehension of the function of lactosamine-galectin interactions has been slow because of an incomplete understanding of the binding preferences of galectins with simple lactosamines, linear PLN and complex branched PLNs. Binding specificities of many galectin family members have been analyzed in some detail using model compounds and, in general, most prefer to bind to linear PLN structures rather than simple lactosamine. Galectin-1 can also bind fucose- and sialic acid-substituted lactosamines but it is unclear whether galectin-1 prefers branched PLN over linear PLN (Brewer 2004, Leppänen et al. 2005, Stowell et al. 2008). Galectin-1 does not bind tetra-antennary glycans in preference to tri-antennary glycans, however (Hirabayashi et al. 2002). Galectin-1 and LEA binding are very similar in that their degree of binding increases as the number of LN repeats increases (Leppänen et al. 2005).

Galectins also affect T cell homeostasis by interacting with N-linked glycans on T cell receptors (TCR). Galectin-1 enhances TCR binding to MHC complexes resulting in negative selection of CD8[+] T cells (Liu et al. 2008). Galectin-1 also negatively regulates proinflammatory cytokine expression, altering the balance of Th1 and Th2 responses (Toscano et al. 2006, 2007). Recent studies also indicate that subsets of regulatory T cells are involved in immunosuppressive activity that can be neutralized by antibodies to galectin-1 (Garín et al. 2007, Ilarregui et al. 2009). Addition of galectin-1 can induce T cell subsets to synthesize interleukin-10, although the mechanism is poorly understood. In addition, selective removal of specific N-glycosylation sites on TCR increases functional avidity resulting in enhanced recognition of tumor cells (Kuball et al. 2009). The use of recombinant galectin-1 in studies of T cell immunosuppression has limitations, however, and its many convincing effects as well as its potential drawbacks has been recently reviewed (Cedeno-Laurent and Dimitroff 2012).

Galectin-1 is also expressed in endothelial cells (ECs) and is upregulated when ECs are stimulated (Baum et al. 1995). In addition, tumor cells secrete galectin-1, which enhances EC activity (Thijssen et al. 2010). Adding exogenous galectin-1 and galectin-3 to EC lines induced VEGFR1 and VEGFR2 phosphorylation and increased angiogenesis; a result believed to be related to a decrease in receptor endocytosis (D'Haene et al. 2013). Recent studies from the Rabinovich laboratory (Croci et al. 2014) confirmed that galectin-1 is able to bind N-glycans on VEGFR2, increasing phosphorylation and leading to enhanced angiogenesis. They showed that in tumors that are refractory to anti-VEGF treatment, ECs have high N-linked β1,6-GlcNAc branches and low α2,6-linked sialic acid. Thus glycosylation of the endothelial cells in blood vessels determines whether tumors are sensitive to anti-VEGF treatment. Analyses indicated that the majority of the galectin-1 reactive glycans on blood vessel ECs were N-linked rather than O-linked. Indeed, blood vessel ECs in mouse brain are highly LEA reactive (see Fig. 2). LEA reactivity on brain ECs is significantly knocked down in *β3GnT2* null mice indicating that PLN expression on mouse ECs is largely N-linked and is regulated by β3GnT2 (Henion and Schwarting 2014). Importantly, these studies reemphasize the contextual nature of glycan function. In this example, expression of N-linked PLN on VEGFR2 and its interaction with galectin-1 plays an important role in ECs of growing tumors, although it is unclear whether they function in a similar capacity during normal development or in adults, since angiogenesis appears normal in galectin-1 knockout mice. Unfortunately, analysis of galectin knockout mice has not added a great deal of clarity to our understanding of galectin function (Poirier 2002). In some cases, one or more galectin family members may compensate for the loss of galectin-1 in knockout mice. For example, endogenous galectin-10 is thought to substitute for the loss of galectin-1 in regulatory T-cell function (Kubach et al. 2007). In the olfactory system, galectin-1 is expressed by glial cells in axon pathways and is capable of mediating axon fasciculation by interacting with LN or PLN on growing axons (Mahanthappa et al. 1994). Galectins-3, -8, and -9 are also expressed in this tissue, however. Analysis of galectin-1, -9 double knockout mice revealed no obvious phenotype in the olfactory system (G.A. Schwarting, unpublished data), despite the fact that galectin-1 single knockout mice were previously reported to have an axon guidance defect (Puche et al. 1996). Although galectins and PLNs are both expressed in many cells and tissues, one reason that galectin knockout mice have so few obvious phenotypes is that the number of proteins expressing branched PLNs with minimal terminal modifications that would function as physiologically relevant galectin ligands *in vivo* may be smaller than the number of galectin ligands described in *in vitro* studies.

Complex N-linked glycans and their interactions with galectins have also been implicated in protein trafficking to specific cell membranes (Vagin et al. 2009, Delacour et al. 2009). Galectin-9 has been shown to play an important role in apical-basal polarity in MDCK cells for example (Mishra et al. 2010). The sialomucin endolyn is targeted to the apical surface of MDCK cells and it was shown that sorting was dependent on sialic acid on N-linked PLN structures and was mediated by galectin-9 (Mo et al. 2012). Neither bisecting GlcNAc nor tetra-antennary structures were required, however, as knockdown of Mgat3 or Mgat5 did not affect endolyn polarity. It would be interesting to determine whether inhibition of β3GnT2 extension or GCNT2 branching would influence trafficking. Recently galectin interactions with N-linked PLN have been shown to mediate protein sorting into exosomes (EMVs), which are membranous particles secreted from most mammalian cell types (Liang et al. 2014). They identified N-linked proteins that reacted with DSA lectin (similar binding specificity to LEA) and colocalized at the cell surface with EMV markers. Together these studies implicate N-linked PLN with galectin-mediated recruitment of specific proteins into selective microdomains of polarized epithelial cells.

Studies Using Animal Models

Production of transgenic mice in which single genes have been mutated has advanced our understanding of many fundamental mechanisms in developmental biology, although progress in glycobiology has been mixed. This is undoubtedly due, at least in part, to redundancies in overlapping expression and enzymatic function of multiple transferases with similar activities. An excellent example is in the polysialyltransferases

ST8SiaII and ST8SiaIV, expressed in the nervous system (Seidenfaden et al. 2000). These enzymes are expressed in partially overlapping locations but have differing time courses. Both ST8SiaII and ST8SiaIV are expressed in embryonic and early postnatal stages. However, expression of ST8SiaIV remains high postnatally whereas ST8SiaII decreases significantly. Furthermore, in the cerebral cortex the two enzymes are differentially expressed. ST8SiaIV is expressed exclusively in mature cortical interneurons whereas ST8SiaII is expressed in immature neurons in the hippocampus and amygdala. Both enzymes are expressed in neuroblasts in the subventricular zone and rostral migratory stream. In these cells, each enzyme can compensate for the loss of the other enzyme. The two enzymes have very similar abilities to synthesize PSA on NCAM, however they differ in their "context- and site-specific regulation of PSA synthesis" (Nacher et al. 2010).

It is more common than not that the loss of expression of a specific glycan in transgenic mice in which a glycosyltransferase has been mutated does not produce an easily detectable phenotype. Such is the case in mice in which the fucosyltransferase *FUT9* is knocked out. In these mice the Lewis X glycan (also known as stage-specific embryonic antigen SSEA-1 and CD15) is not expressed (Kudo et al. 2004). Lewis X is expressed on a LN backbone and has been implicated in several stages of embryonic development, particularly regulation of cell growth, differentiation, cell recognition and adhesion and its misregulation was implicated in tumor invasion. Lewis X is also expressed in later stages of development where it was suspected of playing important roles in neural differentiation (Yamamoto et al. 1985). However, *FUT9* knockout mice have no significant phenotype, development progresses normally, and they have only subtle defects as adults. This is not a case in which compensation by other enzymes preserves the expression of the glycan; mice completely lacking Lewis X are largely normal.

Reassignment of β3GnT1 as β4GAT1, Xylose β1,4-glucuronyltransferase

α-Dystroglycan (α-DG) is a protein characterized by a unique secondary structure that is highly O-glycosylated and although there have been many studies on the structure of the glycans on α-DG, lactosamine or polylactosamine expression has not previously been described. α-DG has a predicted molecular mass of 72 kD but an apparent molecular mass of 120 kD in cortex, 160 kD in muscle and 180 kD in the cerebellum, in each case due to variable amounts of glycosylation. Several congenital disorders of glycosylation (CDGs) are associated with improper synthesis of O-linked glycans on α-DG (Freeze and Haltiwanger 2009). Walker-Warburg syndrome is associated with the deficiency of O-mannosyltransferase POMT1/POMT2 and the failure to glycosylate α-DG properly. Another CDG, muscle-eye-brain disease is associated with a deficiency in POMGNT1, an O-mannosyl-β-1,2-N-acetylglucosaminyltransferase.

Although earlier studies had linked β3GnT1 expression with α-DG in human prostate and breast carcinoma cell lines (Bao et al. 2009) it had not been studied in the nervous system or in muscle and enzyme activity was not analyzed. In several more recent studies, β3GnT1 gene expression was also implicated in glycosylation of α-DG. Wright et al. (2012) demonstrated that glycosylation of α-DG was abnormal in *β3GnT1* mouse mutants. In the developing brain, α-DG was required for radial glial endfoot attachment to the basement membrane and migrating neurons use the glial fibers as guides. Neuronal migration in *β3GnT1* deficient mice was abnormal and closely resembles the defects found in other dystroglycanopathies. Knockdown of β3GnT1 in zebrafish also led to a dystroglycanopathy, muscle degeneration with a loss of sarcolemma integrity (Buysse et al. 2013). Missense mutations in *B3GNT1* lead to Walker-Warburg syndrome, the most severe form of the congenital muscular dystrophies, with abnormalities in white matter, brain stem and cerebellum. Furthermore, α-DG from patient muscle biopsies was unable to bind laminin (Buysse et al. 2013).

Recent studies have convincingly shown that the *B3GNT1* gene is a xylose β1,4-glucuronyltransferase and contributes to the O-mannosyl modification of α-DG (Willer et al. 2014, Praissman et al. 2014). In recognition of this fact it has been renamed BGAT1. The product of BGAT1 is an acceptor for further elongation by LARGE to produce the terminal ligand binding glycan that is critical for fully functional α-DG.

β3GnT2 Knockout Mice

β3GnT2[−/−] mice were studied extensively to determine whether they exhibited an immune defect (Togayachi et al. 2010). T cells and B cells from these mice showed enhanced initiation of immune responses, although there were no differences in the ratio of cell populations in peripheral blood and no changes in distribution of T or B cells. It was concluded that the loss of β3GnT2 does not effect T or B lymphocyte development.

β3GnT2[−/−] mice have an obvious nervous system phenotype, however. Loss of gene expression in the olfactory system leads to an axon guidance phenotype that resembles the phenotype of mice lacking adenylyl cyclase 3 (AC3) (Henion et al. 2005, 2011). AC3 has a predicted molecular mass of 129 kD with 3 potential N-linked PLN glycans that alter its apparent molecular mass to 200–250 kD in olfactory neurons (Bakalyar and Reed 1990). AC3 is heavily N-glycosylated even when expressed in HEK293 cells (Wei et al. 1996). In *β3GnT2* null mice the molecular mass of AC3 is reduced to about 140 kD. In wild-type mice signaling downstream of AC3 transcriptionally regulates expression of several axon guidance cues, including semaphorin 3A and neuropilin-1. Loss of PLN appears to alter the localization of AC3 by specifically eliminating its expression from axons and growth cones (Fig. 4). The extracellular matrix surrounding the axonal but not the somatodendritic compartments is highly enriched in galectin-1 and -9 but whether galectin-PLN interactions participate in the localization of N-linked glycans in olfactory neurons as it does in other epithelial cells is not known. The loss of PLN on AC3 leads to greatly reduced levels of axonal neuropilin-1 expression, which in turn results in defects in the guidance of olfactory axons to targets in the brain (Henion et al. 2011, Knott et al. 2012). Interestingly, there is also a significant

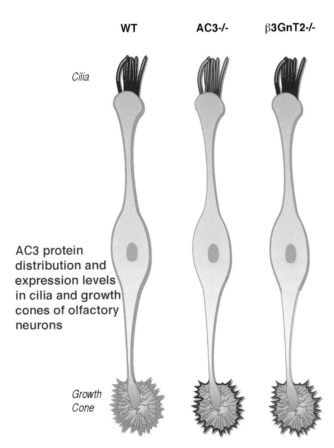

Figure 4. β3GnT2 expression modifies cellular localization of AC3 in olfactory neurons. AC3 is heavily expressed on cilia but is also expressed on dendrites, axons and growth cones of olfactory sensory neurons. Loss of β3GnT2 expression eliminates AC3 from axons and growth cones and causes an axon guidance defect that resembles guidance errors seen in *AC3*[−/−] mice.

phenotype in *β3GnT2*[+/-] mice. In neonatal null mice, neuronal cell death is greatly increased compared to controls and in *β3GnT2* heterozygous mice levels of cell death are midway between controls and mutants (Henion et al. 2005). Western blotting data suggest that intermediate levels of β3GnT2 enzymatic activity results in decreased glycosylation of AC3 and other cell surface proteins, and furthermore, that reduced levels of β3GnT2-dependent glycosylation can have significant effects on cellular function, in this case, on sensory neuron survival.

Another interesting aspect of AC3 regulation is that it is expressed in most neurons in the cerebral cortex where its localization is confined to primary cilia (Bishop et al. 2007). However, because β3GnT2 and GCNT2 are either not expressed or are expressed at very low levels in cortical neurons, AC3 on these cortical neurons is not LEA positive. Thus, AC3 localization, enzymatic activity and signaling function in cortical neurons occur exclusively within the primary cilia but PLN modification is not required for enzymatic activity. The two cell types differ in that PLN[+] AC3 in sensory neurons is localized to cilia, cell soma, and in axons where it performs its downstream signaling function. These results suggest that important cellular functions are often determined by unique glycans on specific proteins in small populations of cells or even at subcellular levels and that teasing out these properties requires structure/function analyses within the specific context of the cellular/subcellular environment in which they occur.

We have also shown that *β3GnT2* mutant mice have an axon guidance defect in the accessory olfactory system (Henion et al. 2013). β3GnT2 is expressed by vomeronasal neurons that send axons to the accessory olfactory bulb (AOB). In *β3GnT2* mutant mice, subsets of axons designated to terminate in the posterior compartment are aberrantly guided to the anterior compartment. The adhesion molecule Kirrel2, which is thought to play an important role in olfactory axon guidance, and is heavily LEA[+], is significantly downregulated on axons projecting to the anterior AOB in *β3GnT2* null mice. There is also a failure to form typically distinct glomeruli (axon terminals) in the anterior AOB. In addition, the guidance cue ephrinA5 is upregulated on axons that project to the anterior AOB. These results demonstrate that N-linked PLN in the accessory olfactory system is required for proper expression of adhesion and guidance molecules, compartmentalization of neuron subsets, and formation of glomeruli.

β3GnT3, β3GnT5 and β3GnT6 Knockout Mice

Lymphocyte homing is mediated by the interaction of L-selectin to 6-sulfo sialyl Lewis X on high endothelial venules (HEV). *β3GnT3* (also named Core1-GnT) was mutated in mice to examine the role of O-glycans in lymphocyte homing. Mice lacking *β3GnT3* retained normal levels of lymphocyte homing suggesting that N-linked glycans on HEV proteins such as CD34 play an important role in L-selectin dependent lymphocyte function (Mitoma et al. 2007).

β3GnT5, also known as Lc3 synthase, initiates the synthesis of neolactoglycolipids containing LN and PLN extensions (Henion et al. 2001, Togayachi et al. 2001). Postnatally, several studies have confirmed β3GnT5 expression in a restricted set of cells and tissues, including lymph nodes, splenic B cells, colon, spleen, and cerebellar Purkinje cells (Henion et al. 2001, Togayachi et al. 2010). In an initial study of mice in which the Lc3 synthase was knocked out, nulls were pre-implantation embryonic lethal (Biellmann et al. 2008). In an independent transgenic mouse model, embryonic development in Lc3 synthase knockout mice was normal but postnatal viability was decreased, with 11% of mice dying within 2 months (Kuan et al. 2010). Null mice also had splenomegaly, reduced fertility, and decreased numbers of splenic B cells. Another *β3GnT5* deficient mouse line developed by Narimatsu's group exhibited alterations in signaling protein composition within glycolipid-enriched microdomain of B-cells, as well as altered thresholds for B-cell receptor activation and lymphocyte proliferation after stimulation (Togayachi et al. 2010). No nervous system phenotype has been reported, however, in any of these models. The discrepancies in viability between the three mouse lines generated may relate to differences in the particular targeting strategies or ES cell lines utilized in the targeting and the genetic background of the strains of mice. In all 3 mouse lines examined, neolacto glycolipid synthesis was abolished, confirming the central role of β3GnT5 in regulating PLN extensions on glycolipids.

β3GnT6 (also named Core3-GnT) is expressed in gastrointestinal epithelial cells and plays an important role in synthesis of O-glycans in the intestinal mucus layer (Iwai et al. 2002). Disruption of the

C3GnT gene in mice eliminated O-glycan structures from the colon (An et al. 2007). These mice exhibited reduced Muc2 expression and were highly susceptible to induced colitis, suggesting that these O-glycans are important for resistance to colonic disease.

CGNT2 Knockout Mice

GCNT2 encodes the β1-6 N-acetyl-GlcNAc transferase that is essential for the synthesis of I-branched glycans on N-linked glycoproteins and on glycolipids. Using an anti-I specific monoclonal antibody, I-branched structures were shown to be absent from most tissues examined including stomach, kidney, bone marrow and cerebellum of GCNT2 knockout mice (Chen et al. 2005). Residual IGnT activity detected in the small intestine with oligosaccharide acceptors was ascribed to C2GnT2 encoded by GCNT3, which is expressed in this tissue and possesses modest I-branching activity (Yeh et al. 1999). A negative rotorod test in null mice suggested that the there were no significant cerebellar abnormalities. The major phenotype described for these mice was that they had a reduced number of lymphocytes, increased vacuolization in kidneys, and renal function was reduced. However, there were no studies carried out to examine abnormalities in sensory neurons where GCNT2 expression is highest. In the absence of *GCNT2*, linear N-linked PLN can still be produced in cells that express β3GnT2, so in the future it will be interesting to determine whether I-branching plays an important role in sensory neuron development.

Mgat5 Knockdown

Studies relating glycosylation and cancer have held a dominant position in glycobiology research since the concept of tumor associated glycans was introduced more than 40 years ago (Meezan et al. 1969). Changes in protein glycosylation such as increased sialylation and fucosylation in tumor cells is well recognized (Schultz et al. 2012, Christiansen et al. 2013). One of the most extensively investigated tumor related glycans is N-linked glycans associated with Mgat5, the gene that encodes the β1-6 N-acetyl-glucosaminyltransferase that catalyzes the addition of GlcNAc to α1,6-mannose on N-linked glycans. It is required for the synthesis of tetra-antennary N-linked glycans (see Fig. 1), and is expressed in most cells and tissues throughout development and in adults.

Increases in the expression of these structures have been implicated in the initial stages of cancer, in the progression of cancer stages, and in metastasis of breast, colon, and hepatocellular carcinoma (Dube and Bertozzi 2005). The association of Mgat5 with malignancy has been reported in many different contexts, but it remains unclear whether it is a causative factor in neoplastic transformation. In one of the first studies of this enzyme, it was shown that Mgat5 deficient cells, selected for by cytotoxic lectin resistance, express lower levels of PLNs (Cummings and Kornfeld 1984). This important study showed that in the absence of tetra-antennary structures, PLN was expressed in tri- and bi-antennary structures. Many studies have been carried out in order to show that Mgat5 is involved in malignant transformation by comparing normal cells to transformed cells and non-metastatic tumor cells to metastatic tumor cells. The results showed that Mgat5 was not necessary for solid tumor growth but was in most cases correlated with metastatic potential and the overall conclusion from this large number of reports was that Mgat5 regulated N-linked PLN expression (Dennis et al. 1987, 1989, Yousefi et al. 1991). It was also concluded that the lectin L-PHA, which recognizes GlcNAc-β1,6mannose, could be used to detect changes in the expression of PLN even though it has negligible reactivity with Gal-β1,4GlcNAc (Laferte and Dennis 1989). *Mgat5* null mice have been extensively analyzed for abnormalities in a variety of systems, primarily related to immune function. In the course of these studies, L-PHA reactivity was the major criterion used to indicate that PLN expression was altered despite the rather indirect connection. *Mgat5*[-/-] mice have delayed cancer progression (Dennis et al. 2002) and increased susceptibility to experimental allergic encephalomyelitis (EAE) due to decreased PLN on T cell receptors (Demetriou et al. 2001). It was also shown that increased E-cadherin-dependent cell-cell adhesion was increased in *Mgat5*[-/-] cells (Guo et al. 2003), although recent studies suggest that Mgat5-dependent glycosylation of E-cadherin may be secondary to the bisecting GlcNAc activity of Mgat3 during epithelial-mesenchymal transitions (Pinho et al. 2009, 2012). Indeed, galectin-regulated growth factor signaling is reduced by Mgat3 expression (Song et al. 2010). This may be due to decreased galectin interactions with complex bisected-GlcNAc glycans, or more likely, that Mgat3-dependent bisected-GlcNAc glycans (see Fig. 1) are poor substrates for Mgat5 and βGalT4 (Fukuta et al. 2000) and express lower amounts of galectin-reactive complex branched PLN structures (Schachter 1986, Yoshimura et al. 1996). It was also shown that Mgat3 modification of proteins such as the α3 integrin subunit counteracts the effects of Mgat5 on the same substrate (Zhao et al. 2006). The fact that there is so little LEA reactive PLN in the mouse central nervous system may, in part, reflect the high levels of expression of Mgat3 in the developing and adult brain (Priatel et al. 1997, Bhattacharyya et al. 2002). In spite of these many caveats, it is generally accepted that Mgat5 influences expression of PLN, at least in the immune system and in relationship to metastatic potential of tumor cells.

A mechanism was proposed suggesting that Mgat5 could play a role in important cellular functions by regulating the amount of N-linked PLN on cell surface glycoproteins (Partridge et al. 2004). It was suggested that the retention of cell surface proteins could be controlled by interaction with one or more PLN-binding molecules, such as galectin family members. Furthermore, this model suggests that by altering expression of N-linked PLN at the cell surface, signaling by cytokines and other active molecules may be affected. As mentioned above, neuronal survival is decreased in *β3GnT2* heterozygous mice, indicating that reduced levels of PLN can affect critical cellular functions in an intact model (Henion et al. 2005). In addition, as shown in Fig. 3, co-expression of β3GnT2 and GCNT2 can further increase N-linked PLN synthesis and expression at the cell surface (Henion and Schwarting 2014). Taken together, these studies suggest that fine-tuning PLN synthesis and expression can have important cellular consequences and that different cells may employ alternate strategies to accomplish that goal. Whether or not levels of PLN expression influence cell functions is likely to be dependent on the cell type in question, the exact receptor, cytokine, or enzyme that is N-glycosylated, the subcellular localization of the protein, its endocytosis and recycling to the cell surface, and the involvement of signaling pathways.

Studies of mice lacking *Mgat5* and/or *Mgat5b*(IX) (a paralog of Mgat5 that synthesizes branches on O-linked glycans in the brain), show that *Mgat5* null brains did not synthesize N-linked β1,6 branched antennas, but they had normal levels of O-linked branched structures (Lee et al. 2012). *Mgat5b* null mice had normal levels of N-linked β1,6 structures. Not unsurprisingly, since there is no evidence that PLN plays a role in α-DG function, loss of both *Mgat5* and *Mgat5b* does not alter the ability of α-DG to bind to laminin (Lee et al. 2012). In fact there does not appear to be any significant structural or functional changes in the nervous system of double knockout mice, indicating that the expression and function of N-linked LN and PLN glycans in the nervous system is independent of Mgat5 and Mgat5b function. In this regard, it is likely that the major regulator of N-linked PLN expression in cells such as olfactory neurons is the co-expression of β3GnT2 and GCNT2 but that in other cells and tissues, Mgat5 may play a role in influencing the levels of N-linked PLN expression (Henion and Schwarting 2014).

Mgat5 knockout mice were also used to study the role of galectin-1 in angiogenesis (Croci et al. 2014). Proteins in *Mgat5*[-/-] mice lack tetra-antennary N-linked glycans and it was shown that there was a decrease in galectin-1 binding to VEGFR2 in null mice. Although Mgat5 siRNA knocked down galectin-1 binding by more than 50%, fluorescent imaging revealed that galectin-1 binding was still quite robust, indicating that PLN expression remained intact. So although loss of Mgat5 expression does not eliminate PLN synthesis, it can influence the level of PLN expression, which in turn, can modulate cellular activity at least in some contexts. It might be informative to carry out similar studies on EC cells from *β3GnT2*[-/-] mice, where LEA-reactive PLN expression is completely knocked down, to look at galectin-1 binding. Interestingly, it was suggested that modulation of angiogenesis, rather than suppression of tumor metastasis (Granovsky et al. 2000), may be an alternative mechanism to explain the reduced tumorigenesis seen in *Mgat5*[-/-] mice.

Conclusions and Future Perspectives

Congenital disorders of glycosylation (CDG) syndromes are a growing family of genetic disorders resulting from defects in the synthesis of O- and N-linked glycans. The nervous system is often affected although other organs are also variably involved (Barone et al. 2014). Analysis of patients with these disorders has proven invaluable in understanding the role of glycans in health and disease. It is interesting that, although 76 different CDGs are known, an unambiguous cancer phenotype has yet to be described. Perhaps this may be part of the reason that all previous attempts to produce antibodies that are clinically useful for various cancer treatments have failed. Interestingly, in March of 2015 Unituxin, humanized antibodies to ganglioside GD2, was FDA-approved as an immunotherapeutic treatment for high-risk neuroblastoma. Unituxin is the first successful immunotherapeutic to target a non-protein antigen. However, because of significant toxicity, second generation antibodies, such as anti-idiotypic antibodies are being generated with the goal of reducing side effects (Yu et al. 2010, Matthay et al. 2012). Using this anti-idiotype approach may be an option for producing other tumor specific anti-glycan therapeutics, such as anti-Neu5Gn (Dalziel et al. 2014).

Many CDGs are caused by defects in the very early events in N-glycan synthesis but a few CDGs result from mutations in glycosyltransferases that are directly involved in synthesis of multi-antennary N-linked glycans. Of these, *MGAT2-CDG* is significant, even though only 4 patients have been described. This syndrome results from mutations in the MGAT2 gene that encodes β-1,2-N-acetylglucosaminyltransferase 2 and is responsible for the synthesis of bi-antennary N-linked glycans. Patients with *MGAT2-CDG* are unable to synthesize more complex tri- and tetra-antennary glycans. These patients have severe defects in development of the nervous system. The have psychomotor retardation, hypotonia, craniofacial dysmorphology, seizures and gastrointestinal problems (Jaeken et al. 1994).

It is said that there is greater potential structural diversity in the glycan repertoire than that generated by all peptides and proteins combined (Ohtsubo and Marth 2006). Although this may be true, the vast majority of glycans that have been structurally characterized have relatively similar core and terminal structures. Furthermore, in most cases, glycans have similar or overlapping functions. They play characteristic roles in many different cell types, such as promotion of protein folding, trafficking, and localization. Functional redundancy tends to limit the deleterious effects of knocking out enzymes responsible for glycan synthesis (Dalziel et al. 2014). Studies of congenital disorders of glycosylation in humans and the production of transgenic animal models have enabled significant advances in our understanding of the function of glycan modification of proteins and lipids, particularly in the nervous system (Schachter 2005, Freeze et al. 2012). Disease models show that synthesis of core glycan structures play similar roles in many cells types, the reason that many of these mutations affect multi-organ systems. Mouse models are critical for establishing the relationship between novel glycans and specific proteins, such as the role of lunatic fringe in transferring O-fucose to Notch proteins during somitogenesis and of POMT1 and 2 and now β4GAT1 in glycosylation of α-dystroglycan during development of the nervous system (Johnston et al. 1997, Willer et al. 2014, Praissman et al. 2014).

Analysis of glycosylation function can be puzzling. The simplest glycans may have the most profound influences on protein function. One simple saccharide, O-GlcNAc, modifies the activity of many cytosolic and nuclear proteins (Hart 2014). O-GlcNAc is enriched in brain, for example, and is believed to modify synaptic plasticity by regulating localization of proteins such as synapsin I to synapses (Cole and Hart 2001, Skorobogatko et al. 2014). Alternatively, extremely complex glycan structures that are expressed at the cell surface may regulate the function of just one or a few specific proteins. For example, sialo-Lewis X expression on leukocytes acts as a selectin ligand (Varki and Gagneux 2012); polysialic acid (PSA) expression on neurons regulates NCAM function (Durbec and Cremer 2001); and O-mannosyl glycans controls α-DG interactions with extracellular matrix proteins (Yoshida-Moriguchi et al. 2010). In cells and tissues in which the synthesis of unique glycans is paired with the expression of a novel protein, it is often the case that an important cellular function is affected. Complex and unusual glycan structure does not guarantee functional significance, however. Knockout of the sulfotransferase that regulates HNK-1 expression in the nervous system has little effect on brain development and only subtle effects on neurological function in adults (Schwarting et al. 1987, Chou et al. 2002, Senn et al. 2002). In contrast, improper heparin sulfate proteoglycan sulfotransferase activity results in misrouting of midline crossing axons in the central nervous system due to aberrant receptor-ligand interactions (Bulow et al. 2008, Conway et al. 2011). In fact, it has been argued by proponents of a 'glycan code' that the function of HSPGs may be determined by variations in the sulfation of the glycan rather than by the core protein itself (Bülow and Hobert 2004).

Although there have been many studies published on LN containing proteins and lipids, only a few reports clearly demonstrate that LN or PLN affect the function of specific proteins in mammals. There are several factors that have contributed to this gap in our understanding: (i), in many reports there is no distinction made between simple LN and linear and branched PLN; (ii), few N- or O-linked PLN structures have been determined, in part due to their size and complexity; and (iii), mouse models in which glycosyltransferases involved in LN and PLN synthesis have been knocked out have only recently begun to reveal interesting phenotypes; (iv) misassignment of one or more glycosyltransferases has lead to confusion which has slowed understanding in this field.

Mutating specific genes in transgenic animals clearly establishes the critical importance of novel glycans modifying protein function. This approach has also recently revealed new functions of LN and PLN glycans during development of the nervous system. However, correct analysis of gene expression and correlation with detailed studies of enzyme activity is key to moving the field rapidly forward. Mutation of the *β3GnT2* gene causes aberrant glycosylation of AC3 and leads to defects in axon guidance of sensory axons in the olfactory system. Similar to the effort directed at understanding the function of the many cytosolic and nuclear proteins that express O-GlcNAc, future studies of PLN function will require in depth genotype/phenotype analyses on a cell by cell and protein by protein basis, using all the techniques available to developmental, molecular, biochemical, neurobiological, cell biological, genetic, and behavioral scientists.

Acknowledgements

This work was supported by the National Institutes of Health grant DC00953. The author thanks Peter Daniel and Timothy Henion for critical reading of the manuscript.

Keywords: Lactosamine, galectin, N-linked glycans, neurons, signaling, axon guidance

References

Amano, M., M. Galvan, J. He and L. G. Baum. 2003. The ST6Gal I sialyltransferase selectively modifies N-glycans on CD45 to negatively regulate galectin-1-induced CD45 clustering, phosphatase modulation, and T cell death. J Biol Chem 278: 7469–7475.

An, G., B. Wei, B. Xia, J. M. McDaniel, T. Ju, R. D. Cummings et al. 2007. Increased susceptibility to colitis and colorectal tumors in mice lacking core 3-derived O-glycans. J Exp Med 204: 1417–1429.

Bakalyar, H. A. and R. R. Reed. 1990. Identification of a specialized adenylyl cyclase that may mediate odorant detection. Science 250: 1403–1406.

Bao, X., M. Kobayashi, S. Hatakeyama, K. Angata, D. Gullberg, J. Nakayama et al. 2009. Tumor suppressor function of laminin-binding alpha-dystroglycan requires a distinct beta3-N-acetylglucosaminyltransferase. Proc Natl Acad Sci USA 106: 12109–12114.

Barone, R., A. Fiumara and J. Jaeken. 2014. Congenital disorders of glycosylation with emphasis on cerebellar involvement. Semin Neurol 34: 357–366.

Baum, L. G., J. J. Seilhamer, M. Pang, W. B. Levine, D. Beynon and J. A. Berliner. 1995. Synthesis of an endogenous lectin, galectin-1, by human endothelial cells is up-regulated by endothelial cell activation. Glycoconj J 12: 63–68.

Bhattacharyya, R., M. Bhaumik, T. S. Raju and P. Stanley. 2002. Truncated, inactive N-acetylglucosaminyltransferase III (GlcNAc-TIII) induces neurological and other traits absent in mice that lack GlcNAc-TIII. J Biol Chem 277: 26300–26309.

Biellmann, F., A. J. Hülsmeier, D. Zhou, P. Cinelli and T. Hennet. 2008. The Lc3-synthase gene B3gnt5 is essential to pre-implantation development of the murine embryo. BMC Dev Biol 8: 109.

Bierhuizen, M. F., M. G. Mattei and M. Fukuda. 1993. Expression of the developmental I antigen by a cloned human cDNA encoding a member of a beta-1,6-N-acetylglucosaminyltransferase gene family. Genes Dev 7: 468–478.

Billiards, S. S., R. L. Haynes, R. D. Folkerth, F. L. Trachtenberg, L. G. Liu, J. J. Volpe et al. 2006. Development of microglia in the cerebral white matter of the human fetus and infant. J Comp Neurol 497: 199–208.

Bishop, G. A., N. F. Berbari, J. Lewis and K. Mykytyn. 2007. Type III adenylyl cyclase localizes to primary cilia throughout the mouse brain. J Comp Neurol 505: 562–571.

Brewer, C. F. 2004. Thermodynamic binding studies of galectin-1, -3 and -7. Glycoconj J 19: 459–465.

Bülow, H. E. and O. Hobert. 2004. Differential sulfations and epimerization define heparan sulfate specificity in nervous system development. Neuron 41: 723–736.

Bülow, H. E., N. Tjoe, R. A. Townley, D. Didiano, T. H. van Kuppevelt and O. Hobert. 2008. Extracellular sugar modifications provide instructive and cell-specific information for axon-guidance choices. Curr Biol 18: 1978–1985.

Buysse, K., M. Riemersma, G. Powell, J. van Reeuwijk, D. Chitayat, T. Roscioli et al. 2013. Missense mutations in β-1,3-N-acetylglucosaminyltransferase 1 (B3GNT1) cause Walker-Warburg syndrome. Hum Mol Genet 22: 1746–1754.

Cedeno-Laurent, F. and C. J. Dimitroff. 2012. Galectin-1 research in T cell immunity: Past, present and future. Clin Immunol 142: 107–116.

Chen, G. Y., H. Muramatsu, M. Kondo, N. Kurosawa, Y. Miyake, N. Takeda et al. 2005. Abnormalities caused by carbohydrate alterations in Ibeta6-N-acetylglucosaminyltransferase-deficient mice. Mol Cell Biol 25: 7828–7838.

Chou, D. K., M. Schachner and F. B. Jungalwala. 2002. HNK-1 sulfotransferase null mice express glucuronyl glycoconjugates and show normal cerebellar granule neuron migration *in vivo* and *in vitro*. J Neurochem 82: 1239–1251.

Christiansen, M. N., J. Chik, L. Lee, M. Anugraham, J. L. Abrahams and N. H. Packer. 2013. Cell surface protein glycosylation in cancer. Proteomics 10.1002/pmic.

Clark, M. C., M. Pang, D. K. Hsu, F. T. Liu, S. de Vos, R. D. Gascoyne et al. 2012. Galectin-3 binds to CD45 on diffuse large B-cell lymphoma cells to regulate susceptibility to cell death. Blood 120: 4635–4644.

Cole, R. N. and G. W. Hart. 2001. Cytosolic O-glycosylation is abundant in nerve terminals. J Neurochem 79: 1080–1089.

Conway, C. D., K. M. Howe, N. K. Nettleton, D. J. Price, J. O. Mason and T. Pratt. 2011. Heparan sulfate sugar modifications mediate the functions of slits and other factors needed for mouse forebrain commissure development. J Neurosci 31: 1955–1970.

Cooling, L. 2010. Polylactosamines, there's more than meets the "Ii": A review of the I system. Immunohematology 26: 133–155.

Croci, D. O., J. P. Cerliani, T. Dalotto-Moreno, S. P. Méndez-Huergo, I. D. Mascanfroni, S. Dergan-Dylon et al. 2014. Glycosylation-dependent lectin-receptor interactions preserve angiogenesis in anti-VEGF refractory tumors. Cell 156: 744–758.

Cummings, R. D. and S. Kornfeld. 1984. The distribution of repeating [Gal beta 1,4GlcNAc beta 1,3] sequences in asparagine-linked oligosaccharides of the mouse lymphoma cell lines BW5147 and PHAR 2.1. J Biol Chem 259: 6253–6260.

Dalziel, M., M. Crispin, C. N. Scanlan, N. Zitzmann and R. A. Dwek. 2014. Emerging principles for the therapeutic exploitation of glycosylation. Science 343: 37–45.

Delacour, D., A. Koch and R. Jacob. 2009. The role of galectins in protein trafficking. Traffic 10: 1405–1413.

Demetriou, M., M. Granovsky, S. Quaggin and J. W. Dennis. 2001. Negative regulation of T-cell activation and autoimmunity by Mgat5 N-glycosylation. Nature 409: 733–739.

Dennis, J. W., S. Laferté, C. Waghorne, M. L. Breitman and R. S. Kerbel. 1987. Beta 1-6 branching of Asn-linked oligosaccharides is directly associated with metastasis. Science 236: 582–585.

Dennis, J. W., K. Kosh, D. M. Bryce and M. L. Breitman. 1989. Oncogenes conferring metastatic potential induce increased branching of Asn-linked oligosaccharides in rat2 fibroblasts. Oncogene 4: 853–860.

Dennis, J. W., J. Pawling, P. Cheung, E. Partridge and M. Demetriou. 2002.UDP-N-acetylglucosamine:alpha-6-D-mannoside beta1,6 N-acetylglucosaminyltransferase V (Mgat5) deficient mice. Biochim Biophys Acta 1573: 414–422.

Dennis, J. W., I. R. Nabi and M. Demetriou. 2009. Metabolism, cell surface organization, and disease. Cell 139: 1229–1241.

D'Haene, N., S. Sauvage, C. Maris, I. Adanja, M. Le Mercier, C. Decaestecker et al. 2013. VEGFR1 and VEGFR2 involvement in extracellular galectin-1- and galectin-3-induced angiogenesis. PLoS One 8: e67029.

Dube, D. H. and C. R. Bertozzi. 2005. Glycans in cancer and inflammation—potential for therapeutics and diagnostics. Nat Rev Drug Discov 4: 477–488.

Durbec, P. and H. Cremer. 2001. Revisiting the function of PSA-NCAM in the nervous system. Mol Neurobiol 24: 53–64.

Earl, L. A., S. Bi and L. G. Baum. 2010. N- and O-glycans modulate galectin-1 binding, CD45 signaling, and T cell death. J Biol Chem 285: 2232–2244.

Feizi, T., R. A. Childs, K. Watanabe and S. I. Hakomori. 1979. Three types of blood group I specificity among monoclonal anti-I autoantibodies revealed by analogues of a branched erythrocyte glycolipid. J Exp Med 149: 975–980.

Feizi, T. 1981. The blood group Ii system: a carbohydrate antigen system defined by naturally monoclonal or oligoclonal autoantibodies of man. Immunol Commun 10: 127–156.

Freeze, H. H. and R. S. Haltiwanger. 2009. Other classes of ER/Golgi-derived glycans. pp. 163–174. *In*: Varki, A., R. D. Cummings, J. D. Esko, H. H. Freeze, P. Stanley, C. R. Bertozzi et al. (eds.). Essentials of Glycobiology, 2nd edition. Cold Spring Harbor Laboratory Press, Cold Spring Harbor, New York, USA.

Freeze, H. H., E. A. Eklund, B. G. Ng and M. C. Patterson. 2012. Neurology of inherited glycosylation disorders. Lancet Neurol 11: 453–466.

Fukuda, M., A. Dell, J. E. Oates and M. N. Fukuda. 1984. Structure of branched lactosaminoglycan, the carbohydrate moiety of band 3 isolated from adult human erythrocytes. J Biol Chem 259: 8260–8273.

Fukuta, K., R. Abe, T. Yokomatsu, F. Omae, M. Asanagi and T. Makino. 2000. Control of bisecting GlcNAc addition to N-linked sugar chains. J Biol Chem 275: 23456–23461.

Galvan, M., S. Tsuboi, M. Fukuda and L. G. Baum. 2000. Expression of a specific glycosyltransferase enzyme regulates T cell death mediated by galectin-1. J Biol Chem 275: 16730–16737.

Garín, M. I., C. C. Chu, D. Golshayan, E. Cernuda-Morollón, R. Wait and R. I. Lechler. 2007. Galectin-1: A key effector of regulation mediated by CD4+CD25+ T cells. Blood 109: 2058–2065.

Goss, P. E., C. L. Reid, D. Bailey and J. W. Dennis. 1997. Phase IB clinical trial of the oligosaccharide processing inhibitor swainsonine in patients with advanced malignancies. Clin Cancer Res 3: 1077–1086.

Granovsky, M., J. Fata, J. Pawling, W. J. Muller, R. Khokha and J. W. Dennis. 2000. Suppression of tumor growth and metastasis in GlcNAc-T V-deficient mice. Nat Med 6: 306–312.

Gu, J., A. Nishikawa, S. Fujii, T. Gasa and N. Taniguchi. 1992. Biosynthesis of blood group I and i antigens in rat tissues. Identification of a novel beta 1-6-N-acetylglucosaminyltransferase. J Biol Chem 267: 2994–2999.

Guo, H. B., I. Lee, M. Kamar and M. Pierce. 2003. N-acetylglucosaminyltransferase V expression levels regulate cadherin-associated homotypic cell-cell adhesion and intracellular signaling pathways. J Biol Chem 278: 52412–54224.

Hart, G. W. 2014. Minireview series on the thirtieth anniversary of research on O-GlcNAcylation of nuclear and cytoplasmic proteins: Nutrient regulation of cellular metabolism and physiology by O-GlcNAcylation. J Biol Chem 289: 34422–34423.

Henion, T. R., D. Zhou, D. P. Wolfer, F. B. Jungalwala and T. Hennet. 2001. Cloning of a mouse beta 1,3 N-acetylglucosaminyltransferase GlcNAc(beta 1,3)Gal(beta 1,4)Glc-ceramide synthase gene encoding the key regulator of lacto-series glycolipid biosynthesis. J Biol Chem 276: 30261–30269.

Henion, T. R., D. Raitcheva, R. Grosholz, F. Biellmann, W. C. Skarnes, T. Hennet et al. 2005. Beta1,3-N-acetylglucosaminyltransferase 1 glycosylation is required for axon pathfinding by olfactory sensory neurons. J Neurosci 25: 1894–1903.

Henion, T. R., A. A. Faden, T. K. Knott and G. A. Schwarting. 2011. β3GnT2 maintains adenylyl cyclase-3 signaling and axon guidance molecule expression in the olfactory epithelium. J Neurosci 31: 6576–6586.

Henion, T. R., P. A. Madany, A. A. Faden and G. A. Schwarting. 2013. β3GnT2 null mice exhibit defective accessory olfactory bulb innervation. Mol Cell Neurosci 52: 73–86.

Henion, T. R. and G. A. Schwarting. 2014. N-linked polylactosamine glycan synthesis is regulated by co-expression of β3GnT2 and GCNT2. J Cell Physiol 229: 471–478.

Hirabayashi, J., T. Hashidate, Y. Arata, N. Nishi, T. Nakamura, M. Hirashima et al. 2002. Oligosaccharide specificity of galectins: A search by frontal affinity chromatography. Biochim Biophys Acta 1572: 232–254.

Hiruma, T., A. Togayachi, K. Okamura, T. Sato, N. Kikuchi, Y. D. Kwon et al. 2004. A novel human beta1,3-N-acetylgalactosaminyltransferase that synthesizes a unique carbohydrate structure, GalNAcbeta1-3GlcNAc. J Biol Chem 279: 14087–14095.

Ilarregui, J. M., D. O. Croci, G. A. Bianco, M. A. Toscano, M. Salatino, M. E. Vermeulen et al. 2009. Tolerogenic signals delivered by dendritic cells to T cells through a galectin-1-driven immunoregulatory circuit involving interleukin 27 and interleukin 10. Nat Immunol 10: 981–991.

Irimura. T. and G. L. Nicolson. 1984. Interaction of pokeweed mitogen with poly(N-acetyllactosamine)-type carbohydrate chains. Carbohydr Res 120: 187–195.

Ishida, H., A. Togayachi, T. Sakai, T. Iwai, T. Hiruma, T. Sato et al. 2005. A novel beta1,3-N-acetylglucosaminyltransferase (beta3Gn-T8), which synthesizes poly-N-acetyllactosamine, is dramatically upregulated in colon cancer. FEBS Lett 579: 71–78.

Iwai, T., N. Inaba, A. Naundorf, Y. Zhang, M. Gotoh, H. Iwasaki et al. 2002. Molecular cloning and characterization of a novel UDP-GlcNAc:GalNAc-peptide beta1,3-N-acetylglucosaminyltransferase (beta 3Gn-T6), an enzyme synthesizing the core 3 structure of O-glycans. J Biol Chem 277: 12802–12809.

Jaeken, J., H. Schachter, H. Carchon, P. De Cock, B. Coddeville and G. Spik. 1994. Carbohydrate deficient glycoprotein syndrome type II: A deficiency in Golgi localised N-acetyl-glucosaminyltransferase II. Arch Dis Child 71: 123–127.

Johnston, S. H., C. Rauskolb, R. Wilson, B. Prabhakaran, K. D. Irvine and T. F. Vogt. 1997. A family of mammalian Fringe genes implicated in boundary determination and the Notch pathway. Development 124: 2245–2254.

Kataoka, K. and N. H. Huh. 2002. A novel beta1,3-N-acetylglucosaminyltransferase involved in invasion of cancer cells as assayed *in vitro*. Biochem Biophys Res Commun 294: 843–848.

Knott, T. K., P. A. Madany, A. A. Faden, M. Xu, J. Strotmann, T. R. Henion et al. 2012. Olfactory discrimination largely persists in mice with defects in odorant receptor expression and axon guidance. Neural Development 7: 17.

Kuan, C. T., J. Chang, J. E. Mansson, J. Li, C. Pegram, P. Fredman et al. 2010. Multiple phenotypic changes in mice after knockout of the B3gnt5 gene, encoding Lc3 synthase—a key enzyme in lacto-neolacto ganglioside synthesis. BMC Dev Biol 10: 114.

Kubach, J., P. Lutter, T. Bopp, S. Stoll, C. Becker, E. Huter et al. 2007. Human CD4+CD25+ regulatory T cells: Proteome analysis identifies galectin-10 as a novel marker essential for their anergy and suppressive function. Blood 110: 1550–1558.

Kuball, J., B. Hauptrock, V. Malina, E. Antunes, R. H. Voss, M. Wolfl et al. 2009. Increasing functional avidity of TCR-redirected T cells by removing defined N-glycosylation sites in the TCR constant domain. J Exp Med 206: 463–475.

Kudo, T., M. Kaneko, H. Iwasaki, A. Togayachi, S. Nishihara, K. Abe et al. 2004. Normal embryonic and germ cell development in mice lacking alpha 1,3-fucosyltransferase IX (Fut9) which show disappearance of stage-specific embryonic antigen 1. Mol Cell Biol 24: 4221–4228.

Laferte, S. and J. W. Dennis. 1989. Purification of two glycoproteins expressing beta 1-6 branched Asn-linked oligosaccharides from metastatic tumour cells. Biochem J 259: 569–576.

Lee, J. K., R. T. Matthews, J. M. Lim, K. Swanier, L. Wells and J. M. Pierce. 2012. Developmental expression of the neuron-specific N-acetylglucosaminyltransferase Vb (GnT-Vb/IX) and identification of its *in vivo* glycan products in comparison with those of its paralog, GnT-V. J Biol Chem 287: 28526–28536.

Leppänen, A., S. Stowell, O. Blixt and R. D. Cummings. 2005. Dimeric galectin-1 binds with high affinity to alpha2,3-sialylated and non-sialylated terminal N-acetyllactosamine units on surface-bound extended glycans. J Biol Chem 280: 5549–5562.

Liang, Y., W. S. Eng, D. R. Colquhoun, R. R. Dinglasan, D. R. Graham and L. K. Mahal. 2014. Complex N-linked glycans serve as a determinant for exosome/microvesicle cargo recruitment. J Biol Chem 289: 32526–32537.

Liu, S. D., C. C. Whiting, T. Tomassian, M. Pang, S. J. Bissel, L. G. Baum et al. 2008. Endogenous galectin-1 enforces class I-restricted TCR functional fate decisions in thymocytes. Blood 112: 120–130.

Magnet, A. D. and M. Fukuda. 1997. Expression of the large I antigen forming beta-1,6-N-acetylglucosaminyltransferase in various tissues of adult mice. Glycobiology 7: 285–295.

Mahanthappa, N. K., D. N. Cooper, S. H. Barondes and G. A. Schwarting. 1994. Rat olfactory neurons can utilize the endogenous lectin, L-14, in a novel adhesion mechanism. Development 120: 1373–1384.

Matthay, K. K., R. E. George and A. L. Yu. 2012. Promising therapeutic targets in neuroblastoma. Clin Cancer Res 2012 18: 2740–2753.

Meezan, E., H. C. Wu, P. H. Black and P. W. Robbins. 1969. Comparative studies on the carbohydrate-containing membrane components of normal and virus-transformed mouse fibroblasts. II. Separation of glycoproteins and glycopeptides by sephadex chromatography. Biochemistry 8: 2518–2524.

Mishra, R., M. Grzybek, T. Niki, H. Hirashima and K. Simons. 2010. Galectin-9 trafficking regulates apical-basal polarity in Madin-Darby canine kidney epithelial cells. Proc Natl Acad Sci USA 107: 17633–17638.

Mitoma, J., X. Bao, B. Petryanik, P. Schaerli, J. M. Gauguet, S. Y. Yu et al. 2007. Critical functions of N-glycans in L-selectin-mediated lymphocyte homing and recruitment. Nat Immunol 2: 409–418.

Mo, D., S. A. Costa, G. Ihrke, R. T. Youker, N. Pastor-Soler, R. P. Hughey et al. 2012. Sialylation of N-linked glycans mediates apical delivery of endolyn in MDCK cells via a galectin-9-dependent mechanism. Mol Bio Cell 23: 3636–3646.

Nacher, J., R. Guirado, E. Varea, G. Alonso-Llosa, I. Röckle and H. Hildebrandt. 2010. Divergent impact of the polysialyltransferases ST8SiaII and ST8SiaIV on polysialic acid expression in immature neurons and interneurons of the adult cerebral cortex. Neuroscience 167: 825–837.

Nguyen, J. T., D. P. Evans, M. Galvan, K. E. Pace, D. Leitenberg, T. N. Bui et al. 2001. CD45 modulates galectin-1-induced T cell death: regulation by expression of core 2 O-glycans. J Immunol 167: 5697–5707.

Ohtsubo, K. and J. D. Marth. 2006. Glycosylation in cellular mechanisms of health and disease. Cell 126: 855–867.

Pace, K. E., H. P. Hahn, M. Pang, J. T. Nguyen and L. G. Baum. 2000. CD7 delivers a pro-apoptotic signal during galectin-1-induced T cell death. J Immunol 165: 2331–2334.

Partridge, E. A., C. Le Roy, G. M. Di Guglielmo, J. Pawling, P. Cheung, M. Granovsky et al. 2004. Regulation of cytokine receptors by Golgi N-glycan processing and endocytosis. Science 306: 120–124.

Pinho, S. S., C. A. Reis, J. Paredes, A. M. Magalhães, A. C. Ferreira, J. Figueiredo et al. 2009. The role of N-acetylglucosaminyltransferase III and V in the post-transcriptional modifications of E-cadherin. Hum Mol Genet 18: 2599–2608.

Pinho, S. S., P. Oliveira, J. Cabral, S. Carvalho, D. Huntsman, F. Gärtner et al. 2012. Loss and recovery of Mgat3 and GnT-III Mediated E-cadherin N-glycosylation is a mechanism involved in epithelial-mesenchymal-epithelial transitions. PLoS One 7: e33191.

Poirier, F. 2002. Roles of galectins *in vivo*. Biochem Soc Symp 69: 95–103.

Praissman, J. L., D. H. Live, S. Wang, A. Ramiah, Z. S. Chinoy, G. J. Boons et al. 2014. B4GAT1 is the priming enzyme for the LARGE-dependent functional glycosylation of α-dystroglycan. Elife 03943.

Priatel, J. J., M. Sarkar, H. Schachter and J. D. Marth. 1997. Isolation, characterization and inactivation of the mouse Mgat3 gene: the bisecting N-acetylglucosamine in asparagine-linked oligosaccharides appears dispensable for viability and reproduction. Glycobiology 7: 45–56.

Puche, A. C., F. Poirier, M. Hair, P. F. Bartlett and B. Key. 1996. Role of galectin-1 in the developing mouse olfactory system. Dev Biol 179: 274–287.

Rabinovich, G. A., L. G. Baum, N. Tinari, R. Paganelli, C. Natoli, F. T. Liu et al. 2002. Galectins and their ligands: amplifiers, silencers or tuners of the inflammatory response? Trends Immunol 23: 313–320.

Sasaki, K., K. Kurata-Miura, M. Ujita, K. Angata, S. Nakagawa, S. Sekine et al. 1997. Expression cloning of cDNA encoding a human beta-1,3-N-acetyllactosaminyltransferase that is essential for poly-N-acetyllactosamine synthesis. Proc Natl Acad Sci USA 94: 14294–14299.

Schachter, H. 1986. Biosynthetic controls that determine the branching and microheterogeneity of protein-bound oligosaccharides. Biochem Cell Biol 64: 163–181.

Schachter, H. 2005. Deficient glycoprotein glycosylation in human and mice. pp. 157–198. *In*: Fukuda, M., U. Rutishauser and R. Schnaar (eds.). Neuroglycobiology. Oxford University Press.

Schultz, M. J., A. F. Swindall and S. L. Bellis. 2012. Regulation of the metastatic cell phenotype by sialylated glycans. Cancer Metastasis Rev 31: 501–518.

Schwarting, G. A., F. B. Jungalwala, D. K. Chou, A. M. Boyer and M. Yamamoto. 1987. Sulfated glucuronic acid-containing glycoconjugates are temporally and spatially regulated antigens in the developing mammalian nervous system. Dev Biol 120: 65–76.

Seidenfaden, R., R. Gerardy-Schahn and H. Hildebrandt. 2000. Control of NCAM polysialylation by the differential expression of polysialyltransferases ST8SiaII and ST8SiaIV. Eur J Cell Biol 79: 680–688.

Senn, C., M. Kutsche, A. Saghatelyan, M. R. Bösl, J. Löhler, U. Bartsch et al. 2002. Mice deficient for the HNK-1 sulfotransferase show alterations in synaptic efficacy and spatial learning and memory. Mol Cell Neurosci 20: 712–729.

Shiraishi, N., A. Natsume, A. Togayachi, T. Endo, T. Akashima, Y. Yamada et al. 2001. Identification and characterization of three novel beta 1,3-N-acetylglucosaminyltransferases structurally related to the beta 1,3-galactosyltransferase family. J Biol Chem 276: 3498–3507.

Skorobogatko, Y., A. Landicho, R. J. Chalkley, A. V. Kossenkov, G. Gallo et al. 2014. O-Linked β-N-Acetylglucosamine (O-GlcNAc) Site Thr-87 Regulates Synapsin I Localization to Synapses and Size of the Reserve Pool of Synaptic Vesicles. J Biol Chem 289: 3602–3612.

Song, Y., J. A. Aglipay, J. D. Bernstein, S. Goswami and P. Stanley. 2010. The bisecting GlcNAc on N-glycans inhibits growth factor signaling and retards mammary tumor progression. Cancer Res 70: 3361–3371.

Stowell, S. R., C. M. Arthur, K. A. Slanina, J. R. Horton, D. F. Smith and R. D. Cummings. 2008. Dimeric Galectin-8 induces phosphatidylserine exposure in leukocytes through polylactosamine recognition by the C-terminal domain. J Biol Chem 283: 20547–20559.

Sutton-Smith, M., N. K. Wong, K. H. Khoo, S. W. Wu, S. Y. Yu, M. S. Patankar et al. 2007. Analysis of protein-linked glycosylation in a sperm-somatic cell adhesion system. Glycobiology 17: 553–567.

Thijssen, V. L., B. Barkan, H. Shoji, I. M. Aries, V. Mathieu, L. Deltour et al. 2010. Tumor cells secrete galectin-1 to enhance endothelial cell activity. Cancer Res 70: 6216–6224.

Togayachi, A., T. Akashima, R. Ookubo, T. Kudo, S. Nishihara, H. Iwasaki et al. 2001. Molecular cloning and characterization of UDP-GlcNAc: Lactosylceramide beta 1,3-N-acetylglucosaminyltransferase (beta 3Gn-T5), an essential enzyme for the expression of HNK-1 and Lewis X epitopes on glycolipids. J Biol Chem 276: 22032–22040.

Togayachi, A., Y. Kozono, A. Kuno, T. Ohkura, T. Sato, J. Hirabayashi et al. 2010. Beta3GnT2 (B3GNT2), a major polylactosamine synthase: Analysis of B3GNT2-deficient mice. Methods Enzymol 479: 185–204.

Toscano, M. A., A. G. Commodaro, J. M. Ilarregui, G. A. Bianco, A. Liberman, H. M. Serra et al. 2006. Galectin-1 suppresses autoimmune retinal disease by promoting concomitant Th2- and T regulatory-mediated anti-inflammatory responses. J Immunol 176: 6323–6332.

Toscano, M. A., G. A. Bianco, J. M. Ilarregui, D. O. Croci, J. Correale, J. D. Hernandez et al. 2007. Differential glycosylation of TH1, TH2 and TH-17 effector cells selectively regulates susceptibility to cell death. Nat Immunol 8: 825–834.

Ujita, M., J. McAuliffe, M. Suzuki, O. Hindsgaul, H. Clausen, M. N. Fukuda et al. 1999a. Regulation of I-branched poly-N-acetyllactosamine synthesis. Concerted actions by I-extension enzyme, I-branching enzyme, and beta1,4-galactosyltransferase I. J Biol Chem 274: 9296–9304.

Ujita, M., J. McAuliffe, O. Hindsgaul, K. Sasaki, M. N. Fukuda and M. Fukuda. 1999b. Poly-N-acetyllactosamine synthesis in branched N-glycans is controlled by complemental branch specificity of I-extension enzyme and beta1,4-galactosyltransferase I. J Biol Chem 274: 16717–16726.

Vagin, O., J. A. Kraut and G. Sachs. 2009. Role of N-glycosylation in trafficking of apical membrane proteins in epithelia. Am J Physiol Renal Physiol 296: F459–469.

Varki, A. and P. Gagneux. 2012. Multifarious roles of sialic acids in immunity. Ann N Y Acad Sci 1253: 16–36.

Wei, J., G. Wayman and D. R. Storm. 1996. Phosphorylation and inhibition of type III adenylyl cyclase by calmodulin-dependent protein kinase II *in vivo*. J Biol Chem 271: 24231–24235.

Wiener, A. S., L. J. Unger, L. Cohen and J. Feldman. 1956. Type-specific cold auto-antibodies as a cause of acquired hemolytic anemia and hemolytic transfusion reactions: biologic test with bovine red cells. Ann Internal Med 44: 221–240.

Willer, T., K. I. Inamori, D. Venzke, C. Harvey, G. Morgensen, Y. Hara et al. 2014. The glucuronyltransferase B4GAT1 is required for initiation of LARGE-mediated α-dystroglycan functional glycosylation. Elife 03941.

Wright, K. M., K. A. Lyon, H. Leung, D. J. Leahy, L. Ma and D. D. Ginty. 2012. Dystroglycan organizes axon guidance cue localization and axonal pathfinding. Neuron 76: 931–944.

Yamamoto, M., A. M. Boyer and G. A. Schwarting. 1985. Fucose-containing glycolipids are stage- and region-specific antigens in developing embryonic brain of rodents. Proc. Natl Acad Sci USA 82: 3045–3049.

Yeh, J. C., E. Ong and M. Fukuda. 1999. Molecular cloning and expression of a novel beta-1, 6-N-acetylglucosaminyltransferase that forms core 2, core 4, and I branches. J Biol Chem 274: 3215–3221.

Yoshida-Moriguchi, T., L. Yu, S. H. Stalnaker, S. Davis, S. Kunz, M. Madson et al. 2010. O-mannosyl phosphorylation of alpha-dystroglycan is required for laminin binding. Science 327: 88–92.

Yoshimura, M., Y. Ihara, A. Ohnishi, N. Ijuhin, T. Nishiura, Y. Kanakura et al. 1996. Bisecting N-acetylglucosamine on K562 cells suppresses natural killer cytotoxicity and promotes spleen colonization. Cancer Res 56: 412–418.

Young, W. W. Jr., J. Portoukalian and S. Hakomori. 1981. Two monoclonal anticarbohydrate antibodies directed to glycosphingolipids with a lacto-N-glycosyl type II chain. J Biol Chem 256: 10967–10972.

Yousefi, S., E. Higgins, Z. Daoling, A. Pollex-Krüger, O. Hindsgaul and J. W. Dennis. 1991. Increased UDP-GlcNAc: Gal beta 1-3GaLNAc-R (GlcNAc to GaLNAc) beta-1, 6-N-acetylglucosaminyltransferase activity in metastatic murine tumor cell lines. Control of polylactosamine synthesis. J Biol Chem 266: 1772–1782.

Yu, A. L., A. L. Gilman, M. F. Ozkaynak, W. B. London, S. G. Kreissman, H. X. Chen et al. 2010. Anti-GD2 antibody with GM-CSF, interleukin-2, and isotretinoin for neuroblastoma. N Engl J Med 363: 1324–1334.

Yu, L. C., Y. C. Twu, M. L. Chou, M. E. Reid, A. R. Gray, J. M. Moulds et al. 2003. The molecular genetics of the human I locus and molecular background explain the partial association of the adult i phenotype with congenital cataracts. Blood 101: 2081–2088.

Zhao, Y., T. Nakagawa, S. Itoh, K. Inamori, T. Isaji, Y. Kariya et al. 2006. N-acetylglucosaminyltransferase III antagonizes the effect of N-acetylglucosaminyltransferase V on alpha3beta1 integrin-mediated cell migration. J Biol Chem 281: 32122–32130.

Zhou, D., A. Dinter, R. Gutiérrez Gallego, J. P. Kamerling, J. F. Vliegenthart, E. G. Berger et al. 1999. A beta-1,3-N-acetylglucosaminyltransferase with poly-N-acetyllactosamine synthase activity is structurally related to beta-1,3-galactosyltransferases. Proc Natl Acad Sci USA 96: 406–411.

CHAPTER 15

Immunoglobulin Glycosylation in Health and Disease

Michelle E. Conroy[1],* and Robert M. Anthony[2],*

Introduction

Immunoglobulins are essential effector proteins of the immune system. They function to pair recognition of foreign threat with immune system response. This requires structural duality of the protein allowing for both diverse target detection and binding to fixed receptors. The precise specificity of antibodies results from programmed genetic rearrangements and mutations. The resultant alterations in protein structure yield marked diversity in antibody recognition. This is the basis for antibody surveillance for innumerable immune system threats. Coupling the detection portion of antibodies to immune system response is critical to this process. As such, the constant region of antibodies, which are invariable and bind specific receptors expressed by various cells of the immune system. Ultimately, antibody interaction with receptors is responsible for the downstream biologic effect of the antibody. Indeed, the interaction of antibody and receptor results in many distinct functions including antibody transport, linking antigen recognition and immune system response, and in controlling the serum half-life of antibodies (Raghavan and Bjorkman 1996).

There are 5 major subtypes of immunoglobulins in mammals, namely IgG, IgA, IgM, IgD, and IgE all of which are produced by B cells. These subclasses are derived from a common pre-cursor with a B cell able to generate each subclass if necessary. Circumstances leading to production of each subclass is complex and involves the antigen itself, local environment and additional signaling (Shroeder and Cavacini 2010). IgM antibodies are associated with acute infection and primary immune responses. In addition, IgM may also have immunoregulatory functions (Boes 2000). IgG is the most abundant of the antibodies with wide distribution and a very long serum half-life. In general, IgG antibodies are potent activators of the complement cascade and also can directly neutralize toxins and viruses (Shroeder and Cavacini 2010). IgA is found in high concentrations at mucosal surfaces and plays a critical role in preventing infection by neutralization and prevention of microbe binding. While IgE is the least abundant of serum antibodies,

[1] Center for Immunology and Inflammatory Diseases, Division of Rheumatology, Allergy, and Immunology, Department of Medicine, 149 13th Street, Room 8.321, Massachusetts General Hospital, Harvard Medical School, Boston, MA, 02129 USA.
 E-mail: meconroy@mgh.harvard.edu
[2] Center for Immunology and Inflammatory Diseases, Division of Rheumatology, Allergy, and Immunology, Department of Medicine, 149 13th Street, Room 8.307, Massachusetts General Hospital, Harvard Medical School, Boston, MA, 02129 USA.
 E-mail: robert.anthony@mgh.harvard.edu
* Corresponding authors

its role in triggering potent allergic reactions is well known. IgD is found on the surface of naive B cells, and its function not well described. Taken together, these classes of antibodies provide surveillance and protection against a wide spectrum of threats. Importantly, all five mammalian antibody types are glycoproteins. While the number of glycosylation sites and types of glycans attached vary depending on the antibody type, recent evidence has demonstrated that glycosylation plays an important and unappreciated role in antibody function.

Overall, antibodies provide a critical aspect of immune system functioning to maintain a healthy host. However, the variable portion of the antibody at times recognizes targets that elicit dysfunction and disease. Many autoimmune diseases, including rheumatoid arthritis, systemic lupus erythematosus, diabetes mellitus, thyroid disease and others, are triggered by antibodies erroneously targeted against host proteins. In addition, autoimmune antibody production has been increasingly implicated in malignancy though causative mechanisms are unclear. Allergic diseases are driven by antibody recognition of what may otherwise be innocuous proteins resulting in food allergy, asthma, and even death from anaphylaxis. Thus, antibody dysfunction can lead to a host of detrimental sequelae. However, despite antibody variability representing a liability in these cases, it can also be potently beneficial. Due to the intrinsic variable nature of antibodies, it has long been known that specificity can be engineered to meet a clinical need. Vaccines deliver pieces of viruses and bacteria and result in generation of specific antibodies to prevent infection. More recently, the therapeutic role of antibodies has expanded exponentially as technology allows for more refined engineering of antibody specificity and downstream responses. Antibody mediated immunotherapy is being increasingly applied to therapeutics for a wide range of diseases. For instance, in cancer antibodies are directed at specific tumor antigens, which can trigger tumor cell death. However, it also seems that the effector portion of these therapeutic antibodies trigger further immune system responses including cellular immunity which may additionally contribute to anti-tumor activity (Michaud et al. 2014). The potential use of antibodies as therapy for a wide range of disorders is becoming increasingly clear. However, optimizing clinical responses clearly rests on combining both aspects of antibody biology: precise recognition of antigen and engagement of host receptors and proteins that trigger desired effector functions.

Antibody Structure

Treatment of IgG with the protease papain revealed two major productions, one that was capable of binding antigen, and another that was crystallizable. These fragments were therefore named the antigen-binding fragments (Fab), and crystallizable fragments (Fc), respectively. Indeed, these basic domains are present on all antibody classes, as the Fab is responsible for the precise recognition of conformational antigens, while the Fc conveys the effector properties of each antibody class. Monomeric structures of antibodies are paired heavy and light chains. Fabs are composed of variable regions at the N-terminus of each chain. A single constant domain in the light chain exists, which pairs with the constant domain 1 of heavy chain. The heavy chain extends to form the antibody Fc, of which different antibody classes determined the number of domains, and also whether the antibodies will form multimers or be monomeric (Fig. 1).

Variable regions are responsible for recognition of antigens, and the minority of immunoglobulins are glycosylated in this region (15–20%). Introduction of glycosylation sites into the variable regions has been observed during somatic hypermutation, the process through which antibodies gain high affinity for antigens (Dudley et al. 2005). It is therefore possible that glycosylation of the Fab is important for antigen-recognition. However, the contribution of glycosylation to antibody effector function will be the focus of this chapter.

IgG and Glycosylation

IgG antibodies are the most prevalent in the circulation, at 10 mg/mL in human sera. IgG antibodies are essential for host defense against infection, and are often the intended outcome of many vaccines. Further, over 30-therapeutic IgG antibodies have been approved for use in humans by regulatory agencies. A number of characteristics of IgG make this antibody class the basis of a useful drug. These antibodies have an extended serum half-life of 21 days, due to the neonatal Fc receptor (FcRn). They often have

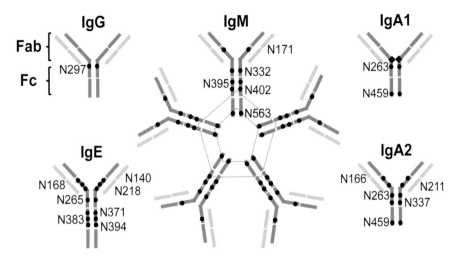

Figure 1. Structures of secreted mammalian antibodies. Light chains (light gray) and heavy chain (gray) pair to form the variable antigen-binding fragments (Fab). The heavy chain extends to the constant crystallizable fragment (Fc). The N-linked glycosylation sites are shown as black circles with amino acid positions are listed. Oligomannose clusters of IgA1 are shown as black diamonds. IgM monomers are linked by the J chain, which is shown as pentagon.

high specificity, and recognize precise structures. Moreover, they can be made recombinantly. Finally, they are potent inducers of inflammation. IgG antibodies engage IgG Fc-specific receptors (FcγRs), which are expressed by leukocytes, thereby linking antibodies with inflammatory cells. IgG can also bind the initiator of the classical complement cascade, C1q.

A single, N-linked glycosylation site is present on all mammalian IgG antibodies, at asparagine-297 in the C_H2 domain of the Fc (Fig. 1). The glycan has a complex, biantennary structure that is highly variable. The Fc glycans face toward the center of the IgG molecule, with the α1,3 arm extending into the cavity between heavy chains, and the α1,6 arm extending along the heavy chain backbone. Indeed, over 30-distinct glycans based on the core biantennary glycan have been identified on IgG Fcs in the sera of healthy individuals. The Fc glycans vary by the presence of fucose attached to the core GlcNAc, bisecting GlcNAc, or by attachment of galactose or sialic acid to the arms (Fig. 2A). Importantly, these variable contributions have marked effects on the biological activity of IgG, as is discussed below.

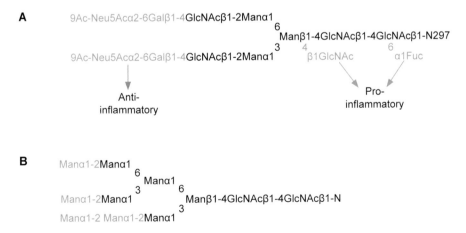

Figure 2. Antibody glycan structures. (A) Complex biantennary N-linked glycan structures found on all antibody types are shown. The core glycan found on all IgG Fc is shown in black, with variable glycan additions in gray. Sialic acid bestows anti-inflammatory activity, while the bisecting GlcNAc and core fucose modulate pro-inflammatory activity. (B) N-linked oligomannose structures are shown, with Man5 core shown in black and Man9 in gray.

Glycosylation through the secretory pathway has been described in detail elsewhere. Briefly, the process begins in the lumen of the endoplasmic reticulum with transfer of a 14 monosaccharide glycan (glucose$_3$mannose$_9$N-acetylglucosamine$_2$ ($Glc_3Man_9GlcNAc_2$)), to aspargine-297 (N297, Fig. 1) on each IgG heavy chain by the enzyme oligosaccharyltransferase. Next, the glycan is trimmed to a high-mannose structure ($Man_{8-9}GlcNAc_2$) by exoglycosidases while the IgG heavy and light chains are assembled together, and the intact IgG molecule is then transported to the Golgi. In the *cis*-Golgi, the mannose residues are trimmed by α1,2 mannosidase-I to yield a $Man_5GlcNAc_2$ glycan. In the *medial*-Golgi, N-acetylglucosamine is added by β1,2-N-acetylglucosaminyltransferase-I forming $GlcNAc_1Man_5GlcNAc_2$, and α1,2 mannosidase-II further removes mannose residues forming the hybrid glycan structure $GlcNAc_1Man_3GlcNAc_2$. Next, the core IgG glycan ($GlcNAc_3Man_3GlcNAc_2$) is generated by the transfer of N-acetylglucosamine by β1,2-N-acetylglucosaminyltransferase-II. Here, the core N-acetylglucosamine is available for fucosylation by α1,6-fucosyltransferase. Bisecting N-acetylglucosamine is attached to the core by N-acetylglucosaminyltransferase-III. As the IgG antibody progresses along the secretory pathway, the glycan can be further modified in the *trans*-Golgi by the addition of galactose and sialic acid to the arms by β1,4 galactosyltransferase and α2,6 sialyltransferase, respectively (Stanley et al. 2009, An 2009).

The single IgG Fc glycan is absolutely required for binding of wild type IgG to FcγRs, as the interaction is lost by de-glycosylating IgG (Feige et al. 2009). The Fc glycan is thought to maintain an open confirmation of the Fc heavy chains required for interactions with FcγRs. The structure of aglycosylated Fcs supports this, as the two heavy chains form a closed conformation, preventing formation of the FcγR binding pocket (Feige et al. 2009). However, mutations in the Fc backbone can be introduced, which presumably mimic appropriate conformation folding, and enable a-glycosylated Fcs to bind FcγRs (Sazinsky et al. 2008). This indicates the Fc glycan primarily affects protein-protein interactions by altering the IgG backbone conformation. However, larger immune complexes formed by a-galactosylated IgG have been demonstrated to be capable of binding to FcγRs, however, whether large, aglycosylated immune complexes are capable of triggering the canonical IgG effector functions is not known (Lux et al. 2013).

Variability in IgG Glycan Structure

With multiple monomeric sugars available as substrates, glycans at the N297 site of IgG can have significant structural variability. For example, approximately 15% of IgG antibodies are sialylated. In addition, in complex glycans of IgG, galactose is the terminal sugar 50% of the time and terminal GlcNAc 35% of the time. A bisecting GlcNAc is present in approximately one third of IgG glycans and a core fucose in almost 70% (Arnold et al. 2007) (Fig. 2a). The determinants of these arrangements are largely based on substrate availability, steric interaction, and glycosylation enzyme availability. In addition, the specifics of the glycan may reflect the genetic and environmental influences on the cell (Maverakis et al. 2015). Within a population, there can be marked variability in the IgG glycome. In a study of over 2000 individuals across three populations, IgG glycome variability was dramatic. Heritability only accounted for about 30–50% of these variations and gender did not play a role. The IgG glycome in this study was three times more variable than the total plasma protein glycome (Pucic et al. 2011). IgG N-linked glycans were generally larger and more complex in children compared to adults. Core fucosylation decreased age. Intriguingly, gender differences were less significant in children than adults (Pucic et al. 2012). However, overall, there seems to be changes in the stability of an individual's glycome over time suggesting temporal uniformity and stability within glycosylation mechanisms (Gornik et al. 2009). A study cohort of both monozygotic and dizygotic female twins suggested the majority of variation in the IgG glycome was attributable to genetic factors. This would suggest that the genetic influence over IgG glycosylation may be significant, perhaps even as compared to the glycome overall. For glycan traits with low heritability, epigenetic associations appeared to play a more significant role (Menni et al. 2013).

As antibodies become increasingly utilized for therapeutics, mass production via non-human mammalian cells lines becomes critical to achieve appropriate quantity. Chinese hamster ovary (CHO) cells lines have become the most common cell host used for this purpose. In 1986, these were initially utilized to generate recombinant tissue plasminogen activator (t-PA). They are now responsible for at least 70% of recombinant protein therapeutics (Kim et al. 2012). Glycosylation can vary significantly between mammalian species. As a result, protein glycosylation in non-human cells might generate glycosylated proteins that trigger an immune response in humans. For example, galactose-α1,3-galactose residues (alpha-gal) can be expressed as a terminal sugar residue not seen in humans. Murine α-1,3-galactosyltransferase produces alpha-gal and many humans have antibodies directed against this sugar, related to prior exposures. Severe anaphylactic reactions occurred in patients in certain U.S. locations upon exposure to a monoclonal antibody with non-human epitopes including alpha-gal (Chung et al. 2008). Murine cells express much higher levels of this enzyme than hamster cells, representing one of several advantages for using CHO cells. While certain glycosylation patterns may prove detrimental to humans, glycoengineering can be utilized to generate advantageous glycan structures. This can be achieved via genetic modifications, such as gene transfection, or use of glycosylation inhibitors (Butler and Spearman 2014). For example, hyperglycosylation of human erythropoietin allowed for increased stability, higher potency, and reduced dosing interval in patients (Elliott et al. 2004).

The composition of the N-glycan can have significant effect on the effector functions of the IgG molecule. Many of these variations have clinical correlations as a result. Several well-studied variations in IgG N-glycans are presented below with associated basic science and clinical findings.

Galactose

Galactose can be added to the glycan arms in β1,4 linkages by β1,4 galactosyltransferase (B4GALT1) in the *trans*-Golgi (Fig. 2a). Altered frequencies of IgG with Fc glycans terminating in galactose have long been observed in various inflammatory diseases, including rheumatoid arthritis. Specifically, reductions in galactosylation, and increases in agalactosylated IgG Fc glycoforms, appear to correlate with ongoing inflammation. Intriguingly, pregnancy-associated remission of inflammatory arthritis was associated with restored levels of galactosylated IgG Fc glycans (van de Geijn et al. 2009). Together, these observations suggest galactose might play a regulatory role. However, enzymatic removal of terminal galactose has no effect on FcγR affinity, serum half-life, or induction of inflammation in induced arthritis and immune thrombocytopenia (ITP) models (Nimmerjahn et al. 2007, Anthony et al. 2008a). Thus, it is likely that galactose itself does not directly attribute to IgG effector properties. Instead, removal of galactose may alter IgG biology by either exposure of GlcNAc on arms, or by reducing sialic acid. Removal of galactose is thought to enhance binding of the mannose-binding lectin, the initiator of the lectin-mediated complement pathway. This has been observed in citrullinated-peptide-specific IgG recovered from RA patients, and also in ANCA-specific IgG recovered from Wegener's granulomatosis patients. Although, highly galactosylated preformed IgG1-immune complexes suppressed inflammation in a mouse model by facilitating the association of the inhibitory receptor FcγRIIB and a C-type lectin-like receptor dectin-1, demonstrating a novel role for terminal galactose on IgG Fc glycans. This association results in inhibition of C5a receptor (C5aR)-mediated inflammatory responses. Intriguingly, the anti-inflammatory activity appears to be subclass specific, as highly galactosylated IgG2a failed to initiate such inhibition (Karsten et al. 2012). Further studies are needed to determine galactosylated IgG1-immune complexes regulation inflammation *in vivo*.

Bisecting GlcNAc

The presence of *N*-acetylglucosamine attached to the bisecting mannose also affects IgG interactions with FcγRs, as the presence of this residue increases affinity to FcγRIIIA (Davies et al. 2001) (Fig. 2a). Consequently, IgGs with bisecting *N*-acetylglucosamine display more potent antibody-dependent cell-mediated cytotoxicity (ADCC) than controls without the linkage. Although, how this linkage is regulated by inflammation is not clear, however increases in addition of bisecting *N*-acetylglucosamine have been reported in Lambert-Eaton myasthenic syndrome, but were found to be unchanged in Myasthenia gravis patients (Selman et al. 2011). Indeed, steric hindrance with the presence of the core fucose is thought to be a determining factor for the addition of bisecting GlcNAc. Intriguingly, analysis of sera from two HIV vaccine trials (RV144 and VAX003) with the same recombinant gp120 differing in amount of immunizations and with a priming consisting of canary pox virus expressing HIV genes (RV144) revealed differences in the GlNAc on the antibodies produced. Although no protection was observed in the VAX003 trial, RV144 offered modest protection of 30%. Analysis of gp120-specific IgG in sera of samples collected from each trial revealed an increase in bisected GlcNAc in RV144 patients (Chung et al. 2014). These results underscore the need for future studies to determine the regulation of bisected GlcNAc on IgG Fc glycans.

Fucose

In humans, the majority of core-fucosylation occurs via an α-1,6 linkage (Fig. 2a). Fucosyltransferase 8 (FUT8), known also as α (1,6) fucosyltransferase, is the sole enzyme responsible for transferring donor fucose to the core N-glycan structure. This modification occurs within the Golgi apparatus (Miyoshi et al. 1999) Core fucose is added to approximately 70% of IgG antibodies (Arnold et al. 2007). When fucose is added to IgG, an alteration in conformation occurs (Matsumiya et al. 2007). This minor alteration in structure results in dramatic reduction in antibody-dependent cell-mediated cytotoxicity (ADCC), a main function of IgG. In the absence of fucose, binding to one of the main ADCC mediating receptors, FcγRIIIA, is greatly increased. Increased hydrogen bonds between the afucosylated glycan and the FcγRIIIA receptor may explain this increased affinity (Ferrara et al. 2011). Removal of fucose to enhance IgG mediated ADCC has been exploited in the application to therapeutics. Cell lines can be specifically hindered from adding fucose to the IgG glycan. This can be achieved by knocking out the enzyme α-1,6-fucosyltransferase, which will lead to generation of afucosylated antibodies (Shields et al. 2002). An antibody for the treatment of T-cell leukemia and lymphoma, generated with these ADCC enhancements, has been recently approved (Beck and Reichert 2012). Mogamulizumab has been used in phase 1–2 clinical trials for the treatment of both peripheral and cutaneous T cell lymphomas with tumor makers associated with poor outcomes. In patients with relapse, mogamulizumab was associated with objective improvement in 1/3 of patients and complete response in 15% (Ogura et al. 2014). Another trial demonstrated a greater than 30% response rate in patients with previously treated cutaneous T cell lymphoma with mostly relatively mild side effects (Duvic et al. 2015).

Anti-CD20 monoclonal antibodies have been used in a wide variety of diseases ranging from autoimmune and dermatologic conditions and have become the cornerstone of treatment for B cell malignancies. CD20 is expressed on the surface of B cells and cross linking this molecule with anti-CD20 appears to have cellular effects including alterations in cell signaling and increased ADCC (Weiner 2010). Despite the overall success of this therapy, many patients do not respond, related to low expression of CD20 (Prevodnik et al. 2011) and down regulation of CD20 during treatment (Davis et al. 1999). Glycoengineered anti-CD20 lacking fucose, has been shown to exhibit increases in both ADCC and B cell depletion (Gasdaska et al. 2012). Trials are ongoing but the application of afucosylation continues to prove valuable. Given the success in anti-CD20 therapies, novel B cell targets continue to be identified. CD19 is a surface receptor expressed on B cells throughout their differentiation. As such, it is an excellent target for a variety of B cell disorders. In developing this monoclonal antibody, reduction in fucose content was a goal from the start. *In vitro* and *in vivo* data suggest that anti-CD19 with low fucose is highly efficient in achieving B cell depletion and ADCC (Breton et al. 2014).

While the absence of fucose on the IgG glycan appears favorable, its presence has been associated with clinical disease. Increased fucose content of anti-citrullinated peptide IgG antibodies (ACPA) has been demonstrated in patients with rheumatoid arthritis, even prior to the onset of symptoms (Rombouts et al. 2015). This leads to the intriguing suggestion that fucosylated ACPA could be an enhanced biomarker to monitor disease activity and may contribute to pathogenesis of the disease.

Fetal or neonatal alloimmune thrombocytopenia (FNAIT) occurs when maternal anti-platelet IgG antibodies cross the placenta. This leads to IgG Fc receptor mediated phagocytic uptake of fetal thrombocytes in the spleen and liver. Thrombocytopenia can be mild or severe with symptoms ranging from skin rash to life threatening intracerebral hemorrhage. As discussed above, the absence of fucose leads to increased ADCC and this is often a favorable condition for immune responses. However, in the case of FNAIT, recent studies suggest afucosylation and resultant amplified ADCC contributes to disease pathogenesis. Specifically, low fucosylation levels on IgG antibodies in maternal FNAIT sera correlated with decreased neonatal platelet counts and increase disease severity. Notably, the majority of FNAIT mothers had marked reductions in fucose compared to controls. In addition, low levels of IgG fucose seemed to persist for a prolonged period after delivery suggesting a possible long-lived mechanism of IgG glycosylation determinants (Kapur et al. 2014a). Similar findings were recently identified in hemolytic disease of the fetus or newborn (HDFN), which occurs due to alloimmunization against paternally inherited red blood cell antigens, typically Rh-D. This can result in fetal anemia, jaundice, hydrops and still-birth (Urbaniak and Greiss 2000). Anti-D specific IgG antibodies mostly consisted of glycoforms lacking fucose in one study. Fetal hemoglobin levels decreased with decreased anti-D IgG fucose content. Notably, fucose content of these specific anti-D antibodies was dramatically reduced as compared to fucose content of total IgG (Kapur et al. 2014b). Taken together, these studies suggest that low fucose and its effects on ADCC can de detrimental in certain circumstances. In addition, assessing glycosylation of IgG may be critical in predicting severity of these conditions and improving outcomes.

Given the role of IgG in the immune response to infections, it seems likely that variation in IgG glycosylation during this time may be clinically relevant. Moreover, given its critical role in global health, further understanding of IgG antibody responses during HIV infection are important. This is especially true given variations in disease trajectory and natural immunity which may provide important clues for vaccine development. IgG glycosylation is significantly impacted and varied during acute HIV infection. Intriguingly, antibodies from so-called "elite controllers" of HIV infection show the most profound changes in the IgG glycan with significantly lower levels of fucose as compared to untreated chronic progressors (Ackerman and Alter 2013). This suggests low fucose content of IgG anti-HIV antibodies may contribute to more potent anti-viral activity and could enhance vaccine protection in the future.

Overall, fucose exerts a potent influence on the function of IgG. Various inflammatory diseases appear to be impacted by both the presence and absence of fucose in the IgG glycan. With increased understanding of the role fucose plays in IgG function, it will serve as a means through which IgG antibodies can be engineered with improved target efficacy.

Sialic Acid

Sialic acid can be added to galactose on each of the extending arms of the biantennary structure of complex glycans (Fig. 2A). B cells express a number of sialyltransferases, but preferentially link sialic acid in α-2,6 linkages to IgG Fc glycans using the enzyme ST6GAL (Arnold et al. 2007). Sialic acid is present in approximately 15% of total IgG (Arnold et al. 2007) yet it appears to have a significant impact on IgG function. Early functional studies noted the addition of sialic acid reduced affinity to canonical FcγRs by 10-fold (Scallon et al. 2007). Indeed, this is true for either 2,3 or 2,6 linkage (Anthony et al. 2008a). Insight into the profound effects of IgG sialylation came with enzymatic removal of sialic acid from intravenous immunoglobulin (IVIG) (Kaneko et al. 2006b). This is a therapeutic preparation of IgG collected from tens of thousands of donors that was originally developed as antibody-replacement therapy in immunocompromised individuals at doses of 400–600 mg/kg. Paradoxically, IVIG exerts immunomodulatory activity when given at a high dose of 1–2 gm/kg and is used clinically to treat a number of inflammatory disorders (Imbach et al. 1981, Jordan et al. 1998, Levy et al. 1999, Negi et al. 2007, Nimmerjahn and Ravetch 2007, 2008). IVIG has been shown in animal models and in clinical use to exert anti-inflammatory effects including ITP (Samuelsson et al. 2001), serum-transfer arthritis (Bruhns et al. 2003), and nephrotoxic arthritis (Kaneko et al. 2006a). Notably, children with ITP had been treated successfully with fusions of only IgG Fc fragments reinforcing the possibility that the Fc was principally responsible for the observed effects of IVIG. With a focus on the Fc portion of IVIG in animal studies, it was consistently noted that removal of terminal sialic acid from the IgG Fc of IVIG lead to reductions in its anti-inflammatory activity. However, restoring IVIG sialic acid content lead to recovery of inflammation mediating properties (Kaneko et al. 2006b). Importantly, sialylation in 2,6-linkage is most responsible for anti-inflammatory IVIG functions. Recombinant human IgG Fc engineered to contain sialic acid with only 2,6-linkages lead to marked reductions in inflammation in a model of murine arthritis. Notably, this effect occurred at a markedly reduced dose relative to IVIG (Anthony et al. 2008a). These studies and others suggested sialic acid conferred IgG with differential properties in order to dramatically alter its downstream biologic activity.

Further studies demonstrated that the addition of sialic acid to the IgG Fc glycan converted receptor-binding properties. As discussed above, sialylated IgGs have reduced binding to canonical, type I FcγRs. However, sialylation results in gain of function interaction with Type II FcγRs, including CD23 and dendritic cell-specific ICAM3 grabbing non-integrin (DC-SIGN, CD209) (Geijtenbeek et al. 2000a, 2000b, Sondermann et al. 2013). Type II FcγRs are C-type lectins that bind constant regions of antibodies in protein-protein interactions. It was demonstrated that the murine orthologue of DC-SIGN, specific ICAM3 grabbing non-integrin, related 1 (SIGN-R1), on macrophages binds sialylated IgG Fcs and is responsible for resultant anti-inflammatory activity (Park et al. 2001, Kang et al. 2003, Anthony et al. 2008b, 2011, 2012). Subsequently, it was demonstrated that the human equivalent to SIGN-R1, DC-SIGN, bound sialylated Fcs with similar efficacy (Anthony et al. 2011). Overall, the presence of sialic acid in the IgG glycome confers a regulatory stimulus to the immune system response via interaction with glycan receptors. As such, sialic acid is a potent modulator of inflammation. Importantly, the anti-inflammatory activity of sialylated IgG has been extended to additional models of autoimmune inflammation and increases of Th2 cytokines including IL-4, IL-13, and IL-33 have been reported as elevated following IVIG infusions in patients (Sharma et al. 2014, Tjon et al. 2014, Washburn et al. 2015, Fiebiger et al. 2015).

With a profound anti-inflammatory role elucidated for sialic acid containing IgG Fcs, clinical correlates of this mechanism have been widely sought. In several autoimmune conditions, reductions in sialic acid content of IgG have been noted. Notably, reductions in sialic acid content of relevant auto-antibodies appears to correlate with disease activity. In patients with granulomatosis polyangiitis (Wegener's granulomatosis), sialic levels were significantly lower during active disease than at times without symptoms (Espy et al. 2011). Similarly, in patients with rheumatoid arthritis, ACPA lack sialic acid residues. This is more prominently noted in synovial fluid samples as compared to serum levels (Scherer et al. 2010). Patients with Sjogren's syndrome also have a reduced level of sialylated IgG compared to healthy controls. This was especially true for the subgroup of Sjogren's patients experiencing extraglandular symptoms such as Raynaud's syndrome and, notably, arthritis (Youinou et al. 1992).

Clinical conditions with variations in sialylated IgG Fcs have not only been described in autoimmune conditions. IVIG is the treatment of choice for Guillan-Barre syndrome (GBS), an immune-mediated disorder that can have devastating effects including progressive muscle weakness and respiratory failure. IgG autoantibodies directed against gangliosides can be found during the acute phase of GBS in about half of patients (van Doorn et al. 2008). This antibody response is likely induced by molecular mimicry from prior infection. During the acute phase of infection, patients demonstrated abnormally low levels of IgG sialylation. Perhaps as notable, persistently low levels of sialylation correlated with delayed or modest clinical improvement (Fokkink et al. 2014).

IgA and Glycosylation

IgA is the second most prevalent immunoglobulin in the circulation, with concentrations of 50–175 mg/dL in human sera, and plays an important role in mucosal immunity (Fig. 1). The two isoforms of IgA (IgA1 and IgA2), exist in three forms, monomeric, dimeric, and secretory. These different forms of IgA occupy distinct niches. Monomer and dimeric IgA are found in the circulation. The same J chain that is responsible for IgM multimerization is dimerizing IgA. Addition of secretory component to IgA enables binding to the polymeric immunoglobulin receptor, which is responsible for transport of secretory IgA (sIgA) across the epithelium, and into mucosal lumen. In human serum, IgA1 accounts for ~85% of total IgA and is predominantly in monomeric form, whereas mucosal IgA primarily exists in polymeric form including dimeric and secretory form.

IgA plays an important role in mucosal immunity by mediating immune exclusion, preventing adhesion of pathogens on the epithelium. Furthermore, IgA can modulate inflammatory activity as a result of triggering either activating or inhibitory signals initiated through FcαRI (CD89) (Monteiro 2010). The diversity of IgA-mediated effector functions is partly attributed to its various structural forms. Additionally, IgA in immune complexes triggers activating ITAM-Syk pathway resulting in pro-inflammatory activity such as ADCC and phagocytosis. On the other hand, monomeric IgA was reported to dampen the inflammatory signal by partially phosphorylate the ITAM on FcRγ that results in recruitment of SHP-1 phosphatase (Bakema and van Egmond 2011).

The glycosylation sites in IgA vary between isotypes and subisotypes. IgA1 has two N-linked complex-type glycosylation sites at N263 on the Cα2 domain and N459 on the tailpiece, and nine O-linked glycosylation sites in the hinge region. In general, fewer than six O-linked sites are glycosylated (Novak et al. 2012). IgA2 has five N-linked glycosylation sites (N166, N211, N263, N337, N459) (Arnold et al. 2007) (Fig. 1).

The importance of N-linked glycans on IgA Fc is currently unclear. One study showed that neither of the N-linked glycans on IgA1 Fc seem to be critical for FcαRI binding; the binding of IgA1 to FcαRI was unaltered by N263A mutation or deletion of C-terminal tailpiece containing N459 (Mattu et al. 1998). However, another study reported that IgA1 binding to FcαRI was abolished when the asparagine residue on the Cα2 domain was mutated to glutamine (Q) (Carayannopolous et al. 1994). Future studies are required to clarify whether N-linked glycans on IgA1 Fc modifies FcαRI binding and the subsequent effector functions. Interestingly, patients with an autoimmune disease that debilitates the exocrine glands, namely primary Sjögren's syndrome, were shown to have an increased level of sialylated monomeric serum IgA1 compared to healthy controls (Basset et al. 2000). The addition of sialic acid was suggested to hinder the clearance of IgA, resulting in excess amount of serum IgA and thus the immune complexes.

In comparison with N-linked glycans, O-linked glycans on the IgA hinge region appear to be important. There are six IgA1 O-linked glycovariants (Arnold et al. 2004) and the predominant forms were shown to be the glycovariants with at least the core GlcNAc and β1,3-linked galactose (76). Aberration in O-linked glycan composition on IgA has been linked to IgA nephropathy.

IgA Glycans and Disease Associations

In humans, IgA1 is the most common form in serum and its extended hinge region is rich with proline, serine and threonine residues. With this amino acid composition, the hinge region is a focus of O-glycosylation, typically at 4–5 sites. These glycans vary in composition with sugars including GalNAc, galactose and sialic acid. Normal serum IgA1 almost never contains galactose deficient glycans (Mattu et al. 1998). IgA nephropathy is the most common cause of primary glomerulonephritis worldwide. Asymptomatic proteinuria and hematuria are common clinical findings and males are predominantly affected. Often exacerbations of this disease are seen after mucosal infections, typically in the upper respiratory tract, but gastroenteritis has been linked as well (Julian et al. 2007). Kidney biopsy is required to make the diagnosis. Pathology demonstrates both IgA and C3 deposits in the mesangial area. IgA1 is the only subtype found in these locations (Conley et al. 1980). Jacalin, a fruit based lectin, binds exclusively to human IgA and not other immunoglobulin subtypes (Roque-Barreira and Campos-Neto 1985). Further, jacalin specifically binds IgA1 due to the presence of terminal galactose in the hinge region (Baenziger and Kornfeld 1974). Notably, in patients with IgA nephropathy, serum IgA binding to jacalin was reduced (Andre et al. 1990). This suggested aberration in IgA1 glycan structure, specifically absence of galactose. There are no alterations in the N-linked glycans of IgA1 in these same patients. C1 inhibitor, a complement regulatory protein which also contains O-glycans and is co-localized in this same condition, did not have alterations in galactose content. Altered glycans of IgA1 in this context have been localized to the hinge region, also consistent with defective O-glycosylation. Changes in the IgA1 glycan may contribute to structural alterations in the antibody leading to decreased clearance (Allen et al. 1995). A subsequent study demonstrated reduction in both galactose and sialic acid in IgA1 isolated renal tissue of patients with IgA nephropathy (Hiki et al. 2001). This provided direct clinical correlation for lectin binding studies. This aberrant IgA1 and O-glycans containing terminal GlcNAc represent novel epitopes to the immune system, resulting in generation of anti-O-glycan antibodies. In turn, immune complexes are generated which accumulate in the mesangium of the kidney. This leads to complement activation and subsequent tissue damage (Suzuki et al. 2011).

IgA1 O-glycan assembly requires GalNAc-transferases given that this sugar is paramount to the core structure of the glycan. As a result, GalNAc-transferases are present in large quantities in IgA1 producing B cells. Production of GalNAc-T14, a specific GalNAc-transferase, is much higher IgA nephropathy patients than in controls. In addition, there is corresponding decreased expression of glycosyltransferases responsible for addition of galactose (Tomana et al. 1999, Suzuki et al. 2014). These alterations in glycosyltransferase expression substantiate the O-glycan alterations seen in IgA1 in these patients. It is intriguing to note that cytokines, including IL-6 and IL-4, act to reduce galactose addition to IgA1 via induced reduction of these same glycosyltransferases (Suzuki et al. 2014). This serves as an explanatory connection between mucosal infections and induction of IgA nephropathy in patients. A multiple hit explanation suggests that a genetically determined elevation in galactose deficient IgA1 is an initial causative factor. Subsequently, anti-glycan antibodies develop and production of these are subsequently exacerbated by infections or other triggers. This leads to excess production of immune complexes, overwhelming renal clearance. Accumulation in the kidney causes mesangial proliferation and ultimately activation of complement (Krzysztof and Novak 2014).

Henoch-Shönlein purpura (HSP) is the most common vasculitis in children. A triad of symptoms including purpuric rash, abdominal and joint pain, are the most common manifesting symptoms. IgA-containing immune complexes accumulating in the walls of small blood vessels including arterioles, capillaries and venules are characteristic of this condition. The majority of episodes are preceded by upper respiratory infections, typically with streptococcus, staphylococcus and parainfluenza (Trnka 2013). Notably, vasculitis involvement of the kidney occurs in about 40% of cases (Saulsbury 1999) and 3% of these children develop end stage renal disease (Delos Santos and Wyatt 2004). Similar to IgA nephropathy, alterations in IgA1 and resultant immune complex formation and mesangial damage have been implicated in HSP (Novak et al. 2007). It has been shown that serum IgA1 in children with HSP has reduced galactose content and that these levels seem to be highly heritable (Krzysztof et al. 2011). This reinforces the role of aberrant IgA glycosylation in immune complex diseases.

IgM and Glycosylation

IgM is the first immunoglobulin class produced during immune responses, is the third most common antibody class in circulation, and is effective at fixing complement. IgM is most frequent formed as a pentameric structure, enabling high avidity binding of antigens. Glycan analysis showed that IgM is highly glycosylated, with five N-linked glycosylation sites including three complex- and two oligomannose-type (Arnold et al. 2007) (Fig. 1). Although GlcNAc-terminating IgM glycoforms bind MBL, the binding is lost when IgM is bound to antigen, suggesting antigen-bound IgM does not trigger complement pathway. The binding of MBL to IgM may facilitate the removal of IgM aggregates by opsonisation (Arnold et al. 2007). Glycosylation of IgM is thought to facility interaction with some C-type lectins. IgM sialylation can engage Siglec2 (CD22) in a B cell intrinsic manner to dampen B cell signaling and activation (Crocker et al. 2007). Also, oligomannose structures on IgM were shown to stabilize interactions with dendritic cells expressing DC-SIGN (CD209) (Coelho et al. 2010).

IgE and Glycosylation

More than one in five individuals worldwide suffers from allergies, asthma, or other allergic disease. IgE antibodies are bound to the surface of mast cells and basophils via the constant fragment, Fc, to high affinity Fc receptors, FcεR1. Cross-linking cell-bound IgE by allergen leads to mast cell activation and, in turn, to canonical symptoms of allergy (Holgate and Church 1982). Almost immediately, preformed mediators including histamine are released causing vascular dilation, vascular permeability, bronchoconstriction, leukocyte extravasation and smooth muscle contractility. Subsequently, a "late phase" reaction can occur due to stimulation of cellular synthetic function. This results in release of mediators including leukotrienes and others.

The IgE antibody is the most heavily glycosylated monomeric immunoglobulin seven N-linked glycans distributed through its constant region (Gould and Sutton 2008) (Fig. 1). IgE is present in limited quantities in the sera (5 ng/ml), making analysis difficult. However, a few studies have examined IgE glycosylation and determined that five glycosylation sites are occupied by complex, bi-antennary glycans. A single N-linked oligo-mannose structure is present in the Cε3 domain at N394 (Fig. 2B), while another glycosylation site in the Cε3 is not glycosylated (Arnold et al. 2004). It is thought the majority of bisecting glycans on IgE are highly processed and sialylated (Arnold et al. 2004, 2007). IgE has two canonical receptors, the aforementioned high affinity receptor, FcεRI, as well as the FcεRII (low affinity and also known as CD23 (Broide 2001, Bruhns et al. 2005). FcεRI is found on the cell surface of mast cells, basophils, and eosinophils and is responsible for binding antigen bound IgE and driving the allergic response. IgE binding to the FcεRI in tissues is responsible for a prolonged half life of 3 weeks as compared to 12 hours in the serum (Gould and Sutton 2008). CD23 is expressed by B cells and antigen presenting cells (Vercelli et al. 1989). CD23 is a C-type lectin structurally unrelated to the FcεRI, but notably of structural similarity to C-type lectins including dendritic cell-specific ICAM3 grabbing non-integrin (DC-SIGN, also known as CD209) (Acharya et al. 2010). In addition, the C-type lectin, galectin-3 was originally identified as ε binding protein because of its ability to bind both IgE and FcεRI. As such, this receptor is also thought to play a role in allergic inflammation (Chen et al. 2006). Galactin-3 recognizes galactose containing glycans, and implication of this receptor in allergic responses indicates that variable glycosylation may contribute to severity of allergic inflammation. One IgE molecule could contain up to 24 exposed galactose residues based on its glycan configuration. As lectin and galactose receptors are known to bind IgE, there is a strong suggestion that IgE glycosylation is critical to allergic disease. Taken together, these various IgE receptors imply that antigen specificity is only one of a number of potential IgE variables determining the mechanisms of allergic inflammation.

As mentioned, IgE is the most heavily glycosylated monomeric human immunoglobulin with 7 N-linked glycosylation sites. Five of these sites are occupied by 5 glycans of complex, bi-antennary structure, composed of various sugars including terminal sialic acid. In addition, one site is occupied by a glycan with an oligomannose structure (Arnold et al. 2007) (Fig. 2b). Structural studies of IgE implicated the Cε3 portion of the IgE Fc as the binding site for the FcεR1. While the IgE Fc is significantly glycosylated, the role of glycosylation in IgE function through receptor binding has been largely dismissed. These assumptions were based on structural studies without correlating functional data. In addition, recombinant proteins were generated in bacterial vectors resulting in aglycosylated Cε3 (Henry et al. 2000). However, given the demonstrated and profound role of glycosylation in other antibody subclasses, subsequent studies sought to decipher its role in IgE biology. A recent study demonstrated that a single oligomannose glycan in the Cε3 domain of IgE is responsible for anaphylaxis. A model of passive cutaneous anaphylaxis was utilized as a functional assessment of IgE function. Mice were immunized with allergen the IgE was delivered intradermal to the ears, devoid of all glycans after enzymatic treatment or with native IgE as a control. The next day they were intravenously challenged with the proper allergen and vascular permeability was measured subsequently. IgE devoid of glycans elicited markedly less allergic inflammation compared to controls. Similar results were seen with bone marrow derived mast cells *in vitro*. Subsequently, a panel of IgE mutants was developed, lacking glycosylation sites in each constant domain. It was determined that mutants lacking glycans in the Cε3 domain had reductions in anaphylaxis. Individual Cε3 site mutants were generated and it was shown that specific removal of the oligomannose lead to abrogation of anaphylaxis while other mutants showed preserved allergic inflammation. Similar findings were seen for human IgE in a humanized mouse model and in human mast cells *in vitro*. As such, the single oligomannose in the Cε3 domain of the IgE Fc was determined as critical for initiation of anaphylaxis (Shade et al. 2015). Notably, the oligomannose glycan is highly conserved across an evolutionary spectrum of species, further reinforcing its importance in IgE function (Shade et al. 2015). Further, this glycosylation site on IgE corresponds to the single site on the IgG Fc, which is responsible for all of its downstream effector functions (Garman et al. 2000). Taken together, these studies suggest IgE Fc glycosylation plays a critical role in its function, in keeping with other immunoglobulin classes.

Conclusions

Antibodies are glycoproteins and accumulating evidence suggests glycosylation acts as an essential regulator of their function. As such, glycosylation is becoming an increasingly important consideration in immunoglobulin biology. The single N-linked glycan on IgG exerts profound effects on IgG biology. It is essential for structural integrity of the IgG Fc, while variable glycosylation determines whether downstream effector function will be pro- or anti-inflammatory. Perturbations in IgG glycosylation have been implicated in a growing number of diseases. Likewise, industry has been able to engineer IgG glycosylation to generate increasing potent therapeutic antibodies to treat a wide variety of diseases. Applications of IgG glycobiology have increased exponentially and this continues to validate the importance of the IgG glycan. Similarly, IgA glycosylation has been well described and alterations also appear to correlate with certain disease phenotypes. The genetics of IgA glycosyltransferase expression have been implicated in various diseases as well. The role of glycosylation in IgE biology is just emerging. Future studies to further dissect the regulatory role of the IgE glycan are underway. In addition, clinical correlations to variations in IgE glycosylation are planned as well. The functional and regulatory significance of IgM glycosylation remains to be fully elucidated.

Defining glycan content and structure across antibody subclasses has been critical to understand their functional significance. However, regulation of glycosylation remains poorly defined. Delineating regulatory aspects of glycosylation machinery is required to develop a comprehensive understanding of glycobiology. With this regulation delineated, applications of glycoengineering can be further applied.

Acknowledgement

The authors are grateful to Kate L. Jeffrey for careful reading of the chapter.

Keywords: IgG, IgA, IgM, IgE, Fc receptor, effector function

References

Acharya, M., G. Borland, A. Edkins, L. MacLellan, J. Matheson, B. Ozanne et al. 2010. Cd23/FceII: Molecular multi-tasking. Clin Exp Immunol 162: 12–23.
Ackerman, M. and G. Alter. 2013. Mapping the journey to an HIV vaccine. N Engl J Med 369(4): 389–91.
Allen, A. C., S. J. Harper and J. Feehally. 1995. Galactosylation of N- and O-linked carbohydrate moieties of IgA1 and IgG in IgA nephropathy. Clin Exp Immunol 100: 470–474.
An, Z. 2009. Therapeutic Monoclonal Antibodies: From Bench to Clinic. John Wiley & Sons, Hoboken, NJ.
Andre, P. M., P. Le Pogamp and D. Chevet. 1990. Impairment of jacalin binding to serum IgA in IgA nephropathy. J Clinical Lab Analysis 4: 115–119.
Anthony, R. M., F. Nimmerjahn, D. J. Ashline, V. N. Reinhold, J. C. Paulson and J. V. Ravetch. 2008a. Recapitulation of IVIG anti-inflammatory activity with a recombinant IgG Fc. Science 320(5874): 373–6.
Anthony, R. M., F. Wermeling, M. C. Karlsson and J. V. Ravetch. 2008b. Identification of a receptor required for the anti-inflammatory activity of IVIG. Proc Natl Acad Sci USA 105(50): 19571–8.
Anthony, R. M., T. Kobayashi, F. Wermeling and J. V. Ravetch. 2011. Intravenous gammaglobulin suppresses inflammation through a novel T(H)2 pathway. Nature 475(7354): 110–3.
Anthony, R. M., F. Wermeling and J. V. Ravetch. 2012. Novel roles for the IgG Fc glycan. Ann N Y Acad Sci 1253: 170–80.
Arnold, J. N., C. M. Radcliffe, M. R. Wormald, L. Royle, D. J. Harvey, M. Crispin et al. 2004. The glycosylation of human serum IgD and IgE and the accessibility of identified oligomannose structures for interaction with mannan-binding lectin. J Immunol 173(11): 6831–40.
Arnold, J. N., M. R. Wormald, R. B. Sim, P. M. Rudd and R. A. Dwek. 2007. The impact of glycosylation on the biological function and structure of human immunoglobulins. Annu Rev Immunol 25: 21–50.
Baenziger, J. and S. Kornfeld. 1974. Structure of the carbohydrate units of IgA1 immunoglobulin. II. Structure of the O-glycosidically linked oligosaccharide units. J Biol Chem 249: 7270–7281.
Bakema, J. E. and M. M. van Egmond. 2011. Immunoglobulin A: A next generation of therapeutic antibodies? J Biol Chem 3: 352–361.
Basset, C. C., V. V. Durand, C. C. Jamin, J. J. Clement, Y. Y. Pennec, P. P. Youinou et al. 2000. Increased N-glycosylation leading to oversialylation of monomeric immunglobulin A1 from patients with Sjogren's syndrome. Scand J Immunol 51: 300–306.
Beck, A. and J. M. Reichert. 2012. Marketing approval of mogamulizumab: A triumph for glyco-engineering, mAbs. Landes Bioscience 419–425.
Boes, M. 2000. Role of natural and immune IgM antibodies in immune responses. Mol Immunol 37: 1141–49.
Breton, C. S., A. Nahimana, D. Aubry, J. Macoin, P. Moretti, M. Bertschinger et al. 2014. A novel anti-CD19 monoclonal antibody (GBR 401) with high killing activity against B cell malignancies. Journal of Hematology and Oncology 7: 33–46.
Broide, D. H. 2001. Molecular and cellular mechanisms of allergic disease. J Allergy Clin Immunol 108(2 Suppl): S65–71.
Bruhns, P., A. Samuelsson, J. W. Pollard and J. V. Ravetch. 2003. Colony-stimulating factor-1-dependent macrophages are responsible for IVIG protection in antibody-induced autoimmune disease. Immunity 18(4): 573–81.
Bruhns, P., S. Fremont and M. Daeron. 2005. Regulation of allergy by Fc receptors. Curr Opin Immunol 17(6): 662–9.

Butler, M. and M. Spearman. 2014. The choice of mammalian cell host and possibilities for glycosylation engineering. Curr Opin Biotechnol 30: 107–12.

Carayannopolous, L., E. E. Max and D. Capra. 1994. Recombinant human IgA expressed in insect cells. Proc Natl Acad Sci USA 91: 8348–8352.

Chen, H., B. Sharma, L. Yu, R. Zuberi, I. Weng, T. Kawakami et al. 2006. Role of galatectin-3 in mast cell functions: galectin-3 deficient mast cells exhibit impaired mediator release and defective JNK expression. J Immunol 177: 4991–7.

Chung, A. W., M. Ghebremichael, H. Robinson, E. Brown, I. Choi, S. Lane et al. 2014. Polyfunctional Fc-effector profiles mediated by IgG subclass selection distinguish RV144 and VAX003 vaccines. Sci Transl Med 6: 228ra38.

Chung, C. H., B. Mirakhur, E. Chan, Q. T. Le, J. Berlin, M. Morse et al. 2008. Cetuximab-induced anapjyalxis and IgE specific for galactose-alpha-1,3-galactose. N Engl J Med 358: 1109–1117.

Coelho, V., S. Krysov, A. M. Ghaemmaghami, M. Emara, K. N. Potter, P. Johnson et al. 2010. Glycosylation of surface Ig creates a functional bridge between human follicular lymphoma and microenvironmental lectins. Proc Natl Acad Sci USA 107: 18587–92.

Conley, M. E., M. D. Cooper and A. F. Michael. 1980. Selective deposition of immunoglobulin A1 in immunoglobulin A nephropathy, anaphylactoid purpura nephritis, and systemic lupus erythematosus. J Clin Invest 66: 1432–1436.

Crocker, P. R., J. C. Paulson and A. Varki. 2007. Siglecs and their roles in the immune system. Nat Rev Immunol 7(4): 255–66.

Davies, J., L. Jiang, L. Z. Pan, M. J. LaBarre, D. Anderson and M. Reff. 2001. Expression of GnTIII in a recombinant anti-CD20 CHO production cell line: Expression of antibodies with altered glycoforms leads to an increase in ADCC through higher affinity for FC gamma RIII. Biotechnol Bioeng 74(4): 288–94.

Davis, T. A., D. K. Czerwinski and R. Levy. 1999. Therapy of B-cell lymphoma with anti-CD20 antibodies can result in loss of CD20 expression. Clin Cancer Res 5: 611–615.

Delos Santos, N. M. and R. J. Wyatt. 2004. Pediatric IgA nephropathies: Clinical aspects and therapeutic approaches. Semin Nephrol 24: 269–286.

Dudley, D. D., J. Chaudhuri, C. H. Bassing and F. W. Alt. 2005. Mechanism and control of V(D)J recombination versus class switch recombination: Similarities and differences. Adv Immunol 86: 43–112.

Duvic, M., L. C. Pinter-Brown, F. M. Foss, L. Sokol, J. L. Jorgensen, P. Challagundia et al. 2015. Phase 1/2 study of mogamulizumab, a defucosylated anti-CCR4 antibody, in previously treated patients with cutaneous T-cell lymphoma. Blood 125: 1883–9.

Elliott, S., J. Egrie, J. Browne, T. Lorenzini, L. Busse, N. Rogers et al. 2004. Control of rHuEPO biological activity: The role of carbohydrate. Exp Hematol 32: 1146–55.

Espy, C., W. Morelle, N. Kavian, P. Grange, C. Goulvestre, V. Viallon et al. 2011. Sialylation levels of anti-proteinase 3 antibodies are associated with the activity of granulomatosis with polyangiitis (Wegener's). Arthritis Rheum 63(7): 2105–15.

Feige, M. J., S. Nath, S. R. Catharino, D. Weinfurtner, S. Steinbacher and J. Buchner. 2009. Structure of the murine unglycosylated IgG1 Fc fragment. J Mol Biol 391(3): 599–608.

Ferrara, C., S. Grau, C. Jager, P. Sondermann, P. Brunker, I. Waldhauer et al. 2011. Unique carbohydrate-carbohydrate interactions are required for high affinity binding between Fc{gamma}RIII and antibodies lacking core fucose. Proc Natl Acad Sci USA 108(31): 12669–74.

Fiebiger, B. M., J. Maamary, A. Pincetic and J. Ravetch. 2015. Protection in antibody- and T cell-mediated autoimmune diseases by antiinflammatory IgG Fcs requires type II FcRs. Proc Natl Acad Sci USA 112: E2385–94.

Fokkink, W. -J.R., M. J. Selman, J. R. Dortland, B. Durmus, K. Kuitwaard, R. Huizinga et al. 2014. IgG Fc N-glycosylation in Guillain-Barre Syndrome treated with immunoglobulins. J Proteome Res 13: 1722–1730.

Garman, S. C., B. A. Wurzburg, S. S. Tarchevskaya, J. P. Kinet and T. S. Jardetsky. 2000. Structure of the Fc fragment of human IgE bound to its high-affinity receptor FceRIa. Nature 406: 259–266.

Gasdaska, J. R., S. Sherwood, J. T. Reagan and L. F. Dickey. 2012. An afucosylated anti-CD20 monoclonal antibody with greater antibody-dependent cellular cytotoxicity and B-cell depletion and lower complement-dependent cytotoxicity than rituximab. Mol Immunol 50: 134–41.

Geijtenbeek, T. B., D. S. Kwon, R. Torensma, S. J. van Vliet, G. C. van Duijnhoven, J. Middel et al. 2000a. DC-SIGN, a dendritic cell-specific HIV-1-binding protein that enhances trans-infection of T cells. Cell 100(5): 587–97.

Geijtenbeek, T. B., R. Torensma, S. J. van Vliet, G. C. van Duijnhoven, G. J. Adema, Y. van Kooyk et al. 2000b. Identification of DC-SIGN, a novel dendritic cell-specific ICAM-3 receptor that supports primary immune responses. Cell 100(5): 575–85.

Gornik, O., J. Wagner, M. Pucic, A. Knezevic, I. Redzic and G. Lauc. 2009. Stability of N-glycan profiles in human plasma. Glycobiology 19: 1547–1553.

Gould, H. J. and B. J. Sutton. 2008. IgE in allergy and asthma today. Nat Rev Immunol 8: 205–17.

Henry, A. J., J. M. McDonnell, R. Ghirlando, B. J. Sutton and H. J. Gould. 2000. Conformation of the isolated Ce3 domain of IgE and its complex with the high-affinity receptor, FceRI. Biochemistry 39: 7406–7413.

Hiki, Y., H. Odani, M. Takahashi, Y. Yasuda, A. Nishimoto, H. Iwase et al. 2001. Mass spectrometry proves under-O-glycosylation of glomerular IgA1 in IgA nephropathy. Kidney Int 59: 1077–1085.

Holgate, S. T. and M. K. Church. 1982. Control of mediator release from mast cells. Clin Allergy 12 Suppl: 5–13.

Imbach, P., S. Barandun, C. Baumgartner, A. Hirt, F. Hofer and H. P. Wagner. 1981. High-dose intravenous gammaglobulin therapy of refractory, in particular idiopathic thrombocytopenia in childhood. Helv Paediatr Acta 36(1): 81–6.

Jordan, S. C., D. Tyan, L. Czer and M. Toyoda. 1998. Immunomodulatory actions of intravenous immunoglobulin (IVIG): potential applications in solid organ transplant recipients. Pediatr Transplant 2(2): 92–105.

Julian, B. A., R. J. Wyatt, K. Matousovic, Z. Moldoveneau, J. Mestecky and J. Novak. 2007. IgA nephropathy: A clinical overview. Contrib Nephrol 157: 19–26.

Kaneko, Y., F. Nimmerjahn, M. P. Madaio and J. V. Ravetch. 2006a. Pathology and protection in nephrotoxic nephritis is determined by selective engagement of specific Fc receptors. J Exp Med 203(3): 789–97.

Kaneko, Y., F. Nimmerjahn and J. V. Ravetch. 2006b. Anti-inflammatory activity of immunoglobulin G resulting from Fc sialylation. Science 313(5787): 670–3.

Kang, Y. S., S. Yamazaki, T. Iyoda, M. Pack, S. A. Bruening, J. Y. Kim et al. 2003. SIGN-R1, a novel C-type lectin expressed by marginal zone macrophages in spleen, mediates uptake of the polysaccharide dextran. Int Immunol 15(2): 177–86.

Kapur, R., L. Della Valle, M. Sonneveld, A. Ederveen, R. Visser, P. Ligthart et al. 2014a. Low anti-RhD IgG-Fc-fucosylation in pregnancy: A new variable in predicting severity in haemolytic disese of the fetus and newborn. British Journal of Haematology 166: 936–945.

Kapur, R., I. Kustiawan, A. Vestrheim, C. A. M. Loeleman, R. Visser, H. K. Einarsdottir et al. 2014b. A prominent lack of IgG1-Fc fucosylation of platelet alloantibodies in pregnancy. Blood 123: 471–480.

Karsten, C. M., M. K. Pandey, J. Figge, R. Kilchenstein, P. R. Taylor, M. Rosas et al. 2012. Anti-inflammatory activity of IgG1 mediated by Fc galactosylation and association of FcgammaRIIB and dectin-1. Nat Med 18(9): 1401–6.

Kim, J. Y., Y. G. Kim and G. M. Lee. 2012. CHO cells in biotechnology for production of recombinant proteins: Current state and further potential. Appl Microbiol Biotechnol 93: 917–930.

Krzysztof, K., Z. Moldoveanu, J. T. Sanders, T. M. Eison, S. Hitoshi, B. A. Julian et al. 2011. Aberrant glycosylation of IgA1 is inherited in pediatric IgA nephropathy and Henoch-Schonlein purpura nephritis. Kidney Int 80: 79–87.

Krzysztof, K. and J. Novak. 2014. The genetics and immunobiology of IgA nephropathy. J Clin Invest 124: 2325–2332.

Levy, Y., Y. Sherer, A. Ahmed, P. Langevitz, J. George, F. Fabbrizzi et al. 1999. A study of 20 SLE patients with intravenous immunoglobulin—clinical and serologic response. Lupus 8(9): 705–12.

Lux, A., X. Yu and F. Nimmerjahn. 2013. Impact of immune complex size and glycosylation on IgG binding to human FcγRs. Journal of Immunology 190: 4315–23.

Matsumiya, S., Y. Yamaguchi, J. -I. Saito, M. Nagano, H. Sasakawa, S. Otaki et al. 2007. Strutural comparison of focusylated and nonfucosylated Fc fragments of human immunoglobulin G1. J Mol Biol 368: 767–779.

Mattu, T. S., R. J. Pleass, A. C. Willis, M. Kilian, M. R. Wormald, A. C. Lellouch et al. 1998. The glycosylation and structure of human serum IgA1, Fab, and Fc regions and the role of N-glycosylation on Fc alpha receptor interactions. J Biol Chem 273: 2260–2272.

Maverakis, E., K. Kim, M. Shimoda, M. Gerschwin, F. Patel, R. Rilken et al. 2015. Glycans in the immune system and the Altered Glycan Theory of Autoimmunity: A critical review. J Autoimmun 5: 1–13.

Menni, C., T. Keser, M. Mangino, J. T. Bell, I. Erte, I. Akmacic et al. 2013. Glycosylation of immunoglobulin G: Role of genetic and epigenetic influences. PLOS One 8: e82558. doi: 10.1371/journal.pone.0082558.

Michaud, H. A., J. F. Eliaou, V. Lafont, N. Bonnefoy and L. Gros. 2014. Tumor antigen-targeting monoclonal antibody-based immunotherapy: Orchestrating combined strategies for the development of long-term antitumor immunity. Oncoimmunology 3: eCollection.

Miyoshi, E., K. Noda, Y. Yamguchi, S. Inoue, Y. Ikeda and W. Wang. 1999. The a-1,6-fucosyltransferase gene and its biological significance. Biochem Biophys Acta 1463: 9–20.

Monteiro, R. C. 2010. The role of IgA and IgA Fc receptors as anti-inflammatory agents. J Clin Immunol 30 Suppl: S61–4.

Negi, V. S., S. Elluru, S. Siberil, S. Graff-Dubois, L. Mouthon, M. D. Kazatchkine et al. 2007. Intravenous immunoglobulin: An update on the clinical use and mechanisms of action. J Clin Immunol 27(3): 233–45.

Nimmerjahn, F. and J. V. Ravetch. 2007. The antiinflammatory activity of IgG: The intravenous IgG paradox. J Exp Med 204(1): 11–5.

Nimmerjahn, F., R. M. Anthony and J. V. Ravetch. 2007. Agalactosylated IgG antibodies depend on cellular Fc receptors for *in vivo* activity. Proc Natl Acad Sci USA 104(20): 8433–7.

Nimmerjahn, F. and J. Ravetch. 2008. Anti-inflammatory actions of intravenous immunoglobulin. Annu Rev Immunol 26: 513–33.

Novak, J., Z. Moldoveanu, M. B. Renfrow, T. Yanagihara, H. Suzuki, M. Raska et al. 2007. IgA nephropathy and Henoch-Schoenlein purpura nephritis: aberrant glycosylation of IgA1, formation of IgA1-containing immune complexes, and activation of mesangial cells. Contrib Nephrol 157: 134–138.

Novak, J. J., B. A. Julian, J. J. Mestecky and M. B. Renfrow. 2012. Glycosylation of IgA1 and pathogenesis of IgA nephropathy. Semin Immunopathol 34: 365–382.

Ogura, M., T. Ishida, K. Hatake, M. Taniwaki, K. Ando, K. Tobinai et al. 2014. Multicenter phase II trial with mogamulizumab (KW-0761), a defucosylated anti-cc chemokine receptor 4 antibody, in patients with relapsed peripheral T-cell lymphoma and cutaneous T-cell lymphoma. J Clin Oncol 32: 1157–63.

Park, C. G., K. Takahara, E. Umemoto, Y. Yashima, K. Matsubara, Y. Matsuda et al. 2001. Five mouse homologues of the human dendritic cell C-type lectin, DC-SIGN. Int Immunol 13(10): 1283–90.

Prevodnik, V. K., J. Lavrencak, M. Horvat and B. J. Novakovic. 2011. The predictive significance of CD20 expression in B-cell lymphomas. Diagn Pathol 6: 33.

Pucic, M., A. Knezevic, S. Vidie, B. Adamezyk, M. Novokmet, O. Polasek et al. 2011. High throughout isolation and glycosylation analysis of IgG-variability and heritability of the IgG glycome in three isolated human populations. Mol Cell Proteomics 10: M111.010090. doi:10.1074/mcp.M111.010090.

Pucic, M., A. Muzinic, M. Novokmet, M. Skledar, N. Pivoc, G. Lauc et al. 2012. Changes in plasma and IgG N-glycome during childhood and adolescence. Glycobiology 22: 975–82.

Raghavan, M. and P. J. Bjorkman. 1996. Fc receptors and their interactions with immunoglobulins. Annu Rev Cell Dev Biol 12: 181–220.

Rombouts, Y., E. Ewing, L. A. van de Stadt, M. J. Selman, L. A. Trouw, A. M. Deelder et al. 2015. Anti-citrullinated protein antibodies acquire a pro-inflammatory Fc glycosylation phenotype prior to onset of rheumatoid arthritis. Ann Rheum Dis 74: 234–41.

Roque-Barreira, M. C. and A. Campos-Neto. 1985. Jacalin: An IgA-binding lectin. J Immunol 134: 1740–1743.

Samuelsson, A., T. L. Towers and J. V. Ravetch. 2001. Anti-inflammatory activity of IVIG mediated through the inhibitory Fc receptor. Science 291(5503): 484–6.

Saulsbury, F. T. 1999. Henoch-Schonlein purpura in children. Report of 100 patients and review of the literature. Medicine 78: 395–409.

Sazinsky, S. L., R. G. Ott, N. W. Silver, B. Tidor, J. V. Ravetch and K. D. Wittrup. 2008. Aglycosylated immunoglobulin G1 variants productively engage activating Fc receptors. Proc Natl Acad Sci USA 105(51): 20167–72.

Scallon, B. J., S. H. Tam, S. G. McCarthy, A. N. Cai and T. S. Raju. 2007. Higher levels of sialylated Fc glycans in immunoglobulin G molecules can adversely impact functionality. Mol Immunol 44(7): 1524–34.

Scherer, H. U., D. van der Woude, A. Ioan-Facsinay, H. el Bannoudi, L. A. Trouw, J. Wang et al. 2010. Glycan profiling of anti-citrullinated protein antibodies isolated from human serum and synovial fluid. Arthritis Rheum 62(6): 1620–9.

Selman, M. H., E. H. Niks, M. J. Titulaer, J. J. Verschuuren, M. Wuhrer and A. M. Deelder. 2011. IgG fc N-glycosylation changes in Lambert-Eaton myasthenic syndrome and myasthenia gravis. J Proteome Res 10(1): 143–52.

Shade, K. -T. C., B. Platzer, N. Washburn, V. Mani, Y. C. Bartsch, M. Conroy et al. 2015. A single glycan on igE is indispensable for intitation of anaphylaxis. J Exp Med 212: 457–467.

Sharma, M., Y. Schoindre, P. Hegde, C. Saha, M. S. Maddur, E. Stephen-Victor et al. 2014. Intravenous immunoglobulin-induced IL-33 is insufficient to mediate basophil expansion in autoimmune patients. Sci Rep 4: 5672.

Shields, R. L., J. Lai, R. Keck, L. Y. O'Connell, K. Hong, Y. G. Meng et al. 2002. Lack of fucose on human IgG1 N-linked oligosaccharide improves binding to human Fcgamma RIII and antibody-dependent cellular toxicity. J Biol Chem 277(30): 26733–40.

Shroeder, H. W. and L. Cavacini. 2010. Structure and function of immunoglobulins. J Allergy Clin Immunol 125: S41–52.

Sondermann, P., A. Pincetic, J. Maamary, K. Lammens and J. V. Ravetch. 2013. General mechanism for modulating immunoglobulin effector function. Proc Natl Acad Sci USA (110): 9868–9872.

Stanley, P., H. Schachter and N. Taniguchi. 2009. N-Glycans. pp. 101–114. *In*: Varki, A., R. D. Cummings, J. D. Esko, H. H. Freeze, P. Stanley, C. R. Bertozzi et al. (eds.). Essentials of Glycobiology, 2 edition. Cold Spring Harbor Laboratory Press, Cold Spring Harbor, New York, NY, USA.

Suzuki, H., K. Kiryluk, J. Novak, Z. Moldoveneau, A. B. Herr, M. B. Renfrow et al. 2011. The pathophysiology of IgA nephropathy. J Am Soc Nephrol 22: 1795–1803.

Suzuki, H., M. Raska, K. Yamada, Z. Moldoveneau, B. A. Julian, R. J. Wyatt et al. 2014. Cytokines alter IgA1 O-glycosylation by dysregulating C1GalT1 and ST6GalNAc-II enzymes. J Biol Chem 289: 5330–5339.

Tjon, A. S., R. van Gent, H. Jaadar, P. Martin van Hagen, S. Mancham, L. J. van der Laan et al. 2014. Intravenous immunoglobulin treatment in humans suppresses dendritic cell function via stimulation of IL-4 and IL-13 production. J Immunol 92: 5625–34.

Tomana, M., J. Novak, B. A. Julian, K. Matousovic, K. Konency and J. Mastecky. 1999. Ciruclating immune complexes in IgA nephropathy consist of IgA1 with galactose-deficient hinge region and antiglycan antibodies. J Clin Invest 104: 73–81.

Trnka, P. 2013. Henoch–Schönlein purpura in children. J Paediatr Child Health 49: 995–1003.

Urbaniak, S. J. and M. A. Greiss. 2000. RhD haemolytic disease of the fetus and newborn. Blood Rev 14: 44–61.

van de Geijn, F. E., M. Wuhrer, M. H. Selman, S. P. Willemsen, Y. A. de Man, A. M. Deelder et al. 2009. Immunoglobulin G galactosylation and sialylation are associated with pregnancy-induced improvement of rheumatoid arthritis and the postpartum flare: results from a large prospective cohort study. Arthritis Res Ther 11(6): R193.

van Doorn, P. A., L. Ruts and B. C. Jacobs. 2008. Clinical features, pathogenesis, and treatment of Guillan-Barre syndrome. Lancet Neurol 7: 939–50.

Vercelli, D., B. Helm, P. Marsh, E. Padlan, R. S. Geha and H. Gould. 1989. The B-cell binding site on human immunoglobulin E. Nature 338(6217): 649–51.

Washburn, N., I. Schwab, D. Ortiz, N. Bhatnagar, J. C. Lansing, A. Medeiros et al. 2015. Controlled tetra-Fc sialylation of IVIg results in a drug candidate with consistent enhanced anti-inflammatory activity. Proc Natl Acad Sci USA 112: E1297–306.

Weiner, G. J. 2010. Rituximab: mechanism of action. Semin Hematol 47: 115–123.

Youinou, P., Y. L. Pennec, R. Casburn-Budd, M. Dueymes, G. Letoux and A. Lemour. 1992. Galactose terminating oligosaccharides of IgG in patients wth primary Sjogren's syndrome. J Autoimmunity 5: 393–400.

CHAPTER 16

Congenital Disorders of Glycosylation

Susan E. Sparks

Introduction

Glycosylation is a process by which sugars are attached to proteins and lipids. Because of the diverse, essential role glycosylation plays in human biology, many inherited disorders of glycosylation are multisystemic and devastating (Jaeken 2003). Since the identification of the first defect on N-linked glycosylation in the 1980s (Jaeken et al. 1984), there are over 100 (Freeze 2013) different congenital disorders of glycosylation. This review encompasses both the medicine and glycobiology of individuals affected with disorders of glycosylation. These include those with defects in the synthetic pathways of N-linked oligosaccharides, O-linked oligosaccharides, dolichol-linked oligosaccharides, glycosylphosphatidylinositol (GPI) anchors and shared substrates of these pathways (Table 1).

Glycosylation Process

Protein glycosylation is defined as the synthesis of glycans and their covalent attachment to proteins. Glycans are also attached to lipids forming glycolipids (glycophospholipids, glycosphingolipids). Approximately 0.5–1% of the transcribed human genome is responsible for the synthesis, degradation, and function of glycoconjugates (Varki and Marth 1995). Since about half of the body proteins are glycoproteins, this is an expansive field of study.

Glycoproteins are classified by the type of linkage of the oligosaccharides to the peptide. This attachment can be either N-linked through the amide group of selected asparagine residues to an *N*-acetylglucosamine (GlcNAc) residue, or O-linked through the hydroxyl group mainly of serine or threonine residues via *N*-acetylgalactosamine (GalNAc), mannose (Man), xylose (Xyl), or other monosaccharide residues.

The biosynthesis of N-linked glycans occurs co-translationally and is spread over the cytosol, the endoplasmic reticulum (ER), and the Golgi compartments. In the cytosol and the ER, monosaccharides are attached in a stepwise fashion to form a lipid-linked oligosaccharide (LLO). The monosaccharide donors are either nucleotide- or dolichol-phosphate-linked sugars synthesized in the cytosol. These are the substrates for specific glycosyltransferases, which sequentially form the progressively growing lipid-linked oligosaccharide (LLO) in the ER ending with three terminal glucose (Glc). In the ER, the completed basic glycan $Glc_3Man_9GlcNAc_2$) is transferred *en bloc* to the asparagine (Asn) which is part

Medical Director, Genetic Diseases, US Medical Affairs, Genzyme, a Sanofi Company, 500 Kendall Street, Cambridge, MA 02142.
E-mail: susan.sparks@genzyme.com

Table 1. Genes Associated with Congenital Disorders of Glycosylation. 1. The original nomenclature used for CDG subtypes includes a Roman numeral, I or II, and a letter (a-i) (Aebi et al. 1999). The Roman numeral is based on transferrin oligosaccharide analytic pattern: Type I and Type II. Letters are assigned in chronologic order of the date of publication of discovery. Current nomenclature involves the gene name followed by "CDG" followed by the original name in parenthesis (Jaeken et al. 2009a). 2. Data are compiled from the following standard references: gene symbol from HGNC; protein name from UniProt. 3. COG = conserved oligomeric Golgi.

CDG Type[1]	Gene Symbol[2]	Protein Name[2]
N-linked glycosylation defects		
PMM2-CDG (*CDG-Ia*)	*PMM2*	Phosphomannomutase 2
MPI-CDG (*CDG-Ib*)	*MPI*	Mannose-6-phosphate isomerase
ALG6-CDG (*CDG-Ic*)	*ALG6*	Dolichyl pyrophosphate Man9GlcNAc2 alpha-1,3-glucosyltransferase
ALG3-CDG (*CDG-Id*)	*ALG3*	Dolichyl-P-Man:Man(5)GlcNAc(2)-PP-dolichyl mannosyltransferase
MPDU1-CDG (*CDG-If*)	*MPDU1*	Mannose-P-dolichol utilization defect 1 protein
ALG12-CDG (*CDG-Ig*)	*ALG12*	Dolichyl-P-Man:Man(7)GlcNAc(2)-PP-dolichyl-alpha-1,6-mannosyltransferase
ALG8-CDG (*CDG-Ih*)	*ALG8*	Probable dolichyl pyrophosphate Glc1Man9GlcNAc2 alpha-1,3-glucosyltransferase
ALG2-CDG (*CDG-Ii*)	*ALG2*	Alpha-1,3-mannosyltransferase ALG2
DPAGT1-CDG (*CDG-Ij*)	*DPAGT1*	UDP-N-acetylglucosamine-dolichyl-phosphate N-acetylglucosamine-phosphotransferase
ALG1-CDG (*CDG-Ik*)	*ALG1/HMT-1*	Chitobiosyldiphosphodolichol beta-mannosyltransferase
ALG9-CDG (*CDG-IL*)	*ALG9*	Alpha-1,2-mannosyltransferase (asparagine-linked glycosylation protein 9 homolog)
RFT1-CDG (*CDG-In*)	*RFT1*	Protein RFT1 homolog
ALG11-CDG (*CDG-Ip*)	*ALG11*	Asparagine-linked glycosylation protein 11 homolog
DDOST-CDG (*CDG-Ir*)	*DDOST*	Oligosaccharyltransferase (dolichyl-diphosphooligosaccharide-protein glycosyltransferase
ALG13-CDG (*CDG-Is*)	*ALG13*	UDP-GlcNAc transferase
PGM1-CDG (*CDG-It*)	*PGM1*	Phosphoglucomutase
MAGT1-CDG	*MAGT1*	Magnesium transporter (oligosaccharyltransferase)
N33/TUSC3-CDG	*N33/TUSC3*	Magnesium transporter (oligosaccharyltransferase subunit)
STT3A-CDG (*CDG-Iw*)	*STT3A*	Catalytic subunit of the oligosaccharide (OST) protein complex
STT3B-CDG (*CDG-Ix*)	*STT3B*	Catalytic subunit of the oligosaccharide (OST) protein complex
SSR4-CDG (*CDG-Iy*)	*SSR4*	
MGAT2-CDG (*CDG-IIa*)	*MGAT2*	Alpha-1,6-mannosyl-glycoprotein 2-beta-N-acetylglucosaminyltransferase
MOGS-CDG (*CDG-IIb*)	*MOGS (GCS1)*	Mannosyl-oligosaccharide glucosidase
B4GALT1-CDG (*CDG-IId*)	*B4GALT1*	Beta-1,4-galactosyltransferase 1
SLC35A1-CDG (*CDG-IIf*)	*SLC35A1*	CMP-sialic acid transporter
ST3GAL3-CDG	*ST3GAL3*	Beta-galactoside-alpha-2,3-sialyltransferase-III

Table 1. contd....

Table 1. contd.

CDG Type[1]	Gene Symbol[2]	Protein Name[2]
O-Mannosylglycan defects		
POMT1-CDG	*POMT1*	Protein-*O*-mannosyltransferase 1
POMT2-CDG	*POMT2*	Protein-*O*-mannosyltransferase 2
POMGnT1-CDG	*POMGnT1*	*O*-mannose β-1,2-*N*-acetylglucosaminyltransferase
POMGnT2-CDG	*POMGnT2*	*O*-mannose β-1,4-*N*-acetylglucosaminyltransferase 2
FKTN-CDG	*FKTN*	Fukutin
FKRP-CDG	*FKRP*	Fukutin-related protein
LARGE-CDG	*LARGE*	N-acetylglucosaminyltransferase-like protein
GNE-CDG	*GNE*	UDP-N-acetylglucosamine-2-epimerase/N-acetylmannosaminekinase
B3GALNT2-CDG	*B3GALNT2*	β1,3-N-acetylgalactosaminyltransferase 2
B4GAT1-CDG	*B4GAT1*	Xylose β1,4-glucuronyltransferase
SGK196/POMK-CDG	*SGK196/POMK*	Protein-O-mannose kinase
TMEM5-CDG	*TMEM5*	Transmembrane protein 5
GMPPB-CDG	*GMPPB*	GDP-mannose pyrophosphorylase beta subunit
ISPD-CDG	*ISPD*	Isoprenoid synthase domain-containing protein
DAG1	*DAG1*	Dystroglycan
O-linked xylose defects		
B4GALT7-CDG	*B4GALT7*	UDP-galactose:O-beta-D-xylosylprotein 4-beta-D-galactosyltransferase
EXT1/EXT2-CDG	*EXT1/EXT2*	Exostosin glycosyltransferase 1 and 2
SLC35D1-CDG	*SLC35D1*	UDP-glucuronic acid/UDP-N-acetylgalactosamine dual transporter
O-linked fucose defects		
B3GALTL-CDG	*B3GALTL*	UDP-Gal:Beta-GlcNAc Beta-1,3-galactosyltransferase-like
LFNG-CDG	*LFNG*	Beta-1,3-N-acetylglucosaminyltransferase
O-GalNAc defects		
GALNT3-CDG	*GALNT3*	UDP-N-Acetyl-alpha-D-galactosamine:polypeptide N-acetylgalactosaminyltransferase 3
C1GALT1-CDG	*C1GLAT1*	Core 1 beta-3-galactosyltransferase
Combined N- and O-linked defects		
GFPT1-CDG	*GFPT1*	glutamine:fructose-6-phosphate transaminase
PGM3-CDG	*PGM3*	Phosphoglucomutase
SLC35C1-CDG (*CDG-IIc*)	*SLC35C1*	GDP-fucose transporter 1
COG7-CDG (*CDG-IIe*)	*COG7*	COG complex subunit 7 [3]
COG1-CDG (*CDG-IIg*)	*COG1*	COG complex subunit 1 [3]
COG8-CDG (*CDG-IIh*)	*COG8*	COG complex subunit 8 [3]

Table 1. contd....

Table 1. contd.

CDG Type[1]	Gene Symbol[2]	Protein Name[2]
Combined N- and O-linked defects		
COG4-CDG (*CDG-IIj*)	COG4	COG complex subunit 4 [3]
COG5-CDG (*CDG-IIj*)	COG5	COG complex subunit 5 [3]
COG6-CDG (*CDG-IIL*)	COG6	COG complex subunit 6 [3]
ATP6V0A2-CDG	ATP6V0A2	ATPase, H+ transporting, lysosomal, V0A2 subunit
Dolichol synthetic defects		
DHDDS-CDG	DHDDS	Dehydrodolichyldiphosphate synthetase (Cis-prenyltransferase CPT)
SRD5A3-CDG	SRD5A3	Probable polyprenol reductase
DPM1-CDG (*CDG-Ie*)	DPM1	Dolichol-phosphate mannosyltransferase
DOLK-CDG (*CDG-Im*)	DOLK (DK1)	Dolichol kinase
DPM3-CDG (*CDG-Io*)	DPM3	Dolichol-phosphate mannosyltransferase subunit 3
DPM2-CDG (*CDG-Iu*)	DPM2	Dolichol-phosphate mannosyltransferase subunit 2
GPI Anchor defects		
PIGA-CDG	PIGA	Phosphatidylinositol glycan A
PIGL-CDG	PIGL	Phosphatidylinositol glycan L
PIGM-CDG	PIGM	Phosphatidylinositol glycan M
PIGN-CDG	PIGN	glycosylphosphatidylinositol (GPI) ethanolamine phosphate transferase-1
PIGV-CDG	PIGV	Phosphatidylinositol glycan V
PIGO-CDG	PIGO	Phosphatidylinositol glycan O
PIGT-CDG	PIGT	Phosphatidylinositol glycan T
PGAP2-CDG	PGAP2	Post-GPI attachment to proteins 2
PIGW-CDG	PIGW	Phosphatidylinositol glycan W
PGAP1-CDG	PGAP1	Post-GPI attachment to proteins 1
Defects of Deglycosylation		
NGLY-1-CDDG	NGLY1	N-glycanase 1

of the consensus sequence on the protein, Asn-X-Serine/Threonine, with X as any amino acid (Kornfeld and Kornfeld 1985). This transfer is catalyzed by the oligosaccharyltransferase complex, a group of 7 subunits (Mohorko et al. 2011).

The glycosylated protein is further processed, within the ER and the Golgi, into a more complex structure by removal of glucose and mannose residues and the addition of GlcNAc, galactose (Gal), fucose (Fuc), and sialic acid (SA) residues by specific glycosidases (Marquardt and Denecke 2003). By far the most abundant and well-studied of the protein hypo-glycosylation defects are the group of disorders known as Congenital Disorders of Glycosylation, or CDG, formerly known as carbohydrate-deficient glycoprotein syndromes. These disorders are caused by defects in the elongation pathway of the biosynthesis of N-glycans that occurs in the ER (type I CDG) and defects in the processing pathway in the ER and Golgi (type II CDG). Due to the utilization of some common enzymes and pools of substrates in the biosynthetic pathways of N- and O-glycans, several of the subtypes of CDG affect O-glycosylation as well.

In contrast, the biosynthesis of O-linked glycans occurs post-translationally and mainly within the Golgi compartment. Of interest, there is no consensus sequence to determine the O-glycosylation sites within a protein. However, since O-linked glycosylation occurs after protein folding; only exposed serine and threonine residues are available for glycosylation. There are seven different types of O-glycan attachments in humans, classified by the first sugar, either (GalNAc, Xyl, GlcNAc, Gal, Man, Glc, or Fuc initially bound to the protein. The mucin-type O-glycoprotein, which begins with the addition of a GalNAc to a serine or threonine of a fully formed protein, and the glycosaminoglycans (GAGs) where a Xyl is the first sugar, are the most common O-linked glycoproteins. Following this initial step, there is elongation and modification of the oligosaccharides (Marquardt and Denecke 2003). Mucin-type O-glycans can be further subdivided into eight core structures depending on the second sugar(s) and/or binding position resulting in at least 50 different oligosaccharide types. GAGs contain 100 or more monosaccharides and their content define different GAG types; with heparin, chondroitin sulfate or dermatan sulfate as examples. The structures of the other 5 O-glycan types show less variability and mostly occur in one conformation (Van den Steen et al. 1998).

A specific type of O-glycosylation involves the attachment of a mannose. While many brain glycoproteins contain O-linked mannose oligosaccharides, only α-dystroglycan has been well characterized (Chai et al. 1999). α-dystroglycan is part of the dystrophin-glycoprotein complex which is important for membrane stability and cell signaling functions in the central nervous system as well as muscle (Ervasti and Campbell 1991). α-Dystroglycan is heavily glycosylated with N-linked oligosaccharides and mucin-type O-linked oligosaccharides. Defects in the glycosylation of α-dystroglycan are called dystroglycanopathies and result in muscular dystrophy with or without brain and eye involvement (Endo 2015).

Historical View of CDG

The first congenital disorder of glycosylation was described by Jaek Jaeken in identical twin sisters with developmental delay, decreased thyroxine-binding globulin levels and increased lysosomal enzyme activities. Further analysis using isoelectric focusing (IEF) of serum transferrin demonstrated a cathodal shift of their transferring IEF profile, which is now considered pathognomonic for the diagnosis of a defect in the synthesis of N-linked oligosaccharide, or CDG in the N-linked pathway (Jaeken and Matthijs 2001). Initially the nomenclature for this group of N-linked glycosylation disorders was CDG followed by the type of transferrin isoelectric focusing pattern (I or II) and the letter in order of the identified gene defect (i.e., CDG-Ia or CDG-IIa). With the identification of many more types of glycosylation defects, this nomenclature was changed with the gene name, followed by "CDG", and the older nomenclature in parenthesis (i.e., PMM2-CDG (*CDG-Ia*) (Jaeken et al. 2009a).

The Clinical Spectrum of N-linked Glycosylation Defects

Below are descriptions of a few exemplary types of N-linked oligosaccharide synthetic disorders which have been reported in the literature. There are many more types, some with only one case reported, and rapidly emerging information about both new types and the spectrum of phenotypic variability in the CDG types discussed.

- **PMM2-CDG (*CDG-Ia*).** This is the most common N-linked CDG, with over 700 patients described worldwide, and is considered the clinical prototype for the group of the CDGs. It is a multisystem disorder characterized by inverted nipples, abnormal subcutaneous fat distribution, and cerebellar hypoplasia, in combination with hypotonia and developmental delay. In infancy, there is failure to thrive with feeding difficulties and gastroesophageal reflux. Serum liver transaminases are elevated and hypoalbuminemia can occur. While most affected newborns survive infancy, some are affected by severe failure to thrive, pronounced hypoalbuminemia, progressive fluid retention with anasarca and death. The frequency of mortality in infancy is 20–25% (Grunewald 2009). Many pro-clotting factors with Factor IX measurable in most clinical labs, can be decreased in affected individuals leading to bleeding following minor trauma or surgery. Decreased levels of Protein C, Protein

S and Antithrombin III can increase risk of thrombosis. Seizures are common and there can be stroke-like episodes. Pericardial effusions, renal cysts, nephrotic syndrome, retinitis pigmentosa, multiple infections and endocrine abnormalities have been described. Adults with PMM2-CDG (*CDG-Ia*) have developmental delay, ataxia, peripheral neuropathy, scoliosis, and hypergonadotropic hypogonadism (Krasnewich et al. 2007). Recent reports have widened the phenotypic spectrum to include hydrops fetalis at the severe end (van de Kamp et al. 2007) and a mild neurologic phenotype in adults with multisystemic involvement at the mild end (Barone et al. 2007, Coman et al. 2007). Clinical presentations tend to be similar in siblings. Reports indicate that the prevalence may be as high as 1:20,000 (Jaeken and Matthijs 2001) and the carrier frequency in the Danish population may be as high as 1:60–1:79 (Matthijs et al. 2000). It is likely that this disorder is under diagnosed.

- **MPI-CDG (*CDG-Ib*).** Protein-losing enteropathy, profound hypoglycemia, failure to thrive, liver fibrosis, and cyclic vomiting, occasionally associated with coagulation disturbances without neurologic involvement, are characteristic of affected individuals. The clinical course is variable even within families. Taken orally, the monosaccharide mannose appears to improve the growth and gastrointestinal manifestations of this disorder. However, there is continued concern about hepatic manifestations even in treated affected individuals and liver transplantation has been successful (de Koning et al. 1998, Niehues et al. 1998, de Lonlay and Seta 2009, Janssen et al. 2014). At least 20 individuals with this diagnosis have been described.

- **ALG6-CDG (*CDG-Ic*).** ALG6-CDG (*CDG-Ic*) was previously classified as carbohydrate-deficient syndrome type V (Korner et al. 1998) and is characterized by mild-to-moderate neurologic involvement with hypotonia, poor head control, developmental delay, ataxia, strabismus, and seizures, ranging from febrile convulsions to epilepsy (Grunewald et al. 2000, Hanefeld et al. 2000). The clinical presentation may be milder than in PMM2-CDG (*CDG-Ia*) and stroke-like episodes and peripheral neuropathy have not been reported. However, retinal degeneration has been demonstrated (Kahook et al. 2006). An adult with ALG6-CDG (*CDG-Ic*) was described with brachydactyly, deep vein thrombosis, pseudotumor cerebri with normal brain MRI, and endocrine abnormalities including hyperandrogenism with virilization (Sun et al. 2005). Pubertal abnormalities have been described in an individual with ALG6-CDG (*CDG-Ic*) (Miller et al. 2011). Over 30 patients with ALG6-CDG (*CDG-Ic*) have been described.

- **ALG3-CDG (*CDG-Id*).** There have been five children described with defects in ALG3. They all had severe psychomotor delay, microcephaly, and intractable seizures. Vision impairment was described in three infants, two with optic atrophy and iris coloboma. Arthrogryposis was described in one of the children. Distinct phenotypes have been reported in siblings, one had significant digestive issues and the other was more neurologically impaired (Stibler et al. 1995, Denecke et al. 2004, 2005). An additional sibling pair had severe developmental delay, failure to thrive, microcephaly, hypotonia, and seizures. Again, one had significant digestive issues; the other was more neurologically impaired (Kranz et al. 2007a).

- **MPDU1-CDG (*CDG-If*).** Five individuals had severe developmental delay, generalized scaly, erythematous skin, and attacks of hypertonia. In addition, short stature, seizures, and vision impairment have been described (Kranz et al. 2001, Schenk et al. 2001).

- **ALG12-CDG (*CDG-Ig*).** Seven individuals had distinctive features, generalized hypotonia, feeding difficulties, moderate to severe developmental delay, progressive microcephaly, frequent upper respiratory tract infections, impaired immunity with decreased immunoglobulin levels, and decreased coagulation factors (Chantret et al. 2002, Grubenmann et al. 2002, Thiel et al. 2002, Zdebska et al. 2003, Di Rocco et al. 2005, Eklund et al. 2005a, Kranz et al. 2007b). Additional features included hypogonadism with or without hypospadias in the males, seizures in two individuals, and cardiac anomalies in two sibs. A skeletal dysplasia phenotype with rhizomelic short stature, talipes equinovarus, platyspondyly and joint dislocations along with marked underossification on radiographs has been described (Murali et al. 2014).

- **ALG8-CDG (*CDG-Ih*).** A four-month-old female had moderate hepatomegaly, severe diarrhea, and hypoalbuminemia from protein-losing enteropathy, normal facial features, and normal development, similar to PMI-CDG (*CDG-Ib*) (Chantret et al. 2003). She had decreased levels of factor XI, protein C, and antithrombin III. Three other affected individuals had cardiorespiratory difficulties with lung hypoplasia, a severe hepatointestinal disorder, and hypotonia (Schollen et al. 2004). Two additional patients were described with hypotonia, edema, seizures and psychomotor delay (Eklund et al. 2005b, Vesela et al. 2009). Most of these reported affected individuals had hematopoietic issues with anemia and thrombocytopenia, and early death between ages three days and 16 months. Two additional siblings with milder disease were described with hypotonia, cognitive impairment, pseudogynecomastia, and ataxia (Stolting et al. 2009).

- **ALG2-CDG (*CDG-Ii*).** A six-year-old had bilateral iris colobomas, unilateral cataract, infantile spasms beginning at age four months, and severe developmental delay; coagulation factors were abnormal (Thiel et al. 2003).

- **DPAGT1-CDG (*CDG-Ij*).** The diagnosis was initially described in an individual with hypotonia, intractable seizures, developmental delay, and microcephaly (Wu et al. 2003). In the subsequent cases, there is a broad phenotype ranging from muscular dystrophy to fetal akineasia deformation sequence (Ganetzky et al. 2015).

- **ALG1-CDG (*CDG-Ik*).** Affected individuals had severe developmental delay, hypotonia, and early-onset seizures, which are difficult to treat and these cases showed early lethality (Grubenmann et al. 2004, Kranz et al. 2004, Schwarz et al. 2004, Morava et al. 2012, Rohlfing et al. 2014). As in ALG3-CDG (*CDG-Id*) and ALG12-CDG (*CDG-Ig*), also caused by mannosyltransferase defects, microcephaly was rapidly progressive. Other features included severe coagulation defects, nephrotic syndrome, liver dysfunction, coagulation abnormalities, cardiomyopathy, and immunodeficiency. Brain imaging showed cerebral atrophy in some individuals, but may also be normal (Morava et al. 2012). Further studies have shown that ALG1-CDG (*CDG-Ik*) and PMI-CDG (*CDG-Ib*) may be the most frequent after PMM2-CDG (*CDG-Ia*) and clinical features present at the severe end of the CDG I spectrum (Dupre et al. 2010, Morava et al. 2012, Rohlfing et al. 2014).

- **ALG9-CDG (*CDG-IL*).** Three children had microcephaly, hypotonia, developmental delay, seizures, and hepatomegaly (Frank et al. 2004, Weinstein et al. 2005, Vleugels et al. 2009a). Two individuals also had failure to thrive and pericardial effusions. Renal cysts and inverted nipples were also described. The phenotype was expanded when mutations in ALG9 were identified in individuals with Gillessen-Kaesbach-Nishimura skeletal dysplasia, a lethal skeletal dysplasia with visceral malformations (Tham et al. 2015).

- **RFT1-CDG (*CDG-In*).** An infant born preterm to unrelated parents had difficulty feeding as a result of an uncoordinated suck and failure to thrive. Myoclonic jerks were noted at three weeks with hypotonia and brisk reflexes progressing to a seizure disorder. Exam was also notable for roving eye movements with a normal ERG and reduced VEP. At age two years the child continues to have marked developmental delay (Imtiaz et al. 2000, Haeuptle et al. 2008, Clayton and Grunewald 2009). Five additional affected individuals have been described (Vleugels et al. 2009b, Jaeken et al. 2009b). The common features in all six children include severe developmental delay, hypotonia, visual disturbances, seizures, feeding difficulties, and sensorineural hearing loss. Also associated are features similar to other types of N-linked CDG including inverted nipples and microcephaly.

- **ALG11-CDG (*CDG-Ip*).** A single infant presented with distinctive features (microcephaly, high forehead, and low posterior hairline), hypotonia, and failure to thrive. She had severe neurologic impairment with frequent and difficult to treat seizures. She developed an unusual fat pattern around 6 months of age. She had persistent vomiting and stomach bleeding and passed away at 2 years of age (Rind et al. 2010).

- **DDOST-CDG (*CDG-Ir*).** A defect in the oligosaccharyltransferase complex (OST) was identified in a 6 month old infant with hypotonia, developmental delay, and liver dysfunction with a deficiency of factor XI, antithrombin III, protein C and protein S (Jones et al. 2012).

- **ALG13-CDG (*CDG-Is*).** Two individuals with ALG13-CDG (*CDG-Is*) have been described. The first was a boy with refractory seizures, microcephaly, optic atrophy with nystagmus. He also had hepatomegaly, swelling of the hands, feet, and eyelids, recurrent infections and increased bleeding tendency. He passed away at 1 year of age (Timal et al. 2012). A 10 year old girl with neonatal feeding issues, hypotonia, seizures and developmental delay was identified. She had macrocephaly and a brain MRI which demonstrated hydrocephalus, delayed myelination and wide sulci. She had distinctive features, small hands and feet, joint contractures, scoliosis, self-mutilation behavior and sleep disturbance (de Ligt et al. 2012). The Epi4K Consortium and Epilepsy Phenome/Genome Project (2013) identified 2 unrelated girls ALG13-CDG (*CDG-Is*). The patients had early onset of seizures at ages 1 and 4 months, respectively. Both had severely delayed psychomotor development after onset of seizures and showed hypsarrhythmia on EEG.

- **PGM1-CDG (*CDG-It*).** PGM1 (phosphoglucomutase 1) deficiency was originally described as a muscle glycogen storage disorder type XIV (Stojkovic et al. 2009). More recently PGM1-CDG has been described and is characterized by a wide range of clinical manifestations and severity. The most common features include cleft lip and bifid uvula, hepatopathy with elevated liver enzymes and sometimes steatosis and fibrosis along with intermittent hypoglycemia. There is short stature. Exercise intolerance along with an increased creatine kinase and even rhabdomyolysis has been described. Less common features include dilated cardiomyopathy and hypogonatoptropic hypogonadism (Timal et al. 2012, Tegtmeyer et al. 2014).

- **MAGT1-CDG.** This is a defect in another subunit of the OST. Reported in a family with two girls with mild cognitive impairment and two boys with more severe cognitive involvement. The mother is reported to have mild cognitive impairment (Molinari et al. 2008).

- **N33/TUSC3-CDG.** Two different kindreds of siblings were described with non-syndromic intellectual disability and had a defect in another subunit of the oligosaccharyltransferase (Molinari et al. 2008, Garshasbi et al. 2008).

- **STT3A-CDG (*CDG-Iw*).** Two siblings with severe developmental delay, microcephaly, failure to thrive, seizures, intractable in one sibling, hypotonia, and cerebellar atrophy have been described (Shrimal et al. 2013).

- **STT3B-CDG (*CDG-Ix*).** One such patient has been reported with severe developmental delay, microcephaly, cerebellar atrophy, seizures, hypotonia, micropenis with hypoplastic scrotum and undescended testes. He had liver dysfunction, thrombocytopenia and passed away at 4 years of age (Shrimal et al. 2013).

- **SSR4-CDG (*CDG-Iy*).** A single patient was described (Losfeld et al. 2014). He is a 16 year old boy who presented at birth with microcephaly and respiratory distress. Distinctive features were described with micrognathia, excess skin around the neck, increased fat pads, mild hypospadias, and clinodactyly of the fourth and fifth toes. He had hypotonia, developmental delay, and mild seizure disorder not requiring therapy.

- **MGAT2-CDG (*CDG-IIa*).** Affected individuals have facial dysmorphism, stereotypic hand movements, seizures, and varying degrees of developmental delay, but no peripheral neuropathy or cerebellar hypoplasia. A bleeding disorder is caused by diminished platelet aggregation (Van Geet et al. 2001). Scoliosis and respiratory compromise can also occur (de Cock and Jaeken 2009).

- **GCS1/MOGS-CDG (*CDG-IIb*).** An infant with generalized hypotonia, distinctive features, hypoplastic genitalia, seizures, feeding difficulties, hypoventilation, and generalized edema died at age 2.5 months (De Praeter et al. 2000).

- **B4GALT1-CDG (*CDG-IId*).** Mild developmental delay, Dandy-Walker malformation, progressive hydrocephalus, coagulation abnormalities, and elevated serum creatine kinase concentration have been observed (Peters et al. 2002). An additional patient was described with normal development, mild hepatic involvement, and coagulation abnormalities (Guillard et al. 2011).

- **SLC35A1-CDG (*CDG-IIf*).** One affected infant presented at age four months with macrothrombocytopenia, neutropenia, and immunodeficiency, and died at age 37 months of complications from bone-marrow transplantation (Martinez-Duncker et al. 2005).

- **ST3GAL3-CDG.** *ST3GAL3* gene encodes beta-galactoside-alpha-2,3-sialyltransferase-III, a Golgi resident membrane protein that forms the sialyl Lewis a (sLe-a) epitope on glycoproteins. ST3GAL3-CDG has been described in individuals with nonsyndromic cognitive impairment (Hu et al. 2011) and infantile epileptic encephalopathy (Edvardson et al. 2013).

The Clinical Spectrum of O-glycosylation Defects

O-mannosylglycan Defects-Dystroglycanopathies

Defective glycosylation of α-dystroglycan, a component of the dystrophin-glycoprotein (DAG) complex, has been implicated in several subtypes of muscular dystrophy, known as the dystroglycanopathies. The DAG complex is a multicomponent complex linking the intracellular cytoskeleton with the extracellular matrix in muscle. Glycosylation of α-dystroglycan is essential for binding to proteins of the extracellular matrix and synaptic molecules, including laminin (Inamori et al. 2012, Goddeeris et al. 2013), agrin (Gee et al. 1994), perlecan (Peng et al. 1998), neurexin (Sugita et al. 2001), pikachurin (Sato et al. 2008), and slit (Wright et al. 2012). α-dystroglycan also plays a role in neuronal migration in addition to its involvement in muscle biology. Thus, patients with severe defective glycosylation of α-dystroglycan demonstrate both muscular dystrophy and central nervous system abnormalities.

The dystroglycanopathies include at the severe end of the phenotypic spectrum, congenital muscular dystrophy-dystroglycanopathy (MDDG) with brain and eye anomalies (type A; MDDGA), previously designated Walker-Warburg syndrome (WWS) or muscle-eye-brain disease (MEB). The intermediate phenotypic spectrum are represented by Fukayama congenital muscular dystrophy (FCMD), which is similar to WWS/MEB, but without eye abnormalities and by congenital muscular dystrophy-dystroglycanopathy with or without cognitive impairment/brain malformations (type B; MDDGB). At the mildest end of the spectrum is the limb-girdle muscular dystrophy (LGMD) phenotype and which is designated type C (MDDGC) (Table 2).

WWS is the most severe of the dystroglycanopathies and is typically associated with death of affected individuals by the age of 2 years. The diagnostic hallmark is the combination of severe brain malformations, typically described as the Cobblestone complex, muscular dystrophy, and structural eye abnormalities, particularly microophthalmia and can include cataracts. The Cobblestone complex is a combination of type II lissencephaly, agenesis of the corpus callosum, cerebellar hypoplasia, and enlarged ventricles (Muntoni et al. 2004, Vajsar and Schachter 2006).

With a slightly milder phenotype than WWS, MEB is characterized by muscular dystrophy, eye involvement (congenital myopia and glaucoma, retinal hypoplasia without congenital cataracts), developmental delay, and structural brain defects ranging from microcephaly to the Cobblestone complex (Yoshida et al. 2001, Muntoni et al. 2004). FCMD is seen almost exclusively in Japan. Like WWS and MEB, FCMD is also characterized by muscle and brain involvement, however, only occasionally are eyes involved (Fukuyama et al. 1981, Muntoni et al. 2004). Congenital muscular dystrophies with or without developmental delay present with congenital weakness, but are less severe than WWS/MEB (Longman et al. 2003, Muntoni et al. 2004, Louhichi et al. 2004, Mercuri et al. 2006a, MacLeod et al. 2007, Clarke et al. 2011).

Table 2. Dystroglycanopathies: CDG type and phenotypic spectrum. MDDGA: muscular dystrophy-dystroglycanopathy type A (congenital onset of muscular dystrophy with brain and eye anomalies, previously designated Walker-Warburg syndrome (WWS) or muscle-eye-brain disease (MEB). MDDGB: muscular dystrophy-dystroglycanopathy type B (congenital onset of muscular dystrophy with or without cognitive impairment/brain malformations; intermediate phenotypic spectrum represented by Fukayama congenital muscular dystrophy (FCMD). MDDGC: muscular dystrophy-dystroglycanopathy type C (mildest end of spectrum, also designated by limb-girdle muscular dystrophy (LGMD).

CDG type	MDDGA (severe)	MDDGB (intermediate)	MDDGC (milder)
POMGnT2-CDG	■		
B3GALNT2-CDG	■		
B4GAT1-CDG	■		
LARGE-CDG	■	■	
TMEM5-CDG	■	■	
POMT1-CDG	■	■	■
POMT2-CDG	■	■	■
POMGnT1-CDG	■	■	■
FKTN-CDG	■	■	■
FKRP-CDG	■	■	■
SGK196/POMK-CDG	■	■	■

Limb-girdle muscular dystrophies resulting from defective glycosylation of α-dystroglycan (DAG1) represent the mildest end of the phenotypic spectrum of the MDDG (type C; MDDGC). The limb-girdle phenotype is characterized by onset of muscular weakness apparent after ambulation is achieved; mental retardation and mild brain anomalies are variable (Balci et al. 2005, Godfrey et al. 2007, Nigro and Savarese 2014).

Specific Disorders of O-linked Mannose Oligosaccharide Synthesis

- **POMT1-CDG (MDDGA1/MDDGB1/MDDGC1(LGMD2K)).** *POMT1* encodes the protein-*O*-mannosyltransferase 1 that catalyzes the first step in *O*-mannosyl glycan synthesis (Willer et al. 2003). Mutations in *POMT1* have been identified in patients with WWS (Beltran-Valero de Bernabe et al. 2002), a milder congenital muscular dystrophy with calf hypertrophy, microcephaly, and cognitive impairment (van Reeuwijk et al. 2006), and in patients with LGMD2K (Balci et al. 2005, Lommel et al. 2010).

- **POMT2-CDG (MDDGA2/MDDGB2/MDDGC2(LGMD2N)).** *POMT2* is a second *O*-mannosyltransferase which complexes with POMT1 for the O-mannosyltransferase activity (Manya et al. 2004, Akasaka-Manya et al. 2006). Mutations in *POMT2* have been described in patients with WWS (van Reeuwijk et al. 2005), a MEB-like phenotype (Mercuri et al. 2006a), a milder congenital muscular dystrophy phenotype (Yanagisawa et al. 2007), and LGMD2N (Biancheri et al. 2007).

- **POMGnT1-CDG (MDDGA3/MDDGB3/MDDGC3(LGMD2O)).** Mutations in the *POMGnT1* gene which encodes the glycosyltransferase, *O*-mannose β-1, 2-*N*-acetylglucosaminyltransferase were identified in patients with MEB (Cormand et al. 1999, Yoshida et al. 2001). Subsequently, mutations in *POMGnT1* were identified in patients with WWS (Bouchet et al. 2007, Godfrey et al. 2007, Teber et al. 2008, Mercuri et al. 2009) and LGMD2O (Clement et al. 2008). *POMGnT1* catalyzes the transfer of *N*-acetylglucosmine to the *O*-linked mannose of glycoproteins including α-dystroglycan.

- **POMGnT2/GTDC2-CDG (MDDGA8).** Defects in POMGnT2 cause a severe WWS phenotype and were described in 3 unrelated families (Manzini et al. 2012). The patients in two families died within the first months of life. In the third family, two affected pregnancies were terminated at 23 and 20 weeks' gestational age due to severe ventricular enlargement.

- **FKTN-CDG (MDDGA4/MDDGB4(FCMD)/MDDGC4(LGMD2M)).** The *fukutin* (*FKTN*) gene was initially identified to cause FCMD (Toda et al. 1993, Kobayashi et al. 1998). *FKTN* mutations have been identified in patients with the more severe phenotype, WWS (Silan et al. 2003, de Bernabe et al. 2003, Godfrey et al. 2007, Cotarelo et al. 2008) as well as milder non-WWS congenital muscular dystrophy (Saredi et al. 2009, Yis et al. 2011) and LGMD2M (Godfrey et al. 2006, Puckett et al. 2009). Mutations in *FKTN* have also been identified in patients with isolated elevations of serum CK (Vuillaumier-Barrot et al. 2009) and cardiomyopathy (Murakami et al. 2006, Arimura et al. 2009). The fukutin protein shares sequence homology to a bacterial glycosyltransferase, but its precise function is unknown (Toda et al. 2003). It has been reported that there is colocalization and molecular interaction of fukutin with POMGnT1, suggesting that fukutin may form a complex with POMGnT1 and modulate its enzymatic activity (Xiong et al. 2006).

- **FKRP-CDG (MDDGA5/MDDGB5/MDDGC5(LGMD2I)).** *FKRP* encodes the fukutin-related protein. Mutations in this gene cause the widest variability in clinical phenotypes, ranging from in utero, severe WWS to very mild LGMD2I (Brockington et al. 2001a, 2001b, De Paula et al. 2003, Mercuri et al. 2003, Louhichi et al. 2004, Mercuri et al. 2006b, MacLeod et al. 2007, van Reeuwijk et al. 2010). Additional features include elevated CK, myalgia, rhabdomyolysis and cardiomyopathy (Mercuri et al. 2003, Poppe et al. 2003, Mathews et al. 2011). Like fukutin, the function of FKRP is unknown, although it shares homology with FKTN and other glycosyltransferases (Kuga et al. 2012).

- **LARGE-CDG (MDDGA6/MDDGB6).** The *LARGE* gene is the fifth largest gene in the human genome, spanning 664 kb of genomic DNA on chromosome 22q12.3-q13.1, and has homology to the glycosyltransferase gene family (Peyrard et al. 1999). It may have bifunctional activity of β1,3 acetylglucosaminyltransferase and α1/3-Xylosyl transferase (Inamori et al. 2012). Mutations in *LARGE* were originally described in MDC1D (Longman et al. 2003, Clarke et al. 2011), however, mutations in LARGE have also been described in patients with the severe congenital muscular dystrophy WWS (van Reeuwijk et al. 2007).

- **GNE-CDG.** *GNE* encodes a bifunctional enzyme (UDP-N-acetylglucosamine 2-epimerase/N-acetylmannosamine kinase) in the biosynthetic pathway of sialic acid, and was identified by linkage analysis to be mutated in hereditary inclusion body myopathy (HIBM) (Keppler et al. 1999, Eisenberg et al. 2001). Mutations in *GNE* cause mostly a distal myopathy, that begins with juvenile onset of muscle weakness which spares the quadriceps and on muscle pathology demonstrates rimmed vacuoles and cytoplasmic and intranuclear inclusions (Argov and Yarom 1984, Sadeh et al. 1993). *GNE* mutations were also described in another distal myopathy with rimmed vacuoles, Nonaka myopathy (Nonaka et al. 1981, Nishino et al. 2002).

- **B3GALNT2-CDG (MDDGA11).** *B3GALNT2* (β1,3-N-acetylgalactosaminyltransferase 2) was identified to be abnormal in six unrelated patients with a WWS/MEB phenotype and abnormal glycosylation of α-dystroglycan (Stevens et al. 2013).

- **B4GAT1-CDG (MDDGA13).** *B4GAT1* (formerly known as B3GNT1) encodesxylose β1,4-glucuronyltransferase (Praissman et al. 2014) and mutations in this gene were identified in a family of East Indian descent in which four siblings had a clinical diagnosis of WWS and abnormal glycosylation of DAG (Buysse et al. 2013). Three pregnancies were terminated and 1 affected son died at 2 years of age. The living patient showed severe hypotonia with increased serum CK and developed intractable seizures. All patients had retinal dysplasia and severe brain malformations, including hydrocephalus, brainstem and cerebellar hypoplasia, nodular heterotopia, and cobblestone lissencephaly. Other more variable abnormalities included thin corpus callosum, absent septum pellucidum, cortical cysts, and Dandy-Walker malformation. Dysplastic kidneys and testicular hypoplasia were seen in one fetus.

- **SGK196/POMK-CDG (MDDGA12/MDDGB12/MDDGC12).** Two siblings were described with a limb-girdle congenital muscular dystrophy phenotype and cognitive impairment (Di Costanzo et al. 2014). Both presented with weakness in infancy and developmental delay, but learned to walk. The older sister at age 25 years had proximal weakness, calf pseudohypertrophy, hyporeflexia and mild facial weakness with an IQ of 80. The 7 1/2 year old brother had milder weakness, could climb stairs without support, but had abnormal posture and gait. His IQ was 83. Both had elevated serum CK and dystrophic muscle biopsies, but normal brain imaging and no eye involvement. Two additional infants were described with a more severe WWS phenotype including abnormal brain MRI and eye abnormalities (Jae et al. 2013, Di Costanzo et al. 2014). These children died at ages 3 and 4 years of age, respectively. One family had a subsequent pregnancy which was terminated at 19 weeks after identification of cerebral ventriculomegaly and a small occipital encephalocele on the 17 week ultrasound. Autopsy showed cerebral anomalies, absence of the falx cerebri and cerebellar tentorium along with bilateral retinal colobomas and cortical cataracts. Two additional siblings were described with progressive congenital muscular dystrophy and severe cognitive impairment (von Renesse et al. 2014). Additional features included mild sensorineural hearing loss and large eyes with decreased visual acuity. At ages 21 and 15 years, the time of the report, both were severely affected and required a wheelchair and had limited functional life skills. One had progressive microcephaly and the other developed scoliosis and required ventilator support.

- **TMEM5-CDG (MDDGA10).** Initially described in nine fetuses from five unrelated families with severe cobblestone lissencephaly (Vuillaumier-Barrot et al. 2012). Additional features included occipital neural tube defects, facial clefts, visceral malformations, retinal dysplasia and gonadal dysgenesis. Subsequently, Jae et al. (2013) described a WWS/MEB phenotype in members of two unrelated families. The first had a newborn male who was large for gestational age with macrocephaly and an occipital encephalocele, right microphthalmia and bilateral opaque cornea. He had severe hypotonia and elevated CK. Due to hydrocephalus, a ventriculoperitoneal shunt was required at 6 weeks of age and the infant passed away at the age of 22 months. The second family had two affected siblings, ages 19 and 21 years who had severe cognitive impairment with autistic features, microcephaly, and were mobile with a broad-based gait. MRI of the older sibling demonstrated brainstem atrophy, ventricular dilatation, diffuse pachygyria and white matter changes consistent with a leukodystrophy.

- **GMPPB-CDG (MDDGA14/MDDGB14/MDDGC14).** The *GMPPB* gene encodes the beta subunit of an essential enzyme, GDP-mannose pyrophosphorylase. This enzyme catalyzes the conversion of mannose-1-phosphate and GTP to inorganic diphosphate and GDP-mannose, a major mannosyl donor for mannose-containing proteins (Ning and Elbein 2000). GDP-mannose is required in four glycosylation pathways, including O-mannosylation of membrane and secretory glycoproteins, such as α-dystroglycan. The whole range of clinical phenotypes with and without cognitive impairment has been described (Messina et al. 2009, Carss et al. 2013). Additional features included seizures, cataracts, ptosis, retinal dysfunction, ataxia, sensorineural hearing loss, cardiomyopathy, cardiac dysrhythmia, and respiratory involvement. One boy had cleft palate and another had microcephaly, ileal atresia, and torticollis (Carss et al. 2013). Brain MRI findings ranged from normal to pontine and cerebellar hypoplasia.

- **ISPD-CDG (MDDGA7/MDDGC7).** ISPD-CDG ranges from WWS phenotype to LGMD phenotype. Two families with two siblings each had childhood onset of proximal muscle weakness affecting the lower extremities more than the upper extremities (Tasca et al. 2013). Two of the sisters in one family initially presented with exercise intolerance with quadriceps muscle pain and myoglobinuria. As adults, all four subjects had scapular winging, tongue and calf hypertrophy and reduced pulmonary function. Three of the patients lost ambulation between 33 and 45 years of age. Brain imaging of two siblings showed discrete gliotic lesions compatible with mild hypoxic-ischemic encephalopathy, but there were no brain malformations. Eighteen patients with WWS/MEB phenotype with brain and eye involvement have been described (Willer et al. 2012, Roscioli et al. 2012). Most died by 2 years of age, but two patients survived past age 2 years and were thus categorized as having MEB. Vuillaumier-Barrot et al. (2012) reported eight fetuses from five unrelated families with ISPD-CDG. The probands were ascertained from a larger study of patients with severe diffuse cobblestone lissencephaly. Additional findings included neural tube defects, limb anomalies, visceral malformations, brain vascular anomalies and retinal dysplasia. One patient had gonadal dysgenesis.

- **DAG1-CDG (MDDGC9 (LGMD2P)).** Initially described in a 16 year old girl with limb girdle muscular dystrophy, cognitive impairment, calf enlargement, ankle contractures and lumbar lordosis (Dincer et al. 2003), a primary defect in DAG1 (dystroglcyan) was identified (Hara et al. 2011). Brain MRI was normal. At 16 years of age she used only 2-word sentences, had a wide-based waddling gait and an IQ of 50.

Clinical Spectrum of O-linked Xylose Oligosaccharide Defects

- **B4GALT7-CDG.** This defect causes a progeroid variant of Ehlers-Danlos syndrome. One patient has been described with premature aging with loose, hyperelastic skin and joint hyperlaxity. In addition, he had developmental delay, macrocephaly, hypotonia, short stature and osteopenia (Marquardt and Denecke 2003). Two additional patients from a large consanguineous family were identified with milder features. There were connective tissue features with skeletal/radiographic findings, short stature, atrophic scarring, sparse hair and wrinkling of the facial skin, although not as classic progeroid. There were additional features of mild developmental delay, microcephaly and distinctive facial features (Faiyaz-Ul-Haque et al. 2004).

- **EXT1/EXT2-CDG.** Defects in the Golgi-localized EXT1/EXT2 complex which has both glucuronyltransferase and *N*-acetyl-D-hexosaminyltransferase activities, cause hereditary multiple exostoses syndrome. EXT1/EXT2-CDG is the most frequent glycosylation defect with an incidence of 1/50,000–100,000 and is inherited in an autosomal dominant fashion. It is characterized by benign osteochondromas on the ends of long bones. These lesions are often present at birth, but not usually diagnosed until childhood, progressively grow through adolescence and stop during adulthood. The risk of progression into sarcoma is about 3% (Marquardt and Denecke 2003).

- **SLC35D1-CDG.** SLC35D1 is a member of the solute carrier family 35 and encodes the ER-localized dual transporter of UDP-glucuronic acid and UDP-N-acetylgalactosamine (Muraoka et al. 2001). Prior to the identification of the genetic defect, SLC35D1-CDG was described as Schneckenbecken dysplasia, a rare lethal skeletal dysplasia with short limb dwarfism and hydrops (Nikkels et al. 2001). Radiographs of individuals with SLC35D1-CDG demonstrate platyspondyly with oval-shaped vertebral bodies, extremely short long bones with a "dumbbell-like" appearance, and small ilia with "snail-like" appearance, due to medial bone projection from the inner iliac margin (Hiraoka et al. 2007, Furuichi et al. 2009).

Clinical Features of O-linked Fucose Oligosaccharide Synthesis Defects

- **B3GALTL-CDG.** Also known as Peters Plus syndrome, this disorder is characterized by abnormalities of the anterior chamber of the eye, of which Peters anomaly is the most common, in combination with other systemic symptoms. Features may include short stature, developmental delay, and craniofacial abnormalities, such as cleft lip with or without cleft palate (Lesnik Oberstein et al. 2006).

- **LFNG-CDG.** *LFNG* encodes a fucose-specific beta-1,3-N-acetylglucosaminyltransferase (Moloney et al. 2000). LFNG-CDG is an autosomal recessive spondylocostal dysostosis phenotype (Sparrow et al. 2006).

Clinical Features of O-GalNAc Oligosaccharide Synthesis Defects

- **GALNT3-CDG.** Defects in the *GALNT3* gene result in familial tumoral calcinosis which is a severe disorder involving hyperphosphatemia and massive calcium deposits in the skin and subcutaneous tissue (Specktor et al. 2006).

- **C1GALT1-CDG.** C1GALT1 is a core 1 beta-3-galactosyltransferase that synthesizes the transfer of galactose from UDP-Gal to GalNAc-alpha-1-R on core 1 O-glycans (Ju et al. 2002). Defects in C1GALT1 result in Tn polyagglutination syndrome, an acquired clonal disorder characterized by the polyagglutination of red blood cells by naturally occurring anti-Tn antibodies following exposure of the Tn antigen on the surface of erythrocytes (Crew et al. 2008).

Clinical Features of Combined N- and O-linked Defects

Many steps of the glycosylation pathways, specifically the sugar transporters and the Golgi trafficking mechanism, are common to both N- and O-linked glycoprotein synthesis, thus defects in these mechanisms affect both pathways. One important protein complex used by both the N-linked and O-linked synthetic pathways is the conserved oligomeric Golgi (COG) complex. The COG complex is evolutionarily conserved and is important for intra-Golgi trafficking. The COG protein complex consists of eight subunits, distributed in two lobes, Lobe A (Cog1–4) and Lobe B (Cog5–8). Defects in the COG complex lead to defects in both N- and O-linked glycosylation along with problems of protein sorting and Golgi integrity (Smith and Lupashin 2008).

- **GFPT1-CDG.** The *GFPT1* gene encodes glutamine:fructose-6-phosphate transaminase, which catalyzes the transfer of an amino group from glutamine onto fructose-6-phosphate, yielding glucosamine 6-phosphate and glutamate. It is the first and rate-limiting enzyme of the hexosamine biosynthetic pathway. Hexosamine is the obligatory source of essential amino sugars for the synthesis of glycoproteins, glycolipids, and proteoglycans. GFPT1-CDG is characterized with a congenital myasthenic syndrome with proximal limb-girdle muscle weakness (Senderek et al. 2011).

- **PGM3-CDG.** Phosphoglucomutase 3 (PGM3) catalyzes the conversion of GlcNAc-6-phosphate into GlcNAc-1-phosphate during synthesis of uridine diphosphate (UDP)-GlcNAc. Three unrelated children with recurrent infections, congenital leukopenia with neutropenia, B cell and T cell lymphopenia and progression to bone marrow failure were identified with *PGM3* mutations by whole-exome sequencing (Stray-Pedersen et al. 2014). Two of the three children had skeletal dysplasias with short stature, brachydactyly, distinctive facial features and cognitive impairment. These features were not seen in the third patient. Two children received hematopoietic stem cell transplantation of cord blood and bone marrow from matched related donors with successful engraftment and correction of neutropenia and lymphopenia.

- **SLC35C1-CDG (*CDG-IIc*).** *SLC35C1* encodes the GDP-fucose transmembrane transporter located in the Golgi apparatus (Luhn et al. 2001, Lubke et al. 2001). SLC35C1-CDG (*CDG-IIc*) presents with severe growth and developmental delay, microcephaly, hypotonia, distinctive features, and recurrent bacterial infections with persistent, highly elevated peripheral blood leukocyte count (Etzioni et al. 2002).

- **COG7-CDG (*CDG-IIe*).** Six affected infants had distinctive features with a small mouth (although one had full lips), microretrognathia, short neck, wrinkled and loose skin, adducted thumbs, and overlapping long fingers; hypotonia; skeletal abnormalities; hepatosplenomegaly; progressive jaundice; seizures; and early death (Wu et al. 2004, Spaapen et al. 2005, Morava et al. 2007, Ng et al. 2007).

- **COG1-CDG (*CDG-IIg*).** An affected infant presented in the first month of life with feeding difficulties, failure to thrive, and hypotonia. She had mild developmental delay, rhizomelic short stature, and progressive microcephaly with slight cerebral and cerebellar atrophy on brain MRI, as well as cardiac abnormalities and hepatosplenomegaly (Foulquier et al. 2006).

- **COG8-CDG (*CDG-IIh*).** Two affected infants were reported who had severe developmental delay, hypotonia, seizures, esotropia, failure to thrive, and progressive microcephaly (Foulquier et al. 2007, Kranz et al. 2007c). More recently, a pair of sibs were described who had a milder presentation with pseudo-gynecomastia, hypotonia, intellectual disability and ataxia (Stolting et al. 2009).

- **COG4-CDG (*CDG-IIj*).** The first child described presented at 4 months with complex seizure that was treated with Phenobarbital. At age 3 years, additional findings included hypotonia, microcephaly, ataxia, brisk uncoordinated movements, absent speech, motor delays and recurrent respiratory infections (Reynders et al. 2009). A second child presented with failure to thrive, frequent and recurrent infections, diarrhea, hypotonia, hepatosplenomegaly, seizures, elevated liver transaminases, and diffuse cerebral atrophy on brain MRI (Miura et al. 2005, Ng et al. 2011).

- **COG5-CDG (*CDG-IIi*).** A single individual was initially described with mild developmental delay in motor and language (Paesold-Burda et al. 2009). Five additional patients were described with variable phenotypes from mild to severe and clinical overlap with COG7-CDG (Rymen et al. 2012).

- **COG6-CDG (*CDG-IIL*).** A single infant presented with severe neurologic disease including vitamin K deficiency, intracranial bleeding, vomiting, intractable seizures and early infant death (Lubbehusen et al. 2010).

- **ATP6V0A2-CDG and other cutis laxa.** Multiple patients with autosomal recessive cutis laxa have subsequently been found to have abnormal transferring isoelectric focusing and mutations in the ATP6V0A2 gene (Van Maldergem et al. 1989, Morava et al. 2005, Kornak et al. 2008).

The Clinical Spectrum of Dolichol Synthetic Defects

Farnesyl diphosphate is a branch step within the mevalonate-cholesterol pathway between ubiquinones and dolichol (Wolfe et al. 2012). The dolichol is phosphorylated by a kinase (DOLK), and Dolichol-phosphate (Dol-P) can then be utilized as the carrier for the oligosaccharide $GlcNAc_2Man_9Glc_3$ or as a carrier for Man and Glc. Dol-P-Man is utilized as a substrate for N-glycosylation, O-mannosylation of proteins (Lommel and Strahl 2009) via the dolichyl-phosphate mannosyltransferase complex (composed of the subunits DMP1, DMP2, and DMP3) and biosynthesis of GPI-anchored proteins (Orlean and Menon 2007).

Specific Disorders of Dolichol Synthesis

- **DHDDS-CDG.** DHDDS, dehydrodolichyldiphosphate synthetase (also known as Cis-prenyltransferase CPT) is the first enzyme dedicated exclusively to dolichol biosynthesis (Endo et al. 2003). Defects in DHDDS were identified in a subgroup of patients with retinitis pigmentosa (Zelinger et al. 2011, Zuchner et al. 2011).

- **SRD5A3-CDG.** SRD5A3 is the reductase that converts polyprenol to dolichol (Cantagrel and Lefeber 2011). Individuals from seven families were identified with common features including congenital eye malformations (ocular colobomas, optic disc hypoplasia, and variable degree of visual loss), nystagmus, hypotonia, and developmental delay/intellectual disability. Dermatologic complications or congenital cardiac defects were identified in some individuals (Cantagrel et al. 2010). An additional 12 individuals from nine families were described with cerebellar ataxia and congenital eye malformations (Morava et al. 2010). Additional mutations in *SRD5A3* have been identified in people with Kahrizi syndrome, which consists of coloboma, cataract, kyphosis, and intellectual disability (Kahrizi et al. 2011).

- **DOLK-CDG (*CDG-Im*).** Dolichol kinase deficiency impairs the phosphorylation of Dolichol to Dolichol-P (Fernandez et al. 2002). Patients with DOLK-CDG have two very different phenotypes. The first is severe with hypotonia, seizures, microcephaly, cardiomyopathy, visual impairment, skin disorder with loss of hair, and infant lethality (Krantz et al. 2007d, Helander et al. 2013). A second phenotype of DOLK-CDG was described in 11 children with dilated cardiomyopathy (DCM) (Lefeber et al. 2011a). In addition to the DCM, a few patients exhibit additional symptoms like ichtyosis, failure to thrive, and mild neurological involvement. Lieu et al. 2013 described a male neonate born to non-consanguineous parents of Palestinian origin presented with dysmorphic features, genital abnormalities, talipes equinovarus, and severe, refractory generalized seizures. Additional multi-systemic manifestations developed including dilated cardiomyopathy, hepatomegaly, severe insulin-resistant hyperglycemia, and renal failure, which were ultimately fatal at age 9 months of age. This patient expands the phenotype of DOLK-CDG (*CDG-Im*) to include anatomic malformations and multi-systemic dysfunction.

- **DPM1-CDG (*CDG-Ie*).** Five individuals had severe developmental delay, microcephaly, seizures, ocular hypertelorism, a "gothic palate," small hands with dysplastic nails, and knee contracture (Imbach et al. 2000, Kim et al. 2000, Orlean 2000, Garcia-Silva et al. 2004). Additionally, two sibs were described with a milder phenotype, consisting of developmental delay, microcephaly, ataxia, and peripheral neuropathy without distinctive features or severe seizures. They had nystagmus and strabismus; one had a retinopathy (Dancourt et al. 2006). An additional infant was described in congenital muscular dystrophy, hypotonia, microcephaly, camptodactyly and severe motor delay (Yang et al. 2013a).

- **DPM3-CDG (*CDG-Io*).** A single described individual diagnosed with DPM3-CDG (*CDG-Io*) at 27 years had a low normal IQ and mild muscle weakness. She presented initially at age 11 years with mild muscle weakness and waddling gait. She was found to have dilated cardiomyopathy without signs of cardiac muscle hypertrophy at age 20 followed by a stroke-like episode at age 21 (Lefeber et al. 2009). In addition to abnormal N-linked glycosylation, there was abnormal O-linked mannosylation of α-dystroglycan (similar to the dystroglycanopathies).

- **DPM2-CDG (*CDG-Iu*).** Two brothers originally reported by Messina et al. (2009) and an additional patient reported by Barone et al. (2012) presented with severe multisystem and neurologic phenotype resulting in early death. Severe hypotonia and distinctive features were noted at birth. Other features included seizures, strabismus, severe joint contractures and scoliosis. Brain imaging demonstrated cerebellar hypoplasia in one infant and loss of periventricular and subcortical white matter in another. All three infants died between 7 and 36 months.

Clinical Spectrum of GPI Anchor Defects

Glycosylphosphatidylinositol (GPI) anchors are lipid based glycans that attach to the cell surface. The common backbone of GPIs is assembled by the sequential additions of sugar and phosphoethanolamine (EtNP) components to phosphatidylinositol in the ER and subsequent remodeling in the Golgi (Gaynor et al. 1999, Brodsky 2008, Maeda and Kinoshita 2011, Kinoshita et al. 2013). The common core structure of GPI consists of a molecule of phosphatidylinositol (PI) and a glycan core that contains glucosamine, 3 mannoses, and an ethanolamine phosphate. Six defects in the biosynthesis of GPI anchors have been identified (Freeze 2013).

Specific Disorders of Defects in GPI Anchor Synthesis

- **PIGA-CDG.** PIG (phosphatidylinositol glycan)-A catalyzes the first step in GPI anchor synthesis, and somatic mutations in the X-linked gene cause paroxysmal nocturnal hemoglobinuria with hemolysis (Bessler et al. 1994, Yang et al. 2013b). Hypomorphic germline mutations have been identified in males with a multiple congenital anomaly with hypotonia and seizure syndrome (Johnston et al. 2012, Swoboda et al. 2014) and infantile epileptic encephalopathy (Belet et al. 2014, Kato et al. 2014).

- **PIGL-CDG.** PIGL carries out the second step of the pathway, de-*N*acetylation of *N*-acetylglucosaminylphosphatidylinositol, and mutations in it cause CHIME syndrome, with ocular coloboma, heart defects, ichthyosis, mental retardation, and ear anomalies (reviewed in Ng et al. 2012).

- **PIGM-CDG.** PIGM is a mannosyltransferase that adds the first mannose to the core GPI. PIGM-CDG is characterized by portal vein thrombosis and hypertension and seizures (Almeida et al. 2006).

- **PIGN-CDG.** *PIGN* encodes the ethanolamine phosphate transferase, which adds the ethanolamine phosphate to the first mannose on the GPI anchor. PIGN-CDG is characterized by multiple congenital anomalies involving the cardiac, urinary, and gastrointestinal systems, developmental delay, hypotonia and seizures (Maydan et al. 2011, Ohba et al. 2014). Additional features include distinctive features and progressive cerebellar atrophy.

- **PIGV-CDG.** PIGV is a mannosyltransferase that adds the second mannose to the GPI core. PIGV-CDG is characterized by hyperphosphatasia and cognitive impairment (Krawitz et al. 2010, Horn et al. 2011, Murakami et al. 2012). Seizures, congenital and skeletal anomalies have been described.

- **PIGO-CDG.** PIGO is involved in the transfer of the phosphatidylethanolamine to the third mannose of the GPI core. PIGO-CDG has a similar phenotype to PIGV-CDG with hyperphosphatasia and cognitive impairment (Krawitz et al. 2012).

- **PIGT-CDG.** PIGT is a subunit of a heteropentameric transamidase complex that catalyzes the attachment of proteins to GPI. PIGT-CDG is characterized by hypotonia, developmental delay, seizures and distinctive features. Additional variable features include anomalies of the renal, cardiac and skeletal systems, endocrine, ophthalmologic and hearing abnormalities (Kvarnung et al. 2013, Lam et al. 2015).

- **PGAP2-CDG.** PGAP2 appears to be involved in maturation of the GPI anchor on GPI-anchored proteins (Tashima et al. 2006). Like other GPI anchor defects, PGAP2-CDG presents with hyperphosphatasia and cognitive impairment (Hansen et al. 2013, Krawitz et al. 2013). Malformations have not been seen.

- **PIGW-CDG.** PIGW acts in the third step of GPI biosynthesis and acylates the inositol ring of phosphatidylinositol. PIGW-CDG is characterized with hyperphosphatasia, cognitive impairment and seizures (Chiyonobu et al. 2014).

- **PGAP1-CDG.** PGAP1 catalyzes the inositol deacylation of GPI. PGAP1-CDG is characterized by developmental delay, seizures, spasticity and brain abnormalities (Murakami et al. 2014, Novarino et al. 2014, Bosch et al. 2015).

The Clinical Spectrum of Defects of Deglycosylation

- **NGLY1-CDDG: a disorder of deglycosylation.** *NGLY1* encodes N-glycanase 1, which catalyzes the deglycosylation of misfolded N-linked glycoproteins by removing the glycan chain before the protein is degraded by the proteasome (Zhou et al. 2006). NGLY1-CDDG is the first defect of deglycosylation and is characterized by developmental delay, hypotonia, refractory seizures, peripheral neuropathy, abnormal involuntary movements, congenital absence of tears and small hands and feet (Need et al. 2012, Enns et al. 2014, Caglayan et al. 2015, He et al. 2015). Abnormal liver function was noted in some and liver biopsy demonstrated inflammatory changes with cytoplasmic accumulation of an amorphous substance. Brain MRI showed prominent perivascular spaces with surrounding gliosis in periarterial white matter and delayed myelination. Urine oligosaccharides were abnormal, showing keratan sulfate, heparan sulfate, and chondroitin sulfate. This is the first described congenital disorder of deglycosylation.

Diagnostic Testing in Congenital Disorders of Glycosylation

Since the identification of a protein glycosylation defect in 1984, isoelectric focusing of serum transferrin is the diagnostic screening test of choice (Jaeken et al. 1984) for N-linked oligosaccharide synthetic disorders. Transferrin has two N-glycosylation sites, but no O-glycosylation sites, thus is a marker defects of N-glycosylation. This method relies on the amount of negative charge on the transferrin related to the number of terminal sialic residues. Type I pattern is characterized by a decrease in the mature tetrasialo-transferrin and an increase of disialo- and asialo-transferrins due to defective assembly of the N-linked glycans in the ER. A type II pattern is characterized by increases of the trisialo- and monosialo-transferrin due to a defect in processing (Jaeken 2003). Since that time, other testing modalities have been employed to recognized deficient glycosylation of serum transferrin including capillary electrophoresis (Carchon et al. 2004) and high-pressure liquid chromatography (HPLC; Helander et al. 2001). The utilization of multiple mass spectrometry methods has expanded the diagnostics and characterization of glycosylation. This allows both determination of the number of glycosylated sites and the variety of N-linked glycan structures. Other methods include electrospray mass spectrometry (ESI-MS; Wada et al. 1992), liquid chromatography (LC) coupled with ESI-MS (Lacey et al. 2001, Bergen et al. 2001), and matrix assisted laser desorption ionization (MALDI)-MS (Wada et al. 1994, Sturiale et al. 2011).

It is important to note that the diagnostic validity of analysis of serum transferrin glycoforms before age three weeks is limited, false negative results may occur, and it is recommended that diagnosis in an infant is delayed until at least 6 weeks of age (Clayton et al. 1992, Stibler and Skovby 1994). The use of Guthrie cards with whole blood samples is not suggested; however, the use of Guthrie cards with blotted serum yields accurate results (Carchon et al. 2006). Rarely, individuals with the diagnosis of PMM enzyme deficiency with normal transferrin glycosylation have been reported (Fletcher et al. 2000, Marquardt and Denecke 2003, Hahn et al. 2006). The possibility that an abnormal transferrin glycoform analysis is the result of a transferrin protein variant can be confirmed with a glycoform analysis of a serum sample from the parents or by a neuraminidase treatment followed by IEF and ESI-TOF MS (Park et al. 2014).

Isoelectric focusing of serum apolipoprotein C-III (APOC3) can be performed to investigate abnormal mucin type O-glycosylation (Wopereis et al. 2005), which can be seen in some of the combined N- and O-linked glycosylation defects. For PGMI-CDG (CDG-It), Tegtmeyer et al. (2014) developed a modified Beutler test using glucose-1-phosphate screening assay. Immunohistochemistry using antibodies to the glycosylated epitope of α-dystroglycan (IIH-6 or VIA4-1) can be utilized to evaluate for dystroglycanopathies (Muntoni et al. 2003, Godfrey et al. 2007, Muntoni et al. 2008, Hewitt 2009) in muscle biopsies, obviously not useful as a screening test. Defects in GPI anchor synthesis can often be identified using antibodies against the GPI anchor itself or more commonly GPI anchored proteins, such as CD59 on leukocytes (Almeida et al. 2006, Murakami et al. 2012). As the field of glycosylation defects expands, newer biomarkers and analyses will be needed both for clinical screening as well as utilization to define the glycobiology defect (Freeze et al. 2014).

Once a defect is suspected, confirmation of variants in a particular gene involved requires molecular analysis. Next-generation sequencing of whole exome and whole genome sequencing has already aided in identifying novel disorders of glycosylation (Lefeber et al. 2011b, Jones et al. 2013, Murali et al. 2014).

Management and Therapy of Individuals Affected with Disorders of Glycosylation

Infants and children with all types of congenital disorders of glycosylation require a multidisciplinary approach. Treatment should be tailored to the individual's complications. Nutrition support providing maximal caloric intake and/or nasogastric or gastrostomy tube feedings may be necessary. A comprehensive multisystem evaluation will help to define optimal care and support for affected individuals. Therapeutic adjuncts including physical, occupational and speech therapy should be utilized to aid in the medical management. Antiepileptic therapy should be used for seizures.

MPI-CDG (*CDG-1b*), which is characterized by hepatic-intestinal disease, is the only type of hypoglycosylation defect where a specific therapy exists. Mannose given as 1 gram per kg body weight per day divided into five oral doses normalized hypoproteinemia and coagulation defects and rapidly improves the hypoglycemia and protein-losing enteropathy (de Lonlay et al. 1999, Harms et al. 2002, Mention et al. 2008). Recurrent episodes of thrombo-embolism and consumptive coagulopathy did not recur in an individual with MPI-CDG (*CDG-Ib*) treated with mannose (Tamminga et al. 2008). In some patients with PMI-CDG (*CDG-Ib*), heparin therapy can be an alternative to mannose in the treatment of the enteropathy (de Lonlay and Seta 2009). A patient who had MPI-CDG (*CDG-Ib*) developed progressive liver fibrosis, despite oral mannose supplementation and repeated fractionated heparin therapy, and progressive respiratory issues resulting in the need for a liver transplant. After transplantation her physical exercise tolerance, pulmonary functions, and metabolic parameters became fully restored and remained well 2 years post-transplant (Janssen et al. 2014).

There has been a report of correction of the infections and improved neutrophil count with fucose treatment in a patient with SLC35C1-CDG (*CDG-IIc*) (Marquardt et al. 1999), a defect in the fucose transporter.

In PGY1-CDG, galactose therapy has shown improved transferrin glycosylation and resolution of hypogonadotropic hypogonadism in 2 girls with delayed puberty (Tegtmeyer et al. 2014).

Butyrate restores GPI expression in PIGM-CDG patients' lymphoblasts and two-week treatment with phenylbutyrate eliminated seizures and improved motor skills in patients with PIGM-CDG (Almeida et al. 2007).

Two children with PGM3-CDG received hematopoietic stem cell transplantation of cord blood and bone marrow from matched related donors with successful engraftment and correction of neutropenia and lymphopenia (Stray-Pedersen et al. 2014).

For the dystroglycanopathies, overexpression of LARGE (Barresi et al. 2004) and galgt2 has been shown to improve glycosylation of α-dystroglycan in cells from patients and animal models of muscular dystrophy (Martin 2007). In addition, patients with dystroglycanopathies have responded to oral steroids with improvement of muscle function (Godfrey et al. 2006).

Conclusions

The field of glycosylation defects has been rapidly expanding due to improved clinical awareness and biochemical diagnostic techniques. The clinical spectrum for defects in both N- and O-linked glycosylation is extremely broad, challenging clinicians to screen for these defects in a variety of settings and disciplines. With some 500 genes involved in the synthesis and function of glycoproteins, it is likely that many more defects have yet to be identified.

Acknowledgements

The author express many thanks to Dr. Donna Krasnewich, National Institute of Health, USA, who provided mentorship and editing support of this review.

Keywords: congenital disorders of glycosylation, dystroglycanopathies, hypoglycosylation, glycoproteins

References

Aebi, M., A. Helenius, B. Schenk, R. Barone, A. Fiumara, E. G. Berger et al. 1999. Carbohydrate-deficient glycoprotein syndromes become congenital disorders of glycosylation: An updated nomenclature for CDG. First International Workshop on CDGS. Glycoconj J 16: 669–71.

Akasaka-Manya, K., H. Manya, A. Nakajima, M. Kawakita and T. Endo. 2006. Physical and functional association of human protein O-mannosyltransferases 1 and 2. J Biol Chem 281: 19339–19345.

Almeida, A. M., Y. Murakami, D. M. Layton, P. Hillmen, G. S. Sellick, Y. Maeda et al. 2006. Hypomorphic promoter mutation in PIGM causes inherited glycosylphatidylinositol deficiency. Nat Med 12: 846–851.

Almeida, A. M., Y. Murakami, A. Baker, Y. Maeda, I. A. Roberts, T. Kinoshita et al. 2007. Targeted therapy for inherited GPI deficiency. N Engl J Med 356: 1641–1647.

Argov, Z. and R. Yarom. 1984. "Rimmed vacuole myopathy" sparing the quadriceps. A unique disorder in Iranian Jews. J Neurol Sci 64: 33–43.

Arimura, T., Y. K. Hayashi, T. Murakami, Y. Oya, S. Funabe, E. Arikawa-Hirasawa et al. 2009. Mutational analysis of fukutin gene in dilated cardiomyopathy and hypertrophic cardiomyopathy. Circ J 73: 158–161.

Balci, B., G. Uyanik, P. Dincer, C. Gross, T. Willer, B. Talim et al. 2005. An autosomal recessive limb girdle muscular dystrophy (LGMD2) with mild mental retardation is allelic to Walker-Warburg syndrome (WWS) caused by a mutation in the *POMT1* gene. Neuromuscul Disord 15: 271–275.

Barone, R., L. Sturiale, A. Fiumara, G. Uziel, D. Garozzo and J. Jaeken. 2007. Borderline mental development in a congenital disorder of glycosylation (CDG) type Ia patient with multisystemic involvement (intermediate phenotype). J Inherit Metab Dis 30: 107.

Barone, R., C. Aiello, V. Race, E. Morava, F. Foulquier, M. Riemersma et al. 2012. DPM2-CDG: A muscular dystrophy-dystroglycanopathy syndrome with severe epilepsy. Ann Neurol 72: 550–558.

Barresi, R., D. E. Michele, M. Kanagawa, H. A. Harper, S. A. Dovico, J. S. Satz et al. 2004. LARGE can functionally bypass alpha-dystroglycan glycosylation defects in distinct congenital muscular dystrophies. Nat Med 10: 696–703.

Belet, S., N. Fieremans, X. Yuan, H. Van Esch, J. Verbeeck, Z. Ye et al. 2014. Early frameshift mutation in PIGA identified in a large XLID family without neonatal lethality. Hum Mutat 35: 350–355.

Beltran-Valero de Bernabe, D., S. Currier, A. Steinbrecher, J. Celli, E. van Beusekom, B. van der Zwaag et al. 2002. Mutations in the O-mannosyltransferase gene *POMT1* give rise to the severe neuronal migration disorder Walker-Warburg syndrome. Am J Hum Genet 71: 1033–1043.

Bergen, H. R., J. M. Lacey, J. F. O'Brien and S. Naylor. 2001. Online single-step analysis of blood proteins: The transferrin story. Anal Biochem 296: 122–129.

Bessler, M., P. J. Mason, P. Hillmen, T. Miyata, N. Yamada, J. Takeda et al. 1994. Paroxysmal nocturnal haemoglobinuria (PNH) is caused by somatic mutations in the *PIG-A* gene. EMBO J 13: 110–117.

Biancheri, R., A. Falace, A. Tessa, M. Pedemonte, S. Scapolan, D. Cassandrini et al. 2007. *POMT2* gene mutation in limb-girdle muscular dystrophy with inflammatory changes. Biochem Biophys Res Commun 363: 1033–1037.

Bosch, D. G., F. N. Boonstra, T. Kinoshita, S. Jhangiani, J. de Ligt, F. P. Cremers et al. 2015. Cerebral visual impairment and intellectual disability caused by PGAP1 variants. Eur J Hum Genet Mar 25 2015 [Epub ahead of print] doi: 10.1038/ejhg.2015.42.

Bouchet, C., M. Gonzales, S. Vuillaumier-Barrot, L. Devisme, C. Lebizec, E. Alanio et al. 2007. Molecular heterogeneity in fetal forms of type II lissencephaly. Hum Mutat 28: 1020–1027.

Brockington, M., Y. Yuva, P. Prandini, S. C. Brown, S. Torelli, M. A. Benson et al. 2001a. Mutations in the fukutin related protein gene (FKRP) identify limb girdle muscular dystrophy 2I as a milder allelic variant of congenital muscular dystrophy MDC1C. Hum Mol Genet 10: 2851–2859.

Brockington, M., D. J. Blake, P. Prandini, S. C. Brown, S. Torelli, M. A. Benson et al. 2001b. Mutations in the fukutin-related protein gene (FKRP) cause a form of congenital muscular dystrophy with secondary laminin alpha-2 deficiency and abnormal glycosylation of alpha-dystroglycan. Am J Hum Genet 69: 1198–1209.

Brodsky, R. A. 2008. Advances in the diagnosis and therapy of paroxysmal nocturnal hemoglobinuria. Blood Rev 22: 65–74.

Buysse, K., M. Riemersma, G. Powell, J. van Reeuwijk, D. Chitayat, T. Roscioli et al. 2013. Missense mutations in beta-1,3-N-acetylglucosaminyltransferase 1 (B3GNT1) cause Walker-Warburg syndrome. Hum Mol Genet 22: 1746–1754.

Caglayan, A. O., S. Comu, J. F. Baranoski, Y. Parman, H. Kaymakcalan, G. T. Akgumus et al. 2015. NGLY1 mutation causes neuromotor impairment, intellectual disability, and neuropathy. Eur J Med Genet 58: 39–43.

Cantagrel, V., D. J. Lefeber, B. G. Ng, Z. Guan, J. L. Silhavy, S. L. Bielas et al. 2010. SRD5A3 is required for converting polyprenol to dolichol and is mutated in a congenital glycosylation disorder. Cell 142: 203–217.

Cantagrel, V. and D. J. Lefeber. 2011. From glycosylation disorders to dolichol biosynthesis defects: A new class of metabolic diseases. J Inherit Metab Dis 34: 859–867.

Carchon, H. A., R. Chevigne, J. B. Falmagne and J. Jaeken. 2004. Diagnosis of congenital disorders of glycosylation by capillary zone electrophoresis of serum transferrin. Clin Chem 50: 101–111.

Carchon, H., C. Nsibu Ndosimao, S. Van Aerschot and J. Jaeken. 2006. Use of serum on guthrie cards in screening for congenital disorders of glycosylation. Clinical Chemistry 52: 774–775.

Carss, K. J., E. Stevens, A. R. Foley, S. Cirak, M. Riemersma, S. Torelli et al. 2013. Mutations in GDP-mannose pyrophosphorylase B cause congenital and limb-girdle muscular dystrophies associated with hypoglycosylation of alpha-dystroglycan. Am J Hum Genet 93: 29–41.

Chai, W., C. T. Yuen, H. Kogelberg, R. A. Carruthers, R. U. Margolis, T. Feizi et al. 1999. High prevalence of 2-mono- and 2,6-di-substituted manol-terminating sequences among O-glycans released from brain glycopeptides by reductive alkaline hydrolysis. Eur J Biochem 263: 879–888.

Chantret, I., T. Dupre, C. Delenda, S. Bucher, J. Dancourt, A. Barnier et al. 2002. Congenital disorders of glycosylation type Ig is defined by a deficiency in dolichyl-P-mannose: Man7GlcNAc2-PP-dolichyl mannosyltransferase. J Biol Chem 277: 25815–25822.

Chantret, I., J. Dancourt, T. Dupre, C. Delenda, S. Bucher, S. Vuillaumier-Barrot et al. 2003. A deficiency in dolichyl-P-glucose: Glc1Man9GlcNAc2-PP-dolichyl alpha3-glucosyltransferase defines a new subtype of congenital disorders of glycosylation. J Biol Chem 278: 9962–9971.

Chiyonobu, T., N. Inoue, M. Morimoto, T. Kinoshita and Y. Murakami. 2014. Glycosylphosphatidylinositol (GPI) anchor deficiency caused by mutations in PIGW is associated with West syndrome and hyperphosphatasia with mental retardation syndrome. J Med Genet 51: 203–207.

Clarke, N. F., S. Maugenre, A. Vandebrouck, J. A. Urtizberea, T. Willer, R. A. Peat et al. 2011. Congenital muscular dystrophy type 1D (MDC1D) due to a large intragenic insertion/deletion, involving intron 10 of the LARGE gene. Eur J Hum Genet 19: 452–457.

Clayton, P. T., B. G. Winchester and G. Keir. 1992. Hypertrophic obstructive cardiomyopathy in a neonate with the carbohydrate-deficient glycoprotein syndrome. J Inherit Metab Dis 15: 857–861.

Clayton, P. T. and S. Grunewald. 2009. Comprehensive description of the phenotype of the first case of congenital disorder of glycosylation due to RFT1 deficiency (CDG In). J Inherit Metab Dis 32: S137–S139.

Clement, E. M., C. Godfrey, J. Tan, M. Brockington, S. Torelli, L. Feng et al. 2008. Mild POMGnT1 mutations underlie a novel limb-girdle muscular dystrophy variant. Arch Neurol 65: 137–141.

Coman, D., J. McGill, R. MacDonald, D. Morris, S. Klingberg, J. Jaeken and D. Appleton. 2007. Congenital disorder of glycosylation type 1a: Three siblings with a mild neurological phenotype. J Clin Neurosci 14: 668–672.

Cormand, B., K. Avela, H. Pihko, P. Santavuori, B. Talim, H. Topaloglu et al. 1999. Assignment of the muscle-eye-brain disease gene to 1p32-p34 by linkage analysis and homozygosity mapping. Am J Hum Genet 64: 126–135.

Cotarelo, R. P., M. C. Valero, B. Prados, A. Pena, L. Rodriguez, O. Fano et al. 2008. Two new patients bearing mutations in the fukutin gene confirm the relevance of this gene in Walker-Warburg syndrome. Clin Genet 73: 139–145.

Crew, V. K., B. K. Singleton, C. Green, S. F. Parsons, G. Daniels and D. J. Anstee. 2008. New mutations in C1GALT1C1 in individuals with Tn positive phenotype. Brit J Haematol 142: 657–667.

Dancourt, J., S. Vuillaumier-Barrot, H. O. de Baulny, I. Sfaello, A. Barnier, C. le Bizec et al. 2006. A new intronic mutation in the DPM1 gene is associated with a milder form of CDG Ie in two French siblings. Pediatr Res 59: 835–839.

de Bernabe, D. B., H. van Bokhoven, E. van Beusekom, W. Van den Akker, S. Kant, W. B. Dobyns et al. 2003. A homozygous nonsense mutation in the fukutin gene causes a Walker-Warburg syndrome phenotype. J Med Genet 40: 845–848.

de Cock, P. and J. Jaeken. 2009. MGAT2 deficiency (CDG-IIa): The Life of J Biochim Biophys Acta 1792: 844–846.

de Koning, T. J., L. Dorland, O. P. van Diggelen, A. M. Boonman, G. J. de Jong, W. L. van Noort et al. 1998. A novel disorder of N-glycosylation due to phosphomannose isomerase deficiency. Biochem Biophys Res Commun 245: 38–42.

de Ligt, J., M. H. Willemsen, B. W. M. van Bon, T. Kleefstra, H. G. Yntema, T. Kroes et al. 2012. Diagnostic exome sequencing in persons with severe intellectual disability. New Eng J Med 367: 1921–1929.

de Lonlay, P., M. Cuer, S. Vuillaumier-Barrot, G. Beaune, P. Castelnau, M. Kretz et al. 1999. Hyperinsulinemic hypoglycemia as a presenting sign in phosphomannose isomerase deficiency: A new manifestation of carbohydrate-deficient glycoprotein syndrome treatable with mannose. J Pediatr 135: 379–383.

de Lonlay, P. and N. Seta. 2009. The clinical spectrum of phosphomannose isomerase deficiency, with an evaluation of mannose treatment for CDG-Ib. Biochim Biophys Acta 1792: 841–843.

De Paula, F., N. Vieira, A. Starling, L. U. Yamamoto, B. Lima, R. de Cassia Pavanello et al. 2003. Asymptomatic carriers for homozygous novel mutations in the FKRP gene: The other end of the spectrum. Europ J Hum Genet 11: 923–930.

De Praeter, C. M., G. J. Gerwig, E. Bause, L. K. Nuytinck, J. F. Vliegenthart, W. Breuer et al. 2000. A novel disorder caused by defective biosynthesis of N-linked oligosaccharides due to glucosidase I deficiency. Am J Hum Genet 66: 1744–1756.

Denecke, J., C. Kranz, D. Kemming, H. G. Koch and T. Marquardt. 2004. An activated 5' cryptic splice site in the human ALG3 gene generates a premature termination codon insensitive to nonsense-mediated mRNA decay in a new case of congenital disorder of glycosylation type Id (CDG-Id). Hum Mutat 23: 477–486.

Denecke, J., C. Kranz, J. Ch. von Kleist-Retzow, K. Bosse, P. Herkenrath, O. Debus et al. 2005. Congenital disorder of glycosylation type Id: clinical phenotype, molecular analysis, prenatal diagnosis, and glycosylation of fetal proteins. Pediatr Res 58: 248–253.

Di Costanzo, S., A. Balasubramanian, H. L. Pond, A. Rozkalne, C. Pantaleoni, S. Saredi et al. 2014. POMK mutations disrupt muscle development leading to a spectrum of neuromuscular presentations. Hum Mol Genet 23: 5781–5792.

Di Rocco, M., T. Hennet, C. E. Grubenmann, S. Pagliardini, A. E. Allegri, C. G. Frank et al. 2005. Congenital disorder of glycosylation (CDG) Ig: report on a patient and review of the literature. J Inherit Metab Dis 28: 1162–1164.

Dincer, P., B. Balci, Y. Yuva, B. Talim, M. Brockington, D. Dincel et al. 2003. A novel form of recessive limb girdle muscular dystrophy with mental retardation and abnormal expression of alpha-dystroglycan. Neuromusc Disord 13: 771–778.

Dupre, T., S. Vuillaumier-Barrot, I. Chantret, H. Sadou Yayé, C. Le Bizec, A. Afenjar et al. 2010. Guanosine diphosphate-mannose: GlcNAc2-PP-dolichol mannosyltransferase deficiency (congenital disorders of glycosylation type Ik): five new patients and seven novel mutations. J Med Genet 47: 729–735.

Edvardson, S., A. -M. Baumann, M. Muhlenhoff, O. Stephan, A. W. Kuss, A. Shaag et al. 2013. West syndrome caused by ST3Gal-III deficiency. Epilepsia 54: e24–e27.

Eisenberg, I., N. Avidan, T. Potikha, H. Hochner, M. Chen, T. Olender et al. 2001. The UDP-N-acetylglucosamine 2-epimerase/N-acetylmannosamine kinase gene is mutated in recessive hereditary inclusion body myopathy. Nat Genet 29: 83–87.

Eklund, E. A., J. W. Newell, L. Sun, N. S. Seo, G. Alper, J. Willert et al. 2005a. Molecular and clinical description of the first US patients with congenital disorder of glycosylation Ig. Mol Genet Metab 84: 25–31.

Eklund, E. A., L. Sun, V. Westphal, J. L. Northrop, H. H. Freeze and F. Scaglia. 2005b. Congenital disorder of glycosylation (CDG)-Ih patient with a severe hepato-intestinal phenotype and evolving central nervous system pathology. J Pediatr 147: 847–850.

Endo, S., Y. -W. Zhang, S. Takahashi and T. Koyama. 2003. Identification of human dehydrodolichyl diphosphate synthase gene. Biochim Biophys Acta 1625: 291–295.

Endo, T. 2015. Glycobiology of α-dystroglycan and muscular dystrophy. J Biochem 157: 1–12.

Enns, G. M., V. Shashi, M. Bainbridge, M. J. Gambello, F. R. Zahir, T. Bast et al. 2014. Mutations in NGLY1 cause an inherited disorder of the endoplasmic reticulum-associated degradation pathway. Genet Med 16: 751–758.

Epi4K Consortium and Epilepsy Phenome/Genome Project. 2013. *De novo* mutations in epileptic encephalopathies. Nature 501: 217–221.

Ervasti, J. M. and K. P. Campbell. 1991. Membrane organization of the dystrophin-glycoprotein complex. Cell 66: 1121–1131.

Etzioni, A., L. Sturla, A. Antonellis, E. D. Green, R. Gershoni-Baruch, P. M. Berninsone et al. 2002. Leukocyte adhesion deficiency (LAD) type II/carbohydrate deficient glycoprotein (CDG) IIc founder effect and genotype/phenotype correlation. Am J Med Genet 110: 131–135.

Faiyaz-Ul-Haque, M., S. H. E. Zaidi, M. Al-Ali, M. S. Al-Mureikhi, S. Kennedy, G. Al-Thani et al. 2004. A novel missense mutation in the galactosyltransferase-I (B4GALT7) gene in a family exhibiting facioskeletal anomalies and Ehlers-Danlos syndrome resembling the progeroid type. Am J Med Genet 128A: 39–45.

Fernandez, F., P. Shridas, S. Jiang, M. Aebi and C. J. Waechter. 2002. Expression and characterization of a human cDNA that complements the temperature sensitive defect in dolichol kinase activity in the yeastsec59-1 mutant: the enzymatic phosphorylation of dolichol and diacylglycerol are catalyzed by separate CTP mediated kinase activities in Saccharomyces cerevisiae. Glycobiology 12: 555–562.

Fletcher, J. M., G. Matthijs, J. Jaeken, E. Van Schaftingen and P. V. Nelson. 2000. Carbohydrate-deficient glycoprotein syndrome: beyond the screen. J Inherit Metab Dis 23: 396–398.

Foulquier, F., E. Vasile, E. Schollen, N. Callewaert, T. Raemaekers, D. Quelhas et al. 2006. Conserved oligomeric Golgi complex subunit 1 deficiency reveals a previously uncharacterized congenital disorder of glycosylation type II. Proc Natl Acad Sci USA 103: 3764–3769.

Foulquier, F., D. Ungar, E. Reynders, R. Zeevaert, P. Mills, M. T. García-Silva et al. 2007. A new inborn error of glycosylation due to a Cog8 deficiency reveals a critical role for the Cog1-Cog8 interaction in COG complex formation. Hum Mol Genet 16: 717–730.

Frank, C. G., C. E. Grubenmann, W. Eyaid, E. G. Berger, M. Aebi and T. Hennet. 2004. Identification and functional analysis of a defect in the human ALG9 gene: definition of congenital disorder of glycosylation type IL. Am J Hum Genet 75: 146–150.

Freeze, H. H. 2013. Understanding human glycosylation disorders: Biochemistry leads the charge. J Biol Chem 288: 6936–6945.

Freeze, H. H., J. X. Chong, M. J. Bamshad and B. G. Ng. 2014. Solving glycosylation disorders: Fundamental approaches reveal complicated pathways. Am J Hum Genet 94: 161–175.

Fukuyama, Y., M. Osawa and H. Suzuki. 1981. Congenital progressive muscular dystrophy of the Fukuyama type - clinical, genetic and pathological considerations. Brain Dev 3: 1–29.

Furuichi, T., H. Kayserili, S. Hiraoka, G. Nishimura, H. Ohashi, Y. Alanay et al. 2009. Identification of loss-of-function mutations of SLC35D1 in patients with Schneckenbecken dysplasia, but not with other severe spondylodysplastic dysplasias group diseases. J Med Genet 46: 562–568.

Ganetzky, R., K. Izumi, A. Edmondson, C. C. Muraresku, E. Zackai, M. Deardorff et al. 2015. Fetal akinesia deformation sequence due to a congenital disorder of glycosylation. Am J Med Genet A 2015 May. doi: 10.1002/ajmg.a.37184 [Epub ahead of print].

Garcia-Silva, M. T., G. Matthijs, E. Schollen, J. C. Cabrera, J. Sanchez del Pozo, M. Marti Herreros et al. 2004. Congenital disorder of glycosylation (CDG) type Ie. A new patient. J Inherit Metab Dis 27: 591–600.

Garshasbi, M., V. Hadavi, H. Habibi, K. Kahrizi, R. Kariminejad, F. Behjati et al. 2008. A defect in the TUSC3 gene is associated with autosomal recessive mental retardation. Am J Hum Genet 82: 1158–1164.

Gaynor, E. C., G. Mondesert, S. J. Grimme, S. I. Reed, P. Orlean and S. D. Emr. 1999. MCD4 encodes a conserved endoplasmic reticulum membrane protein essential for glycosylphosphatidylinositol anchor synthesis in yeast. Mol Biol Cell 10: 627–648.

Gee, S. H., F. Montanaro, M. H. Lindenbaum and S. Carbonetto. 1994. Dystroglycan-alpha, adystrophin-associated glycoprotein, is a functional agrin receptor. Cell 77: 675–686.

Goddeeris, M. M., B. Wu, D. Venzke, T. Yoshida-Moriguchi, F. Saito, K. Matsumura et al. 2013. LARGE glycans on dystroglycan function as a tunable matrix scaffold to prevent dystrophy. Nature 503: 136–140.

Godfrey, C., D. Escolar, M. Brockington, E. M. Clement, R. Mein, C. Jimenez-Mallebrera et al. 2006. Fukutin gene mutations in steroid-responsive limb girdle muscular dystrophy. Ann Neurol 60: 603–610.

Godfrey, C., E. Clement, R. Mein, M. Brockington, J. Smith, B. Talim et al. 2007. Refining genotype phenotype correlations in muscular dystrophies with defective glycosylation of dystroglycan. Brain 130: 2725–2735.

Grubenmann, C. E., C. G. Frank, S. Kjaergaard, E. G. Berger, M. Aebi and T. Hennet. 2002. ALG12 mannosyltransferase defect in congenital disorder of glycosylation type Ig. Hum Mol Genet 11: 2331–2339.

Grubenmann, C. E., C. G. Frank, A. J. Hulsmeier, E. Schollen, G. Matthijs, E. Mayatepek et al. 2004. Deficiency of the first mannosylation step in the N-glycosylation pathway causes congenital disorder of glycosylation type Ik. Hum Mol Genet 13: 535–542.

Grunewald, S., T. Imbach, K. Huijben, M. E. Rubio-Gozalbo, A. Verrips, J. D. de Klerk et al. 2000. Clinical and biochemical characteristics of congenital disorder of glycosylation type Ic, the first recognized endoplasmic reticulum defect in N-glycan synthesis. Ann Neurol 47: 776–781.

Grunewald, S. 2009. The clinical spectrum of phosphomannomutase 2 deficiency (CDG-Ia). Biochim Biophys Acta 1792: 827–34.

Guillard, M., E. Morava, J. de Ruijter, T. Roscioli, J. Penzien, L. van den Heuvel et al. 2011. B4GALT1-congenital disorders of glycosylation presents as a non-neurologic glycosylation disorder with hepatointestinal involvement. J Pediatr 159: 1041–1043.

Haeuptle, M. A., F. M. Pujol, C. Neupert, B. Winchester, A. J. Kastaniotis, M. Aebi et al. 2008. Human RFT1 deficiency leads to a disorder of N-linked glycosylation. Am J Hum Genet 82: 600–606.

Hahn, S. H., S. J. Minnich and J. F. O'Brien. 2006. Stabilization of hypoglycosylation in a patient with congenital disorder of glycosylation type Ia. J Inherit Metab Dis 29: 235–237.

Hanefeld, F., C. Korner, U. Holzbach-Eberle and K. von Figura. 2000. Congenital disorder of glycosylation-Ic: case report and genetic defect. Neuropediatrics 31: 60–62.

Hansen, L., H. Tawamie, Y. Murakami, Y. Mang, S. Rehman, R. Buchert et al. 2013. Hypomorphic mutations in PGAP2, encoding a GPI-anchor-remodeling protein, cause autosomal-recessive intellectual disability. Am J Hum Genet 92: 575–583.

Hara, Y., B. Balci-Hayta, T. Yoshida-Moriguchi, M. Kanagawa, D. Beltran-Valero de Bernabe, H. Gundesli et al. 2011. A dystroglycan mutation associated with limb-girdle muscular dystrophy. N Engl J Med 364: 939–946.

Harms, H. K., K. P. Zimmer, K. Kurnik, R. M. Bertele-Harms, S. Weidinger and K. Reiter. 2002. Oral mannose therapy persistently corrects the severe clinical symptoms and biochemical abnormalities of phosphomannose isomerase deficiency. Acta Paediatr 91: 1065–1072.

He, P., J. E. Grotzke, B. G. Ng, M. Gunel, H. Jafar-Nejad, P. Cresswell et al. 2015. A congenital disorder of deglycosylation: Biochemical characterization of N-glycanase 1 deficiency in patient fibroblasts. Glycobiology 2015 Apr 21.

Helander, A., G. Eriksson, H. Stibler and J. O. Jeppsson. 2001. Interference of transferrin isoform types with carbohydrate-deficient transferrin quantification in the identification of alcohol abuse. Clin Chem 47: 1225–1233.

Helander, A., T. Stodberg, J. Jaeken, G. Matthijs, M. Eriksson and G. Eggertsen. 2013. Dolichol kinase deficiency (DOLK-CDG) with a purely neurological presentation caused by a novel mutation. Molec Genet Metab 110: 342–344.

Hewitt, J. E. 2009. Abnormal glycosylation of dystroglycan in human genetic disease. Biochim Biophys Acta 1792: 853–861.

Hiraoka, S., T. Furuichi, G. Nishimura, S. Shibata, M. Yanagishita, D. L. Rimoin et al. 2007. Nucleotide-sugar transporter SLC35D1 is critical to chondroitin sulfate synthesis in cartilage and skeletal development in mouse and human. Nature Med 13: 1363–1367.

Horn, D., P. Krawitz, A. Mannhardt, G. C. Korenke and P. Meinecke. 2011. Hyperphosphatasia-mental retardation syndrome due to PIGV mutations: expanded clinical spectrum. Am J Med Genet 155A: 1917–1922.

Hu, H., K. Eggers, W. Chen, M. Garshasbi, M. M. Motazacker, K. Wrogemann et al. 2011. ST3GAL3 mutations impair the development of higher cognitive functions. Am J Hum Genet 89: 407–414.

Imbach, T., B. Schenk, E. Schollen, P. Burda, A. Stutz, S. Grunewald et al. 2000. Deficiency of dolichol-phosphate-mannose synthase-1 causes congenital disorder of glycosylation type Ie. J Clin Invest 105: 233–239.

Imtiaz, F., V. Worthington, M. Champion, C. Beesley, J. Charlwood, P. Clayton et al. 2000. Genotypes and phenotypes of patients in the UK with carbohydrate-deficient glycoprotein syndrome type 1. J Inherit Metab Dis 23: 162–174.

Inamori, K., T. Yoshida-Moriguchi, Y. Hara, M. E. Anderson, L. Yu and K. P. Campbell. 2012. Dystroglycan function requires xylosyl- and glucuronyltransferase activities of LARGE. Science 335: 93–96.

Jae, L. T., M. Raaben, M. Riemersma, E. van Beusekom, V. A. Blomen, A. Velds et al. 2013. Deciphering the glycosylome of dystroglycanopathies using haploid screens for lassa virus entry. Science 340: 479–483.

Jaeken, J., H. G. van Eijk, C. van der Heul, L. Corbeel, R. Eeckels and E. Eggermont. 1984. Sialic acid-deficient serum and cerebrospinal fluid transferrin in a newly recognized genetic syndrome. Clin Chim Acta 144: 245–247.

Jaeken, J. and G. Matthijs. 2001. Congenital disorders of glycosylation. Annu Rev Genomics Hum Genet 2: 129–151.

Jaeken, J. 2003. Komrower Lecture. Congenital disorders of glycosylation (CDG): It's all in it! J Inherit Metab Dis 26: 99–118.

Jaeken, J., T. Hennet, G. Matthijs and H. H. Freeze. 2009a. CDG nomenclature: Time for a change! Biochim Biophys Acta 1792: 825–826.

Jaeken, J., W. Vleugels, L. Regal, C. Corchia, N. Goemans, M. A. Haeuptle et al. 2009b. RFT1-CDG: Deafness as a novel feature of congenital disorders of glycosylation. J Inherit Metab Dis 32: S335–S338.

Janssen, M. C., R. H. de Kleine, A. P. van den Berg, Y. Heijdra, M. Van Scherpenzeel, D. J. Lefeber et al. 2014. Successful liver transplantation and long-term follow-up in a patient with MPI-CDG. Pediatrics 134: e279–e283.

Johnston, J. J., A. L. Gropman, J. C. Sapp, J. K. Teer, J. M. Martin, C. F. Liu et al. 2012. The phenotype of a germline mutation in PIGA: the gene somatically mutated in paroxysmal nocturnal hemoglobinuria. Am J Hum Genet 90: 295–300.

Jones, M. A., B. G. Ng, S. Bhide, E. Chin, D. Rhodenizer, P. He et al. 2012. DDOST mutations identified by whole-exome sequencing are implicated in congenital disorders of glycosylation. Am J Hum Genet 90: 363–368.

Jones, M. A., D. Rhodenizer, C. da Silva, I. J. Huff, L. Keong, L. J. Bean et al. 2013. Molecular diagnostic testing for congenital disorders of glycosylation (CDG): Detection rate for single gene testing and next generation sequencing panel testing. Mol Genet Metab 110: 78–85.

Ju, T., K. Brewer, A. D'Souza, R. D. Cummings and W. M. Canfield. 2002. Cloning and expression of human core 1 beta-1,3-galactosyltransferase. J Biol Chem 277: 178–186.

Kahook, M. Y., N. Mandava, J. B. Bateman and J. A. Thomas. 2006. Glycosylation type Ic disorder: Idiopathic intracranial hypertension and retinal degeneration. Br J Ophthalmol 90: 115–116.

Kahrizi, K., C. H. Hu, M. Garshasbi, S. S. Abedini, S. Ghadami, R. Kariminejad et al. 2011. Next generation sequencing in a family with autosomal recessive Kahrizi syndrome (OMIM 612713) reveals a homozygous frameshift mutation in SRD5A3. Eur J Hum Genet 19: 115–117.

Kato, M., H. Saitsu, Y. Murakami, K. Kikuchi, S. Watanabe, M. Iai et al. 2014. PIGA mutations cause early-onset epileptic encephalopathies and distinctive features. Neurology 82: 1587–1596.

Keppler, O. T., S. Hinderlich, J. Langner, R. Schwartz-Albiez, W. Reutter and M. Pawlita. 1999. UDP-GlcNAc 2-epimerase: A regulator of cell surface sialylation. Science 284: 1372–1376.

Kim, S., V. Westphal, G. Srikrishna, D. P. Mehta, S. Peterson, J. Filiano et al. 2000. Dolichol phosphate mannose synthase (DPM1) mutations define congenital disorder of glycosylation Ie (CDG-Ie). J Clin Invest 105: 191–198.

Kinoshita, T., Y. Maeda and M. Fujita. 2013. Transport of glycosylphosphatidylinositol-anchored proteins from the endoplasmic reticulum. Biochim Biophys Acta 1833: 2473–2478.

Kobayashi, K., Y. Nakahori, M. Miyake, K. Matsumura, E. Kondo-Iida, Y. Nomura et al. 1998. An ancient retrotransposal insertion causes Fukuyama-type congenital muscular dystrophy. Nature 394: 388–392.

Kornak, U., E. Reynders, A. Dimopoulou, J. van Reeuwijk, B. Fischer, A. Rajab et al. 2008. Impaired glycosylation and cutis laxa caused by mutations in the vesicular H+-ATPase subunit ATP6V0A2. Nat Genet 40: 32–34.

Korner, C., R. Knauer, U. Holzbach, F. Hanefeld, L. Lehle and K. von Figura. 1998. Carbohydrate-deficient glycoprotein syndrome type V: deficiency of dolichyl-P-Glc: Man9GlcNAc2-PP-dolichyl glucosyltransferase. Proc Natl Acad Sci USA 95: 13200–13205.

Kornfeld, R. and S. Kornfeld. 1985. Assembly of asparagine-linked oligosaccharides. Ann Rev Biochem 54: 631–634.

Kranz, C., J. Denecke, M. A. Lehrman, S. Ray, P. Kienz, G. Kreissel et al. 2001. A mutation in the human MPDU1 gene causes congenital disorder of glycosylation type If (CDG-If). J Clin Invest 108: 1613–1619.

Kranz, C., J. Denecke, L. Lehle, K. Sohlbach, S. Jeske, F. Meinhardt et al. 2004. Congenital disorder of glycosylation type Ik (CDG-Ik): a defect of mannosyltransferase I. Am J Hum Genet 74: 545–551.

Kranz, C., L. Sun, E. A. Eklund, D. Krasnewich, J. R. Casey and H. H. Freeze. 2007a. CDG-Id in two siblings with partially different phenotypes. Am J Med Genet A 143A: 1414–1420.

Kranz, C., A. A. Basinger, M. Gucsavas-Calikoglu, L. Sun, C. M. Powell, F. W. Henderson et al. 2007b. Expanding spectrum of congenital disorder of glycosylation Ig (CDG-Ig): sibs with a unique skeletal dysplasia, hypogammaglobulinemia, cardiomyopathy, genital malformations, and early lethality. Am J Med Genet A 143A: 1371–1378.

Kranz, C., B. G. Ng, L. Sun, V. Sharma, E. A. Eklund, Y. Miura et al. 2007c. COG8 deficiency causes new congenital disorder of glycosylation type IIh. Hum Mol Genet 16: 731–741.

Kranz, C., C. Jungeblut, J. Denecke, A. Erlekotte, C. Sohlbach, V. Debus et al. 2007d. A defect in dolichol phosphate biosynthesis causes a new inherited disorder with death in early infancy. Am J Hum Genet 80: 433–440.

Krasnewich, D., K. O'Brien and S. Sparks. 2007. Clinical features in adults with congenital disorders of glycosylation type Ia (CDG-Ia). Am J Med Genet C Semin Med Genet 145C: 302–306.

Krawitz, P. M., M. R. Schweiger, C. Rodelsperger, C. Marcelis, U. Kolsch, C. Meisel et al. 2010. Identity-by-descent filtering of exome sequence data identifies PIGV mutations in hyperphosphatasia mental retardation syndrome. Nature Genet 42: 827–829.

Krawitz, P. M., Y. Murakami, J. Hecht, U. Kruger, S. E. Holder, G. R. Mortier et al. 2012. Mutations in PIGO, a member of the GPI-anchor-synthesis pathway, cause hyperphosphatasia with mental retardation. Am J Hum Genet 91: 146–151.

Krawitz, P. M., Y. Murakami, A. Riess, M. Hietala, U. Kruger, N. Zhu et al. 2013. PGAP2 mutations, affecting the GPI-anchor-synthesis pathway, cause hyperphosphatasia with mental retardation syndrome. Am J Hum Genet 92: 584–589.

Kuga, A., M. Kanagawa, A. Sudo, Y. M. Chan, M. Tajiri, H. Manya et al. 2012. Absence of post-phosphoryl modification in dystroglycanopathy mouse models and wild-type tissues expressing non-laminin binding form of alpha-dystroglycan. J Biol Chem 287: 9560–9567.

Kvarnung, M., D. Nilsson, A. Lindstrand, G. C. Korenke, S. C. C. Chiang, E. Blennow et al. 2013. A novel intellectual disability syndrome caused by GPI anchor deficiency due to homozygous mutations in PIGT. J Med Genet 50: 521–528.

Lacey, J. M., H. R. Bergen, M. J. Magera, S. Naylor and J. F. O'Brien. 2001. Rapid determination of transferrin isoforms by immunoaffinity liquid chromatography and electrospray mass spectrometry. Clin Chem 47: 513–518.

Lam, C., G. A. Golas, M. Davids, M. Huizing, M. S. Kane, D. M. Krasnewich et al. 2015. Expanding the clinical and molecular characteristics of PIGT-CDG, a disorder of glycosylphosphatidylinositol anchors. Mol Genet Metab 115: 128–140.

Lefeber, D. J., J. Schonberger, E. Morava, M. Guillard, K. M. Huyben, K. Verrijp et al. 2009. Deficiency of Dol-P-Man synthase subunit DPM3 bridges the congenital disorders of glycosylation with the dystroglycanopathies. Am J Hum Genet 85: 76–86.

Lefeber, D. J., A. P. de Brouwer, E. Morava, M. Riemersma, J. H. Schuurs-Hoeijmakers, B. Absmanner et al. 2011a. Autosomal recessive dilated cardiomyopathy due to DOLK mutations results from abnormal dystroglycanO-mannosylation. PLoS Genet 7: e1002427.

Lefeber, D. J., E. Morava and J. Jaeken. 2011b. How to find and diagnose a CDG due to defective N-glycosylation. J Inherit Metab Dis 34: 849–852.

Lesnik Oberstein, S. A., M. Kriek, S. J. White, M. E. Kalf, K. Szuhai, J. T. den Dunnen et al. 2006. Peters Plus syndrome is caused by mutations in B3GALTL, a putative glycosyltransferase. Am J Hum Genet 79: 562–566.

Lieu, M. T., B. G. Ng, J. S. Rush, T. Wood, M. J. Basehore, M. Hegde et al. 2013. Severe, fatal multisystem manifestations in a patient with dolichol kinase-congenital disorder of glycosylation. Mol Genet Metab 110: 484–489.

Lommel, M. and S. Strahl. 2009. Protein O-mannosylation: conserved from bacteria to humans. Glycobiology 19: 816–828.

Lommel, M., S. Cirak, T. Willer, R. Hermann, G. Uyanik, H. van Bokhoven et al. 2010. Correlation of enzyme activity and clinical phenotype in POMT1-associated dystroglycanopathies. Neurology 74: 157–164.

Longman, C., M. Brockington, S. Torelli, C. Jimenez-Mallebrera, C. Kennedy, N. Khalil et al. 2003. Mutations in the human LARGE gene cause MDC1D, a novel form of congenital muscular dystrophy with severe mental retardation and abnormal glycosylation of alpha-dystroglycan. Hum Mol Genet 12: 2853–2861.

Losfeld, M. E., B. G. Ng, M. Kircher, K. J. Buckingham, E. H. Turner, A. Eroshkin et al. 2014. A new congenital disorder of glycosylation caused by a mutation in SSR4, the signal sequence receptor 4 protein of the TRAP complex. Hum Mol Genet 23: 1602–1605.

Louhichi, N., C. Triki, S. Quijano-Roy, P. Richard, S. Makri, M. Méziou et al. 2004. New FKRP mutations causing congenital muscular dystrophy associated with mental retardation and central nervous system abnormalities. Identification of a founder mutation in Tunisian families. Neurogenetics 5: 27–34.

Lubbehusen, J., C. Thiel, N. Rind, D. Ungar, B. H. Prinsen, T. J. de Koning et al. 2010. Fatal outcome due to deficiency of subunit 6 of the conserved oligomeric Golgi complex leading to a new type of congenital disorders of glycosylation. Hum Mol Genet 19: 3623–3633.

Lubke, T., T. Marquardt, A. Etzioni, E. Hartmann, K. von Figura and C. Korner. 2001. Complementation cloning identifies CDG-IIc, a new type of congenital disorders of glycosylation, as a GDP-fucose transporter deficiency. Nature Genet 28: 73–76.

Luhn, K., M. K. Wild, M. Eckhardt, R. Gerardy-Schahn and D. Vestweber. 2001. The gene defective in leukocyte adhesion deficiency II encodes a putative GDP-fucose transporter. Nature Genet 28: 69–72.

MacLeod, H., P. Pytel, R. Wollmann, E. Chelmicka-Schorr, K. Silver, R. B. Anderson et al. 2007. A novel FKRP mutation in congenital muscular dystrophy disrupts the dystrophin glycoprotein complex. Neuromuscul Disord 17: 285–289.

Maeda, Y. and T. Kinoshita. 2011. Structural remodeling, trafficking and functions of glycosylphosphatidylinositol anchored proteins. Prog Lipid Res 50: 411–424.

Manya, H., A. Chiba, A. Yoshida, X. Wang, Y. Chiba, Y. Jigami et al. 2004. Demonstration of mammalian protein O-mannosyltransferase activity: coexpression of POMT1 and POMT2 required for enzymatic activity. Proc Natl Acad Sci USA 101: 500–505.

Manzini, M. C., D. E. Tambunan, R. S. Hill, T. W. Yu, T. M. Maynard, E. L. Heinzen et al. 2012. Exomesequencing and functional validation in zebrafish identify GTDC2 mutations as a cause of Walker-Warburg syndrome. Am J Hum Genet 91: 541–547.

Marquardt, T., K. Luhn, G. Srikrishna, H. H. Freeze, E. Harms and D. Vestweber. 1999. Correction of leukocyte adhesion deficiency type II with oral fucose. Blood 94: 3976–3985.

Marquardt, T. and J. Denecke. 2003. Congenital disorders of glycosylation: review of their molecular bases, clinical presentations and specific therapies. Eur J Pediatr 162: 359–379.

Martin, P. T. 2007. Congenital muscular dystrophies involving the O-mannose pathway. Curr Mol Med 7: 417–425.

Martinez-Duncker, I., T. Dupre, V. Piller, F. Piller, J. J. Candelier, C. Trichet et al. 2005. Genetic complementation reveals a novel human congenital disorder of glycosylation of type II, due to inactivation of the Golgi CMP-sialic acid transporter. Blood 105: 2671–2676.

Mathews, K. D., C. M. Stephan, K. Laubenthal, T. L. Winder, D. E. Michele, S. A. Moore et al. 2011. Myoglobinuria and muscle pain are common in patients with limb-girdle muscular dystrophy 2I. Neurology 76: 194–195.

Matthijs, G., E. Schollen, C. Bjursell, A. Erlandson, H. Freeze, F. Imtiaz et al. 2000. Mutations in PMM2 that cause congenital disorders of glycosylation, type Ia (CDG-Ia). Hum Mutat 16: 386–394.

Maydan, G., I. Noyman, A. Har-Zahav, Z. B. Neriah, M. Pasmanik-Chor, A. Yeheskel et al. 2011. Multiple congenital anomalies-hypotonia-seizures syndrome is caused by a mutation in PIGN. J Med Genet 48: 383–389.

Mention, K., F. Lacaille, V. Valayannopoulos, S. Romano, A. Kuster, M. Cretz et al. 2008. Development of liver disease despite mannose treatment in two patients with CDG-Ib. Mol Genet Metab 93: 40–43.

Mercuri, E., M. Brockington, V. Straub, S. Quijano-Roy, Y. Yuva, R. Herrmann et al. 2003. Phenotypic spectrum associated with mutations in the fukutin-related protein gene. Ann Neurol 53: 537–542.

Mercuri, E., A. D'Amico, A. Tessa, A. Berardinelli, M. Pane, S. Messina et al. 2006a. *POMT2* mutation in a patient with 'MEB-like' phenotype. Neuromuscul Disord 16: 446–448.

Mercuri, E., H. Topaloglu, M. Brockington, A. Berardinelli, A. Pichiecchio, F. Santorelli et al. 2006b. Spectrum of brain changes in patients with congenital muscular dystrophy and *FKRP* gene mutations. Arch Neurol 63: 251–257.

Mercuri, E., S. Messina, C. Bruno, M. Mora, E. Pegoraro, G. P. Comi et al. 2009. Congenital muscular dystrophies with defective glycosylation of dystroglycan: a population study. Neurology 72: 1802–1809.

Messina, S., G. Tortorella, D. Concolino, M. Spano, A. D'Amico, C. Bruno et al. 2009. Congenital muscular dystrophy with defective alpha-dystroglycan, cerebellar hypoplasia, and epilepsy. Neurology 73: 1599–1601.

Miller, B. S., H. H. Freeze, G. F. Hoffmann and K. Sarafoglou. 2011. Pubertal development in ALG6 deficiency (congenital disorder of glycosylation type Ic). Mol Genet Metab 103: 101–103.

Miura, Y., S. K. Tay, M. M. Aw, E. A. Eklund and H. H. Freeze. 2005. Clinical and biochemical characterization of a patient with congenital disorder of glycosylation (CDG) IIx. J Pediatr 147: 851–853.

Mohorko, E., R. Glockshuber and M. Aebi. 2011. Oligosaccharyltransferase: The central enzyme of N-linked protein glycosylation. J Inherit Metab Dis 34: 869–878.

Molinari, F., F. Foulquier, P. S. Tarpey, W. Morelle, S. Boissel, J. Teague et al. 2008. Oligosaccharyltransferase-subunit mutations in nonsyndromic mental retardation. Am J Hum Genet 82: 1150–1157.

Moloney, D. J., V. M Panin, S. H. Johnston, J. Chen, L. Shao, R. Wilson et al. 2000. Fringe is a glycosyltransferase that modifies Notch. Nature 406: 369–375.

Morava, E., S. Wopereis, P. Coucke, G. Gillessen-Kaesbach, T. Voit, J. Smeitink et al. 2005. Defective protein glycosylation in patients with cutis laxa syndrome. Eur J Hum Genet 13: 414–421.

Morava, E., R. Zeevaert, E. Korsch, K. Huijben, S. Wopereis, G. Matthijs et al. 2007. A common mutation in the COG7 gene with a consistent phenotype including microcephaly, adducted thumbs, growth retardation, VSD and episodes of hyperthermia. Eur J Hum Genet 15: 638–645.

Morava, E., R. A. Wevers, V. Cantagrel, L. H. Hoefsloot, L. Al-Gazali, J. Schoots et al. 2010. A novel cerebello-ocular syndrome with abnormal glycosylation due to abnormalities in dolichol metabolism. Brain 133: 3210–3220.

Morava, E., J. Vodopiutz, D. J. Lefeber, A. R. Janecke, W. M. Schmidt, S. Lechner et al. 2012. Defining the phenotype in congenital disorder of glycosylation due to ALG1 mutations. Pediatrics 130: e1034–e1039.

Muntoni, F., B. Valero de Bernabe, R. Bittner, D. Blake, H. van Bokhoven, M. Brockington et al. 2003. 114th ENMC International Workshop on Congenital Muscular Dystrophy (CMD) 17–19 January 2003, Naarden, The Netherlands: (8th Workshop of the International Consortium on CMD; 3rd Workshop of the MYO-CLUSTER project GENRE). Neuromuscul Disord 13: 579–588.

Muntoni, F., M. Brockington, S. Torelli and S. C. Brown. 2004. Defective glycosylation in congenital muscular dystrophies. Curr Opin Neurol 17: 205–209.

Muntoni, F., S. Torelli and M. Brockington. 2008. Muscular dystrophies due to glycosylation defects. Neurotherapeutics 5: 627–632.

Murakami, T., Y. K. Hayashi, S. Noguchi, M. Ogawa, I. Nonaka, Y. Tanabe et al. 2006. Fukutin gene mutations cause dilated cardiomyopathy with minimal muscle weakness. Ann Neurol 60: 597–602.

Murakami, Y., N. Kanzawa, K. Saito, P. M. Krawitz, S. Mundlos, P. N. Robinson et al. 2012. Mechanism for release of alkaline phosphatase caused by glycosylphosphatidylinositol deficiency in patients with hyperphosphatasia mental retardation syndrome. J Biol Chem 287: 6318–6325.

Murakami, Y., H. Tawamie, Y. Maeda, C. Buttner, R. Buchert, F. Radwan et al. 2014. Null nutation in PGAP1 impairing Gpi-anchor maturation in patients with intellectual disability and encephalopathy. PLoS Genet 10: e1004320.

Muraoka, M., M. Kawakita and N. Ishida. 2001. Molecular characterization of human UDP-glucuronic acid/UDP-N-acetylgalactosamine transporter, a novel nucleotide sugar transporter with dual substrate specificity. FEBS Lett 495: 87–93.

Murali, C., J. T. Lu, M. Jain, D. S. Liu, R. Lachman, R. A. Gibbs et al. 2014. Diagnosis of ALG12-CDG by exome sequencing in a case of severe skeletal dysplasia. Mol Genet Metab Rep 1: 213–219.

Need, A. C., V. Shashi, Y. Hitomi, K. Schoch, K. V. Shianna, M. T. McDonald et al. 2012. Clinical application of exome sequencing in undiagnosed genetic conditions. J Med Genet 49: 353–361.

Ng, B. G., C. Kranz, E. E. Hagebeuk, M. Duran, N. G. Abeling, B. Wuyts et al. 2007. Molecular and clinical characterization of a Moroccan Cog7 deficient patient. Mol Genet Metab 91: 201–204.

Ng, B. G., V. Sharma, L. Sun, E. Loh, W. Hong, S. K. Tay et al. 2011. Identification of the first COG-CDG patient of Indian origin. Mol Genet Metab 102: 364–367.

Ng, B. G., K. Hackmann, M. A. Jones, A. M. Eroshkin, P. He, R. Wiliams et al. 2012. Mutations in the glycosylphosphatidylinositol gene PIGL cause CHIME syndrome. Am J Hum Genet 90: 685–688.

Niehues, R., M. Hasilik, G. Alton, C. Körner, M. Schiebe-Sukumar, H. G. Koch et al. 1998. Carbohydrate-deficient glycoprotein syndrome type Ib. Phosphomannose isomerase deficiency and mannose therapy. J Clin Invest 101: 1414–1420.

Nikkels, P. G., R. H. Stigter, I. E. Knol and H. J. van der Harten. 2001. Schneckenbecken dysplasia, radiology, and histology. Pediat Radiol 31: 27–30.

Nigro, V. and M. Savarese. 2014. Genetic basis of limb-girdle muscular dystrophies: the 2014 update. Acta Myol 33: 1–12.

Ning, B. and A. D. Elbein. 2000. Cloning, expression and characterization of the pig liver GDP-mannose pyrophosphorylase. Evidence that GDP-mannose and GDP-Glc pyrophosphorylases are different proteins. Eur J Biochem 267: 6866–6874.

Nishino, I., S. Noguchi, K. Murayama, A. Driss, K. Sugie, Y. Oya et al. 2002. Distal myopathy with rimmed vacuoles is allelic to hereditary inclusion body myopathy. Neurology 59: 1689–1693.

Nonaka, I., N. Sunohara, S. Ishiura and E. Satoyoshi. 1981. Familial distal myopathy with rimmed vacuole and lamellar (myeloid) body formation. J Neurol Sci 51: 141–155.

Novarino, G., A. G. Fenstermaker, M. S. Zaki, M. Hofree, J. L. Silhavy, A. D. Heiberg et al. 2014. Exome sequencing links corticospinal motor neuron disease to common neurodegenerative disorders. Science 343: 506–511.

Ohba, C., N. Okamoto, Y. Murakami, Y. Suzuki, Y. Tsurusaki, M. Nakashima et al. 2014. PIGN mutations cause congenital anomalies, developmental delay, hypotonia, epilepsy, and progressive cerebellar atrophy. Neurogenetics 15: 85–92.

Orlean, P. 2000. Congenital disorders of glycosylation caused by defects in mannose addition during N-linked oligosaccharide assembly. J Clin Invest 105: 131–132.

Orlean, P. and A. K. Menon. 2007. Thematic review series: lipid posttranslational modifications. GPI anchoring of protein in yeast and mammalian cells, or: how we learned to stop worrying and love glycophospholipids. J Lipid Res 48: 993–1011.

Paesold-Burda, P., C. Maag, H. Troxler, F. Foulquier, P. Kleinert, S. Schnabel et al. 2009. Deficiency in COG5 causes a moderate form of congenital disorders of glycosylation. Hum Mol Genet 18: 4350–4356.

Park, J. H., A. Zuhlsdorf, Y. Wada, C. Roll, S. Rust, I. Du Chesne et al. 2014. The novel transferrin E592A variant impairs the diagnostics of congenital disorders of glycosylation. Clin Chim Acta 436: 135–139.

Peng, H. B., A. A. Ali, D. F. Daggett, H. Rauvala, J. R. Hassell and N. R. Smalheiser. 1998. The relationship between perlecan and dystroglycan and its implication in the formation of the neuromuscular junction. Cell Adhes Commun 5: 475–489.

Peters, V., J. M. Penzien, G. Reiter, C. Körner, R. Hackler, B. Assmann et al. 2002. Congenital disorder of glycosylation IId (CDG-IId)—a new entity: Clinical presentation with Dandy-Walker malformation and myopathy. Neuropediatrics 33: 27–32.

Peyrard, M., E. Seroussi, A. C. Sandberg-Nordqvist, Y. G. Xie, F. Y. Han, I. Fransson et al. 1999. The human LARGE gene from 22q12.3-q13.1 is a new, distinct member of the glycosyltransferase gene family. Proc Natl Acad Sci USA 96: 598–603.

Poppe, M., L. Cree, J. Bourke, M. Eagle, L. V. B. Anderson, D. Birchall et al. 2003. The phenotype of limb-girdle muscular dystrophy type 2I. Neurology 60: 1246–1251.

Praissman, J. L., D. H. Live, S. Wang, A. Ramiah, Z. S. Chinoy, G. -J. Boons et al. 2014. B4GAT1 is the priming enzyme for the LARGE-dependent functional glycosylation of α-dystroglycan. eLife 3: e03943.

Puckett, R. L., S. A. Moore, T. L. Winder, T. Willer, S. G. Romansky, K. K. Covault et al. 2009. Further evidence of Fukutin mutations as a cause of childhood onset limb-girdle muscular dystrophy without mental retardation. Neuromuscul Disord 19: 352–356.

Reynders, E., F. Foulquier, E. Leao Teles, D. Quelhas, W. Morelle, C. Rabouille et al. 2009. Golgi function and dysfunction in the first COG4-deficient CDG type II patient. Hum Mol Genet 18: 3244–3256.

Rind, N., V. Schmeiser, C. Thiel, B. Absmanner, J. Lübbehusen, J. Hocks et al. 2010. A severe human metabolic disease caused by deficiency of the endoplasmatic mannosyltransferase hALG11 leads to congenital disorder of glycosylation-Ip. Hum Mol Genet 19: 1413–1424.

Rohlfing, A. K., S. Rust, J. Reunert, M. Tirre, I. Du Chesne, S. Wemhoff et al. 2014. ALG1-CDG: a new case with early fatal outcome. Gene 534: 345–351.

Roscioli, T., E. J. Kamsteeg, K. Buysse, I. Maystadt, J. van Reeuwijk, C. van den Elzen et al. 2012. Mutations in ISPD cause Walker-Warburg syndrome and defective glycosylation of alphadystroglycan. Nat Genet 44: 581–585.

Rymen, D., L. Keldermans, V. Race, L. Regal, N. Deconinck, C. Dionisi-Vici et al. 2012. COG5-CDG: expanding the clinical spectrum. Orphanet J Rare Dis 7: 94.

Sadeh, M., N. Gadoth, H. Hadar and E. Ben-David. 1993. Vacuolar myopathy sparing the quadriceps. Brain 116: 217–232.

Saredi, S., A. Ruggieri, E. Mottarelli, A. Ardissone, S. Zanotti, L. Farina et al. 2009. Fukutin gene mutations in an Italian patient with early onset muscular dystrophy but no central nervous system involvement. Muscle Nerve 39: 845–848.

Sato, S., Y. Omori, K. Katoh, M. Kondo, M. Kanagawa, K. Miyata et al. 2008. Pikachurin, a dystroglycan ligand, is essential for photoreceptor ribbon synapse formation. Nat Neurosci 11: 923–931.

Schenk, B., T. Imbach, C. G. Frank, C. E. Grubenmann, G. V. Raymond, H. Hurvitz et al. 2001. MPDU1 mutations underlie a novel human congenital disorder of glycosylation, designated type If. J Clin Invest 108: 1687–1695.

Schollen, E., C. G. Frank, L. Keldermans, R. Reyntjens, C. E. Grubenmann, P. T. Clayton et al. 2004. Clinical and molecular features of three patients with congenital disorders of glycosylation type Ih (CDG-Ih) (ALG8 deficiency). J Med Genet 41: 550–556.

Schwarz, M., C. Thiel, J. Lubbehusen, B. Dorland, T. de Koning, K. von Figura et al. 2004. Deficiency of GDP-Man: GlcNAc2-PP-dolichol mannosyltransferase causes congenital disorder of glycosylation type Ik. Am J Hum Genet 74: 472–481.

Senderek, J., J. S. Muller, M. Dusl, T. M. Strom, V. Guergueltcheva, I. Diepolder et al. 2011. Hexosamine biosynthetic pathway mutations cause neuromuscular transmission defect. Am J Hum Genet 88: 162–172.

Shrimal, S., B. G. Ng, M. E. Losfeld, R. Gilmore and H. H. Freeze. 2013. Mutations in STT3A and STT3B cause two congenital disorders of glycosylation. Hum Molec Genet 22: 4638–4645.

Silan, F., M. Yoshioka, K. Kobayashi, E. Simsek, M. Tunc, M. Alper et al. 2003. A new mutation of the fukutin gene in a non-Japanese patient. Ann Neurol 53: 392–396.

Smith, R. D. and V. V. Lupashin. 2008. Role of the conserved oligomeric Golgi (COG) complex in protein glycosylation. Carbohydrate Research 343: 2024–2031.

Spaapen, L. J., J. A. Bakker, S. B. van der Meer, H. J. Sijstermans, R. A. Steet, R. A. Wevers et al. 2005. Clinical and biochemical presentation of siblings with COG-7 deficiency, a lethal multiple O- and N-glycosylation disorder. J Inherit Metab Dis 28: 707–714.

Sparrow, D. B., G. Chapman, M. A. Wouters, N. V. Whittock, S. Ellard, D. Fatkin et al. 2006. Mutation of the lunatic fringe gene in humans causes spondylocostal dysostosis with a severe vertebral phenotype. Am J Hum Genet 78: 28–37.

Specktor, P., J. G. Cooper, M. Indelman and E. Sprecher. 2006. Hyperphosphatemic familial tumoral calcinosis caused by a mutation in GALNT3 in a European kindred. J Hum Genet 51: 487–490.

Stevens, E., K. J. Carss, S. Cirak, A. R. Foley, S. Torelli, T. Willer et al. 2013. Mutations in B3GALNT2 cause congenital muscular dystrophy and hypoglycosylation of alpha-dystroglycan. Am J Hum Genet 92: 354–365.

Stibler, H. and F. Skovby. 1994. Failure to diagnose carbohydrate-deficient glycoprotein syndrome prenatally. Pediatr Neurol 11: 71.

Stibler, H., U. Stephani and U. Kutsch. 1995. Carbohydrate-deficient glycoprotein syndrome—a fourth subtype. Neuropediatrics 26: 235–237.

Stojkovic, T., J. Vissing, F. Petit, M. Piraud, M. C. Orngreen, G. Andersen et al. 2009. Muscle glycogenosis due to phosphoglucomutase 1 deficiency. (Letter) New Eng J Med 361: 425–427.

Stolting, T., H. Omran, A. Erlekotte, J. Denecke, J. Reunert and T. Marquardt. 2009. Novel *ALG8* mutations expand the clinical spectrum of congenital disorder of glycosylation type Ih. Mol Genet Metab 98: 305–309.

Stray-Pedersen, A., P. H. Backe, H. S. Sorte, L. Morkrid, N. Y. Chokshi, H. C. Erichsen et al. 2014. PGM3 mutations cause a congenital disorder of glycosylation with severe immunodeficiency and skeletal dysplasia. Am J Hum Genet 95: 96–107.

Sturiale, L., R. Barone and D. Garozzo. 2011. The impact of mass spectrometry in the diagnosis of congenital disorders of glycosylation. J Inherit Metab Dis 34: 891–899.

Sugita, S., F. Saito, J. Tang, J. Satz, K. Campbell and T. C. Sudhof. 2001. A stoichiometric complex of neurexins and dystroglycan in brain. J Cell Biol 154: 435–445.

Sun, L., E. A. Eklund, J. L. Van Hove, H. H. Freeze and J. A. Thomas. 2005. Clinical and molecular characterization of the first adult congenital disorder of glycosylation (CDG) type Ic patient. Am J Med Genet A 137: 22–26.

Swoboda, K. J., R. L. Margraf, J. C. Carey, H. Zhou, T. M. Newcomb, E. Coonrod et al. 2014. A novel germline PIGA mutation in Ferro-Cerebro-Cutaneous syndrome: a neurodegenerative X-linked epileptic encephalopathy with systemic iron-overload. Am J Med Genet 164A: 17–28.

Tamminga, R. Y., D. J. Lefeber, W. A. Kamps and F. J. Spronsen. 2008. Recurrent thrombo-embolism in a child with a congenital disorder of glycosylation (CDG) type Ib and treatment with mannose. Pediatr Hematol Oncol 25: 762–768.

Tasca, G., F. Moro, C. Aiello, D. Cassandrini, C. Fiorillo, E. Bertini et al. 2013. Limb-girdle muscular dystrophy with alpha-dystroglycan deficiency and mutations in the ISPD gene. Neurology 80: 963–965.

Tashima, Y., R. Taguchi, C. Murata, H. Ashida, T. Kinoshita and Y. Maeda. 2006. PGAP2 is essential for correct processing and stable expression of GPI-anchored proteins. Molec Biol Cell 17: 1410–1420.

Teber, S., T. Sezer, M. Kafali, M. C. Manzini, B. Konuk Yüksel et al. 2008. Severe muscle-eye-brain disease is associated with a homozygous mutation in the *POMGnT1* gene. Eur J Paediatr Neurol 12: 133–136.

Tegtmeyer, L. C., S. Rust, M. van Scherpenzeel, B. G. Ng, M. E. Losfeld, S. Timal et al. 2014. Multiple phenotypes in phosphoglucomutase 1 deficiency. New Eng J Med 370: 533–542.

Tham, E., E. A. Eklund, A. Hammarsjo, P. Bengtson, S. Geiberger, K. Lagerstedt-Robinson et al. 2015. A novel phenotype in N-glycosylation disorders: Gillessen-Kaesbach-Nishimura skeletal dysplasia due to pathogenic variants in ALG9. Eur J Hum Genet 2015 May 13. doi: 10.1038/ejhg.2015.91 [Epub ahead of print].

Thiel, C., M. Schwarz, M. Hasilik, U. Grieben, F. Hanefeld, L. Lehle et al. 2002. Deficiency of dolichyl-P-Man: Man7GlcNAc2-PP-dolichyl mannosyltransferase causes congenital disorder of glycosylation type Ig. Biochem J 367: 195–201.

Thiel, C., M. Schwarz, J. Peng, M. Grzmil, M. Hasilik, T. Braulke et al. 2003. A new type of congenital disorders of glycosylation (CDG-Ii) provides new insights into the early steps of dolichol-linked oligosaccharide biosynthesis. J Biol Chem 278: 22498–22505.

Timal, S., A. Hoischen, L. Lehle, M. Adamowicz, K. Huijben, J. Sykut-Cegielska et al. 2012. Gene identification in the congenital disorders of glycosylation type I by whole-exome sequencing. Hum Mol Genet 21: 4151–4161.

Toda, T., M. Segawa, Y. Nomura, I. Nonaka, K. Masuda, T. Ishihara et al. 1993. Localization of a gene for Fukuyama type congenital muscular dystrophy to chromosome 9q31-33. Nat Genet 5: 283–286.

Toda, T., K. Kobayashi, S. Takeda, J. Sasaki, H. Kurahashi, H. Kano et al. 2003. Fukuyama-type congenital muscular dystrophy (FCMD) and alpha-dystroglycanopathy. Congenit Anom (Kyoto) 43: 97–104.

van de Kamp, J. M., D. J. Lefeber, G. J. Ruijter, S. J. Steggerda, N. S. den Hollander, S. M. et al. 2007. Congenital disorder of glycosylation type Ia presenting with hydrops fetalis. J Med Genet 44: 277–280.

Van den Steen, P., P. M. Rudd, R. A. Dwek and G. Opendenakker. 1998. Concepts and principles of O-linked glycosylation. Crit Rev Biochem Mol Biol 33: 151–208.

Van Geet, C., J. Jaeken, K. Freson, T. Lenaerts, J. Arnout, J. Vermylen et al. 2001. Congenital disorders of glycosylation type Ia and IIa are associated with different primary haemostatic complications. J Inherit Metab Dis 24: 477–492.

Van Maldergem, L., G. Ogur and M. Yuksel. 1989. Facial anomalies in congenital cutis laxa with retarded growth and skeletal dysplasia. Am J Med Genet 32: 265.

van Reeuwijk, J., M. Janssen, C. van den Elzen, D. Beltran-Valero de Bernabe, P. Sabatelli, L. Merlini et al. 2005. *POMT2* mutations cause alpha-dystroglycan hypoglycosylation and Walker-Warburg syndrome. J Med Genet 42: 907–912.

van Reeuwijk, J., S. Maugenre, C. van den Elzen, A. Verrips, E. Bertini, F. Muntoni et al. 2006. The expanding phenotype of *POMT1* mutations: from Walker-Warburg syndrome to congenital muscular dystrophy, microcephaly, and mental retardation. Hum Mutat 27: 453–459.

van Reeuwijk, J., P. K. Grewal, M. A. Salih, D. Beltran-Valero de Bernabe, J. M. McLaughlan, C. B. Michielse et al. 2007. Intragenic deletion in the *LARGE* gene causes Walker-Warburg syndrome. Hum Genet 121: 685–690.

van Reeuwijk, J., M. J. Olderode-Berends, C. Van den Elzen, O. F. Brouwer, T. Roscioli, M. G. Van Pampus et al. 2010. A homozygous *FKRP* start codon mutation is associated with Walker-Warburg syndrome, the severe end of the clinical spectrum. Clin Genet 78: 275–281.

Vajsar, J. and H. Schachter. 2006. Walker-Warburg syndrome. Orphanet J Rare Dis 1: 29.

Varki, A. and J. Marth. 1995. Oligosaccharides in vertebrate development. Dev Biol 6: 127–138.

Vesela, K., T. Honzik, H. Hansikova, M. A. Haeuptle, J. Semberova, Z. Stranak et al. 2009. A new case of ALG8 deficiency (CDG Ih). J Inherit Metab Dis 32: 259–264.

Vleugels, W., L. Keldermans, J. Jaeken, T. D. Butters, J. C. Michalski, G. Matthijs et al. 2009a. Quality control of glycoproteins bearing truncated glycans in an ALG9-defective (CDG-IL) patient. Glycobiology 19: 910–917.

Vleugels, W., M. A. Haeuptle, B. G. Ng, J. C. Michalski, R. Battini, C. Dionisi-Vici et al. 2009b. RFT1 deficiency in three novel CDG patients. Hum Mutat 30: 1428–1434.

von Renesse, A., M. V. Petkova, S. Lutzkendorf, J. Heinemeyer, E. Gill, C. Hubner et al. 2014. POMK mutation in a family with congenital muscular dystrophy with merosin deficiency, hypomyelination, mild hearing deficit and intellectual disability. J Med Genet 51: 275–282.

Vuillaumier-Barrot, S., S. Quijano-Roy, C. Bouchet-Seraphin, S. Maugenre, P. Peudenier, P. Van den Bergh et al. 2009. Four Caucasian patients with mutations in the fukutin gene and variable clinical phenotype. Neuromuscul Disord 19: 182–188.

Vuillaumier-Barrot, S., C. Bouchet-Seraphin, M. Chelbi, L. Devisme, S. Quentin, S. Gazal et al. 2012. Identification of mutations in TMEM5 and ISPD as a cause of severe cobblestone lissencephaly. Am J Hum Genet 91: 1135–114.

Wada, Y., A. Nishikawa, N. Okamoto, K. Inui, H. Tsukamoto, S. Okada et al. 1992. Structure of serum transferrin in carbohydrate-deficient glycoprotein syndrome. Biochem Biophys Res Commun 189: 832–836.

Wada, Y., J. Gu, N. Okamoto and K. Inui. 1994. Diagnosis of carbohydrate-deficient glycoprotein syndrome by matrix-assisted laser desorption time-of-flight mass spectrometry. Biol Mass Spectrom 23: 108–109.

Weinstein, M., E. Schollen, G. Matthijs, C. Neupert, T. Hennet, C. E. Grubenmann et al. 2005. CDG-IL: an infant with a novel mutation in the ALG9 gene and additional phenotypic features. Am J Med Genet A 136: 194–197.

Willer, T., M. C. Valero, W. Tanner, J. Cruces and S. Strahl. 2003. O-mannosyl glycans: From yeast to novel associations with human disease. Curr Opin Struct Biol 13: 621–630.

Willer, T., H. Lee, M. Lommel, T. Yoshida-Moriguchi, D. B. de Bernabe, D. Venzke et al. 2012. ISPD loss of function mutations disrupt dystroglycan O-mannosylation and cause Walker-Warburg syndrome. Nat Genet 44: 575–580.

Wolfe, L. A., E. Morova, M. He, J. Vockley and K. M. Gibson. 2012. Heritable disorders in the metabolism of dolichols: A bridge from sterol biosynthesis to molecular glycosylation. Am J Med Genet C Semin Med Genet 160C: 322–328.

Wopereis, S., E. Morava, S. Grunewald, M. Adamowicz, K. M. Huijben, D. J. Lefeber et al. 2005. Patients with unsolved congenital disorders of glycosylation type II can be subdivided in six distinct biochemical groups. Glycobiology 15: 1312–1319.

Wright, K. M., K. A. Lyon, H. Leung, D. J. Leahy, L. Ma and D. D. Ginty. 2012. Dystroglycan organizes axon guidance cue localization and axonal pathfinding. Neuron 76: 931–944.

Wu, X., J. S. Rush, D. Karaoglu, D. Krasnewich, M. S. Lubinsky, C. J. Waechter et al. 2003. Deficiency of UDP-GlcNAc: Dolichol Phosphate N-Acetylglucosamine-1 Phosphate Transferase (DPAGT1) causes a novel congenital disorder of Glycosylation Type Ij. Hum Mutat 22: 144–150.

Wu, X., R. A. Steet, O. Bohorov, J. Bakker, J. Newell, M. Krieger et al. 2004. Mutation of the COG complex subunit gene *COG7* causes a lethal congenital disorder. Nat Med 10: 518–523.

Xiong, H., K. Kobayashi, M. Tachikawa, H. Manya, S. Takeda, T. Chiyonobu et al. 2006. Molecular interaction between fukutin and POMGnT1 in the glycosylation pathway of alpha-dystroglycan. Biochem Biophys Res Commun 350: 935–941.

Yanagisawa, A., C. Bouchet, P. Y. Van den Bergh, J. M. Cuisset, L. Viollet, F. Leturcq et al. 2007. New *POMT2* mutations causing congenital muscular dystrophy: identification of a founder mutation. Neurology 69: 1254–1260.

Yang, A. C., B. G. Ng, S. A. Moore, J. Rush, C. J. Waechter, K. M. Raymond et al. 2013a. Congenital disorder of glycosylation due to DPM1 mutations presenting with dystroglycanopathy-type congenital muscular dystrophy. Mol Genet Metab 110: 345–351.

Yang, H. S., M. Yang, X. Li, S. Tugulea and H. Dong. 2013b. Diagnosis of paroxysmal nocturnal hemoglobinuria in peripheral blood and bone marrow with six-color flow cytometry. Biomarkers Med 7: 99–111.

Yis, U., G. Uyanik, P. B. Heck, M. Smitka, H. Nobel, F. Ebinger et al. 2011. Fukutin mutations in non-Japanese patients with congenital muscular dystrophy: less severe mutations predominate in patients with a non-Walker-Warburg phenotype. Neuromuscul Disord 21: 20–30.

Yoshida, A., K. Kobayashi, H. Manya, K. Taniguchi, H. Kano, M. Mizuno et al. 2001. Muscular dystrophy and neuronal migration disorder caused by mutations in a glycosyltransferase, POMGnT1. Dev Cell 1: 717–724.

Zdebska, E., B. Bader-Meunier, P. O. Schischmanoff, T. Dupre, N. Seta, G. Tchernia et al. 2003. Abnormal glycosylation of red cell membrane band 3 in the congenital disorder of glycosylation Ig. Pediatr Res 54: 224–229.

Zelinger, L., E. Banin, A. Obolensky, L. Mizrahi-Meissonnier, A. Beryozkin, D. Bandah-Rozenfeld et al. 2011. A missense mutation in DHDDS, encoding dehydrodolichyl diphosphate synthase, is associated with autosomal-recessive retinitis pigmentosa in Ashkenazi Jews. Am J Hum Genet 88: 207–215.

Zhou, X., G. Zhao, J. J. Truglio, L. Wang, G. Li, W. J. Lennarz et al. 2006. Structural and biochemical studies of the C-terminal domain of mouse peptide-N-glycanase identify it as a mannose-binding module. Proc Nat Acad Sci 103: 17214–17219.

Zuchner, S., J. Dallman, R. Wen, G. Beecham, A. Naj, A. Farooq et al. 2011. Whole-exome sequencing links a variant in DHDDS to retinitis pigmentosa. Am J Hum Genet 88: 201–206.

CHAPTER 17

Antibodies to Hyaluronic Acid in Preeclampsia

M.M. Ziganshina,[1,a,]* *N.V. Shilova,*[2,h] *N.R. Khasbiullina,*[2,i]
M.E. Navakouski,[2,j] *M.A. Nikolaeva,*[1,b] *N.E. Kan,*[1,c] *O.V. Vavina,*[1,d]
A.V. Nikolaeva,[1,e] *V.L. Tyutyunnik,*[1] *N.V. Tyutyunnik,*[1,f] *I. Bot,*[3]
G.T. Sukhikh[1,g] *and N.V. Bovin*[2,k]

Introduction

Pre-eclampsia (PE) is a multisystem pathological state with clinical signs being displayed after week 20 of pregnancy. The symptoms are characterized with arterial hypertension in combination with proteinuria (≥ 0.3 g/l in daily urine), often with edemas, and manifestations of multiorgan/multisystemic failures (Magee et al. 2014). PE can be complicated with eclampsia, HELLP-syndrome, acute renal failure, pulmonary edema, stroke, intrauterine growth retardation, abruption of placenta and antenatal intrauterine fetal death (Chaiworapongsa et al. 2014). PE is one of the main causes of maternal and perinatal morbidity and mortality

[1] Federal State Budget Institution «Research Center for Obstetrics, Gynecology and Perinatology» of Ministry of Healthcare of the Russian Federation, Moscow, 117997, Oparin street, 4.
  E-mail: med@oparina4.ru
[a] E-mail: mmz@mail.ru
[b] E-mail: MNikolaeva@oparina4.ru
[c] E-mail: n_kan@oparina4.ru
[d] E-mail: o_vavina@oparina4.ru
[e] E-mail: a_nikolaeva@oparina4.ru
[f] E-mail: n_tyutyunnik@oparina4.ru
[g] E-mail: g_sukhikh@oparina4.ru
[2] M.M. Shemyakin and Y.A. Ovchinnikov Institute of Bioorganic Chemistry, Russian Academy of Sciences, 117997, Russian Federation, Moscow, GSP-7, Miklukho-Maklaya,16/10.
  E-mail: office@ibch.ru
[h] E-mail: pumatnv@gmail.com
[i] E-mail: crosbreed@list.ru
[j] E-mail: maxushob@gmail.com
[k] E-mail: professorbovin@yandex.ru
[3] Leiden Academic Centre for Drug Research, Leiden University, Einsteinweg 55, 2333 CC, Leiden, The Netherlands.
  E-mail: i.bot@lacdr.leidenuniv.nl
* Corresponding author

worldwide. PE complicates 2–8% of total pregnancies in developed countries (USA and Western Europe) (Ramma and Ahmed 2011, Uzan et al. 2011, von Dadelszen and Magee 2014), affecting negatively health quality of mother and newborn. About 63000 women die annually of PE and its complications. 9% of deaths occurs in Asia and Africa and up to 25% to Latin America and Caribbean countries (Smith et al. 2013). The importance of the problem can be illustrated by the following example: about 5000 people died of Ebola virus in March–October 2014, whereas about 30000 women died of PE during this period (Brown 2014).

At present there is no any test with suitable sensitivity and specificity particularities that would provide early diagnostics/revealing of PE development risks. A combination of tests, including ultrasound dopplerometry of uterus arteries, ultrasound evaluation of placenta structure, and several biochemistry tests listed in Table 1 are considered as an addition to anamnestic data and data of external evaluation (mean, BP, BMI, first pregnancy, or PE in anamnesis).

Table 1. Biochemical markers used in diagnostics/prediction of PE.

Parameter	Interpretation	Source
PAPP-A (pregnancy related plasma protein A)	Decrease in the first trimester < 5th percentile	(Di Lorenzo et al. 2012)
AFP (alpha fetoprotein)	Increase in the second trimester unexplained by other authors	(Barton and Sibai 2008)
hCG (horionic gonadotropin)	Increase in the second trimester > 3 MoM	(Towner et al. 2006)
Inhibin A	Increase in the first or second trimester	(Giguere et al. 2010)
sFlt-1/PlGF	Increase of sFlt-1 level is fixed 5 weeks before clinical signs of preeclampsia. These changes are preceded by low plasma concentration of free PlGF, noted at weeks 13–16 of pregnancy	(Leaños-Miranda et al. 2012, Verlohren et al. 2012)
PP13 (galectin 13)	Decrease in the first trimester	(Huppertz et al. 2013)
P-selectin	Increase in the first trimester	(Muller-Deile and Schiffer 2014)

Antibodies are prospective biomarkers for pregnancy pathology: alloantibodies produced in response to fetus alloantigens, and autoantibodies divided in preexisting natural autoantibodies and disease-associated autoantibodies. Determination of specificity of latter ones would help to understand the reasons/mechanisms of the disease development. Additionally, the level of circulating antibodies could be a parameter indirectly reflecting activation/suppression of immune response, which is also significant for the study of the mechanisms of the disease development.

According to numerous studies, hyperactivation of immune system is developed during PE, whereas the activity of immune system is decreased during normal pregnancy (Schiessl 2007, Chaouat et al. 2010, Leber et al. 2011). Hyperactivation is caused by the development of systemic inflammation response and endothelial dysfunction (Borzychowski et al. 2006, Germain et al. 2007, Powe et al. 2011), which is the sequence of chronic endothelium activation and can lead to irreversible cell lesion, apoptosis, and necrosis (Germain et al. 2007). There are only occasional reports on the presence of antiendothelial antibodies (AECA) in patients with PE (Yamamoto et al. 1998, Mendonca et al. 2000), however their epitope specificity is unknown and target antigens have been characterized only partially (Youinou 2005, Servettaz et al. 2008a,b).

Pro-inflammation action on endothelial cells obviously should affect molecular architecture of glycocalix. This is manifested as the change in presentation of functional carbohydrate residues of glycocalix and as shedding of its components in blood. Structural changes of glycocalix can lead to formation of Danger Associated Molecular Patterns (DAMP) (Laresgoiti-Servitje 2013, Gaudet and Popovich 2014, Heil and Land 2014), i.e., combinations of tightly and regularly arranged normal molecules, which can induce appearance of auto-antibodies. This can shift homeostatic balance in the pool of natural antibodies. A considerable part of human natural antibodies is directed to cell surface glycans (Bovin 2013). In case of pathologies repertoire of these antibodies becomes changed, this being true for antigens targeted to glycans of glycocalix too. It is known that the targets for AECA, which can fulfill regulatory function (Servettaz et al. 2008b), and be the key unit in humoral response against endothelium during pathologies, also include carbohydrate molecules (Cieslik et al. 2008).

The aim of this work was the study of repertoire of antibodies towards glycans of glycocalix in peripheral blood of patients with PE and their potential ling to AECA.

Methods

A prospective *case-control* study was performed. The main cohort consisted of 28 patients with PE in the third trimester of pregnancy. Reference cohort included 30 conditionally healthy patients; the exclusion criteria were: severe obstetrics and extragenital pathologies, acute inflammation diseases, hemotransfusion and organ transplantation in anamnesis, immunoglobulin therapy, administration of preparations affecting antibody production.

Microarrays containing 374 glycans printed as described in (Blixt et al. 2004), including hyaluronic acid with degree of polymerization ~12, were used for determination of antiglycan antibodies in peripheral blood. Microarrays were incubated with the samples of studied sera as described in (Huflejt et al. 2009). Then antibodies bound with glycans were developed by secondary antibodies against IgG or IgM fluorescence labeled with Alexa555 and Alexa647, respectively (Invitrogen, USA). Signals were red using fluorescence scanner ScanArray Gx (Perkin Elmer, USA). The results were processed using software ScanArrayExpress 4.0 with the fixed rings method, diameter 70 μm. Fluorescence values exceeding background signal (i.e., the signal from the surface not containing the ligand) five-fold.

Cell line EA.hy926 (ATCC, CRL-2922, USA) obtained by hybridization of the primary cell line of human endothelial cells (HUVEC) with lung carcinoma cells A-549 (Edgell et al. 1983). The used cells reproduce all major morphological, phenotypic and functional characteristics inherent to endothelial cells of macrovessels.

The study of binding activity of AECA presented by immunoglobulins of classes M and G was performed by flow cytometry on FACSCalibur (Becton Dickinson, USA), as described in (Ziganshina et al. 2015). Cells were incubated with sera on study followed by development of antibodies bound with cells using fluorescence labeled secondary antibodies specific to Fc fragment of human IgG or μ-chain of human IgM (Sigma, USA). Then the samples were washed; propidium iodide was added and the samples were assayed with flow cytometer. Activity of endothelial antibodies binding with surface antigens was characterized by concurrent evaluation of several parameters: percentage of living cells that bind antibodies from blood sample (FCM, %); MFI, mean fluorescence intensity of cells covered with antibodies labeled with fluorescein isothiocyanate, expressed in relative fluorescence units (RFU); median RFU—the value characterizing call distribution by fluorescence intensity; moda RFU—parameter, which characterizes the position of the channel linked to maximum amount of stained AECA-labeled cells.

Statistical analysis of results was performed using electronic tables Microsoft Office Excel, application package IBM SPSS Statistics Standard for Windows and software R (developer: The R Foundation for Statistical Computing). Normalcy of distribution was evaluated using Shapiro-Wilk test. Significance of differences between values was evaluated using Wilcoxon-Mann-Whitney test (WMW test). Differences were considered significant at confidence level $p < 0.05$. Data are reported as median ± absolute deviation for median.

Results and Discussion

It is supposed that humans have a conservative repertoire of natural antibodies, which execute regulatory function, control activation of endothelial cells, manifest anti-inflammation and antithrombotic effect and act as factors that inhibit endothelial cell proliferation (Tseng et al. 2007, Servettaz et al. 2008b, Kimura et al. 2015). In this study AECA were detected in two cohorts of pregnant women. The first one included patients with preeclampsia (main group) and the second one—individuals with physiological pregnancy (reference group). In parallel the repertoire of serum Ab to glycans was profiled. This study was performed using a microarray including glycans typical for mammalian glycoproteins and glycolipids. It is known that Ab to heparin are a component of the pool of AECA in humans and mice (Harper and Savage 1998, Renaudineau et al. 1998, Cieslik et al. 2008). This permitted expecting that Ab to hyaluronic acid reported earlier by Fattal et al. (2010), and Bovin (2013) are also the component of the pool of AECA, because hyaluronic acid is core structure of proteoglycans.

AECA were revealed in both cohorts. This is evidenced by significant differences in a number of parameters determined by flow cytometry (Table 2), however their content in ill individuals was higher[1] relative to healthy pregnant women (Fig. 1A, B), though this is true only for Ab of G class.

Table 2. Binding of antibodies from peripheral blood of patients with physiological pregnancy and PE with endothelial cells (EA hy.926).

Parameter	Ab subclass	Main group	Reference group	p (WMW-test)
FCM,%	IgM	89.4 ± 12.9	93.8 ± 5.6	0.34
MFI, RFU	IgM	74.4 ± 43.1	86.2 ± 32.0	0.80
median, RFU	IgM	55.8 ± 26.6	57.0 ± 13.6	0.56
moda, RFU	IgM	52.0 ± 26.7	57.0 ± 16.3	0.39
FCM,%	IgG	6.9 ± 3.3	6.1 ± 2.7	0.18
MFI, RFU	IgG	26.4 ± 9.2	22.2 ± 6.8	**0.02**
median, RFU	IgG	14.3 ± 3.9	12.0 ± 2.0	**0.012**
moda, RFU	IgG	14.5 ± 5.2	11.0 ± 1.5	**0.02**

(FCM, %) percentage of living cells that bind antibodies from blood sample;
MFI—mean fluorescence intensity of with fluorescein labeled antibodies bound cells, expressed in relative fluorescence units (RFU);
median RFU—the value characterizing call distribution by fluorescence intensity;
moda RFU—parameter, which characterizes the position of the channel linked to maximum amount of dyed cells.
Reference group—conditionally healthy patients with physiological pregnancy.

Antibodies to about 120 glycans of both IgG and IgM were observed in healthy pregnant women (374 glycans are printed on a chip), whereas this number reached about 180 in PE group. So, antiglycan Ab not observed during normal pregnancy are produced during PE. Significant differences between two cohorts were observed for several antibodies, notably, for Ab to glycans with terminal αGal-, and βGlcNAc- residues (Fig. 2).

Of particular interest are Ab to glycans, which are the components of glycocalix of endothelial cells, because we suppose that they are the targets for AECA. In this report we focus only for Ab to hyaluronic acid [-4GlcAβ1-3GlcNAcβ1-]$_n$, demonstrating significantly increased titer (p = 0.0027) in patients with PE relative to reference cohort (Fig. 3).

Additionally, Ab to disaccharide GlcAβ1-3GlcNAcβ repeating unit of this regular polysaccharide were also elevated (p = 0.0022). Significant decrease of titer was observed only for Ab of IgG class (Fig. 2). Direct correlation between these two specificities should be noted: in reference cohort r_s = 0,677, p = 0.0006, and in PE cohort r_s = 0.784, p = 0.00001. By this we consider Ab binding with polymer and its fragment to be identical or, at least, similar by epitope specificity.

By chemical composition hyaluronic acid is related to linear nonsulfated glycosaminoglycans. It is one of the main components of extracellular matrix including endothelial glycocalix (Hascall and Esco 2009). Structure unit of hyaluronic acid is D-glucuronic acid 1–3 bound to N-acetylglucosamine. This biopolymer is anchored in membrane or exists in unbound state in glycocalix or it can form a complex with hyaluronate-

---

[1] It is more correct to use the term titer as the measured value is a multiple of concentration (amount) of Ab to their affinity.

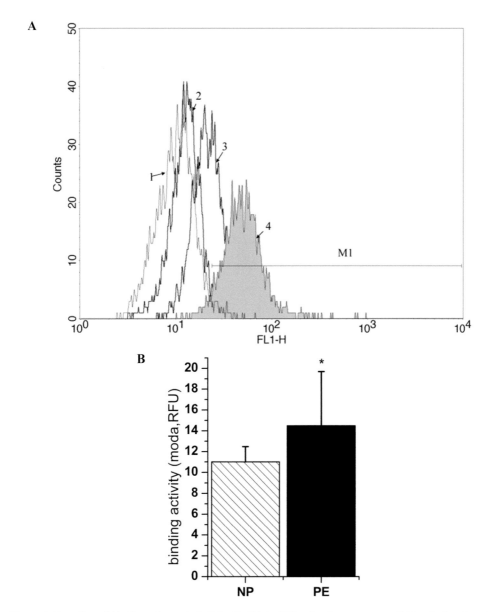

Figure 1. Revealing of Ab directed to endothelial cells (EA hy.926) using flow cytometry. (A) Incubation: 1—with PBS-BSA; 2—pooled sera of healthy donors, blood group AB; 3—serum of a patient with physiological pregnancy; 4—serum of a patient with preeclampsia. The cursor M1 divides positive and negative cells. (B) titers of AECA in blood of patients with physiological pregnancy (white bar) and preeclampsia (black bar). *- differences from reference group are significant p = 0,022.

binding proteins, of which more than a dozen has been reported, the most known is CD44 (Hascall and Esco 2009, Lipowsky et al. 2012, Salmon and Satchell 2012). Due to negative charge it has conformation of extended helix. This shape together with high molecular weight allow the anchored form of HA to pierce glycocalix and thus become available for interaction with blood proteins, including Ab.

Correlation between the titers of AECA and titers of several antiglycan antibodies (Table 3) was observed in reference cohort. Direct correlation was observed for the titer of Ab to Galα-terminated glycans (Table 3, line 1–4), including blood group B antigens (Table 3, lines 1–4).

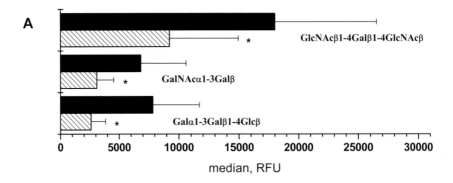

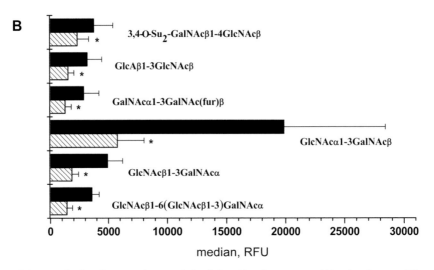

Figure 2. Antiglycan antibodies, demonstrating correlation links with reference group (A) and main group (B). Error is given as MAD/2. * - differences from reference group are significant $p < 0.05$.

No.	Glycan structure	Trivial name
1	GlcNAcβ1-4Galβ1-4GlcNAcβ	GN4LN
2	GalNAcα1-3Galβ	A_{di}
3	Galα1-3Galβ1-4Glcβ	αGal epitope
4	3,4-O-Su$_2$-GalNAcβ1-4GlcNAcβ	LacdiNAc3',4'Su2
5	GlcAβ1-3GlcNAcβ	GUb3GN
6	GalNAcα1-3GalNAc(fur)β	Fs(f)-2
7	GlcNAcα1-3GalNAcβ	GNa3AN
8	GlcNAcβ1-3GalNAcα	core 3
9	GlcNAcβ1-6(GlcNAcβ1-3)GalNAcα	core 4

Significant negative correlations between the titer of AECA and anti-hyaluronic and a number of other antiglycan Ab (Table 3) were observed in the patients of PE cohort. We suppose that physiological role of antihyalouronic Ab is down-regulation of the ability of hyaluronic acid to activate alloimmunity (Tesar et al. 2006), which is of particular importance during pregnancy. Importantly, significant differences between the two cohorts by titer of antibodies to most of the noted glycans (Fig. 2A, B) have been revealed.

Reverse correlation between AECA and antiglycan Ab can be explained by an additional the third factor, presumably, the presence of free hyaluronic acid. We suppose that AEAC of G class, which titer

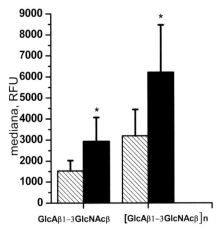

Figure 3. Revealing of IgG Ab to repeating unit GlcAβ1-3GlcNAcβ- of HA and polymer [GlcAβ1-3GlcNAcβ]$_n$ of HA (n ~ 12). White bars: Ab at physiological pregnancy; black bars: Ab at preeclampsia. Error is given as MAD/2. Median, RFU—is given in relative units. * - differences from reference group are significant, p < 0.035.

Table 3. Correlation link between antiglycan and antiendothelial IgG Ab.

No.	parameters	Glycan structure	Trivial name	r_s	P	Cohort
1	Moda antiendothelial Ab vs antiglycan Ab	Galα1-3Galβ1-4Glcβ-	αGal epitope	0.356	0.054	healthy pregnant
2		Galα1-3(Fucα1-2)Galβ1-3GalNAcα-	B type 3	0.419	0.021	healthy pregnant
3		Galα1-3(Fucα1-2)Galβ1-3GalNAcβ-p	B type 4	0.390	0.033	healthy pregnant
4		Galα1-3(Fucα1-2)Galβ-	B_{tri}	0.371	0.044	healthy pregnant
5		GalNAcα1-3Galβ-	A_{di}	0.412	0.024	healthy pregnant
6		GlcNAcβ1-4Galβ1-4GlcNAcβ-	-	0.352	0.057	healthy pregnant
7	FCM,%antiendothelial Ab vs antiglycan Ab	GlcAβ1-3GlcNAcβ		–0.443	0.019	preeclampsia
8		GlcNAcβ1-6(GlcNAcβ1-3)GalNAcα		–0.435	0.022	preeclampsia
9		GlcNAcβ1-3GalNAcα		–0.428	0.024	preeclampsia
10		GlcNAcα1-3GalNAcβ		–0.394	0.038	preeclampsia
11		3,4-O-Su$_2$-GalNAcβ1-4GlcNAcβ		–0.392	0.040	preeclampsia
12		[GlcAβ1-3GlcNAcβ]$_n$	Hyaluronic acid (HA)	–0.369	0.054	preeclampsia

is increased in PE patients injure endothelial cells. At the same time, IgG possibly hinder cytotoxic effect of AECA, but due to destruction of glycocalix during inflammation response and increase in amount of circulating hyaluronic acid protective action of antiglycan Ab is leveled. It should be noted once more that hyaluronic acid is not necessarily bound to glycocalix: it has been observed in a free state. Its concentration in lymph reaches 100 μg/l in blood (Engstrom-Laurent 1989, Banerji et al. 1999, Fraser et al. 1988); increase in its content is observed during pathologies (Grundmann et al. 2012, Padberg et al. 2014), including PE (Berg et al. 2001, Hofmann-Kiefer et al. 2013). As circulating polymer masks antibodies, in reality Ab level must be increased even more notably than we observed. This is indirectly supported by the fact that only the level of IgG is increased in PE patients. This can be explained by preferential neutralization of immunoglobulins M by circulating multivalent hyaluronic acid.

Notably increased titer of antibodies to HA observed in patients with PE can be the evidence of, firstly, the impairment of the process of trophoblast invasion to spiral uterine arteries, the main pathogenetic factor of PE development (Uzan et al. 2011, Chaiworapongsa et al. 2014), because Ab can serve as inhibitors of cell-cell and cell-matrix interaction. Despite the consideration that main stages of morphogenesis of placenta are finished before the third trimester of pregnancy, the belonging of Ab to IgG class confirms the presence of preceding immunopathologic process. Secondly, the increased titer can reflect the impaired processes of organization of endothelial cell glycocalix being the evidence of disruption of mechanotransduction in cardio-vascular of PE patients. Thirdly, the presence of Ab to HA obviously affects the biological effect of circulating HA, influencing their regulatory function. Fourthly, the link between AECA (IgG) and antiglycan (IgG) Ab observed in this study allows us to suppose participation of the latter in binding of AECA with endothelial cell. Probably, the increased generation of antibodies to HA in PE patients is not specific for this pathology but is the result of excessive systemic inflammatory response, however, giving evidence of manifestation of endothelial activation and could be significant in pathogenesis of PE.

Thus, the observed humoral response to antigens of endothelial cells, revealed during this study is the confirmation of expressed endothelial activation, which is one of the principal pathogenetic factors of PE development. The data obtained allows us to make a hypothesis on role of glycocalix in pathogenesis of the disease, because the main stages of pathogenesis, i.e., (1) impaired invasion of trophoblast cells in spiral uterine arteries leading to inadequate perfusion of feto-placental system and ischemia and (2) endothelial dysfunction, which is the reason of endotheliosis and increased vascular tone in patients with PE, are both related to the impaired intercellular interactions and loss the ability to execute their functions by the cells. In this connection hyaluronic acid, as one of the structure units of glycocalix may be significant for cell locomotion during its interaction with receptors and the processes of mechanotransduction regulating vascular tone. Destabilization and desquamation of glycocalix in case of excessive systemic inflammation response critically changes the response of endothelial cells to mechanical stimuli because decrease of glycocalix layer decreases mechanosensitivity of endothelial cells, which causes vasoconstrictive effect in conditions of increased circulation and increases the permeability of glomerular filter, which is manifested by proteinuria. So, glycocalix can be the main point of application of impairing factors. We believe that it is the principal candidate for morphological substrate during PE because its impairment can lead to manifestation of clinical signs. The presence of circulating antibodies to hyaluronic acid, which executes the function of organization and stabilization of 3D structure of glycocalix, can potentially be bad prognostic factor not only to patients with PE, but also with hypertension disorders also without pregnancy. High risk of development of cardiovascular diseases in patients having PE in anamnesis can be related to the presence of autoantibodies to hyaluronic acid, which can block regeneration of glycocalix to physiological norm. The obtained data can extend the knowledge on pathogenesis of PE and have realization in practice for diagnostics and prognosis of the disease.

Acknowledgements

The work was done within the frames of State Contract of the Russian Ministry of Education and Science "Study of molecular-genetic, proteomic and mitochondrial determinants of the development of preeclampsia" RK No. 114040970024.

Keywords: preeclampsia, anti-glycan antibodies, glycocalyx, antiendothelial cells antibodies (AECA), glycochip, antibodies to hyaluronic acids

References

Banerji, S., J. Ni, S. -X. Wang, S. Clasper, J. Su, R. Tammi et al. 1999. LYVE-1, a new homologue of the CD44 glycoprotein, is a lymph-specific receptor for hyaluronan. J Cell Biol 144: 789–801.
Barton, J. R. and B. M. Sibai. 2008. Prediction and prevention of recurrent preeclampsia. Obstet Gynecol 112: 359–372.
Berg, S., A. Engman, S. Holmgren, T. Lundahl and T. C. Laurent. 2001. Increased plasma hyaluronan in severe pre-eclampsia and eclampsia. Scand J Clin Lab Invest 61: 131–137.

Blixt, O., S. Head, T. Mondala, C. Scanlan, M. E. Huflejt, R. Alvarez et al. 2004. Printed covalent glycan array for ligand profiling of diverse glycan binding proteins. Proc Natl Acad Sci 101: 17033–17038.

Borzychowski, A. M., I. L. Sargent and C. W. Redman. 2006. Inflammation and pre-eclampsia. Semin Fet Neonat Med 11: 309–316.

Bovin, N. V. 2013. Natural antibodies to glycans. Biochemistry (Moscow) 78: 1008–1022.

Brown, M. A. Pre-eclampsia in 2014: Seven ways to make a difference. 2014. Pregnancy Hypertension: An Intern J Women's Cardiovascular Health 4: 249–252.

Chaiworapongsa, T., P. Chaemsaithong, L. Yeo and R. Romero. 2014. Pre-eclampsia part 1: current understanding of its pathophysiology. Nat Rev Nephrol 10: 466–480.

Chaouat, G., M. Petitbarat, S. Dubanchet, M. Rahmati and N. Ledee. 2010. Tolerance to the foetal allograft? Amer J Reprod Immunol 63: 624–636.

Cieslik, P., A. Hrycek and P. Klucinski. 2008. Vasculopathy and vasculitis in systemic lupus erythematosus. Pol Arch Med Wewn 118: 57–63.

Di Lorenzo, G., M. Ceccarello, V. Cecotti, L. Ronfani, L. Monasta, L. Vecchi Brumatti et al. 2012. First trimester maternal serum PlGF, free β-hCG, PAPP-A, PP-13, uterine artery Doppler and maternal history for the prediction of preeclampsia. Placenta 33: 495–501.

Edgell, C. J., C. C. McDonald and J. B. Graham. 1983. Permanent cell line expressing human factor VIII-related antigen established by hybridization. Proc Natl Acad Sci 80: 3734–3737.

Engstrom-Laurent, A. 1989. Changes in hyaluronan concentration in tissues and body fluids in disease states. Ciba Found Symp 143: 233–240.

Fattal, I., N. Shental, D. Mevorach, J. M. Anaya, A. Livneh, P. Langevitz et al. 2010. An antibody profile of systemic lupus erythematosus detected by antigen microarray. Immunology 130: 337–343.

Fraser, J. R., W. G. Kimpton, T. C. Laurent, R. N. Cahill and N. Vakakis. 1988. Uptake and degradation of hyaluronan in lymphatic tissue. Biochem J 256: 153–158.

Gaudet, A. D. and P. G. Popovich. 2014. Extracellular matrix regulation of inflammation in the healthy and injured spinal cord. Exp Neurol 258: 24–34.

Germain, A. M., M. C. Romanik, I. Guerra, S. Solari, M. S. Reyes, R. J. Johnson et al. 2007. Endothelial dysfunction: A link among preeclampsia, recurrent pregnancy loss, and future cardiovascular events? Hypertension 49: 90–95.

Giguere, Y., M. Charland, E. Bujold, N. Bernard, S. Grenier, F. Rousseau et al. 2010. Combining biochemical and ultrasonographic markers in predicting preeclampsia: A systematic review. Clin Chem 56: 361–375.

Grundmann, S., K. Fink, L. Rabadzhieva, N. Bourgeois, T. Schwab, M. Moser et al. 2012. Perturbation of the endothelial glycocalyx in post cardiac arrest syndrome. Resuscitation 83: 715–720.

Harper, L. and C. O. S. Savage. 1998. Anti-heparin antibodies: part of the repertoire of anti-endothelial cell antibodies (AECA). Lupus 7: 68–72.

Hascall, V. and J. D. Esco. 2009. Hyaluronan. pp. 219–228. *In*: Varki, A. (ed.). Essentials of Glycobiology, 2nd ed. Cold Spring Harbor Lab. Press, New York, USA.

Heil, M. and W. G. Land. 2014. Danger signals—damaged-self recognition across the tree of life. Front Pl Sci 5: A.578.1–16.

Hofmann-Kiefer, K. F., D. Chappell, J. Knabl, H. G. Frank, N. Martinoff, P. Conzen et al. 2013. Placental syncytiotrophoblast maintains a specific type of glycocalyx at the fetomaternal border: the glycocalyx at the fetomaternal interface in healthy women and patients with HELLP syndrome. Reprod Sci 20: 1237–1245.

Huflejt, M. E., M. Vuskovic, D. Vasiliu, H. Xu, P. Obukhova, N. Shilova et al. 2009. Anti-carbohydrate antibodies of normal sera: Findings, surprises and challenges. Mol Immunol 46: 3037–3049.

Huppertz, B., H. Meiri, S. Gizurarson, G. Osol and M. Sammar. 2013. Placental protein 13 (PP13): a new biological target shifting individualized risk assessment to personalized drug design combating pre-eclampsia. Hum Reprod Update 19: 391–405.

Kimura, A., T. Sakurai, A. Yoshikura, Y. Hayashi, H. Ohtaki, M. Chousa et al. 2015. Identification of target antigens of antiendothelial cell antibodies against human brain microvascular endothelial cells in healthy subjects. Curr Neurovasc Res 12: 25–30.

Laresgoiti-Servitje, E. 2013. A leading role for the immune system in the pathophysiology of preeclampsia. J Leukoc Biol 94: 247–257.

Leaños-Miranda, A., I. Campos-Galicia, I. Isordia-Salas, R. Rivera-Leaños, J. F. Romero-Arauz, J. A. Ayala-Méndez et al. 2012. Changes in circulating concentrations of soluble fms-like tyrosine kinase-1 and placental growth factor measured by automated electrochemiluminescence immunoassays methods are predictors of preeclampsia. J Hypertens 30: 2173–2181.

Leber, A., M. L. Zenclussen, A. Teles, N. Brachwitz, P. Casalis, T. El-Mousleh et al. 2011. Pregnancy: Tolerance and suppression of immune responses. Methods Mol Biol 677: 397–417.

Lipowsky, H. H., L. Gao and A. Lescanic. 2012. Shedding of the endothelial glycocalyx in arterioles, capillaries, and venules and its effect on capillary hemodynamics during inflammation. Amer J Physiol 301: 2235–2245.

Magee, L. A., A. Pels, M. Helewa, E. Rey and P. von Dadelszen. 2014. Diagnosis, evaluation, and management of the hypertensive disorders of pregnancy. Pregnancy Hypertension: An Intern J Women's Cardiovasc Health 4: 105–145.

Mendonca, L. L., M. A. Khamashta, M. J. Cuadado, M. L. Bertolaccini and G. R. Hughes. 2000. Natural immune response involving anti-endothelial cell antibodies in normal and lupus pregnancy. Arthr Rheum 43: 1511–1515.

Muller-Deile, J. and M. Schiffer. 2014. Preeclampsia from a renal point of view: Insides into disease models, biomarkers and therapy. World J Nephrol 3: 169–181.

Padberg, J. S., A. Wiesinger, G. S. di Marco, S. Reuter, A. Grabner, D. Kentrup et al. 2014. Damage of the endothelial glycocalyx in chronic kidney disease. Atherosclerosis 234: 335–343.

Powe, C. E., R. J. Levine and S. A. Karumanchi. 2011. Preeclampsia, a disease of the maternal endothelium: the role of antiangiogenic factors and implications for later cardiovascular disease. Circulation 123: 2856–2869.

Ramma, W. and A. Ahmed. 2011. Is inflammation the cause of preeclampsia? Adv Cell Mol Biol Angiogenesis 39: 1619–1627.

Renaudineau, Y., R. Revelen, A. Bordron, D. Mottier, P. Youinou and R. Le Corre. 1998. Two populations of endothelial cell antibodies cross-react with heparin. Lupus 7: 86–94.

Salmon, A. H. and S. C. Satchell. 2012. Endothelial glycocalyx dysfunction in disease: Albuminuria and increased microvascular permeability. J Pathol 226: 562–574.

Schiessl, B. 2007. Inflammatory response in preeclampsia. Mol Asp Med 28: 210–219.

Servettaz, A., P. Guilpain, L. Camoin, P. Mayeux, C. Broussard, M. C. Tamby et al. 2008a. Identification of target antigens of antiendothelial cell antibodies in healthy individuals: A proteomic approach. Proteomics 8: 1000–1008.

Servettaz, A., P. Guilpain, N. Tamas, S. V. Kaveri, L. Camoin and L. Mouthon. 2008b. Natural anti-endothelial cell antibodies. Autoimmun Rew 7: 426–430.

Smith, J. M., R. F. Lowe, J. Fullerton, S. M. Currie, L. Harris and E. Felker-Kantor. 2013. An integrative review of the side effects related to the use of magnesium sulfate for pre-eclampsia and eclampsia management. BMC Rregn Childbirth 13: 34.

Tesar, B. M., D. Jiang, J. Liang, S. M. Palmer, P. W. Noble and D. R. Goldstein. 2006. The role of hyaluronan degradation products as innate alloimmune agonists. Am J Transplant 6: 2622–2635.

Towner, D., S. Gandhi and D. El Kady. 2006. Obstetric outcomes in women with elevated maternal serum human chorionic gonadotropin. Amer J of Obster Gynecol 194: 1676–1681.

Tseng, J. -C., L. -Y. Lu, R. J. Hu, C. K. Kau, H. H. Cheng, P. R. Lin et al. 2007. Elevated serum anti-endothelial cell autoantibodies titer is associated with lupus nephritis in patients with systemic lupus erythematosus. J Microbiol Immun Infect 40: 50–55.

Uzan, J., M. Carbonnel, O. Piconne, R. Asmar and J. -M. Ayoubi. 2011. Pre-eclampsia: Pathophysiology, diagnosis, and management. Vasc Health Risk Manag 7: 467–474.

Verlohren, S., H. Stepan and R. Dechend. 2012. Angiogenic growth factor in the diagnosis and prediction of pre-eclampsia. Clin Sci 122: 43–52.

von Dadelszen, P. and L. A. Magee. 2014. Pre-eclampsia: An update. Curr Hypertens Rep 16: 454.

Yamamoto, T., Y. Geshi, S. Kuno, N. Kase and H. Mori. 1998. Anti-endothelial cell antibody in preeclampsia: Clinical findings and serum cytotoxicity to endothelial cell. Nihon Rinsho Meneki Gakkai Kaishi 21: 191–197.

Youinou, P. 2005. New target antigens for anti-endothelial cell antibodies. Immunobiology 210: 789–797.

Ziganshina, M. M., M. A. Nikolaeva, E. O. Stepanova, L. V. Krechetova, N. E. Kan, D. I. Sokolov et al. 2015. Detection of antibodies *in vitro* binding to endothelial cells in sera from women with normal pregnancy and preeclampsia. Bull Exp Biol Med 159: 475–478.

Index